Erin,

To a fellow "rehabite" who knows & supports our efforts in the ICU. Keep up the good work.

Linda Machy

Erin -
May we all continue to learn and teach for the betterment of persons with BI

Phyllis Chapman

Erin,
To a fellow clinician, I hope this book is all you need. Please enjoy, Thank you.

Tom Mosp

Maximizing Brain Injury Recovery: Integrating Critical Care and Early Rehabilitation

Linda E. Mackay, MA, CCC-Sp
Manager, Brain Injury Programs
Saint Francis Hospital and Medical Center
The Rehabiliation Hospital of Connecticut
and Instructor of Clinical Surgery
University of Connecticut School of Medicine
Farmington, Connecticut

Phyllis E. Chapman, BS, RPT
Manager, Medical/Surgical Rehabilitation Program
Saint Francis Hospital and Medical Center
The Rehabilitation Hospital of Connecticut
Hartford, Connecticut

Anthony S. Morgan, MD, FACS
Chief, Trauma Services
Vice Chairman, Department of Surgery
Director, Trauma Research and Education Center
and Professor of Surgery
University of Connecticut School of Medicine
Farmington, Connecticut

AN ASPEN PUBLICATION®
Aspen Publishers, Inc.
Gaithersburg, Maryland
1997

Library of Congress Cataloging-in-Publication Data

Mackay, Linda E.
Maximizing brain injury recovery: integrating critical care and early rehabilitation/
Linda E. Mackay, Phyllis E. Chapman, Anthony Morgan.
p. cm.
Includes bibliographical references and index.
ISBN 0-8342-0655-2. — ISBN 0-8342-0655-2
1. Brain damage—Treatment. 2. Brain damage—Patients—Rehabilitation.
3. Neurological intensive care. I. Chapman, Phyllis E. II. Morgan, Anthony. III. Title.
[DNLM: 1. Brain Injuries—rehabilitation. 2. Brain Injuries—complications.
3. Critical Care. WL 354 M153m 1998]
RC387.5.M33 1997
616.8 ' 046—DC21
DNLM/DLC
for Library of Congress
97-21586
CIP

Orders: (800) 638-8437
Customer Service: (800) 234-1660

About Aspen Publishers • For more than 35 years, Aspen has been a leading professional publisher in a variety of disciplines. Aspen's vast information resources are available in both print and electronic formats. We are committed to providing the highest quality information available in the most appropriate format for our customers. Visit Aspen's Internet site for more information resources, directories, articles, and a searchable version of Aspen's full catalog, including the most recent publications: **http://www.aspenpub.com**
Aspen Publishers, Inc. • The hallmark of quality in publishing
Member of the worldwide Wolters Kluwer group

The authors have made every effort to ensure the accuracy of the information herein. However, appropriate information sources should be consulted, especially for new or unfamiliar procedures. It is the responsibility of every practitioner to evaluate the appropriateness of a particular opinion in the context of actual clinical situations and with due considerations to new developments. Authors, editors, and the publisher cannot be held responsible for any typographical or other errors found in this book.

Editorial Resources: Bill Fogle
Library of Congress Catalog Card Number: 97-21586
ISBN: 0-8342-0655-2

Printed in the United States of America

1 2 3 4 5

This book is dedicated to the memory of our friend, Marietta Kelly.

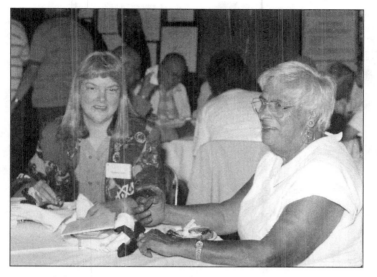

To my mom and dad and Sand_, an unending source of support and encouragement
   for me;
To Steth, my source of strength and love;
To Drew, who unknowingly instilled in me the motivaton for pursuing a profes-
   sion and passion for brain injury.
To Mathew and the Kosbobs, who showed me that no matter how difficult the
   path, there is no substitute for the love of a family.

Linda E. Mackay

To my sister, Marilyn, for her support and encouragement during the writing of
   this book;
To the staff who supported and encouraged me through this endeavor.

Phyllis E. Chapman

To my mother, who encouraged me to pursue wisdom and knowledge for the rest
   of my life;
To my sons, Sean and Eric, who are what is best in me;
To the Witness, who has shown me that two spirits can possess the same soul.

Anthony S. Morgan

Chapter Contributors

Chapter 1	Linda E. Mackay, Anthony S. Morgan
Chapter 2	Linda E. Mackay, Linda C. Degutis, Phyllis E. Chapman
Chapter 3	Anthony S. Morgan, Mary Ita Malone, John Calogero
Chapter 4	Carlos Barba, Mary Ita Malone, Anthony S. Morgan
Chapter 5	Phyllis E. Chapman, Linda E. Mackay, Anthony S. Morgan
Chapter 6	Rehka Singh
Chapter 7	Phyllis E. Chapman
Chapter 8	Phyllis E. Chapman
Chapter 9	Anthony S. Morgan, Louise M. Thomas, Carlos Barba, Rehka Singh
Chapter 10	Judith Pepe, Anthony S. Morgan, Linda E. Mackay
Chapter 11	Linda E. Mackay, Jacqueline Magennis
Chapter 12	Bette Kitik
Chapter 13	Catherine F. Bontke, Anthony S. Morgan
Chapter 14	Linda E. Mackay
Chapter 15	Linda E. Mackay, John Calogero, Anthony S. Morgan

Carlos Barba, MD
Associate Director, Trauma and
  Surgical Critical Care
Saint Francis Hospital and Medical
  Center
Hartford, Connecticut
Assistant Professor of
  Surgery
University of Connecticut School of
  Medicine
Farmington, Connecticut

Catherine F. Bontke, MD
System Medical Director
The Rehabilitation Hospital of
  Connecticut
Hartford, Connecticut

John Calogero, MD
Senior Attending Neurosurgery
Saint Francis Hospital and Medical
  Center
Hartford, Connecticut

Phyllis E. Chapman, BS, RPT
Manager, Medical/Surgical Rehabilitation Program
Saint Francis Hospital and Medical Center
The Rehabilitation Hospital of Connecticut
Hartford, Connecticut

Linda C. Degutis, DrPH, MSN, BS
Co-Director, New Haven Regional Injury Prevention Program
Assistant Professor, Yale University School of Medicine, Department of Surgery, Section of Emergency Medicine
New Haven, Connecticut

Bette Kitik, MS, CCC-A
Clinical Audiologist
Saint Francis Hospital and Medical Center,
Hartford, Connecticut

Linda E. Mackay, MA, CCC-Sp/L
Manager, Brain Injury Programs
Saint Francis Hospital and Medical Center
The Rehabilitation Hospital of Connecticut
Hartford, Connecticut
and Instructor of Clinical Surgery
University of Connecticut School of Medicine
Farmington, Connecticut

Jacqueline Magennis, MS, CCC-SLP
Speech/Language Pathologist
Saint Francis Hospital and Medical Center
The Rehabilitation Hospital of Connecticut
Hartford, Connecticut

Mary Ita Malone, MD, MPH
Attending Physiatrist
Saint Francis Hospital and Medical Center
Hartford, Connecticut

Anthony S. Morgan, MD, FACS
Chief, Trauma Services
Vice Chairman, Department of Surgery
Director, Trauma Research and Education Center
Saint Francis Hospital and Medical Center
Hartford, Connecticut
and Professor of Surgery
University of Connecticut School of Medicine
Farmington, Connecticut

Judith Pepe, MD
Associate Director, Surgical Critical Care and Trauma
Director of Nutritional Services
Saint Francis Hospital and Medical Center
Hartford, Connecticut
Assistant Professor of Surgery
University of Connecticut School of Medicine
Farmington, Connecticut

Rehka Singh, MD
Attending General Surgery and Surgical Critical Care
New Britain General Hospital
New Britain, Connecticut
Assistant Professor of Surgery
University of Connecticut School of Medicine
Farmington, Connecticut

Louise Thomas, RRT
Registered Respiratory Therapist
Saint Francis Hospital and Medical Center
Hartford, Connecticut

Contents

Foreword ix

Preface xi

Acknowlegments xiii

Chapter 1—Trauma Systems: A Continuum of Care for the Severely Brain
   Injured 1

  Epidemiology of Brain Injury 1
  The Evolution of Trauma Care 5
  Primary Prevention 7
  Prehospital Care 12
  Trauma Centers 13
  Impact of Regionalized Systems of Trauma Care 20
  Functional Outcomes 22
  Current Status in the Progress of Trauma Systems 29
  Health Care Reform and the Economic Status of Trauma Systems 31
  Summary 33
  Appendix 1–A Essential and/or Desirable Characteristics for the
    Four Levels of Trauma Centers 44

Chapter 2—Team-Focused Intervention within Critical Care 56

  Team Organization 57
  Benefits of Using a Team Approach 58
  Team Members 59

Team Effectiveness 73
Summary 76

**Chapter 3—Basic Knowledge of the Brain and the Clinical Ramifications
Post Injury 80**

Overview of Neuroanatomy 80
Blood Supply 106
The Physiology/Pathophysiology of Brain Injury and Its Management
    and Treatment 108
Summary 127

Chapter 4—Cranial Nerve, Maxillofacial, and Blunt Carotid Injuries 135

Anatomy and Physiology of the Cranial Nerves 135
Diagnosis and Management of Cranial Nerve Injuries 159
Maxillofacial Injuries 166
Management of Maxillofacial Injuries 167
Blunt Injury to the Carotid Artery 171

Chapter 5—Implications of Patient Data and Use of Technology 177

Implications of Patient Data 177
Use of Technology 194
The Unstable Patient 207
Summary 211

Chapter 6—Management of Complicating Associated Injuries 215

Spinal Cord Injury 215
Musculoskeletal Injuries 236
Thoracic and Cardiovascular Trauma 250
Abdominal Injuries 260

Chapter 7—Physical Therapy in the Intensive Care Unit 271

Assessment 272
Focus of Physical Therapy Services 280
Treatment 280
Complications 297

Interactions with the Family 300
Summary 300

Chapter 8—Occupational Therapy for Severe Brain Injury **304**

Assessment 305
Occupational Therapy Goals 315
Treatment 316
Interactions with the Family 327
Summary 328

Chapter 9—Respiratory Management of the Brain-Injured Patient **331**

Pulmonary Function and Respiratory Support 331
Pulmonary Complications 349
Conclusion 383

**Chapter 10—The Metabolic Response to Acute Traumatic Brain Injury
and Associated Complications** **396**

Metabolic Response to Acute Traumatic Brain Injury 396
Nutritional Support for Acute Traumatic Brain Injury 403
Electrolyte Abnormalities Associated with Traumatic Brain Injury 413
Cardiovascular Complications of Acute Traumatic Brain Injury 417
Nosocomial Infections: Extracranial and Intracranial 420
Conclusion 433

**Chapter 11—The Contributions of Speech/Language Pathology
in Critical Care** **444**

Patient Equipment and Monitoring Devices 445
Patient Observation 446
Assessment 447
Formal Assessment Tools 451
Treatment 451
Vocal Cord Integrity 458
Swallowing 468
Family Involvement 475
Conclusion 476

Chapter 12—Audiological Issues in Critical Care **483**

Mechanisms of Damage to the Ear and Appropriate Patient Selection 483
Chart Review 486
Test Rationale and Methodology 487
Assessment of Hearing Acuity 490
Conclusion 497

**Chapter 13—Pharmacologic Management of Persons with Severe
Brain Injury** **503**

The Role of Neurotransmitters 504
Medications that Facilitate or Hinder Recovery 506
Treatment of Specific Medical Problems in the ICU 512
Conclusion 521

Chapter 14—Crisis Intervention: Care and Involvement of the Family ..530

Anatomy of a Crisis 531
Historical Development of Crisis Theory 532
Factors that Influence a Crisis 533
Assessment 535
Intervention 538
Key Family Needs 545
Special Needs of Children or Siblings 558
Cultural Diversity in the Context of Critical Care 558
Conclusion 561
Appendix 14–A State Brain Injury Associations and Affiliates 566

**Chapter 15—The Benefits of Combining Rehabilitation
with Critical Care: Future Focus in Therapy and Medications** **572**

Benefits of Secondary Medical Prevention 572
Future Medical Advances 574
Benefits of Rehabilitative Interventions 579
Transfer Planning 586
Conclusion 590

Index **603**

Foreword

I am often asked to review books and to write a foreword, and most often I decline. But, when Linda Mackay, Dr. Anthony S. Morgan, and Phyllis Chapman asked me to review their new textbook and reference book, *Maximizing Brain Injury Recovery: Integrating Critical Care and Early Rehabilitation*, I had no hesitancy at all. I knew it would be comprehensive, up to date, useful, and well written.

As President of the Brain Injury Association, I am always looking for reference material that is useful for our constituents. The Brain Injury Association consists of professionals in all fields of brain injury treatment, research, and prevention; family members; persons with brain injury; and providers of rehabilitation.

What I find so appealing about *Maximizing Brain Injury Recovery: Integrating Critical Care and Early Rehabilitation* is that this book uses an interdisciplinary approach to working with persons with severe brain injury. This approach combines the efforts of multiple specialists and therapists. The book, while containing highly technical information, also contains much basic information and many charts, graphs, and cartoons that are helpful and easy to understand. I found this text to be well written and organized and to contain the most current information available from a medical and rehabilitative perspective. No other text currently exists that provides the basic science and clinical data for this unique and effective intervention approach.

The premise of this textbook and reference book is that aggressive rehabilitation should begin as soon as possible to maximize the potential for the person with severe brain injury to return to a productive healthy life in the family and community. The Brain Injury Association supports this approach.

I am particularly pleased with the chapters "Crisis Intervention: Care and Involvement of the Family" and "The Benefits of Combining Rehabilitation with Critical Care: Future Focus in Therapy and Medications." The Brain Injury Association was founded by family members and key professionals in the field back in 1980. I am a strong advocate of the inclusion of the family and the person with brain injury in designing rehabilitation and other programs.

This is a very comprehensive book that every practitioner can learn from and should own.

George A. Zitnay, PhD
President and Chief Executive Officer
Brain Injury Association
Washington, DC

Preface

One aspect of brain injury makes it unparalleled among all forms of disease and injury. The brain is the only organ that, when diseased or injured, can produce a total absence of consciousness. And in particular, during the recovery process, one's own identity may be transiently or permanently lost.

The charge of modern medicine is to develop methods and strategies for returning the person with severe brain injury to some degree of normalcy. In the last few decades, the critical care management of the person with severe brain injury has developed to the point that clinical management decisions can be based on relevant physiologic variables with the application of sound neurotrauma intensive care principles.

In many respects, rehabilitation medicine has paralleled the evolution of neurotrauma intensive care medicine. Beginning with Cope and Hall, the administrators of acute rehabilitation hospitals began to realize that the sooner rehabilitation is implemented, the better the functional outcome. More recently, our own work has demonstrated that rehabilitation should begin even sooner: that whenever possible, aggressive early rehabilitation must take place within the intensive care unit setting. It is clear that the benefits of this approach will result in less morbidity, better functional outcomes, fewer inpatient hospital days, and lower costs.

We have attempted to design a textbook and reference book that will educate the reader on the current acceptable guidelines and standards of practice in critical care and rehabilitation medicine. The essential theme of this text is the necessity of an interdisciplinary approach to treating persons with severe brain injury that combines the efforts of multiple specialists and therapists. This approach guided the book's organization. To demonstrate the integration of critical care and rehabilitation medicines, we have placed the rehabilitation therapy chapters not in a separate section, but next to chapters on related medical issues. The book's final chapter brings together the issues discussed, highlighting the benefits of medical, pharmacologic, and rehabilitative interventions and laying the groundwork for future advances.

Because both basic and highly technical information is presented, the book should appeal to a wide audience, from students of critical care and rehabilitation medicine to highly specialized physicians, nurses, and therapists in the field of brain injury. We hope that the information will prove useful for those confronted with the clinical and scientific problems of the severely brain injured.

Linda E. Mackay
Phyllis E. Chapman
Anthony S. Morgan

Acknowledgments

We would like to thank Dan Aitchison, Lisa Marie Anderson, Flo Hidalgo, Bette Kitik, Vivian Lane, and Joe Milhomens for their invaluable assistance and input into this book. Much appreciation is given to Linda Tanukis for her patience and talents in creating this textbook's artwork. We would also like to acknowledge Sandra Greenfield, OTR/L, for her assistance with the occupational therapy chapter.

CHAPTER 1

Trauma Systems: A Continuum of Care for the Severely Brain Injured

EPIDEMIOLOGY OF BRAIN INJURY

Trauma is the leading cause of death in the first four decades of life, resulting in more than 150,000 deaths annually.[1] In 1990, an estimated 9 million disabling injuries occurred, with 340,000 resulting in permanent impairment.[1] In 1966, a report by the National Academy of Sciences–National Research Council (NAS-NRC) characterized trauma as the "neglected disease of modern society."[2]

Brain injury is the leading cause of trauma-related deaths. Brain injuries occur every seven seconds and result in death every five minutes. The annual incidence of brain injury in the United States ranges from a low of 180 per 100,000[3] to an estimated high of 400 to 600 per 100,000,[4-6] according to extrapolations from studies. Major brain injury carries a mortality rate of 30% to 50%.[4] Of the 500,000 people who are permanently impaired or die from trauma, approximately 200,000 sustain major brain injury. For the entire US population, there is a conservative estimate of 500,000 new cases of brain injury per year.[7] Annual direct and indirect costs associated with brain injury are estimated at $39 billion.[7]

In no other category of trauma are young people so well represented. The peak age range for occurrence of brain injury is 15 to 24 years.[3] Increases are also noted in both sexes for those aged over 70 years.[3] Males are at greater risk of brain injury than females, with 3:1 ratios reported (Figure 1–1).

Mild brain injuries account for almost three quarters of all hospital admissions for brain injuries (approximately 73%). Moderate and severe brain injuries each account for approximately 16%, and 11% are reported as immediate deaths.[3]

The rate of brain injury deaths varies by geographical region. The highest incidence is reported in the West, a rate of 18.3 per 100,000 residents.[8] Other areas, including the South, Midwest, and Northeast, have reported incidences of 17.8, 16.0, and 15.6 per 100,000 respectively.[8]

1

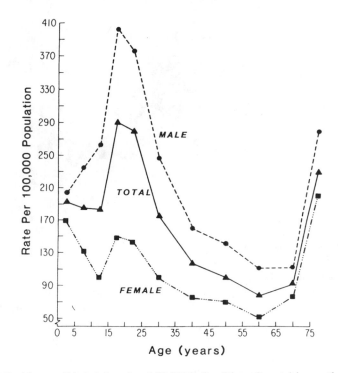

Figure 1–1 Incidence of brain injury (per 100,000 in San Diego County) by gender and age factors. *Source:* Reprinted with permission from J.F. Kraus, et al., *American Journal of Epidemiology,* Vol. 119, No. 2, p. 192, © 1984, The Johns Hopkins University School of Hygiene and Public Health.

External causes of brain injuries also differ by region. Figure 1–2 summarizes those causes within San Diego County.[3] Transport-related causes account for the highest percentage, followed by falls, assaults, sports/recreational activities, firearms, and blunt forces (eg, machinery). Sosin and colleagues,[8] using data from the National Center for Health Statistics, reported that brain injury–associated deaths are most often related to motor vehicles (57%), firearms (14%), and falls (12%). Within certain geographical areas, however, including nine states and the District of Columbia, firearms are now responsible for more fatalities than motor vehicle crashes.[9,10]

In 1992, violence was declared a public health emergency.[11] Violence has now extended beyond the urban environment and is not limited to certain ages, genders, or socioeconomic groups. Violence involving firearms is both a preventable illness and a major and worsening public health problem. Firearm injuries kill

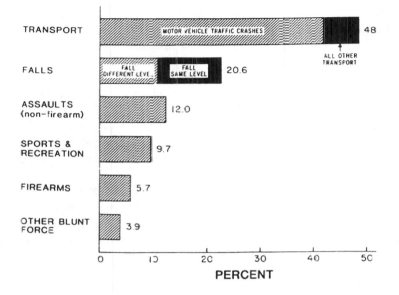

Figure 1–2 Categories of external causes of brain injury in San Diego County. *Source:* Reprinted with permission from J F. Kraus, et al., *American Journal of Epidemiology,* Vol. 119, No. 2, p. 194, © 1984, The Johns Hopkins University School of Hygiene and Public Health.

40,000 and injure 240,000 annually in the United States.[2] From 1970–1974, more Americans were killed by firearms in the United States than during the entire Vietnam conflict.[13] An estimated 200 million firearms are in circulation.[14,15] Nearly half of all households have one or more firearms, and one in four contains a handgun.[14] Handguns are the cause of approximately two thirds of homicides in the United States.[16]

Gunshot wounds to the head are the most lethal of all firearm injuries. Mortality rates vary from a low of 54% to a high of 88%.[16–23] Survivors of gunshot wounds to the head constitute less than 10% of patients with brain injury who survive.[24] In Los Angeles, a large proportion (72%) of gunshot wounds to the head in children and young adults is gang related.[25] Other metropolitan areas are also seeing significant rises in gang-related firearm violence.[26]

Suicide rates for children and adolescents have more than doubled in the past 30 years, primarily due to increased use of firearms.[27,28] Fifty-nine percent of all suicides are caused by firearms.[29] Having a firearm within a household increases the risk for a suicide severalfold.[30,31]

The estimated annual hospital cost associated with treatment of firearm-related injuries is greater than $1 billion.[32] The majority of victims of firearm injuries are uninsured.[33] Firearm-related injuries result in an estimated yearly economic burden, from lost wages and benefits and so forth, of $19 billion.[34]

In the 1980s, more than 40,000 deaths in the United States were caused by motorcycle crashes,[35–37] and upwards of 4,400 deaths per year continue to occur.[38] Motorcycle crash fatality rates are just below 80 per 100,000 registered motorcycles[39] and represent the highest rate of fatalities among all road vehicle accidents.[39] For each fatality, 90 other motorcyclists are injured severely enough to seek medical evaluation.[40] Brain injuries are the primary cause of those deaths and severe injuries.[29,41,42]

Bicycle crashes cause nearly 1,000 deaths in the United States per year and 550,000 cases of related injuries treated in emergency departments (ED).[35,43–46] Brain injuries are the primary cause of death and severe injury in bicycle-related crashes,[29,47–56] accounting for 62% to 64% of bicycle-related deaths, 33% of bicycle-related ED visits, and 67% of bicycle-related hospital admissions.[43,44,48,53,55–58] Frontal and temporal lobe contusions are the most common cause of fatal brain injury, followed by subdural hematomas.[57] As with other types of brain injury, death and injury rates are higher among males, with a male-to-female death ratio of approximately 4:1.[59] Collisions with motor vehicles account for nearly 90% of bicycle-related brain injury deaths.[48] Motor vehicle collisions, however, account for less than 25% of nonfatal bicycle-related brain injuries. Other causes include falls, striking fixed objects, and collisions with other bicyclists.[58,60] The annual societal cost of bicycle-related injuries and deaths is approximately $8 billion.[61]

Mechanisms of injury differ among various age groups. Among transport-related brain injuries, the percentage of pedestrian/vehicle collisions is highest in the younger-than-10-year age range and with bicyclists in the 5- to 15-year age range.[3,48,62] The single most common cause of serious brain injury in children younger than age 15 is bicycle accidents.[63] Nearly one quarter of all brain injuries in children younger than 15 years are bicycle related.[64] Falls generally occur most frequently in persons younger than 5 years and older than 65 years of age.[3] Assaults are most frequent between 15 and 24 years, and sports/recreational brain injuries are most frequent between 10 and 14 years of age.[3]

Brain injury deaths vary among racial groups. Motor vehicle–related deaths are reportedly 39% higher for whites than for blacks, whereas firearm-related deaths are 39% higher for blacks than for whites.[8] The percentage of firearm-related deaths is higher for blacks than for whites at all ages through 54 years.[8] However, the peak age range for firearm-related homicides for both blacks and whites is 25 to 34 years.[8] For whites, suicides account for 72% of firearm-related deaths, and homicides account for 21%.[8] For blacks, suicides account for 21% of firearm-related deaths, and homicides account for 72%.[8]

Regardless of the cause or incidence, several factors differentiate brain injuries from other forms of trauma. Compared with other types of trauma, such as visceral or musculoskeletal, traumatic brain injuries (TBIs) are more complex to treat. A lack of knowledge regarding the recovery process and a lack of treatment modalities that protect neuronal cell function contribute to this complexity. The degree of recovery and length of the recovery period are also unique with brain injuries. This silent epidemic not only involves extensive medical intervention but also necessitates months of inpatient rehabilitation followed by months or years of outpatient treatment and, often, transitional and vocational training. These individuals and their families must make a lifelong commitment to face the new and ongoing challenges that brain injury brings upon them.

The tragedy is that much of this mortality and morbidity can be prevented. Evidence has accumulated showing that organized approaches to treatment translate into decreased mortality, morbidity, and disability due to injuries.[65-85] For more than a decade, organizations such as the American College of Surgeons' Committee on Trauma (ACSCOT) and the American College of Emergency Physicians (ACEP) have supported the establishment of comprehensive trauma systems. Both have put forth guidelines to assist regions in planning, implementing, and evaluating all aspects of a trauma care system.

THE EVOLUTION OF TRAUMA CARE

During the late 1960s and early 1970s, the need for a systematic approach to trauma care became apparent. Early efforts were based on identifying patient needs by the type of injury (eg, burn, spinal cord injury).[86] The application of a systems approach called for the expansion of in-hospital techniques and technology to the prehospital and interhospital phases. The state of Illinois initiated statewide regionalization of emergency care for multiple and critical injuries in 1971. This system matured over time, initiating a program of patient transfer and care for burn patients to specific burn units, including a major burn center in Chicago.[87] Other programs, including one for spinal cord injuries, established in 1972,[88] were developed. The Illinois trauma program and the Maryland Institute for Emergency Medicine, established in 1973,[89] became the pioneering catalysts for the development of future regional trauma/emergency medical services (EMS) systems.

The Committee on Trauma is the oldest standing committee of the American College of Surgeons (ACS). Established in 1922 and initially called the Committee on the Treatment of Fractures, it became the Committee on Trauma in 1949. In

1976, the committee published the first document establishing guidelines for the care of the injured patient.[90] Although these guidelines have been revised on many occasions, they stand today as the benchmark for state trauma systems. The present guidelines include all aspects of a trauma system, including prehospital and hospital resources, rehabilitation, prevention, and quality improvement.[91]

In 1986, ACEP's Trauma Committee published guidelines identifying the components, providers, and settings for trauma care systems,[92] complementing those previously established by ACSCOT. In September 1992, these guidelines were updated.[93] This policy statement reviews the guidelines for system management, prehospital care, trauma care facilities, rehabilitation, injury control, and quality improvement. To portray the comprehensive trauma system, it employs a three-dimensional model encompassing four providers and nine components in two settings (Figure 1–3).

In 1990, Congress passed the Trauma Care Systems Planning and Development Act, which proposed a model trauma care system.[94] The act recognized injury as a public health problem and established a plan to serve the needs of all patients regardless of the severity of the injury. The model called for an all-inclusive trauma system integrating the EMS system into the coordinated sequence of events. In the plan, the trauma center is the central clinical institution, with other strategic components complementing a comprehensive system of care.

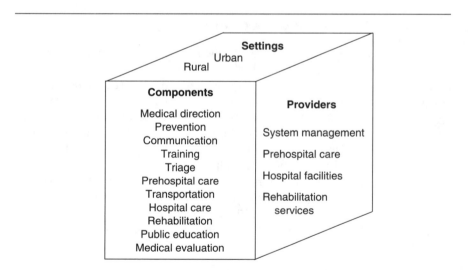

Figure 1–3 Three-dimensional model of a trauma care system. *Source*: Reprinted with permission from *Annals of Emergency Medicine,* Vol. 21, No. 6, p. 100, © 1992, The American College of Emergency Physicians.

In a systems approach to trauma, hospitals, skilled personnel, and public service agencies all work in concert to restore an individual's productive role in society. Once an injury occurs, the systems approach begins in the field, progresses to the hospital phase, and continues throughout rehabilitation and community reentry. A trauma system is not just a series of places (field, trauma center, rehabilitation facility) or a collection of specialists (EMS, emergency medicine, critical care medicine, trauma, rehabilitation) or concepts (preventive, educational, rehabilitative). A trauma system is all of these and more. It is how these components *work together* that results in a successful system of care for the injured patient.

PRIMARY PREVENTION

ACSCOT requires that trauma centers participate in preventative efforts. It is clearly recognized that the most effective and definitive intervention is still prevention. Three major approaches to prevention are automatic protection from and elimination of environmental hazards, legislation, and education. Programs established by trauma centers should focus on issues relevant to community needs and their high-risk populations (eg, violence, drunk driving). Trauma centers, in collaboration with public and private agencies, can successfully encourage use of preventative equipment, such as seat belts, air bags, and helmets. Automatic protection through product engineering is the most cost-effective intervention technique and can be quite effective in reducing the incidence of brain injury.

Safety Belts

The safety belt, specifically the lap-shoulder belt, is designed to protect occupants from ejection and to mitigate interior impact by restraining the upper body. New York State became the first state, in 1984, to pass a mandatory seat belt law, with 15 other states following within one year. In the United States, from 1980 to 1990, safety belt usage increased from 11% to 49%, primarily due to enactment of state laws.[95,96] Currently, 43 states, the District of Columbia, and Puerto Rico have passed mandatory seat belt laws. The national rate of safety belt usage has increased to 62%.[97] The National Highway Traffic Safety Administration estimates that lap and shoulder safety belts (three-point seat belts) reduce deaths to front-seat passengers by 45% and moderate to critical injuries by 50%.[98]

The head is one of the most commonly and most seriously injured areas in the unbelted patient,[99,100] with the majority of fatalities caused by brain injuries.[101] The incidence of brain injury is reduced when seat belts are used.[102,103] Additionally, hospital admissions, lengths of stay, mean hospital charges, and frequency of surgery are lower among belted patients.[102,104-106]

Although safety belt laws have been effective in increasing compliance, continued public education and enforcement of current laws are vital. The federal government estimates that approximately 10,000 lives could be saved per year by increasing safety belt compliance to 85%.[107] Unbelted persons are younger than belted persons and are more likely to be male and to have consumed alcohol.[106,108] They are more likely to be involved in head-on or rollover crashes.[106] Alcohol use is a factor in about half of all motor vehicle fatalities and results in more severe injuries in survivors.[109–111] Some racial and ethnic minority groups have lower rates of seat belt usage than whites.[112–114] These identified risk factors should be addressed when developing prevention programs for targeted populations.[114]

Air Bags

The air bag is designed to protect occupants by providing excellent interior impact mitigation and load distribution. It is designed to deploy when deceleration along the main vehicle axis exceeds a specified threshold. Air bags are most beneficial in frontal impacts. The recent implementation of side-impact air bags is expected to improve outcome in other types of collisions. Air bags provide a reported 12% to 19% additional increase in fatality prevention when coupled with seat belt usage[115–119] and may reduce serious brain injuries to belted drivers.[117] It appears that the combined efforts of seat belts and air bags provide more optimal protection against death and injury from motor vehicle accidents (MVAs) (Figure 1–4).[120–124]

Federal regulations require cars produced after 1990 to be equipped with automatic restraints.[125] These requirements, phased in over three years, stipulate either

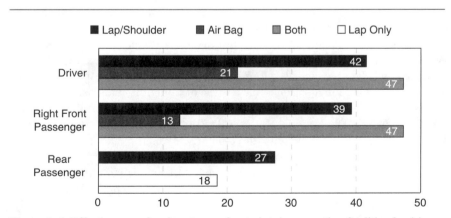

Figure 1–4 Effectiveness of various types of restraints in preventing fatalities for drivers, right front passengers, and rear passengers. *Source:* Data from references 121–125.

automatic safety belts or air bags. It takes about 15 years for a new technology to phase into current use. Lap-shoulder belts, introduced in the 1960s, are standard on virtually all passenger vehicles. By 1990, fewer than 4 million vehicles were equipped with driver-side air bags, but this number increased to approximately 5.5 million by 1991. Air bag usage does not have the obstacles to compliance that seat belt usage does.

Motorcycle Helmets

Helmet use lowers death rates as well as preventing and reducing the severity of brain injury from motorcycle crashes. Despite this fact debate continues to ensue in medical literature, public forums, and the media from proponents on both sides of mandated helmet-use laws. Studies demonstrate that the overall rate of brain injury increases two- to threefold or more in patients not wearing a helmet.[42,126-142] In one study, the frequency of brain injury in helmeted riders was 38%, compared to 66% for nonhelmeted riders.[143]

Methodologically sound studies exist demonstrating that states with full helmet-use laws have consistently lower brain injury–associated death rates than states without such laws.[126,127,129-131,138] States such as California, Louisiana, Nebraska, Texas, and Washington have studied the trends in brain injury–associated deaths and injuries secondary to enactment of mandatory helmet laws.[126,127,129,138] Of all fatally injured riders, the proportion with severe brain injury decreased 20% to 57%.[127,129,138] Declines of 22% in smaller studies and 30% to 55% in larger studies were noted for nonfatally injured riders.[126,127,129,131]

In 1967, the federal government issued standards requiring states to have motorcycle helmet–use laws to qualify for certain federal highway funds. Thirty-seven states enacted such laws within two years after the passage of this legislation. In 1976, Congress removed the financial penalty provisions, and within two years, 26 states had removed or reduced the requirements for helmet use. Currently, only 24 states and the District of Columbia have full mandatory helmet laws. A 1980 study estimated that $61 million could be saved annually if all states adopted mandatory helmet laws.[144]

Bicycle Helmets

Bicycle helmets reduce the incidence of fatal and nonfatal bicycle-related brain injuries up to 85%.[48-58,145-148] A study in Australia comparing 1,710 victims revealed at least a 39% reduced risk for brain injury with approved helmets; when cases of helmet dislodgment were excluded, the risk reduction was 45%.[149,150] Almost half of the impact points associated with head and face injuries were within the areas that would have been protected by a helmet. The largest prospective case-control study to date, completed in 1996, demonstrated a protective effect of 69% to 74% for helmets for three categories of head injury (any head injury, brain injury, and severe brain injury).[151] Additionally, helmets were equally effective in preventing brain injuries in crashes involving motor vehicles and those not involving motor vehicles.

In the year following enactment of mandatory bicycle helmet legislation in Victoria, Australia, 48% fewer brain injury admissions and deaths were noted. In the second year, a 70% decrease in admission and deaths was noted.[152] Several states and local municipalities have enacted laws requiring helmets, including California, Connecticut, Georgia, Massachusetts, New Jersey, New York, Oregon, Pennsylvania, Tennessee, several counties in Maryland, and the city of Beechwood, Ohio.

Although bicycle helmets provide protection against brain injury, only approximately 18% of bicyclists wear helmets all or most of the time.[61] The Centers for Disease Control and Prevention (CDC) have developed guidelines for state and local agencies and organizations planning brain injury prevention programs regarding the use of bicycle helmets.[43,44] Several studies have demonstrated the benefit of community bicycle helmet campaigns in increasing helmet usage.[153–159] Programs are most effective when conducted on a local or community level, adjusting to the needs of a specific community. Civic and public service organizations, local businesses, and hospitals can provide incentives, such as discount coupons or giveaways for bicycle helmets.

Other prevention efforts to reduce bicycle-related brain injuries include bicycle safety education,[160] designed to increase safe bicycling behaviors and improved design and manufacturing of bicycle helmets.[161–163] Some investigators have advocated separation of bicycles and motor vehicles through the design of bicycle lanes independent of roadways. Although this idea is appealing, it may be economically and geographically difficult or prohibitive.[160] Because most bicycle-related deaths are not due to collisions with motor vehicles, other efforts may be more effective in reducing the occurrence of brain injuries.

Firearms and Violence

Violence, including firearm usage, is a major public health problem in the United States. The Department of Health and Human Services has made prevention of suicide, homicide, and accidents a national priority.[107] Gunshot wounds to the head are the most lethal of all body wounds, accounting for 75% to 80% of deaths.[164,165] Handguns are the cause of two thirds of homicides. In 1988, handguns accounted for 75% of homicides, compared with shotguns (10%), assault weapons (8%), and rifles (7%).[166] Studies have demonstrated that access to guns promotes suicide, homicide, and accidents.[167–173]

One form of prevention includes legislation for improved gun control. Like other prevention strategies, however, gun control has been met with opposition by organizations such as the National Rifle Association.[174] In 1993, Congress passed the Brady Handgun Violence Prevention Act 18 USC §921, which mandates a five-day waiting period and requires background checks on handgun purchasers prior to gun purchase.[175] This legislation is only a first step. A nationwide computer system is expected to be implemented that will instantly complete a criminal background check and negate the need for the waiting period requirement. However, this requirement expires in 1998, regardless of whether the computerized system is in place.

Implementation of a national firearm control program has been recommended that would potentially restrict firearms to those who can rigorously justify a purpose for owning or selling guns and can ensure minimal standards of safety and training.[27,176] Currently, the United States has more gun dealers than gas stations.[177] A gun dealer's license costs only $10 and is easily available, allowing the new dealer to purchase firearms wholesale and to avoid waiting periods.[178] Most states have few, if any, restrictions on the number of guns an individual can purchase. Virginia has passed a law limiting handgun purchase to one per month. Legislation has been proposed to extend this law nationally. Other suggestions to reduce the number of guns in circulation include increasing the sales tax on firearms and ammunition for civilian use and expanding incentives for gun return programs.

Other preventative efforts include improving design modifications and expanding the use of firearm safety devices. Electronic trigger locks, which recognize owner fingerprints, are under development. This measure has the potential to reduce intentional/unintentional firearm use by family members, as well as to render stolen weapons inoperable.[175,179] A cooperative effort between a trauma center and a retailer resulted in consumer purchase of 850 trigger locks over a three-month period.[180]

Public education again surfaces as a viable means to reduce the incidence of violence and gun-related injuries. Education and prevention programs must be targeted appropriately to different groups. Those programs successful for adults may not be appropriate for adolescents, and programs geared toward minorities must differ from those geared toward Caucasians.[181] The high likelihood of repeated injury from interpersonal intentional violence warrants "postvention" in addition to prevention.[182] Trauma centers frequently sponsor or participate in prevention programs. Those programs can focus on drinking and driving, conflict resolution and violence prevention, and increased use of safety equipment.[183]

Education must also include accurate data, which are presently limited. Efforts to increase data on firearm injuries and death are needed. The state of Massachusetts established the first statewide surveillance system in the country requiring medical providers to report all gunshot wounds and intentional knife or sharp instrument wounds to police.[184] The Weapon-Related Injury Surveillance System is a three-year program sponsored by a grant from the CDC. Data from the project, shared with violence prevention groups, hospitals, and policy makers, has heightened prevention awareness within the state. The data have been used to help create victim services programs, teen violence prevention brochures, mentoring programs, and expanded education topics for residents.

PREHOSPITAL CARE

The 1966 NAS-NRC monograph entitled *Accidental Death and Disability: The Neglected Disease of Modern Society*[2] became the catalyst for the organization of the EMS system approach to care of the trauma patient.[185] In 1973, the NAS-NRC produced recommendations for appropriate strategies for developing and implementing a national system. Those recommendations facilitated the passage of the Emergency Medical Services System Act of 1973.[186] As a result of its passage, great emphasis, as well as funding, was given to developing regional EMS systems. New prehospital care professionals were developed: the emergency medical technician (EMT) and the paramedic. The act identified 15 components that would assist in establishing comprehensive, areawide, and regional EMS programs: personnel, training, communication, transportation, emergency facilities, critical care units, public safety, consumer participation, improved access to care, patient transfer, standardized recordkeeping, public information and education, system review and evaluation, disaster, and mutual aid. However, it failed to include the issue of medical direction.

Since that time, revisions have modernized these components to emphasize additional areas.[187] The revised components are training, communication, prehospital transport agencies, interfacility transport agencies, receiving facilities, specialty care units, public information and education, audit and quality assurance, disaster, mutual aid, protocols (triage, treatment, transport transfer), financing, dispatch, and medical direction. Between 1974 and 1981, more than $244 million was spent in the United States to establish and improve EMS systems.

As previously mentioned, the EMS system was integrated into an inclusive trauma system on November 16, 1990, when President George Bush signed into law the Trauma Care Systems Planning and Development Act.[94]

Prehospital management remains one of the most important factors in the acute care of an individual with brain injury, often influencing the final outcome. It begins with evaluation and treatment at the scene and continues until the patient is admitted to an appropriate facility. The best outcomes have been achieved by minimizing the amount of time spent in the prehospital phase. Currently, the prehospital phase of care consists of two levels of care: basic life support (BLS) and advanced life support (ALS).[188-190] Emergency medical technicians trained in BLS provide cardiopulmonary resuscitation, airway management, hemorrhage control, stabilization of fractures, and immobilization of the spine. EMT paramedics trained in ALS may perform more sophisticated procedures, including insertion of endotracheal tubes and intravenous lines.

The responsibility for EMS system development and funding is currently that of individual states. Not all states subsidize EMS systems, resulting in discrepancies between states in terms of education, training, and availability of certain prehospital personnel.[189]

Regardless of individual state discrepancies, improved outcomes have been associated with advancements in prehospital care during the last two decades.[69,190,191] What has become commonly known as the ABCs of trauma management—airway, breathing, and circulation—contributes to minimizing the secondary effects of hypoxia and hypotension by restoring adequate oxygen supply and preserving brain function. By minimizing risks and maximizing function, prehospital care can ensure that a patient with brain injury enters the trauma center with the best possible chances for an optimal recovery.

TRAUMA CENTERS

Optimal care for brain injury survivors requires the resources of highly specialized institutions called *trauma centers*. Trauma centers are part of a network of categorized and designated facilities equipped and staffed to deliver timely and specialized therapeutic intervention. The establishment of trauma centers has resulted in improved survival and functional outcome.[65,68,75,85,89,192,193] The provision of such specialized care requires both institutional and personal commitment. Institutions must commit by making available state-of-the-art facilities and equipment, including EDs, laboratories, operating rooms, radiology services, and intensive care units (ICUs), and by staffing these areas appropriately. Personal commitment is demonstrated by the support from hospital trustees and administration and by the training and dedication of the health care professionals involved in the treatment of trauma patients.

ACSCOT's publication *Resources for Optimal Care of the Injured Patient* outlines institutional guidelines for four levels of trauma centers.[91] These guidelines are listed in Exhibit 1–1. Essential versus desirable characteristics for the various levels have also been determined and are listed in Appendix 1–A.

Through the ACS's verification/consultation programs, trauma centers undergo an evaluatory process to assess their capability and performance in providing care to trauma patients. This verification process, established in 1987, includes completion of a questionnaire and a two-day on-site review of the trauma center and its medical, professional, and administrative staff by a team of ACS trauma

Exhibit 1–1 Guidelines for Four Levels of Trauma Centers

LEVEL I

The Level I facility is a regional resource trauma center that is a tertiary care facility central to the trauma care system. Ultimately, all patients who require the resources of the Level I center should have access to it. This facility must have the capability of providing leadership and total care for every aspect of injury, from prevention through rehabilitation. In its central role, the Level I center must have adequate depth of resources and personnel. Essential areas that distinguish Level I from Level II centers are as follows:

Clinical capabilities

- Cardiac surgery
- Hand surgery
- Microvascular surgery (replantation)
- Infectious disease
- Pediatric surgeons
- In-house general surgeon

Facilities/resources

- Cardiopulmonary bypass
- Operating microscope
- Acute hemodialysis
- Nuclear scanning
- Neuroradiology

Because of the large personnel and facility resources required for patient care, education, and research, most Level I trauma centers are university-based teaching hospitals. Other hospitals willing to commit these resources, however, may meet the criteria for Level I recognition.

In addition to acute care responsibilities, Level I trauma centers have the major responsibility of providing leadership in education, research, and system planning. This responsibility extends to all hospitals caring for injured patients in their region.

Medical education programs include postgraduate training in trauma for physicians, nurses, and prehospital providers. Education can be accomplished through a variety of mechanisms, including classic continuing medical education (CME), preceptorships, personnel exchanges, and other approaches appropriate to the local situation. Research and prevention programs, as defined in this document, are essential for a Level I trauma center.

LEVEL II

The Level II trauma center is a hospital that is also expected to provide initial definitive trauma care regardless of severity of injury. Depending on geographical location, patient volume, personnel, and resources, however, the Level II trauma center may not be able to provide the same comprehensive care as a Level I trauma center. Therefore, patients with more complex injuries may have to be transferred to a Level I center (for example, patients requiring advanced and extended surgical critical care). Level II trauma centers may be the most prevalent facility in a community, managing the majority of trauma patients.

continues

Exhibit 1–1 continued

The Level II trauma center can be an academic institution or a public or private community facility located in an urban, suburban, or rural area. Educational outreach, research, and prevention programs are similar to those required by a Level I trauma center. However, research is NOT an essential criterion for a Level II center. In some areas where a Level I center does not exist, the Level II center should take on the responsibility for education and system leadership.

LEVEL III

The Level III trauma center serves communities that do not have immediate access to a Level I or II institution. Level III trauma centers can provide prompt assessment, resuscitation, emergency operations, and stabilization and also arrange for possible transfer to a facility that can provide definitive trauma care. Prompt availability of general surgeons is required in a Level III facility. Planning for care of injured patients in these hospitals requires transfer agreements and standardized treatment protocols. Level III trauma centers are generally not appropriate in an urban or suburban area with adequate Level I and/or Level II resources.

LEVEL IV

Level IV trauma facilities provide advanced trauma life support prior to patient transfer in remote areas where no higher-level care is available. Such a facility may be a clinic rather than a hospital and may or may not have a physician available. Because of geographic isolation, however, the Level IV trauma facility is the de facto primary care provider. If willing to make the commitment to provide optimal care, given its resources, the Level IV trauma facility should be an integral part of the inclusive trauma system. As at Level III trauma centers, treatment protocols for resuscitation, transfer protocols, data reporting, and participation in system quality improvement (QI) are essential.

A Level IV trauma facility must have a good working relationship with the nearest Level I, II, or III trauma center. This relationship is vital to the development of a rural trauma system in which realistic standards must be based on available resources. Optimal care in rural areas can be provided by skillful use of existing professional and institutional resources supplemented by guidelines that result in enhanced education, resource allocation, and appropriate designation for all levels of providers. Also, it is essential for the Level IV facility to have the involvement of a committed health care provider, who can provide leadership and sustain the affiliation with other centers.

An inclusive system should leave no facility without direct linkage to a Level I or II trauma center. This association should facilitate expeditious transfer of seriously injured patients who require a higher level of care. Exchange of medical personnel between Level I/II and Level III/IV facilities may be an excellent way to develop this relationship. The Level I and II trauma centers have an obligation to extend their

continues

Exhibit 1–1 continued

educational outreach to the rural areas in the form of professional education, consultation, or community outreach. A mechanism should also be in place to deliver to the referring hospital feedback about individual patient care and outcome analysis.

Source: Reprinted with permission from *Resources for Optimal Care of the Injured Patient,* pp. 3–4, © 1993, American College of Surgeons.

surgeons. Following review and approval of the site by the Review Committee, ACSCOT may issue a verification certificate. This certificate remains valid for a maximum duration of three years.

The verification/consultation program is, as it states, a verification of the capabilities and qualifications of a particular facility. The *designation* of trauma centers is a separate political process involving specified government bodies. The development of trauma systems, including facility designation and role assignment within the system, lies within the jurisdiction of local, regional, or state health care system agencies. These agencies are responsible for anticipating the volume of major trauma cases and assessing available resources to determine the optimal number and level of trauma centers in a given area. Factors taken into consideration include geographical location, patient volume, personnel, and resources.

Once trauma centers are designated, the trauma system must strive to ensure that the "right patient" gets to the "right facility" to maximize cost-effectiveness and functional outcome. Little has been published on the extent to which regionalized systems achieve this goal. In 1990, MacKenzie et al[194] described criteria to identify patients who should be treated at trauma centers. The criteria were established by a panel of eight recognized experts in the delivery of trauma care. When the criteria were applied to all 1988 hospital trauma discharges in a state with regionalized trauma care, only 66% of patients who should have been treated at a trauma center received that level of care. Of patients identified as not requiring care at a trauma center, 66% were actually treated at non–trauma center hospitals. Despite some methodological limitations, this study provides insight regarding identification of patients at risk for receiving care that is not adequate to the extent of their overall injuries. The authors suggest continued development of guidelines for patient triage and transfer.

Rehabilitation

ACSCOT recognizes the necessity of including rehabilitation in a trauma system. *Resources for Optimal Care of the Injured Patient*[91] outlines relevant training for rehabilitation staff at Level I and II trauma centers regarding the acute care needs of critically injured patients. The prereview application does not specify requirements for individual therapies or the timing of initiation of services. However, it does request information on the relationship between trauma services and rehabilitation and requires that specific therapies in the ICU be identified (Exhibit 1–2). Trauma center verification at all levels requires establishment of contacts and protocols for the transfer of patients to rehabilitation facilities.

Rehabilitation standards are the weakest and most vague standards within the ACSCOT guidelines. Great variations in rehabilitative service provision exist within Level I trauma centers. In 1994, Mackay and Chapman surveyed ACS-verified Level I trauma centers. The purpose of the study was to identify referral and treatment patterns for rehabilitative services with patients with severe brain injuries. A total of 82 of 197 surveys were completed, representing hospitals in 32 different states. Information was obtained from staff within the rehabilitation departments on seven major areas:

1. therapy involvement
2. use of dedicated staff
3. means of referral
4. participation in interdisciplinary rounds
5. number of days from admission to therapy referral
6. percentage of patients treated in the ICU
7. frequency of therapy

Data are outlined in Table 1–1. Results of the study revealed that approximately two thirds of the trauma centers used treatment teams involving physical therapy (PT), occupational therapy (OT), and speech/language pathology (SLP). A physiatrist was included as a direct team member in approximately one third of the hospitals surveyed. The majority of hospitals initiated therapy services on an individual basis rather than using blanket orders (ie, ordering a TBI consult, which includes PT, OT, and SLP) or ordering a physiatrist consult. Other consult services available in the trauma center included audiology (46%), neuropsychology (40%), and psychology (33%).

The most common program characteristics identified were

- patient referral for rehabilitation services within 1 to 5 days post injury
- provision of ongoing physical, occupational, and SLP services during acute admission
- variations in initiation of therapies, with PT often initiated first
- provision of therapists' treatment to a mixed caseload of patients (ie, trauma and nontrauma patients), versus provision to only TBI or trauma patients

Exhibit 1–2 Rehabilitation Subsection of the American College of Surgeons Committee on Trauma's Prereview Questionnaire

---

Rehabilitative Services

1. Who is your Chief of Rehabilitation?

_____

   (Have Curriculum Vitae available during review)
   a. Board Certification? ____Yes ____No
   If yes, what specialty?

_____

   b. Describe the role and relationship of rehabilitation services to the trauma
      service.

_____

_____

_____

2. Are rehabilitative consultations routinely obtained while the trauma patient is in
   the ICU?
   ____Yes ____No
   If yes, who responds?

_____

3. What services are provided in the ICU?
   physical therapy ____Yes ____No
   occupational therapy ____Yes ____No
   speech therapy ____Yes ____No
   Other—please list

_____

_____

4. Have available (during review) the transfer protocols for acute or long-term
   disabilities.

Source: Reprinted with permission from *Pre-Review Questionnaire,* p. 13, © American College of Surgeons.

- daily treatment by all therapies involved
- involvement in trauma rounds on a weekly basis

Although the above model is that most commonly used, variations do exist. For example, the number of days from admission to referral for rehabilitation therapy

Table 1–1 Characteristics of Rehabilitation Services Provided within Level I Trauma Centers in the United States

Rehabilitation Services Provided within Level I Trauma Centers

Treating Discipline[a]	PT, OT, SLP	PT, OT, SLP, Phy	PT					Total
	53	28	1					82

Staff Caseload[b]	Dedicated	Mixed						Total
	26	40						66

Days to Referral[c]	1–2 days	3–5 days	6–10 days	>10 days				Total
	30	32	6	2				70

Referral Procedure[d]	Individual	Blanket	Physiatry	Standing order				Total
	54	13	7	7				81

% ICU Therapy[e]	100%	95–99%	90%	80–89%	70–75%	50%	<10%	Total
	32	5	10	10	7	10	1	75

Frequency Therapy[f]	1–2×/day	3–5×/week						Total
	64	11						75

Frequency Rounds[g]	1×/week	Daily	None	2×/week				Total
	48	7	15	4				74

[a] Therapies that provide ongoing treatment for patients with brain injuries while in the trauma center; PT = physical therapy; OT = occupational therapy; SLP = speech/language pathology; Phy = physiatry.

[b] Dedicated = therapist providing services only to trauma patients; Mixed-therapist providing services to both trauma and nontrauma patients.

[c] Number of days from admission to first rehabilitation referral.

[d] Individual = each discipline is ordered on an individual basis; Blanket = multiple therapies are ordered via one order (ie, TBI consult); Physiatry = physiatry consult obtained first, and physiatrist then orders rehabilitation therapies as needed; Standing order = Automatic on admission rehabilitation orders (either on individual or blanket basis).

[e] Percentage of patients with severe brain injury whose therapy was started in the ICU.

[f] Frequency of therapy sessions.

[g] Frequency of multidisciplinary rounds in which rehabilitation professionals participate.

spanned from one to more than 10 days. The percentage of patients whose therapy was initiated in the ICU varied from 100% to less than 10%. The frequency of therapy varied from twice a day to once or twice a week. The extent to which these variations affect patient outcome has not been extensively studied. A review of studies on the benefits of early intervention is provided in Chapter 15.

IMPACT OF REGIONALIZED SYSTEMS OF TRAUMA CARE

Several studies have reported on the impact of regionalized trauma systems. Some of these have used comparisons of mortality rates before and after institution of regionalized trauma care.[67,68,70,75,76,82,85,195] A series of articles investigating the impact of regionalized trauma care in California was published between 1979 and 1985. The first study, by West et al,[65] reviewed 90 fatalities in Orange County and 92 deaths in San Francisco County secondary to MVAs. Within Orange County, these patients were taken to the closest receiving hospital. Within San Francisco County, patients were brought to a centrally located trauma facility. Deaths were classified as preventable, potentially preventable, or not preventable, following calculation of Injury Severity Score (ISS)[196] scores and review of death certificates, coroner's reports, and autopsy data. Hospital records were also available for review within San Francisco County only. Of the 92 San Francisco County fatalities, only 1 was judged to be potentially preventable. In Orange County, as many as 73% of non–central nervous system (non-CNS) related deaths and 28% of CNS-related deaths were judged to be preventable. In San Francisco County, the majority of deaths occurred in the older-than- 50-year age range, whereas the majority of deaths in Orange County occurred in the 10- to 40-year age range.

In 1980, Orange County implemented a regionalized system of trauma care. West et al[67] compared the MVA fatalities occurring during this first year to those in their previous study, using the "autopsy method"[66] of evaluation. The results indicate a large reduction in the percentage of potentially preventable non–CNS-related deaths, from 73% to 9%. In 1983, Cales,[68] using a different patient cohort and methodology within the same county, compared 58 pre–trauma system MVA deaths to 60 post–trauma system MVA deaths. These fatalities included both CNS- and non–CNS-related diagnoses. A reduction in potentially salvageable deaths from 34% to 15% indicates that the implementation of a regionalized trauma system has a major impact on the quality of care for patients.

San Diego County incorporated a regionalized system of trauma care in 1984. Shackford et al[76] reported on an analysis of hospital records and coroner's reports for patients with Trauma Scores[197] less than or equal to 8 who were admitted during the first year of regionalization. Survival probability, determined using the TRISS method[198,199] (Trauma Score, Injury Severity Score, and age), was compared with that of the most recent coefficients of an index population (Major Trauma Outcome Study [MTOS]).[200,201] Results indicated significantly better survival of severely injured trauma patients. Forty patients were predicted to survive, and 67 did survive. No deaths within this study were judged to be preventable; all were secondary to lethal head injuries or a lethal combination of injuries.

In 1989, Guss et al[82] compared trauma deaths in San Diego County during 1986 to those occurring in 1979[202] before regionalization. This study used the same group of physician reviewers as the 1979 study, employing consistent methodology and variables. Physician reviewers were also blinded to the treating physician and hospital. The study reported a decline in preventable trauma deaths from 11.4% to less than 1%. The overall decline was largely due to non–CNS-related deaths. The authors do note, however, that other factors may have contributed to the decline in preventable deaths, including increased advanced trauma certification and improved prehospital care.

Similar results were also reported in 1990 by Smith et al,[203] who demonstrated significantly fewer complications and lower mortality rates for trauma victims treated in trauma versus nontrauma centers. In 1992, Kane et al[204] demonstrated statistically significant improvements in survival among MVA victims with ISSs between 26 and 50 following activation of a trauma system in Los Angeles County. In 1993, Thoburn et al[84] reported a reduction in non–CNS-related preventable deaths from 22.6% to 7% following the implementation of a regionalized system of trauma care in Florida. In 1994, Mullins et al[85] reported a one-third reduction in the adjusted rate of mortality at the designated trauma centers following implementation of a trauma system within Oregon.

Data from before the implementation of regionalized trauma systems continue to be collected in counties, states, and even countries. Sampalis and colleagues[83] reported on 355 severely injured patients (CNS and non-CNS) in a metropolitan area in Canada without regionalized trauma care. Results revealed 81% excess mortality following standardization to the MTOS population. Reduced excess mortality was seen in Level I– or II–compatible hospitals compared to Level III facilities. Additionally, there was a 30-fold increase in the standardized odds of dying associated with prehospital times exceeding 60 minutes.

West Germany is an example of a country that has instituted regional trauma care and has perhaps the most impressive system in the world today.[77, 205] Particularly impressive is the prehospital care; no patient is more than 30 minutes from a designated trauma center. Trauma centers have been established along the main highways, or autobahns. More important than the prehospital system, however, is the integration of trauma care within the hospitals, which are categorized and designated according to their capability to care for trauma patients. The German system has a very strong rehabilitation program as well, whose primary goal is to get the accident victim back to gainful employment. Since the inception of this integrated system in 1970, the mortality from MVAs has experienced a remarkable drop of 25%, from 16,000 to 12,000 per year.

FUNCTIONAL OUTCOMES

The focus of outcome studies that explore the benefits of trauma systems is mostly limited to issues of mortality and preventable deaths (Table 1–2). Certainly, decreased mortality has a positive impact on society from both an economic and a social perspective. However, there is a dearth of literature available on functional outcomes. Such information could greatly expand the knowledge base regarding the impact of trauma systems. True reflections of benefit should be measured in terms of length of stay, cost, individual functional skills, independence, and return to work and social activities.

In 1988, MacKenzie et al[206] reported on physical outcomes and return to work status one year post injury. They prospectively followed 479 trauma patients discharged from two Level I hospitals between July 1982 and March 1983. Severity of injury was quantified using the Abbreviated Injury Scale[207] and ranged from mild to severe. Of 147 patients with brain injuries, 52% had severe injury, 25% moderate injury, and 23% mild injury. At one year post injury, 39% of patients with severe brain injury had limitations with self-care, 13% had mobility or physical activity limitations, and 48% reported none of these limitations. Of patients with severe brain injury who had been premorbidly employed full time, 45% had returned to full-time employment at one year post injury. However, 33% were still convalescing, and 22% remained unemployed for other reasons. Cognitive impairments had a large influence on this persistent unemployment. Other factors that influenced but did not specifically prevent return to work were higher educational level, white-collar employment, higher preinjury income, and the presence of supportive family and friends.

Outcomes between the two facilities were not differentiated. However, significant differences in patient characteristics were noted. Seventy percent of all patients were discharged from one facility. That facility also had a higher percentage of patients who were white (83% vs 23%), had been employed before the injury (69% vs 42%), and were high school educated (67% vs 46%) than did the second facility. Also, 53% of patients discharged from that facility had sustained head or spine injuries (vs 12% in the other facility).

This study is significant in that it addresses the issue of functional outcome as it relates to physical mobility and self-care. However, the impact of other deficits, such as cognitive/language skills, was not studied. Studying such deficits is especially important for individuals with brain injuries, whose most common residual deficit is in short-term memory recall. This study also did not identify whether

Table 1–2 Review of the Effectiveness of Trauma Systems in Published Studies from 1979 to 1994

Author	Year	Time Period for Data Collection	Geographic Area	No. of Patients	Sample Description	Purpose/ Design	Results
West et al[65]	1979	1974–1975	Orange & San Francisco Counties	182	MVA deaths, excluding prehospital deaths	Compare % of preventable deaths for MVA victims in regions with and without trauma system	73% non-CNS and 28% CNS deaths in region without trauma system judged preventable
West[66]	1982	7/77–7/78	Orange County	100	MVA deaths, excluding prehospital deaths	Compare % of preventable deaths for non-CNS injuries using autopsy method versus hospital record method	71% of non-CNS deaths judged preventable by autopsy method as compared to 85% by hospital record; no false positives
West et al[67]	1983	6/80–6/81	Orange County	29	MVA deaths, including prehospital and CNS deaths	Compare trauma survival with and without trauma system by identifying	No. of preventable deaths decreased from 73% and 71% (pre–trauma

continues

Table 1–2 continued

Author	Year	Time Period for Data Collection	Geographic Area	No. of Patients	Sample Description	Purpose/ Design	Results
						and comparing % of preventable deaths (compare to West et al, 1979, and West, 1982)	system) to 9% (with trauma system); 4/6 preventable deaths for patients taken to nontrauma center
Cales[68]	1984	7/77–6/78 7/80–6/81	Orange County	118	MVA deaths, excluding burns without other injury, prehospital cardiac arrests, and late deaths unrelated to initial injury	Evaluate effect of implementation of trauma system by identifying potentially salvageable deaths before and after implementation	Proportion of salvageable deaths decreased from 34% to 15% and was associated with increase in age and severity of injury; MVA death rate dropped

Reference	Year	Dates	Location	N	Population	Purpose	Results
Shackford et al[76]	1987	8/84–7/85	San Diego Co	249	All trauma patients with TS ≤ 8 triaged to trauma center	Identify impact of regionalized trauma care on outcome for patients with TS ≤ 8 by comparing survival probability of patients to MTOS data	Observed survival rate for blunt injury (29%) significantly higher than predicted rate of 18%; for penetration injuries, observed survival rate 20% compared with predicted rate of 9%
Guss et al[82]	1989	1979 1986	San Diego Co	211	All in-hospital trauma deaths 1 hour post admission (CNS and non-CNS)	Measure impact of regionalized trauma system on preventable trauma deaths (comparing to previous 1979 study)	Decline in preventable deaths from 11.4% to <1%; significant decline in non-CNS; non-significant decline in CNS-related preventable deaths
Smith et al[100]	1990	PA: 1985 MD: 1986–1987	Western PA and MD	1,332	Femoral fractures with OR (non-CNS injuries)	Evaluate difference in LOS, complications, and deaths	Patients in trauma center showed significantly fewer complications (21% vs 33%)

continues

Table 1-2 continued

Author	Year	Time Period for Data Collection	Geographic Area	No. of Patients	Sample Description	Purpose/ Design	Results
						between trauma and nontrauma centers for patients with femoral fractures taken to OR	and lower mortality rate ($p<.05$)
Kane et al[204]	1992	9/82–11/82 9/84–11/84	Los Angeles Co	1,424	Patients with ISS >15, admitted to 1 of 57 hospitals in study; injury not limited to anoxic/ hypoxic injury or spontane- ous pathologic fracture	Ascertain if there was a decline in mortality rates following implementation of trauma system	Significant improve- ment in adjusted odds of survival with MVA victims with multiple serious injuries following imple- mentation of trauma system

Author	Year	Dates	Location	N	Sample	Methods	Results
Sampalis et al[83]	1992	4/87–3/88	Montreal	355	Sample patients with severe trauma admitted to hospital (CNS and non-CNS)	Apply Flora's Z statistic and indirect standardization to MTOS in non–trauma system study sample and to identify association between prehospital and hospital components and a standardized mortality ratio	81% excess mortality compared to MTOS data; reduced excess mortality in Levels I and II versus III; significant increase in excess mortality when prehospital time >60 minutes
Thoburn et al[84]	1993	10/89–4/91	Florida	504	Trauma deaths, including isolated CNS, drowning, and thermal injuries and prehospital deaths	Evaluate effect of implementation of trauma system on preventable death rate by comparing post–trauma system data to 1984 study (pre–trauma system)	Decrease in preventable trauma death rate from 23% to 7% following implementation of trauma system

continues

Table 1–2 continued

Author	Year	Time Period for Data Collection	Geographic Area	No. of Patients	Sample Description	Purpose/ Design	Results
Mullins et al[85]	1994	1984–1985 presystem 1986–1987 early 1990–1991 established	Portland, OR		All trauma patients admitted during identified time periods (CNS and non-CNS)	Ascertain if there was a reduction in risk of death or mortality following implementation of trauma system	Patients with ISS ≥16—77% admitted to Level I; patients with ISS <16—72% admitted to nontrauma center; risk of death at Level I declined after implementation of truama system

rehabilitation services had been received. The presence or absence and frequency of rehabilitative services could have influenced the reported outcomes.

In 1988, Rhodes et al[208] reported on long-term outcomes of individuals admitted to a Level I trauma center via helicopter. Of the 302 survivors, extremity and pelvic injuries were most common, followed by injuries to the chest, head/neck, abdomen, and face. At 6 months post injury, 17 patients had severe disability, 34 had moderate disability, and 251 had good recovery, according to the Glasgow Outcome Scale.[209] Of the patients with good recovery, the most common injury was to the extremities or pelvis. Of the patients with moderate or severe disability, approximately half had serious injuries to the head or neck, the extremities or pelvis, or both. Of 292 previously employed individuals, 220 had returned to work by six months. At follow-up three to four years post injury, 26 of the 72 remaining individuals had returned to work, 3 were looking for employment, 26 were not employed, 1 was deceased, and 16 could not be contacted.

Although these studies did address functional outcome, they did not compare pre- and post-trauma system outcomes or outcomes between institutions with and without intact trauma systems. One cannot ascertain if outcomes would have been similar if patients had been admitted to hospitals that were not within a trauma system.

CURRENT STATUS IN THE PROGRESS OF TRAUMA SYSTEMS

The majority of states in the United States have no formalized system of care for the trauma patient. Progression in the development of state and county systems has been reported in several published articles. In 1988, West et al[210] reported on a survey conducted with state EMS directors or health departments having responsibility over emergency and trauma planning. States were identified as having a regional trauma system when they complied with eight essential components identified by the authors. These components, based on criteria set forth by the ACS, are as follows:

1. established legal authority to designate trauma centers
2. established formal designation process
3. use of ACS standards for trauma centers
4. use of outside survey team for trauma center designation
5. number of trauma centers, based on volume and population
6. written triage criteria for bypassing nontrauma centers
7. ongoing monitoring systems
8. statewide trauma center coverage

Results identified only two states, Maryland and Virginia, complying with all essential components. Nineteen states and the District of Columbia had systems but did not meet all eight components. Twenty-nine states, at that time, had not initiated the process of trauma center designation.

In 1995, Bazzoli et al[211] published data updating the study of West et al. The study, examining the status of trauma system development in 1993, stands as the most current publication of data. The authors noted an increasing interest among state agencies in developing trauma systems, stemming from the increased availability of funds through the Trauma Care System Planning and Development Act of 1990. Through this public law, 19 states were awarded grants in 1993 to initiate development of trauma systems, and an additional 16 states received grants to refine existing programs.

Bazzoli et al identified 43 regional and state organizations with legal authority to administer trauma systems and to designate trauma centers: 13 regional organizations within the state of California; 8 regional and 2 state organizations within the states of Florida and Massachusetts; 18 state organizations within Delaware; Georgia; Illinois; Missouri; Nevada; New Jersey; New Mexico; New York; North Carolina; Oregon; South Carolina; Tennessee; Utah; Virginia; Washington, DC; and West Virginia; and 2 state public and private organizations within Maryland and Pennsylvania. According to the eight essential components identified by West et al, five states (Florida, Maryland, Nevada, New York, and Oregon) in 1993 now met the criteria for a regional trauma system, compared with two in 1987 (Maryland and Virginia). Virginia no longer limited the number of designated trauma centers and therefore no longer met the eight components. In October 1995, the state of Connecticut instituted a statewide trauma system.

One significant finding of the Bazzoli et al study is that most trauma systems do not have policies to limit the number of designated trauma centers. Of the 20 states and Washington, DC, with organizations for designation of trauma centers, only 5 imposed these limitations. The primary reason for limiting designation is that trauma centers are thereby ensured adequate numbers of patients and are better able to maintain proficiency. Mullins and colleagues[85] substantiated a decline in the risk of death at Level I trauma centers when the number of seriously injured patients treated at those facilities was increased. It was suggested that this increase improved proficiency and facilitated the development of better protocols.

In 1990, Smith et al[212] analyzed data on 1,643 severely injured trauma patients to determine the relationship between volume and mortality rates. Results indicated an inverse relationship between volume and mortality. The authors stated that "certain minimum numbers of seriously injured patients are needed to be seen by each trauma center to insure optimal performance."[212 (p1074)]

Published data exist demonstrating reductions in morbidity and mortality through the implementation of trauma systems. Nonetheless, progress in implementing regional trauma systems continues to be slow. Many factors influence the rate of progression, including health care reform–related issues.

HEALTH CARE REFORM AND THE ECONOMIC STATUS OF TRAUMA SYSTEMS

Despite enthusiastic support for trauma systems from groups like the ACS, several common obstacles affect their development[213]:

1. Many states lack the statutory framework for overseeing the implementation process. This backing of public authority is vital for an effective trauma system.
2. Trauma system development is not immune to political opposition. Individual hospitals may have concerns regarding the effect of redirecting patients to other trauma centers. Volunteer ambulance organizations, fire chiefs, and sheriffs may be skeptical about supporting state-organized systems.
3. Financial concerns continue to plague hospitals. Trauma centers incur large costs in establishing and maintaining equipment and providing adequate staffing and education. Financial burdens vary depending upon many factors, including the adequacy of the state's Medicaid program, the availability of reimbursement for uninsured and indigent patients, the degree to which the state enforces mandatory automobile insurance laws, the distribution of patients, and the general economic status of the community.

The problem of uncompensated care is a key factor in the overall financial equation affecting trauma care. Uncompensated care has been identified as one of the primary reasons that trauma centers close.[214] By 1990, 66 trauma centers across 14 states and the District of Columbia had closed. Areas where trauma center closures were most common included Los Angeles; Dade County, Florida; and Chicago.[215]

Trauma Care Reimbursement

Many payers, including Medicare and some Medicaid programs, use a diagnosis-related group (DRG) system for reimbursement. This prospective payment system is based on fixed allocation, with no consideration for individual hospital service. Thus, each DRG category has a set payment rate independent of the actual services rendered by the hospital.

A study by Schwab et al[216] in 1988 reported that prospective payment fee levels are inadequate to meet the costs of successful trauma care. They reported that as severity of injury (according to ISS group) increased, cost, length of stay, and mortality increased. Although reimbursement also increased, it was not proportionate with trauma center costs, resulting in substantial financial loss for all ISS groups, with greater losses incurred with more seriously injured patients.

Other systems of reimbursement exist, including private health insurance, automobile insurance, workers' compensation, and an increasing number of managed-care systems. In 1994, Eastman et al[217] reported on a survey of 313 trauma centers from 48 states, identifying the present economic issues confronting trauma centers. Sixty-nine percent of respondents providing financial data reported financial losses. Fifty-eight percent of trauma centers reported serious financial problems, and 36% reported minor financial problems. The most frequently reported cause was increasing numbers of uninsured patients. The percentage of reimbursement varied dependent upon payer class, with ranges from 54% loss to 24% surplus. Those payers whose reimbursement resulted in a loss for the trauma centers included self-pay, county, Medicaid, and Medicare. These four payers accounted for 49.4% of all patients. Total reimbursement for all payer classes resulted in an average 8.4% loss. Varying rates of surplus or loss were identified by service areas, with urban areas experiencing an 11.8% loss; suburban areas, a 5.7% loss; and rural areas, a 3.7% surplus.

Some states use automobile insurance as an important source of reimbursement. States vary greatly, however, in the proportion of trauma center revenue recouped from automobile insurance. Ranges vary from highs of 50% to lows of 7% or lower. Trauma centers in states that use "no-fault" insurance policies and have high volumes of motor vehicle accidents are most successful in using this form of insurance as a source of reimbursement.

Physician Support

Trauma centers also face difficulties in maintaining the support of trauma physicians. Problems include financial concerns and staff commitment for on-call scheduling. The unwillingness of physicians to be on call for trauma can seriously affect the quality of services provided.[214] Recruitment of physician staff, including trauma physicians, can be difficult.[214,217]

Cost Containment

Trauma centers are not immune to the economic pressures of cost containment. Measures such as reducing staffing, eliminating unnecessary procedures, and controlling unnecessary use of supplies are occurring across the nation. Physicians are pressured to minimize lengths of stay to reduce hospital losses. Trauma centers are not the only institutions faced with the issues of cost containment. Rehabilitation facilities face similar difficulties, and this can negatively affect the trauma center. Lack of funding sources can delay or prevent the transfer of patients to rehabilitation facilities. Managed-care providers frequently dictate approved rehabilitation facilities, often reducing a patient's options and sometimes resulting in admission delays to those facilities. Trauma centers also experience difficulties in placing patients with specific needs (eg, ventilator dependency, quadraparesis, or persistent coma).

SUMMARY

Health care reform, spurred by the 1992 presidential election and continuing increases in cost, has made changes in the provision of health care inevitable. Even in the face of difficult economic conditions, advances in provision of trauma care can prove to be cost-effective and beneficial to the community. Long-term solutions will involve cooperative agreement and support between institutions and state and federal agencies. Injury prevention programs and public education must become integral components of trauma systems. Those programs must address issues relative to community needs, including increases in interpersonal and domestic violence. The most certain means of cost containment remains prevention.

With the advent of trauma systems, a reshifting of patient care has occurred. Level I and II trauma centers receive higher-acuity trauma patients with significantly higher ISS scores. The establishment of trauma centers has also resulted in improved survival and outcome. Patients who in the past would have succumbed to their injuries are now surviving with improved chances for a good outcome. The ED and ICU become the primary arenas to stabilize a brain injury and prevent secondary complications. Approaches that can maximize outcomes for persons with severe brain injuries must be identified and thoroughly researched. Interventions, specifically in the ICU, fostered by good teamwork are the rate-limiting steps in minimizing secondary injuries and maximizing functional outcome.

REFERENCES

1. National Safety Council. *Accident Facts*. Chicago, Ill: National Safety Council; 1991.

2. National Academy of Sciences–National Research Council. *Accidental Death and Disability: The Neglected Disease of Modern Society*. Washington, DC: National Academy of Sciences; 1966:195.

3. Kraus JF, Black MA, Hessol N, Ley P, et al. The incidence of acute brain injury and serious impairment in a defined population. *Am J Epidemiol*. 1984;119:186–201.

4. Frankowski RF, Annegers JF, Whitman S. Epidemiology and descriptive studies 1. The descriptive epidemiology of head trauma in the United States. In: Becker DB, Povlishock JT, eds. *Central Nervous System Trauma: Status Report*. Bethesda, Md: National Institutes of Health; 1985.

5. Jagger J, Levine JL, Jane JA, Rimel RW. Epidemiologic features of head injury in a predominately rural population. *J Trauma*. 1984;24:40–44.

6. Marshall SB, Marshall LF, Vos HR, Chesnut RM. *Neuroscience Critical Care: Pathophysiology*. Philadelphia, Pa: WB Saunders Co; 1990.

7. Zitnay GA. SCI's silent partner: mild brain injury. *Adv Directors Rehabil*. 1995;4:6. Guest Editorial.

8. Sosin DM, Sacks JJ, Smith SM. Head injury–associated deaths in the United States from 1979 to 1986. *JAMA*. 1989;262:2251–2255.

9. Recktenwalk W. Guns lead a deadly race: more Illinoisans die from bullets than car crashes. *Chicago Tribune*. November 1, 1993;1:4.

10. Centers for Disease Control and Prevention. Deaths resulting from firearm and motor vehicle related injuries: United States, 1968–1991. *MMWR*. 1994;43:37–42.

11. Novello AC, Shosky J, Froehlke R. From the Surgeon General, US Public Health Service: a medical response to violence. *JAMA*. 1992;267:3007.

12. Voelker R. Taking aim at handgun violence. *JAMA*. 1995;273:1739–1740.

13. Adelson L. The gun and the sanctity of human life; or the bullet as pathogen. *Pharos*. 1980;43:15–25.

14. Cook PJ. Notes on the availability and prevalence of firearms. *Am J Prev Med.* 1993;9:33–37.

15. Council on Scientific Affairs, American Medical Association. Assault weapons as a public health hazard in the United States. *JAMA*. 1992;267:3067–3070.

16. Kaufman HH. Civilian gunshot wounds to the head. *Neurosurgery.* 1993;32:962–964.

17. Deshmukh VD, Laneve L, Fallon WF Jr. Violent brain injuries by gunshot in Duval County, Florida, 1989–1991. *Arch Neurol*. 1992;49:588. Letter.

18. Levi L, Linn S, Feinsod M. Penetrating craniocerebral injuries in civilians. *Br J Neurosurg.* 1991;5:241–247.

19. Benzel EC, Day WT, Kesterson L, Willis BK. Civilian craniocerebral gunshot wounds. *Neurosurgery*. 1991;29:67–71.

20. Siccardi D, Cavaliere R, Pau A, Lubinu F, et al. Penetrating craniocerebral missile injuries in civilians: a retrospective analysis of 314 cases. *Surg Neurol.* 1991;35:455–460.

21. Mancuso P, Chiarmonte I, Passanisi M, Guarnera F, et al. Craniocerebral gunshot wounds in civilians: report on 40 cases. *J Neurosurg Sci.* 1988;32:189–194.

22. Cavaliere R, Cavenago L, Siccardi D, Viale GL. Gunshot wounds of the brain in civilians. *Acta Neurochir (Wien)*. 1988;94:133–136.

23. Clark WC, Muhlbauer MS, Watridge CB, Ray MW. Analysis of 76 civilian craniocerebral gunshot wounds. *J Neurosurg*. 1986;65:9–14.

24. Grafman J, Salazar A. Methodological considerations relevant to the comparison of recovery from penetrating and closed head injuries. In: Levin HS, Grafman J, Eisenberg HM, eds. *Neurobehavioral Recovery from Head Injury*. New York, NY: Oxford University Press; 1987:43–54.

25. Levy ML, Masri LS, Levy KM, Johnson FL. Penetrating craniocerebral injury resultant from gunshot wounds: gang-related injury in children and adolescents. *Neurosurgery*. 1993;33:1018–1024.

26. Stone JL, Lichtor T, Fitzgerald LF, Barrett JA, et al. Demographics of civilian cranial gunshot wounds: devastation related to escalating semiautomatic usage. *J Trauma*. 1995;38:851–854.

27. Koop CE, Lundberg GD. Violence in America: a public health emergency. *JAMA*. 1992;267:3075–3076.

28. Seltzer F. Trend in mortality from violent deaths: suicide and homicide, United States, 1960–1991. *Stat Bull Metropolitan Insurance Co.* 1994;75:10–18.

29. Baker S, O'Neill B, Ginsburg M, Li G, eds. *The Injury Fact Book.* 2nd ed. New York, NY: Oxford University Press; 1992.

30. Kellermann AL, Rivara FP, Rushforth NB, Banton JG. Gun ownership as a risk factor for homicide in the home. *N Engl J Med.* 1993;329:1084–1091.

31. Kellermann AL, Rivara FP, Somes G, Reay DT. Suicide in the home in relation to gun ownership. *N Engl J Med.* 1992;327:467–472.

32. Martin MJ, Hunt TK, Hulley SB. The cost of hospitalization for firearm injuries. *JAMA.* 1988;260:3048–3050.

33. Clancy TV, Misick LN, Covington D, Churchill MP, et al. The financial impact of intentional violence on community hospitals. *J Trauma.* 1994;37:1–4.

34. Max W, Rice DP. Data watch. Shooting in the dark: estimating the cost of firearm injuries. *Health Aff (Millwood).* 1993;12:171–185.

35. National Highway Traffic Safety Administration. *Fatal Accident Reporting System: 1989.* Washington, DC: US Dept of Transportation; 1990. Publication DOT-HS 809-507.

36. Zettas JP, Zettas P, Thanasophon B. Injury patterns in motorcycle accidents. *J Trauma.* 1979;19:833–836.

37. Andrew TA. A six-month review of motorcycle accidents. *Injury.* 1978;10:317–320.

38. National Highway Traffic Safety Administration. *Fatal Accident Reporting System—1985.* Washington, DC: US Dept of Transportation; 1987. Publication (DO) HS 807-071.

39. Kraus JF, Peek C, McArthur DL. Williams A. The effect of the 1992 California motorcycle helmet use law on motorcycle crash fatalities and injuries. *JAMA.* 1994;272:1506–1511.

40. Barancik JI, Chatterjee BF, Greene-Cradden YC, Michenzi EM. Motor vehicle trauma in northeastern Ohio: I. Incidence and outcome by age, sex, and road-use category. *Am J Epidemiol.* 1986;123:846–861.

41. Russo PK. Easy rider—hard facts. *N Engl J Med.* 1978;299:1074–1076.

42. Sarkar S, Peek C, Kraus JF. Fatal injuries in motorcycle riders according to helmet use. *J Trauma.* 1995;38:242–245.

43. Centers for Disease Control and Prevention. Injury control recommendations for bicycle helmets. *J Sch Health.* 1995;65:133–139.

44. Centers for Disease Control and Prevention. Injury-control recommendations: bicycle helmets. *MMWR.* 1995;44(RR-1):1–17.

45. National Center for Health Statistics. *Vital Statistics Mortality Data, Multiple Causes of Death Detail, 1984–1988.* Hyattsville, Md: US Dept of Health and Human Services, Centers for Disease Control. Machine-readable public-use tapes.

46. National Safety Council. *Accident Facts.* Chicago, Ill: National Safety Council; 1982:45–91.

47. Bicycle helmet promotion programs: Canada, Australia, and United States. *MMWR.* 1993;42:203–210.

48. Sacks JJ, Holmgreen P, Smith SM, Sosin DM. Bicycle-associated head injuries and deaths in the United States from 1984 through 1988: how many are preventable? *JAMA.* 1991;266:3016–3018.

49. Cass DT, Gray AJ. Paediatric bicycle injuries. *Aust NZ J Surg.* 1989;59:719–724.

50. Nixon J, Clacher R, Pearn J, Corcoran A. Bicycle accidents in childhood. *Br Med J.* 1987;294:1267–1269.

51. Waters EA. Should pedal cyclists wear helmets? A comparison of head injuries sustained by pedal cyclists and motor cyclists in road traffic accidents. *Injury.* 1986;17:372–375.

52. McDermott FT, Klug GL. Injury profile of pedal and motor cyclist casualties in Victoria. *Aust NZ J Surg.* 1985;55:477–483.

53. Friede AM, Azzara CV, Gallagher SS, Guyer B. The epidemiology of injuries to bicycle riders. *Pediatr Clin North Am.* 1985;32:141–151.

54. Thorson J. Pedal cycle accidents. *Scand J Soc Med.* 1984;2:121–126.

55. Fife D, Davis J, Tate L, Wells JK, et al. Fatal injuries to bicyclists: the experience in Dade County, Florida. *J Trauma.* 1983;23:745–755.

56. Guichon DM, Myles ST. Bicycle injuries: one-year sample in Calgary. *J Trauma.* 1975;15:504–506.

57. Bjornstig U, Ostrom M, Eriksson A, Sonntag-Ostrom E. Head and face injuries in bicyclists, with special reference to possible effects of helmet use. *J Trauma.* 1992;33:887–893.

58. Thompson RS, Rivara FP, Thompson DC. A case-control study of the effectiveness of bicycle safety helmets. *N Engl J Med.* 1989;320:1361–1367.

59. Baker SP, O'Neil B, Karpf RS. *The Injury Fact Book.* Lexington, Mass: Lexington Books; 1984:265–267.

60. Belongia E, Weiss H, Bowman M, Rattanassiri P. Severity and types of head trauma among adult bicycle riders. *Wis Med J.* 1988;87:11–14.

61. Rodgers GB. *Bicycle and Bicycle Helmet Use Patterns in the United States: A Description and Analysis of National Survey Data.* Washington, DC: US Consumer Product Safety Commission; 1993.

62. Gerberich SG, Parker D, Dudzik M. Bicycle-motor vehicle collisions: epidemiology of related injury incidence and consequences. *Minn Med.* 1994;77:27–31.

63. Ivan LP, Choo SH, Ventureyra EC. Head injuries in childhood: a 2-year survey. *Can Med Assoc J.* 1983;128:281–284.

64. Kraus JF, Fife D, Cox P, Ramstein K. Incidence, severity, and external causes of pediatric brain injury. *Am J Dis Child.* 1986;140:687–693.

65. West JG, Trunkey DD, Lim RC. Systems of trauma care: a study of two counties. *Arch Surg.* 1979;114:455–460.

66. West JG. Validation of autopsy method for evaluating trauma care. *Arch Surg.* 1982;117:1033–1035.

67. West JG, Cales RH, Cazzaniga AB. Impact of regionalization: the Orange County experience. *Arch Surg.* 1983;118:740–744.

68. Cales RH. Trauma mortality in Orange County: the effect of implementation of a regional trauma system. *Ann Emerg Med.* 1984;13:1–10.

69. Jacobs LM, Sinclair A, Beiser A, D'Agostino RB. Prehospital advanced life support: benefits in trauma. *J Trauma.* 1984;24:8–13.

70. Cales RH, Anderson PG, Heilig RW Jr. Utilization of medical care in Orange County: the effect of implementation of a regional trauma system. *Ann Emerg Med.* 1985;14:853–858.

71. Cales RH, Trunkey DD. Preventable trauma deaths: a review of trauma care systems development. *JAMA.* 1985;254:1059–1063.

72. National Highway Traffic Safety Administration. *Emergency Medical Services Program and Its Relationship to Highway Safety.* US Dept of Transportation technical report, publication DOT HS 806. Washington, DC: Government Printing Office; 1985:832.

73. Ornato JP, Craren EJ, Nelson NM, Kimball KF. Impact of improved emergency medical services and emergency trauma care on the reduction in mortality from trauma. *J Trauma.* 1985;25:575–579.

74. Alexander RH, Pons PT, Krischer J, Hunt P. The effect of advanced life support and sophisticated hospital systems on motor vehicle mortality. *J Trauma.* 1984;24:486–490.

75. Shackford SR, Hollingsworth-Fridlund P, Cooper GF, Eastman AB. The effect of regionalization upon the quality of trauma care as assessed by concurrent audit before and after institution of a trauma system: a preliminary report. *J Trauma.* 1986;26:812–820.

76. Shackford SR, Mackersie RC, Hoyt DB, Baxt WG, et al. Impact of a trauma system on outcome of severely injured patients. *Arch Surg.* 1987,122:523–527.

77. *Congressional Record.* January 6. 1938;133.

78. Committee on Labor and Human Resources. *Report on Emergency Medical Services and Trauma Care Improvement Act of 1988.* 1988:100–504.

79. Zoler ML. Trauma care. *Med World News.* June 13, 1988:69.

80. *Congressional Record.* January 25, 1989;135.

81. Emergency Medical Services and Trauma Care Improvement Act of 1989. 101st Congress, 1st session (Jan. 25, 1989).

82. Guss DA, Meyer FT, Neuman TS, Baxt WG, et al. The impact of a regionalized trauma system on trauma care in San Diego County. *Ann Emerg Med.* 1989;18:1141–1145.

83. Sampalis JS, Lavoie A, Williams JI, Mulder DS, et al. Standardized mortality ratio analysis on a sample of severely injured patients from a large Canadian city without regionalized trauma care. *J Trauma.* 1992;33:205–211.

84. Thoburn E, Norris P, Flores R, Goode S, et al. System care improves trauma outcome: patient care errors dominate reduced preventable death rate. *J Emerg Med.* 1993;11:135–139.

85. Mullins RJ, Veum-Stone J, Helfand M, Zimmer-Gembeck M, et al. Outcome of hospitalized injured patients after institution of a trauma system in an urban area. *JAMA.* 1994;271:1919–1924.

86. Boyd D, Edlich RD, Micik SH. *Systems Approach to Emergency Medical Care.* Norwalk, Conn: Appleton-Century-Crofts; 1983.

87. Ogilivie RB. *Special Message on Health Care.* Springfield, Ill: State of Illinois Printing Office; 1971.

88. Meyer P, Rosen HB, Hall W. Fracture dislocations of the cervical spine: transportation, assessment, and immediate management. *An Acad Orthop Surg.* 1976;25:171–183.

89. Cowley RA. Trauma center: a new concept for the delivery of critical care. *J Med Soc NJ.* 1977;74:979–986.

90. American College of Surgeons. *Hospital and Prehospital Resources for Optimal Care of the Injured Patient.* Chicago, Ill: American College of Surgeons; 1976:3–4.

91. American College of Surgeons. *Resources for Optimal Care of the Injured Patient.* Chicago, Ill: American College of Surgeons, 1993.

92. American College of Emergency Physicians. Guidelines for trauma care systems. *Ann Emerg Med.* 1987;16:459–463.

93. American College of Emergency Physicians. *Guidelines for Trauma Care Systems.* Dallas, Tex: American College of Emergency Physicians; 1992.

94. Trauma Care Systems Planning and Development Act of 1990. 42 USC §§300d-11, 300d-31.

95. National Highway Traffic Safety Administration. *Occupant Protection Facts*. Washington, DC: US Dept of Transportation; 1991.

96. Increased safety-belt use: United States, 1991. *MMWR*. 1992;41:421–423.

97. National Highway Traffic Safety Administration. *Card Announces Record Year for Highway Safety* [news release]. Washington, DC: US Dept of Transportation; December 1992.

98. National Highway Traffic Safety Administration. *1991 Occupant Protection Facts*. Washington, DC: US Dept of Transportation; 1992.

99. Sato TB. Effects of seat belts and injuries resulting from improper use. *J Trauma*. 1987;27:754–758.

100. Daffner RH, Deeb ZL, Lupetin AR, et al. Patterns of high-speed impact injuries in motor vehicle occupants. *J Trauma*. 1988;28:498–501.

101. Mackay M. Mechanisms of injury and biomechanics: vehicle design and crash performance. *World J Surg*. 1992;16:420–427.

102. Redelmeier DA, Blair PJ. Survivors of motor vehicle trauma: an analysis of seat belt use and health care utilization. *J Gen Intern Med*. 1993;8:199–203.

103. Lestina DC, Williams AF, Lund AK, Zador P, et al. Motor vehicle crash injury patterns and the Virginia seat belt law. *JAMA*. 1991;265:1409–1413.

104. Marine WM, Kerwin EM, Moore EE, Lezotte DC, et al. Mandatory seatbelts: epidemiologic, financial, and medical rationale from the Colorado matched pairs study. *J Trauma*. 1994;36:96–100.

105. Reath DB, Kirby J, Lynch M, Maull KI. Injury and cost comparison of restrained and unrestrained motor vehicle crash victims. *J Trauma*. 1989;29:1173–1176.

106. Public health focus: impact of safety-belt use on motor-vehicle injuries and costs—Iowa, 1987–1988. *MMWR*. 1993;42:704–706.

107. US Dept of Health and Human Services. *Healthy People 2000: National Health Promotion and Disease Prevention Objectives*. Washington, DC: US Government Printing Office; 1990.

108. Bueno MM, Redeker N, Norman EM. Analysis of motor vehicle crash data in an urban trauma center: implications for nursing practice and research. *Heart Lung*. 1992;21:558–567.

109. National Committee for Injury Prevention and Control. *Injury Prevention: Meeting the Challenge*. New York, NY: Oxford University Press; 1989.

110. National Research Council (US) Committee on Trauma Research. *Injury in America: A Continuing Public Health Problem*. Washington, DC: National Academy Press; 1985.

111. Table reporting alcohol involvement in fatal motor-vehicle crashes. *JAMA*. 1992;268:317–318.

112. Council FM. *Seat Belts: A Follow-Up Study of Their Use under Normal Driving Conditions*. Chapel Hill, NC: University of North Carolina Highway Safety Research Center; 1969.

113. Hunter WW, Campbell BJ, Stewart JR. Seat belts pay off: the evaluation of a community-wide incentive program. *J Safety Res*. 1986;17:23–31.

114. Colon I. Race, belief in destiny, and seat belt usage: a pilot study. *Am J Public Health*. 1992;82:875–877.

115. Viano DC. Restraint effectiveness, availability and use in fatal crashes: implications to injury control. *J Trauma*. 1995;38:538–546.

116. Zador PL, Ciccone MA. Automobile driver fatalities in frontal impacts: air bags compared with manual belts. *Am J Public Health*. 1993;83:661–666.

117. Lund AK, Ferguson SA. Driver fatalities in 1985–1993 cars with airbags. *J Trauma*. 1995;38:469–475.

118. National Highway Traffic Safety Administration. *Evaluation of the Effectiveness of Occupant Protection: Federal Motor Vehicle Safety Standard 208.* Washington DC: US Dept of Transportation; 1992.

119. Kahane CJ. Fatality reduction by automatic occupant protection in the United States. Presented at 14th International Technical Conference on Enhanced Safety of Vehicles; September 1994; Munich, Germany.

120. Evans L. The effectiveness of safety belts in preventing fatalities. *Accident Anal Preven.* 1986;18:229–241.

121. Evans L. *Traffic Safety and the Driver.* New York, NY: Van Nostrand Reinhold; 1991.

122. Evans L, Frick MC. Potential fatality reductions through eliminating occupant ejection from cars. *Accident Anal Preven.* 1989;21:169–182.

123. Zador P, Ciccone M. *Driver Fatalities in Frontal Impacts: Comparison between Cars with Airbags and Manual Belts.* Arlington, Va: Insurance Institute for Highway Safety; 1991.

124. Viano DC. Crash injury prevention: a case study of fatal crashes of lap-shoulder belted occupants. In: Society of Automotive Engineers, ed. *Proceedings of the 1992 Stapp Car Crash Conference.* Warrendale, Pa: Society of Automotive Engineers; 1992.

125. 49 CFR §5 571.208.

126. Mock CN, Maier RV, Boyle E, Pilcher S, et al. Injury prevention strategies to promote helmet use decrease severe head injuries at a Level I trauma center. *J Trauma.* 1995;39:29–33.

127. Kraus JF, Peek C, McArthur DL, Williams A. The effect of the 1992 California motorcycle helmet use law on motorcycle crash fatalities and injuries. *JAMA.* 1994;272:1506–1511.

128. Orsay EM, Muelleman RL, Peterson TD, Jurisic DH, et al. Motorcycle helmets and spinal injuries: dispelling the myth. *Ann Emerg Med.* 1994;23:802–806.

129. Fleming NS, Becker ER. The impact of the Texas 1989 motorcycle helmet law on total and head-related fatalities, severe injuries, and overall injuries. *Med Care.* 1992;30:832–845.

130. Sosin DM, Sacks JJ. Motorcycle helmet-use laws and head injury prevention. *JAMA.* 1992;267:1649–1651.

131. Muelleman RL, Mlinek EJ, Collicott PE. Motorcycle crash injuries and costs: effect of an enacted comprehensive helmet use law. *Ann Emerg Med.* 1992;21:266–272.

132. Kelly P, Sanson T, Strange G, Orsay E. A prospective study of the impact of helmet usage on motorcycle trauma. *Ann Emerg Med.* 1991;20:852–856.

133. Sosin DM, Sacks JJ, Holmgreen P. Head injury-associated deaths from motorcycle crashes: relationship to helmet-use laws. *JAMA.* 1990;264 2395–2399.

134. McSwain NE Jr, Belles A. Motorcycle helmets: medical costs and the law. *J Trauma.* 1990;30:1189–1199

135. Shankar BS, Dischinger PC, Ramzy AL, et al. Helmet use, patterns of injury and medical outcome among motorcycle drivers in Maryland. In: Association for the Advancement of Automotive Medicine, ed. *34th Annual Proceedings of the Association for the Advancement of Automotive Medicine.* Des Plaines, Ill: Association for the Advancement of Automotive Medicine; 1990: 13–34.

136. Bachulis BL, Sangster W, Gorrell GW, Long WB. Patterns of injury in helmeted and nonhelmeted motorcyclists. *Am J Surg.* 1988;155:708–711.

137. Evans L, Frick MC. Helmet effectiveness in preventing motorcycle driver and passenger fatalities. *Accident Anal Preven.* 1988;20:447–458.

138. McSwain NE, Willey AB. *Impact of the Re-enactment of the Motorcycle Helmet Law in Louisiana: Final Report for National Highway Traffic Safety Administration.* New Orleans, La: Tulane University School of Medicine; 1984.

139. McSwain NE Jr, Petrucelli E. Medical consequences of motorcycle helmet nonusage. *J Trauma.* 1984;24:233–236.

140. Heilman DR, Weisbuch JB, Blair RW, Graf LL. Motorcycle-related trauma and helmet usage in North Dakota. *Ann Emerg Med.* 1982;11:659–664.

141. Luna GK, Copass MK, Oreskovich MR, Carrico CJ. The role of helmets in reducing head injuries from motorcycle accidents: a political or medical issue? *West J Med.* 1981;135:89–92.

142. Watson GS, Zador PL, Wilks A. Helmet use, helmet use laws, and motorcyclist fatalities. *Am J Public Health.* 1981;71:297–300.

143. Offner PJ, Rivara FP, Maier RV. The impact of motorcycle helmet use. *J Trauma.* 1992;32:636–641.

144. Muller A. Evaluation of the costs and benefits of motorcycle helmet laws. *Am J Public Health.* 1980;70:586–592.

145. Wasserman RC, Waller JA, Monty MJ, Emery AB, et al. Bicyclists, helmets and head injuries: a rider-based study of helmet use and effectiveness. *Am J Public Health.* 1988;78:1220–1221.

146. Worell J. Head injuries in pedal cyclists: how much will protection help? *Injury.* 1987;18:5–6.

147. Dorsch MM, Woodward AJ, Somers RL. Do bicycle helmets reduce severity of head injury in real crashes? *Accident Anal Preven.* 1987;19:183–190.

148. Wasserman RC, Buccini RV. Helmet protection from head injuries among recreational bicyclists. *Am J Sports Med.* 1990;18:96–97.

149. McDermott FT. Bicyclist head injury prevention by helmets and mandatory wearing legislation in Victoria, Australia. *Ann R Coll Surg Engl.* 1995;77:38–44.

150. McDermott FT, Lane JC, Brazenor GA, Debney EA. The effectiveness of bicyclist helmets: a study of 1710 casualties. *J Trauma.* 1993;34:834–844.

151. Thompson DC, Rivara FP, Thompson RS. Effectiveness of bicycle satety helmets in preventing head injuries. *JAMA.* 1996;276:1968–1973.

152. Cameron MH, Vulcan AP, Finch CF, Newstead SW. Mandatory bicycle helmet use following a decade of voluntary promotion in Victoria, Australia: an evaluation. *Accident Anal Preven.* 1994;26:325–337.

153. DiGuiseppi CG, Rivara FP, Koepsell TD, Polissar L. Bicycle helmet use by children: evaluation of community-wide helmet campaign. *JAMA.* 1989;262:2256–2261.

154. Vulcan AP, Cameron MH, Heiman L. Evaluation of mandatory bicycle helmet use in Victoria, Australia. Presented at the 36th Annual Meeting of the Association for the Advancement of Automotive Medicine; May 1992; Portland, Ore.

155. Cote TR, Sacks JJ, Lambert-Huber DA, Dannenberg AL, et al. Bicycle helmet use among Maryland children: effect of legislation and education. *Pediatrics.* 1992;89:1216–1220.

156. Dannenberg AL, Gielen AC, Beilenson PL, Wilson MH, et al. Bicycle helmet laws and educational campaigns: an evaluation of strategies to increase children's helmet use. *Am J Public Health.* 1993;83:667–674.

157. Rodgers LW, Bergman AB, Rivara FP. Promoting bicycle helmets to children: a campaign that worked. *J Musculoskeletal Med.* 1991;8:64–77.

158. Rivara FP, Thompson DC, Thompson RS, Rogers LW, et al. The Seattle children's bicycle helmet campaign: changes in helmet use and head injury admissions. *Pediatrics.* 1994;93:567–569.

159. Morris BA, Trimble NE. Promotion of bicycle helmet use among school children: a randomized clinical trial. *Can J Public Health.* 1991;82:92–94.

160. Weiss BD. Bicycle-related head injuries. *Clin Sports Med.* 1994;13:99–112.

161. Ryan GA. Improving head protection for cyclists, motorcyclists, and car occupants. *World J Surg.* 1992;16:398–402.

162. Resnick MP, Ross M, Schmidt TA, Wiest J Jr, et al. Helmets and preventing motorcycle and bicycle injuries: comments and a correction. *JAMA.* 274:939. Letter to editor.

163. Hadden TA, Benzel EC. Preventive aspects of helmet safety. *Western J Med.* 1993;158:69–70. Letter to editor.

164. Awasthi D, Hickey J, Carey ME. Civilian gunshot wounds to the head: a demographic study. Presented at 60th Annual Meeting, American Association of Neurological Surgeons; April 11–16, 1992; San Francisco, Calif.

165. Lee RK, Waxweiler RJ, Dobbins JG, Paschetag T. Incidence rates of firearm injuries in Galveston, Texas, 1979–1981. *Am J Epidemiol.* 1991;134:511–521.

166. Council on Scientific Affairs, American Medical Association. Assault weapons as a public health hazard in the United States. *JAMA.* 1992;267:3067–3070.

167. Blackman PH. Firearm access and suicide. *JAMA.* 1992;267:3026–3027.

168. Brent DA, Perper JA, Allman CJ, Moritz GM, et al. The presence and accessibility of firearms in the homes of adolescent suicides: a case-control study. *JAMA.* 1991;266:2989–2995.

169. Cotton P. Gun-associated violence increasingly viewed as public health challenge. *JAMA.* 1992;267:1171–1174.

170. Loftin C, McDowall D, Wiersema B, Cottey TJ. Effects of restrictive licensing of handguns on homicide and suicide in the District of Columbia. *N Engl J Med.* 1991;325:1615–1620.

171. Taubes G. Violence epidemiologists test the hazards of gun ownership. *Science.* 1992;258:213–215.

172. National Center for Environmental Health and Injury Control, Centers for Disease Control. Unintentional firearm-related fatalities among children, teenagers: United States, 1982–1988. *JAMA.* 1992;268:451–452.

173. Webster DW, Chaulk CP, Teret SP, Wintemute GJ. Reducing firearm injuries. *Issues Sci Technol.* 1991;7:73–79.

174. Voelker R. NRA fires at CDC gun injury research. *Am Med News.* May 20, 1991:6.

175. Culcross P. Legislative strategies to address firearm violence and injury. *J Fam Pract.* 1996;42:15–17.

176. Committee on Public Health, New York Academy of Medicine. Firearm violence and public health: limiting the availability of guns. *JAMA.* 271;1281–1283.

177. Violence Policy Center. *More Gun Dealers Than Gas Stations: A Study of Federally Licensed Firearms Dealers in America.* Washington, DC: Violence Policy Center; 1992.

178. Teret SP, Wintemute GJ. Policies to prevent firearm injuries. *Health Aff (Millwood).* 1993;12:96–108.

179. American College of Physicians. Preventing firearm violence: a public health imperative. *Ann Intern Med.* 1995;122:311–313.

180. Flinn RJ, Allen LG. Trigger locks and firearm safety: one trauma center's prevention campaign. *J Emerg Nurs.* 1995;21:296–298.

181. Rodriguez MA, Brindis CD. Violence and Latino youth: Prevention and methodological issues. *Public Health Rep.* 1995;110:260–267.

182. Schwarz DF, Grisso JA, Miles CG, Holmes JH, et al. A longitudinal study of injury morbidity in an African-American population. *JAMA*. 1994;271:755–760.

183. Lane-Reticker A, Weiner AL, Morgan AS, Griffin A. Violence prevention program targeting Connecticut adolescents: description and preliminary results. *Conn Med*. 1996;60:15–19.

184. Ozonoff VV, Barber CW, Spivak H, Hume B, et al. Weapon-related injury surveillance in the emergency department. *Am J Public Health*. 1994;84:2024–2025.

185. O'Rourke B. Emergency medical services system legislation. In: Cleary VL, Wilson P, Super G, eds. *Prehospital Care: Administration and Clinical Management*. Rockville, Md: Aspen Publishers, Inc; 1987:3–8.

186. Emergency Medical Services System Act of 1973. 42 USC §§5g-9, 300d.

187. Roush WR, McDowell RM. Emergency medical services system. In: Roush WR, ed. *Principles of EMS Systems: A Comprehensive Text for Physicians*. Dallas, Tex: American College of Emergency Physicians; 1989:9–17.

188. Morgan AS. The trauma center as a continuum of care for persons with severe brain injury. *J Head Trauma Rehabil*. 9;1994:1–10.

189. Lee RW. Education of prehospital personnel. In: Roush WR, ed. *Principles of EMS Systems: A Comprehensive Text for Physicians*. Dallas, Tex: American College of Emergency Physicians; 1989:181–187.

190. Drake L, Thompson M. System design and human resources. In: Cleary VL, Wilson P, Super G, eds. *Prehospital Care: Administration and Clinical Management*. Rockville, Md: Aspen Publishers, Inc; 1987:9–23.

191. Fortner GS, Oreskovich MR, Copass MK, Carrico CJ. The effects of prehospital trauma care on survival from a 50-meter fall. *J Trauma*. 1983;23:976–981.

192. Mackay LE, Bernstein BA, Chapman PE, Morgan AS, et al. Early intervention program in severe head injury: long term benefits of a formalized program. *Arch Phys Med Rehabil*. 1992;73:635–641.

193. Morgan AS, Chapman P, Tokarski L. Improved care of the traumatically brain injured. Presented at First Annual Conference of the Eastern Association for Surgery of Trauma; January 1988; Longboat Key, Fla.

194. MacKenzie EJ, Steinwachs DM, Ramzy AI. Evaluating performance of statewide regionalized systems of trauma care. *J Trauma*. 1990;30:681–688.

195. Rutledge R, Fakhry SM, Meyer A, Sheldon GF, et al. An analysis of the association of trauma centers with per capita hospitalizations and death rates from injury. *Ann Surg*. 1993;218:512–524.

196. Baker SP, O'Neill B, Haddon W Jr, Long WB. The Injury Severity Score: a method for describing patients with multiple injuries and evaluating emergency care. *J Trauma*. 1974;14:187–196.

197. Moreau M, Gainer PS, Champion HR, Sacco WJ. Application of the trauma score in the prehospital setting. *Ann Emerg Med*. 1985;14:1049–1054.

198. Champion HR, Sacco WJ, Carnazzo AJ, Copes W, et al. Trauma score. *Crit Care Med*. 1981;9:672–676.

199. American College of Surgeons, Committee on Trauma. Quality assessment and assurance in trauma care. *Bull Am Coll Surg*. 1986;71:4–23.

200. Champion HR, Gainer PS, Yackee E. A progress report on the trauma score in predicting a fatal outcome. *J Trauma*. 1986;26:927–931.

201. Champion HR, Frey CF, Sacco WJ. Determination of national normative outcomes for trauma. *J Trauma.* 1984;24:651. Abstract.

202. Neuman TS, Bockman MA, Moody P, Danford JV. An autopsy study of traumatic deaths: San Diego County—1979. *Am J Surg.* 1982;144:722–727.

203. Smith JS Jr, Martin LF, Young WW, Macioce DP. Do trauma centers improve outcome over non-trauma centers: The evaluation of regional trauma care using discharge abstract data and patient management categories. *J Trauma.* 1990;30:1533–1538.

204. Kane G. Wheeler NC, Cook S, Englehardt R, et al. Impact of the Los Angeles County trauma system on the survival of seriously injured patients. *J Trauma.* 1992;32:576–583.

205. Trunkey DD. Predicting the community's needs. In: West JG, ed. *Trauma Care Systems.* New York, NY: Praeger Publishers; 1983:5–10.

206. MacKenzie EJ, Siegel JH, Shapiro S, Moody M, et al. Functional recovery and medical costs of trauma: an analysis by type and severity of injury. *J Trauma.* 1988;28:281–295.

207. American Association for Automotive Medicine, Committee on Injury Scaling. *The Abbreviated Injury Scale—1985 Revision.* Des Plaines, Ill: American Association for Automotive Medicine; 1985.

208. Rhodes M, Aronson J, Moerkirk G. Petrash E. Quality of life after the trauma center. *J Trauma.* 1988;28:931–937.

209. Jennett B, Bond M. Assessment of outcome after severe brain damage: a practical scale. *Lancet.* 1975;1:430–484.

210. West JG, Williams MJ, Trunkey DD, Wolferth CC Jr. Trauma systems: current status—future challenges. *JAMA.* 1988;259:3597–3600.

211. Bazzoli GJ, Madura KJ, Cooper GF, Mackenzie EJ, et al. Progress in the development of trauma systems in the United States. *JAMA* 1995;273:395–401.

212. Smith RF, Frateschi L, Sloan EP, Campbell L, et al. The impact of volume on outcome in seriously injured trauma patients: two years' experience of the Chicago trauma system. *J Trauma.* 1990;30:1066–1075.

213. Mendeloff JM, Cayten CG. Trauma systems and public policy. *Annu Rev Public Health.* 1991;12:401–424.

214. Dailey JT, Teter H, Cowley RA. Trauma center closures: a national assessment. *J Trauma.* 1992;33:539–547.

215. Uzych L. Trauma care systems. *Am J Emerg Med.* 1990;8:71–75.

216. Schwab CW, Young G, Civil I, Ross SE, et al. DRG reimbursement for trauma: the demise of the trauma center (the use of ISS grouping as an early predictor of total hospital cost). *J Trauma.* 1988;28:939–946.

217. Eastman AB, Bishop GS, Walsh JC, Richardson JD, et al. The economic status of trauma centers on the eve of health care reform. *J Trauma.* 1994;36:835–846.

Essential and/or Desirable Characteristics for the Four Levels of Trauma Centers

Source: Reprinted with permission from *Resources for Optimal Care of the Injured Patient,* pp. 119–124, © 1993, American College of Surgeons.

HOSPITAL CRITERIA CHECKLIST

The following table shows levels of categorization and their essential (E) or desirable (D) characteristics.

	I	II	III	IV	Checklist for your hospital Yes	No
		Levels				
A. HOSPITAL ORGANIZATION						
1. Trauma Service	E	E	E	—	☐	☐
2. Trauma Service Director	E	E	E	—	☐	☐
3. Trauma Multidisciplinary Committee	E	E	D	—	☐	☐
4. Hospital Departments/Divisions/ Sections						
a. General Surgery	E	E	E	D	☐	☐
b. Neurologic Surgery	E	E	D	—	☐	☐
c. Orthopaedic Surgery	E	E	D	—	☐	☐
d. Emergency Services	E	E	E	D	☐	☐
e. Anesthesia	E	E	E	—	☐	☐
B. CLINICAL CAPABILITIES						
Specialty Availability						
1. In-house 24 hours a day:						
a. General Surgery	E[1]	E[1]	—	—	☐	☐
b. Neurologic Surgery	E[2]	E[2]	—	—	☐	☐
c. Emergency Medicine	E[3]	E[3]	E[4]	—	☐	☐
d. Anesthesiology	E[5]	E[5,6]	—	—	☐	☐
2. On call and promptly available:[7]						
a. Anesthesiology	—	—	E[3]	D	☐	☐
b. Cardiac Surgery	E	D	—	—	☐	☐
c. Cardiology	E	E	D	—	☐	☐
d. General Surgery	—	—	E[9]	D	☐	☐
e. Hand Surgery	E	D	—	—	☐	☐
f. Infectious Disease	E	D	—	—	☐	☐
g. Internal Medicine	E[10]	E[10]	E[10]	—	☐	☐
h. Microvascular Surgery (replant/flaps)	E	D	—	—	☐	☐
i. Neurologic Surgery	—	—	D	—	☐	☐
j. Obstetric/Gynecologic Surgery	E	E	D	—	☐	☐
k. Ophthalmic Surgery	E	E	D	—	☐	☐
l. Oral/Maxillofacial Surgery	E	E	—	—	☐	☐

	Levels				Checklist for your hospital	
	I	II	III	IV	Yes	No
m. Orthopaedic Surgery	E	E	D	—	☐	☐
n. Pediatric Surgery[11]	E	D	—	—	☐	☐
o. Pediatrics[10]	E	E	D	—	☐	☐
p. Plastic Surgery	E	E	D	—	☐	☐
q. Pulmonary Medicine	E	E	—	—	☐	☐
r. Radiology	E	E	D	D	☐	☐
s. Thoracic Surgery	E[12]	E[12]	—	—	☐	☐
t. Urologic Surgery	E	E	D	—	☐	☐

C. FACILITIES/RESOURCES/CAPABILITIES

1. Emergency department (ED)
   a. Personnel

	I	II	III	IV	Yes	No
1) Designated physician director	E	E	E	D	☐	☐
2) Physician who has special competence in care of critically injured and who is a designated member of the trauma team and is physically present in the ED 24 hours a day	E[3]	E[3]	E	—	☐	☐
3) Nursing personnel with special capability in trauma care who provide continual monitoring of the trauma patient from hospital arrival to disposition in ICU, OR, or patient care unit	E	E	E	D	☐	☐

   b. Equipment for resuscitation of patients of **all ages** shall include but not be limited to:

	I	II	III	IV	Yes	No
1) Airway control and ventilation equipment, including laryngo-scopes and endotracheal tubes of all sizes, bag-mask resuscit-ator, pocket masks, and oxygen	E	E	E	E	☐	☐
2) Pulse oximetry	E	E	E	D	☐	☐
3) End-tidal CO_2 determination	E	E	D	D	☐	☐
4) Suction devices	E	E	E	E	☐	☐

	I	II	III	IV	Checklist for your hospital Yes	No
5) Electrocardiograph-oscillo-scope-defibrillator	E	E	E	E	☐	☐
6) Apparatus to establish central venous pressure monitoring	E	E	E	D	☐	☐
7) Standard intravenous fluids and administration devices, including large-bore intravenous catheters	E	E	E	E	☐	☐
8) Sterile surgical sets for						
a) Airway control/cricothyrotomy	E	E	E	E	☐	☐
b) Thoracotomy	E	E	E	D	☐	☐
c) Vascular access	E	E	E	E	☐	☐
d) Chest decompression	E	E	E	E	☐	☐
9) Gastric decompression	E	E	E	E	☐	☐
10) Drugs necessary for emergency care	E	E	E	E	☐	☐
11) X-ray availability, 24 hours a day	E	E	E	D	☐	☐
12) Two-way communication with vehicles of emergency transport system	E	E	E	E	☐	☐
13) Skeletal traction devices, including capability for cervical traction	E	E	E	D	☐	☐
14) Arterial catheters	E	E	D	D	☐	☐
15) Thermal control equipment						
a) For patient	E	E	E	E	☐	☐
b) For blood and fluids	E	E	E	D	☐	☐
2. Operating suite						
a. Personnel and operating room Operating room adequately staffed in-house and immediately available 24 hours a day	E	E	D	—	☐	☐
b. Equipment for **all ages** shall include but not be limited to						
1) Cardiopulmonary bypass capability	E	D	—	—	☐	☐

	Levels				Checklist for your hospital	
	I	II	III	IV	Yes	No
2) Operating microscope	E	D	—	—	☐	☐
3) Thermal control equipment						
a) For patient	E	E	E	—	☐	☐
b) For blood and fluids	E	E	E	—	☐	☐
4) X-ray capability including c-arm image intensifier available 24 hours a day	E	E	D	—	☐	☐
5) Endoscopes	E	E	D	—	☐	☐
6) Craniotomy instruments	E	E	D	—	☐	☐
7) Equipment appropriate for fixation of long-bone and pelvic fractures	E	E	D	—	☐	☐
3. Postanesthetic recovery room (surgical intensive care unit is acceptable)						
a. Registered nurses and other essential personnel 24 hours a day	E	E	E	—	☐	☐
b. Equipment for the continuous monitoring of temperature, hemodynamics, and gas exchange	E	E	E	—	☐	☐
c. Equipment for the continuous monitoring of intracranial pressure	E	E	D	—	☐	☐
d. Pulse oximetry	E	E	E	—	☐	☐
e. End-tidal CO_2 determination	E	E	D	—	☐	☐
f. Thermal control	E	E	E	—	☐	☐
4. Intensive care units (ICUs) for trauma patients						
a. Personnel						
1) Designated surgical director of trauma patients	E	E	E	—	☐	☐
2) Physician, with privileges in critical care and approved by the trauma director, on duty in ICU 24 hours a day or immediately available in hospital	E	E[1]	D	—	☐	☐
b. Equipment Appropriate monitoring and resuscitation equipment	E	E	E	—	☐	☐

		Levels			Checklist for your hospital	
	I	II	III	IV	Yes	No
c. Support services Immediate access to clinical diagnostic services	E[13]	E[13]	E[13]	—	☐	☐
5. Acute hemodialysis capability	E	D	—	—	☐	☐
6. Organized burn care	E	E	E	E	☐	☐
a. Physician-directed burn center staffed by nursing personnel trained in burn care and equipped properly for care of the extensively burned patient OR						
b. Transfer agreement with burn center						
7. Acute spinal cord/head injury management capability	E	E	E	E	☐	☐
a. In circumstances in which a designated spinal cord injury rehabilitation center exists in the region, early transfer should be considered; transfer agreements should be in effect OR						
b. In circumstances in which a head injury center exists in the region, transfer should be considered in selected patients; transfer agreements should be in effect						
8. Radiological special capabilities						
a. In-house radiology technician 24 hours a day	E	E	E[14]	—	☐	☐
b. Angiography	E	E	D	—	☐	☐
c. Sonography	E	E	D	—	☐	☐
d. Nuclear scanning	E	D	D	—	☐	☐
e. Computed tomography (CT)	E	E	D	—	☐	☐
f. In-house CT technician 24 hours a day	E[14]	E[14]	D	—	☐	☐
g. Neuroradiology	E	D	—	—	☐	☐
9. Rehabilitation						
a. Rehabilitation service staffed by personnel trained in rehabili-						

	I	II	III	IV	Checklist for your hospital Yes	No
tation care and equipped properly for acute care of the critically injured patient	E	E	D	—	☐	☐
b. Full in-house service or transfer agreement to a rehabilitation service for long-term care	E	E	E	E	☐	☐
10. Clinical laboratory service (available 24 hours a day)						
a. Standard analyses of blood, urine, and other body fluids	E	E	E	D	☐	☐
b. Blood typing and cross-matching	E	E	E	D	☐	☐
c. Coagulation studies	E	E	E	D	☐	☐
d. Comprehensive blood bank or access to a community central blood bank and adequate storage facilities	E	E	E	D	☐	☐
e. Blood gases and pH determinations	E	E	E	D	☐	☐
f. Microbiology	E	E	E	D	☐	☐
g. Drug and alcohol screening	E	E	D	D	☐	☐
D. QUALITY IMPROVEMENT						
1. Quality improvement programs	E	E	E	E	☐	☐
2. Trauma registry	E	E	E	E	☐	☐
3. Special audit for all trauma deaths	E	E	E	E	☐	☐
4. Morbidity and mortality review	E	E	E	E	☐	☐
5. Trauma conference, multidisciplinary	E	E	E	D	☐	☐
6. Medical nursing audit, utilization review, tissue review	E	E	E	E	☐	☐
7. Review of prehospital trauma care	E	E	E	D	☐	☐
8. Published on-call schedule must be maintained for surgeons, neurosurgeons, orthopaedic surgeons, and other major specialists	E	E	E	D	☐	☐
9. Times of and reasons for trauma-related bypass must be documented and reviewed by quality improvement program	E	E	E	—	☐	☐

	I	II	III	IV	Checklist for your hospital Yes	No
		Levels				

	I	II	III	IV	Yes	No
10. Quality improvement personnel dedicated to and specific for the trauma program	E	E	D	D	☐	☐

E. OUTREACH PROGRAM

	I	II	III	IV	Yes	No
Telephone and on-site consultations with physicians of the community and outlying areas	E	E	—	—	☐	☐

F. PREVENTION/PUBLIC EDUCATION

	I	II	III	IV	Yes	No
1. Epidemiology research						
a. Conduct studies in injury control	E	D	—	—	☐	☐
b. Collaborate with other institutions in research	E	D	D	D	☐	☐
c. Monitor progress of prevention programs	E	D	D	D	☐	☐
d. Consult with qualified researchers on evaluation measures[15]	E	D	D	D	☐	☐
2. Surveillance						
a. Special ED and field collection projects[16]	E	D	—	—	☐	☐
b. Expanded trauma registry data[17]	E	D	D	—	☐	☐
c. Minimal trauma registry data	E	E	E	D	☐	☐
3. Prevention						
a. Designated prevention coordinator[18]	E	E	D	—	☐	☐
b. Outreach activities and program development	E	E	D	—	☐	☐
c. Information resource	E	E	D	—	☐	☐
d. Collaboration with existing national, regional, and state programs	E	E	D	D	☐	☐

G. TRAUMA RESEARCH PROGRAM[19]

	I	II	III	IV	Yes	No
1. Organized program with designated director	E	D	—	—	☐	☐
2. Regular meeting of research group	E	D	—	—	☐	☐
3. Evidence of productivity						
a. Proposals reviewed by IRB	E	D	—	—	☐	☐

	Levels				Checklist for your hospital	
	I	II	III	IV	Yes	No
b. Presentation at local/regional/ national meetings	E	D	—	—	☐	☐
c. Publications in peer-reviewed journals	E	D	—	—	☐	☐

H. CONTINUING EDUCATION
Formal programs in continuing education provided by hospital for:

	I	II	III	IV	Yes	No
1. Staff physicians	E	E	D	—	☐	☐
2. Nurses	E	E	E	D	☐	☐
3. Allied health personnel	E	E	E	D	☐	☐
4. Community physicians	E	E	D	—	☐	☐

I. TRAUMA SERVICE SUPPORT PERSONNEL

	I	II	III	IV	Yes	No
Trauma coordinator	E	E	D	D	☐	☐

J. ORGAN PROCUREMENT ACTIVITY

	I	II	III	IV	Yes	No
	E	E	E	—	☐	☐

K. TRANSFER AGREEMENTS

	I	II	III	IV	Yes	No
1. As transferring facility	D	E	E	E	☐	☐
2. As receiving facility	E	E	D	—	☐	☐

NOTES

[1] The Committee on Trauma believes the active involvement of the trauma surgeon is crucial to optimal care of the injured patient in all phases of management, including resuscitation, identification and prioritization of injuries, therapeutic decisions, and operative procedures.

In both Level I and II facilities the 24-hour in-house availability of the attending trauma surgeon is the most direct method for providing this involvement. However, alternative methods for providing immediate availability of the attending surgeon are also acceptable.

In hospitals with residency programs, evaluation and treatment may be started by a team of surgeons that will include a PGY4 or more senior surgical resident who is a member of that hospital's residency program. This may allow the attending surgeon to take calls from outside the hospital. In this case, local criteria must be established to define conditions requiring the attending surgeon's immediate hospital presence. The attending surgeon's participation in major therapeutic decisions, presence in the emergency department for major resuscitations, and presence at operative procedures are mandatory. Compliance with these criteria and their appropriateness must be monitored by the hospital's trauma QI program.

In Level II hospitals without residency programs, local conditions may allow the surgeons to be rapidly available on short notice. Under these circumstances local criteria must be established that allow the general surgeon to take calls from outside the hospital, but with the clear commitment on the part of the hospital and the surgical staff that the general surgeon will be present in the emergency department at the time of arrival of the trauma patient to supervise resuscitation and major therapeutic decisions, provide operative treatment, and be available to care for trauma patients in the ICU. Compliance with this requirement and applicable criteria must be monitored by the hospital's QI program.

[2] An attending neurosurgeon must be promptly available and dedicated to that hospital's trauma service. The in-house requirement may be fulfilled by an in-house neurosurgeon or surgeon who has special competence, as judged by the chief of neurosurgery, in the care of patients with neurotrauma and who is capable of initiating measures directed toward stabilization of the patient and initiating diagnostic procedures.

[3] In Level I and Level II institutions, requirements may be fulfilled by emergency medicine chief residents capable of assessing emergency situations in trauma patients and providing any indicated treatment. When chief residents are used to fulfill availability requirements, the staff specialist on call will be advised and be promptly available. In those institutions without emergency medicine coverage, a surgical resident PGY2 working under the direction of the physician director of the emergency department may also fulfill this requirement.

[4] This requirement may be fulfilled by a physician who is credentialed by the hospital to provide emergency medical services.

[5] Requirements may be fulfilled by anesthesiology chief residents PGY4/CA4 who are capable of assessing emergent situations in trauma patients and of providing any indicated treatment, including initiation of surgical anesthesia. When anesthesiology chief residents are used to fulfill availability requirements, the staff anesthesiologist on call will be advised and be promptly available.

[6] Requirements may be fulfilled when local conditions assure that the staff anesthesiologist will be in the hospital at the time of the patient's arrival. During the interim period prior to the arrival of the staff anesthesiologist, an in-house certified registered nurse anesthetist (CRNA) capable of assessing emergent situations in trauma patients and of initiating and providing any indicated treatment will be

available. In some hospitals without a CRNA in-house, local conditions may allow anesthesiologists to be rapidly available on short notice. Under these circumstances, local criteria must be established to allow anesthesiologists to take calls from outside the hospital without CRNA availability, but with the clear commitment that anesthesiologists will be immediately available for airway emergencies and operative management. The availability of the anesthesiologist and the absence of delays in airway control or operative anesthesia must be documented by the hospital QI process.

[7] The staff specialists on call will be notified immediately and will be promptly available. This availability will be continuously monitored by the trauma quality improvement program.

[8] May be provided by a CRNA under physician supervision.

[9] Communication should be such that the general surgeon will be present in the emergency department at the time of arrival of the major trauma patient.

[10] The patient's primary care physician should be notified at an appropriate time.

[11] A pediatric surgeon is defined as a surgeon who has been granted privileges by the hospital to provide surgical care for the injured child.

[12] A general trauma surgeon is presumed to be qualified and should have privileges to provide thoracic surgical care to patients with thoracic injuries. In facilities where the trauma on-call general surgeon does not have privileges to provide thoracic surgical care, a board-certified thoracic surgeon should be available.

[13] Blood gas measurements, hematocrit level, and chest X-ray studies should be available within 30 minutes of request. This capability will be continuously monitored by the quality improvement program.

[14] If this requirement is fulfilled by technicians not in-house 24 hours a day, quality improvement must verify that the procedure is promptly available.

[15] An epidemiologist or biostatistician should be available.

[16] This includes the capability of doing special data collection projects as need is identified, such as monitoring bicycle helmet use in the community.

[17] This includes expanded data on prevention, such as blood alcohol levels, toxic agent presence, use of restraint systems, helmet utilization, and so on.

[18] This activity may be part of the trauma care coordinator effort.

[19] A trauma research program should be designed to produce new knowledge applicable to the care of injured patients. This research may be conducted in a number of ways, including traditional laboratory and clinical research, reviews of clinical series, and epidemiologic or other studies. Regardless of the approach, the study design must include the development and testing of a clearly defined hypothesis. Consistent publication of articles focused on a clinical problem in peer-reviewed journals is the distinguishing feature of an effective research program. A trauma research program should have an organizational structure that fosters and

monitors such ongoing productivity. In addition to the publications mentioned above, presentation of results at local, regional, and national society meetings and ongoing studies approved by local human and animal research review boards are expected from productive programs.

CHAPTER 2

Team-Focused Intervention within Critical Care

Brain injury can be an isolated system injury, yet it can have numerous multisystem effects. These multisystem problems create a greater need for a team approach to care. This approach minimizes the use of hospital resources—a benefit especially important in today's environment of managed care—and maximizes patient outcome. Consequently, trauma centers must work creatively to develop it.

Teams can be described as multidisciplinary, interdisciplinary, or transdisciplinary. Since the prefix *multi-* means "of or having many or several," a *multidisciplinary* approach is one in which persons from several disciplines deliver services, with each team member assuming responsibilities related only to his or her own discipline.[1,2] Team members have minimal direct effect on one another. This approach is frequently used in medicine when individually consulted physicians evaluate and treat a patient in the context of their areas of specialty. Collaborative efforts at planning are not made.

In an *interdisciplinary* approach, different disciplines with different branches of expertise are responsible for individual decisions but also work as team members toward a common goal by sharing responsibilities.[2] Since *inter-* means "between, among, and with each other," the core strength of this team lies in communication, collaboration, and consolidation of knowledge. Trauma and rehabilitation teams use this approach when they coordinate the activities of the different disciplines in addressing the comprehensive needs of individuals who have sustained central nervous system injuries.

In a *transdisciplinary* team, the boundaries between professions are to some extent transcended (*trans-* meaning "over, across, or beyond"). Representatives from various disciplines work together in evaluating and establishing treatment plans and use cross-trained professionals for total service delivery. Such an approach is often used in early childhood intervention, in which a multiskilled professional may provide services established through consultation among specific team members.

Teams can be described not only by how they perform tasks but also by the way they interact with each other. "It is how, when faced with a crisis, [team members] interact and react as a group that determines their success."[3(p27)] Harmonious collaboration among team members is not always innate, yet it is vital in the critical care setting. Communication, knowledge, trust, respect, and ongoing effort on the part of all team members are essential. Each member must understand his or her responsibilities, freedoms, and limitations, as well as those of other team members. Roles must be defined in relation to both individual professional practices and the demands of the specific environment. Delineation of roles is important to avoid confusion, overlap, and even confrontation in patient management. An understanding of roles enables all team members to form realistic expectations of each other's contributions toward achieving the best results for persons with brain injury.

TEAM ORGANIZATION

Industrial and psychologic research supports the premise that clear organization and task allocation can greatly enhance a team's performance.[4,5] Organization and task allocation can be described as either vertical or horizontal. Under horizontal organization, team members carry out individual tasks simultaneously,[6,7] whereas under vertical organization they carry out prioritized tasks sequentially. Different stages in the management of trauma patients lend themselves to different types of task allocation. For example, research demonstrates that resuscitation times can be significantly reduced by using prioritized task allocation and horizontal organization.[8] To an untrained observer, the initial resuscitation of trauma patients in the emergency department (ED) appears to be a pandemonium of isolated events performed in a random sequence. In reality, it is a highly orchestrated sequence of events occurring simultaneously under the direction of one senior member, usually the traumatologist or other designated physician. As with all teams, members must not only know "the game plan" but also be aware of protocols and algorithms.[3] Protocols for assessment and treatment are vital. Without them, chaos would quickly ensue as individual health care professionals blindly determined interventions, placing the patient at risk for a poor outcome.

Rehabilitation generally uses an interdisciplinary model in which outcomes produced by the whole team are more important than those produced by each discipline's efforts. In fact, a comprehensive treatment team is the foundation of modern rehabilitation.[9–13] Coordinating efforts of a variety of disciplines is a central concept in rehabilitation[14] transcending the traditional boundaries of physical therapy, occupational therapy, and speech/language pathology. The focus is on the physiologic, psychologic, social, educational, vocational, and medical needs of the patient.

Rehabilitation teams encourage the patient to become an active participant in the recovery process. They do activities "with" the patient, rather than "for" the patient, at least to the extent that the patient's activity level allows. The German philosopher Immanuel Kant theorized that one should respect an individual as "a rational determiner of his or her own destiny."[15] This value of respect is central to the rehabilitative approach of empowering the patient.[16] For these reasons, rehabilitation professionals tend to assimilate easily and naturally into a team model.

BENEFITS OF USING A TEAM APPROACH

Literature is available that demonstrates benefits from the implementation and use of teams within health care.[17–22] Researchers have identified collaboration as a vital factor in patient outcomes.[17]

The use of a multidisciplinary team can improve outcomes for patients with head and neck cancer.[18] Such patients are often referred to an individual physician who provides treatment, then refers them to another specialist for additional therapy. The lack of cooperation among a variety of specialists reduces the benefit of the *whole* to the knowledge and experience of the *one*. This approach commonly prolongs treatment regimes and, ultimately, satisfactory rehabilitation. The use of a multidisciplinary team is reported to reduce post-treatment morbidity by shortening the length of recovery and rehabilitation.[18]

Positive outcomes secondary to the implementation of an acute multidisciplinary team for patients with spinal cord injuries have also been reported.[20] Statistically significant reductions in lengths of stay have been noted. The use of multidisciplinary teams also results in statistically significant increases in stabilization procedures, decreases in decompression, and decreases in the average number of febrile days. Other benefits include improved interactions among staff, improved consistency of care, improved comprehensiveness in documentation, and team development of protocols designed to expedite appropriate treatment.

Neurologically impaired patients with dysphagia also benefit from the use of a multidisciplinary management program.[19] Reported results include improved patient safety, significant weight gain, and increased caloric intake.

The uses and benefits of a team approach are strongly supported in the area of nutrition. Hundreds of institutions have developed nutritional support teams consisting of physicians, dietitians, pharmacists, nurses, respiratory therapists, and, at times, speech/language pathologists. Team roles vary between institutions, with some being consultative and others involving direct intervention and management. Regardless of the model used, nutritional support teams positively influence patient outcomes,[23–28] including reductions in catheter insertion complications and catheter-related sepsis,[29–32] incidence of metabolic complications,[25,29,32–34] and adjusted mortality rate, length of stay, and readmission rate.[35] These teams are also more likely to evaluate, document, and subsequently meet a patient's nutritional requirements.[29] Financial benefits are reflected in reduced numbers of units of total parenteral nutrition (TPN) mixed, reduced TPN bags wasted, and reductions secondary to the reductions in complications listed above.[24,30,36–41] These improvements are the direct result of an organized, goal-directed team approach. Nutritional support teams set guidelines and protocols for the preparation, administration, and monitoring of prescribed nutrients, and serve in a quality control capacity, standardizing materials and formulas.[27,42,43] They recommend not only the most beneficial therapy for a patient but also the most economical. They also evaluate and monitor patients, working toward established nutritional goals. The strength of this team approach lies in the combined contributions of team members.

The use of ventilatory management teams in the intensive care unit (ICU) is another team approach that is cost-effective.[44–48] It results in decreased days of mechanical ventilation, decreased ICU length of stay, and reduced numbers of arterial blood gases and numbers of indwelling arterial catheters.[44] These reductions result in substantial cost savings per episode of mechanical ventilation.[44]

The literature is replete with studies examining the effects of an acute care team approach on the outcome of individuals with brain injuries. Some studies have examined outcomes of brain injury secondary to trauma center approaches but include the use of a team approach as one of many factors.[49] What is lacking in trauma center literature has been well studied in literature on the later rehabilitation and community-entry stages of recovery. Here, as in other areas of patient care, team approaches have demonstrated positive effects on patient outcome.

TEAM MEMBERS

Team Constellations

The makeup of an ICU team is influenced by injury severity, concomitant injuries, and the structure and availability of specialty areas of medicine within a given trauma center. However, certain team members are necessary to maximize prognosis and outcome for patients with traumatic brain injury (TBI). This core team is outlined in Figure 2–1. All members are represented as equal contributors to the recovery process. Family members are also considered part of this team, with their own unique contributions to and impact on recovery and outcome.

Several different members of a discipline may be represented on a team. For example, the specific number of physicians involved in a team varies by degree and type of injuries as well as the location of the patient within the hospital. Both

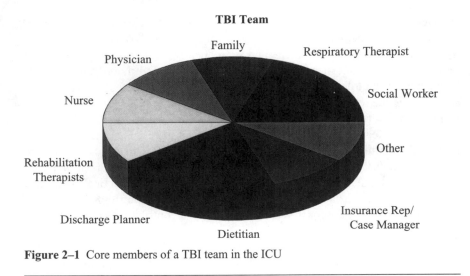

Figure 2–1 Core members of a TBI team in the ICU

primary physicians and potential secondary consults are outlined in Exhibit 2–1. With few exceptions, the makeup of the primary team should be the same in all trauma centers. The traumatologist and neurosurgeon interact with the patient at all stages of care within the trauma center. The roles of the emergency physician and neurotrauma intensivist are "place specific" within the system of care.

Exhibit 2–1 Primary and Potential Secondary Physicians on a TBI Team

PHYSICIANS	
PRIMARY TEAM	*SECONDARY CONSULTS* *(dependent on injury/complication)*
Traumatologist	Infectious Disease Physician
Emergency Physician	Neurologist
Neurosurgeon	Neuro-Ophthalmologist
Neurotrauma Intensivist	Optometrist
(Critical Care Intensivist)	Oral Maxillofacial Surgeon
Surgical House Staff	Orthopaedic Surgeon
	Otolaryngologist
	Plastic Surgeon
	Psychiatrist
	Urologist

Exhibit 2–2 Various Types of Nurses on a TBI Team within a Trauma Center

---

NURSING

PRIMARY TEAM
Emergency Nurse
Critical Care Nurse
Medical/Surgical Nurse
Neurotrauma Nurse
Trauma Nurse Coordinator

Nurses are always primary team members in a TBI team, but the specific types of nurses and their roles are also "place specific." The various types of nurses are listed in Exhibit 2–2. The trauma nurse coordinator remains the one nurse whose primary function is to follow the patient from admission to discharge. In some institutions, rehabilitation nurses provide input to the team to improve and maximize care relative to the rehabilitative needs of the patient.

Rehabilitation medicine specialists are primary team members within the critical care environment (Exhibit 2–3). Currently, state-of-the-art intervention includes the involvement of physical therapy, occupational therapy, and speech/language pathology. The availability and involvement of a physiatrist will vary among institutions. In some institutions, the social worker is part of the rehabilitation department. Secondary consults may include audiological evaluation or neuropsychological or psychological intervention. Again, the availability and involvement of these services will vary among institutions.

With variations in team constellation, additional team members are added to meet the needs of a particular patient or a particular system of care. Other potential team members are listed in Exhibit 2–4.

Exhibit 2–3 Rehabilitation Medicine Specialists on a TBI Team

---

REHABILITATION

PRIMARY TEAM	*SECONDARY CONSULTS*
Physiatrist	Audiologist
Physical Therapist	Neuropsychologist/Psychologist
Occupational Therapist	
Speech/Language Pathologist	
Rehabilitation Social Worker	

Three team members whose roles are expanding with changes related to health care reform are the social worker, the discharge planner, and the insurance representative or case manager. The emphasis on cost-effectiveness and reductions in length of stay has bearing upon the expediency of transfer to a rehabilitation facility or extended-care facility. The social worker and the discharge planner (who may be a nurse or a social worker) must work together to facilitate the internal plan for the patient, as well as the anticipated needs post discharge. Some institutions have implemented a case management position to oversee these aspects, as well as all aspects of efficient, yet comprehensive provision of care. The early and active involvement of an insurance company representative or case manager assists in this facilitation. All of these professionals are active team members during the ICU phase of care.

The critical nature of patient care in the ICU calls for unique and innovative interventions. As a result, some disciplines' involvement expands beyond what is perceived as their traditional scope of services. Rehabilitation therapists, for example, must have a working knowledge of critical care issues, including mechanical ventilation and the purpose and placement of physiologic monitoring devices. The speech/language pathologist's role in the ICU extends beyond the traditional areas of speech, language, cognition, and dysphagia to include participation in tracheostomy management. Other team members' roles may be more predictable but encompass expanded duties unique to caring for persons with severe brain injury. For instance, the critical care nurse assumes responsibilities, such as neurologic assessment and intracranial pressure (ICP) monitoring, that are unique to central nervous system disorders.

The roles of various rehabilitative disciplines (physical and occupational therapy, speech/language pathology, and audiology) are described in Chapters 7, 8, 11, and 12. The roles of four other team members, with unique contributions to

---

Exhibit 2–4 Other Potential Professionals on a TBI Team

OTHER
Pharmacist
Substance Abuse Counselor
Trauma Registrar
Reference Librarian
Clergy

the patient with severe brain injury (nurse, trauma nurse coordinator, physiatrist, and social worker) are described in this chapter.

The Role and Contributions of Nursing

Within the ICU, it is critical that the physician and nurse coordinate the efforts of all team members. It is the primary nurse, however, who bears the responsibility of 24-hour care, maintains the most current information on patient status and treatment, and keeps other team members apprised of interventions and outcomes. The primary nurse must always maintain a global view of the overall plan of care. The goals of nursing care in the ICU for the person with a severe brain injury should include

- stabilization of the patient's condition
- prevention of further injury
- prevention of complications
- carryover of rehabilitation
- involvement of the family/significant others in the plan of care

To provide optimal care, nursing staff should have a basic understanding of neuroanatomy, neuroassessment, and treatment modalities as they relate to central nervous system injuries.

Initial Assessment and Stabilization

Before definitive treatment of an injury can begin, it is necessary to stabilize the patient's condition and establish that vital physiologic functions are intact. A review of ED and/or operating room procedures must be completed. Information gleaned from these areas may include estimated blood loss and the units of blood received, hypotensive episodes noted in the field or following admission, medications administered, surgical procedures, and type of anesthesia used. Initial assessment of the patient with a brain injury begins with an assessment of airway, breathing, and circulation. An awareness of the specific airway adjuncts that are used at a particular institution is essential, since there are a number of methods of establishing and maintaining an airway. Ongoing reassessment of patient status that includes these parameters is important. Most frequently, it is the nurse at the bedside who first identifies changes in the patient's condition that warrant physician notification and corresponding changes in treatment.[50] A perceptive, educated nurse can potentially thwart complications that may impede maximal outcomes.

Airway and Breathing

Airway adjuncts frequently used in patients with injuries include endotracheal tubes, cricothyroidotomy, and tracheostomy.[51] The choice of airway adjunct is dependent upon the patient's condition on arrival at the hospital and on changes in the patient's condition that occur over time. Endotracheal tubes are often placed in the prehospital setting in patients who are critically injured. Paramedics have extensive training and experience in the placement of these airways and have a high rate of successful placement. Most endotracheal tubes will be placed through the mouth, although occasionally a nasotracheal tube will be placed. Intubation may not be possible due to massive facial fractures. When it is not possible to intubate the patient, a cricothyroidotomy is the airway of choice. A cricothyroidotomy may remain the airway of use for the short term but should be converted to a tracheostomy secondary to concerns that complications, such as tracheal stenosis, may arise if a cricothyroidotomy is left in place. Early tracheostomy is performed in patients who will require long-term ventilatory support and assistance with pulmonary toilet. A more recent development in the tracheostomy technique is percutaneous tracheostomy, which may be done at the bedside. Regardless of the method used, it is important that the site of the airway be clean and free from infection.

Breathing and respiratory effort should be assessed on a continuous basis. Documentation of mode of mechanical ventilation, Fio_2, tidal volume, positive end expiratory pressure (PEEP), and spontaneous breaths should be maintained.

Circulation

An adequate blood volume is essential to maintain perfusion of vital organs, including the brain. If the patient is hypovolemic, cerebral perfusion pressure may be inadequate, thus increasing the risk of further injury to the brain. Conversely, excessive fluid resuscitation can be detrimental to the patient with a brain injury in that it can increase cerebral edema. Fluid balance, therefore, must be carefully maintained.

Monitoring the patient's circulatory status can be done in several modes, depending upon the patient's condition. The monitoring of blood pressure and heart rate determines if pressure is adequate to meet brain tissue perfusion requirements.[51] Blood pressure and pulse will provide a basic assessment of circulatory function, as well as resuscitation status. These parameters may be measured manually, with an automatically cycling monitoring device, or using invasive monitoring techniques, such as arterial lines. In addition, a patient who has severe hemodynamic instability may be monitored using a Swan-Ganz catheter to assess central pressures. As with respiratory assessment, these parameters must be monitored on a regular basis, and trends that are indicative of changes in the patient's condition should be noted. Specific alterations in circulatory patterns that result from brain injury must also be identified. For example, increased ICP may lead to decreased blood pressure, along with bradycardia. The parameters that should be documented include blood pressure, heart rate, and mean arterial pressure. Central pressures may or may not be monitored.

Neurologic Assessment

The Glasgow Coma Scale (GCS)[52] is a method of assessing neurologic function using three parameters: eye opening, motor response, and verbal response (Table 2–1). An advantage to using the GCS is that it provides a standardized method of monitoring neurologic function. The patient is given a score for each of the three parameters, and these scores are totaled for a final GCS. The score for each area is the best function observed at the time of the assessment. The scores for the GCS range from 3 to 15, with 3 representing complete unresponsiveness and 15 representing a patient who is awake, alert, oriented, and able to follow commands.

In addition to GCS parameters, other aspects of neurologic function that should be measured include pupillary response and motor and sensory function. Pupils are assessed according to three parameters: size, shape, and reactivity. Abnormal changes can be indicative of neurologic deterioration, such as transtentorial herniation. The normal pupil averages 3 mm in diameter. The primary issue in assessment of size is notable differences between the pupils. Approximately 11% to

---

Table 2–1 Components and Scoring of the Glasgow Coma Scale

Parameter	Score
Eye Opening	
Spontaneous	4
To voice	3
To pain	2
Does not open eyes	1
Motor Response	
Obey commands	6
Localizes to pain	5
Flexes and withdraws to pain	4
Abnormal flexion (decorticate posturing)	3
Abnormal extension (decerebrate posturing)	2
No response to pain (flaccid)	1
Verbal Response	
Oriented	5
Disoriented but coherent	4
Inappropriate words	3
Incoherent words or sounds	2
No verbal response	1
Total Maximum Score	**15**

16% of individuals have anisocoria (inequality of pupil diameter), but the difference is most often less than 1 mm.[51] Pupillary asymmetry of 1 mm or more is significant and warrants medical attention.

The normal pupil is round and regular. The progression from a round to an oval-shaped pupil is significant and often forewarns of progression to a fixed and dilated pupil.[53] Irregularly shaped pupils are associated with upper brainstem (midbrain) compression.

A normal pupil reacts briskly to light by constricting (*direct response*). An indirect reaction to light, called a *consensual response*, involves the constriction of the contralateral pupil. Absent or sluggish pupillary responses are significant. The absence of a direct response indicates midbrain compression of the oculomotor nerve (cranial nerve III) or an optic nerve lesion (cranial nerve II). An oculomotor nerve lesion will result in the absence of both direct and indirect pupillary responses. Small, reactive pupils are due to metabolic or hypothalamic dysfunction.[51] Small, unreactive pupils are associated with lower brainstem (pons) dysfunction.[51]

Accurate assessment of neurologic functioning involves collaborative efforts between nursing and rehabilitation staff. Sharing input regarding spontaneous and volitional movements is important because patient responses fluctuate. Ongoing efforts to collaborate also facilitate carryover of therapeutic techniques throughout the 24-hour day. Cooperative efforts between the nurse and speech/language pathologist on swallowing and tracheostomy management reduce the risk of aspiration and respiratory complications. Carryover of positioning and equipment recommendations (eg, splints) from the physical and occupational therapists can reduce tone and posturing, thereby maximizing range of motion.

Intracranial Pressure Monitoring

The detection and control of intracranial hypertension is a central activity of nursing care in the ICU. Intracranial pressure may be monitored in several ways, including intraparenchymal fiber-optic catheters, subarachnoid screws, epidural monitors, and subarachnoid catheters.[51] The use of these devices presents a risk of infection that varies depending upon the type of device. Nursing care should focus on monitoring the pressure, ensuring that the monitoring device is intact, and preventing infection of the site. Nursing therapies based upon sound clinical judgment can be used to reduce ICP through caregiving tasks and minimizing or reducing stimulations known to increase ICP. Endotracheal suctioning, known to increase hypoxia and hypercarbia, thereby increases ICP. Suctioning techniques including limiting length of time per pass, limiting the number of passes, and providing hyperventilation and preoxygenation before and between catheter insertions should be routinely used with patients with brain injury.[51] Head elevation to 15 to 30 degrees is another technique used to reduce ICP. Proper positioning, especially in the presence of decerebrate or decorticate posturing, can also help control ICP. Minimizing the frequency of other noxious activities associated with increases in ICP, such as needle punctures, tube insertion, and painful stimulation, is an ongoing nursing responsibility.[51] Chapter 3 discusses normal ranges for ICP and cerebral perfusion pressure.

Sedation and Paralysis

It is sometimes necessary to sedate the patient with a brain injury. In addition, paralytic agents may be used in highly agitated patients. One difficulty with sedating or paralyzing the patient is that it interferes with the ability to perform a neurologic examination to monitor the patient's progress.[51] The nurse, in conjunction with the physician, coordinates medication administration to allow for periodic assessment of the patient's neurologic status. It is the role of the nursing staff to facilitate an environment for the patient that minimizes the need for sedating medications.

Agitated and aggressive patients place additional demands on nursing staff. An important focus is to maintain a safe environment for the patient.[54] Promotion of safety includes consistent use of side rails, frequent orientation to decrease confusion, bedside use of essential equipment only, positioning of access lines and tubes out of reach of the patient, and frequent monitoring of the patient. Restraints should be used only when issues of self-injury arise. The use of restraints often increases, rather than decreases, agitation in patients with brain injury. Coordination of therapy sessions and family visits with needed periodic rest periods can reduce the extended need for restraints. The nurse can educate family members regarding agitated behaviors and appropriate interactions, potentially allowing temporary removal of restraints.

Prevention of Complications

Infection is a major complication in the ICU. One of the major benefits of ongoing nursing assessment in the ICU is the early detection of actual or impending complications.[55] Specific infectious processes are discussed in Chapter 10. Nursing interventions can be very effective in decreasing infection rates in ICU patients. Simple measures such as using protective clothing and gloves when caring for patients and adequate handwashing before and after completing interventions are quite effective in preventing the spread of infection. Close attention must be paid to wounds and sites of invasive lines and airways to reduce the possibility of contamination. Infection risks should be a factor in determining nursing care assignments. Patients with systemic infection and those with significant infections should not be assigned to the same nurse.

Aggressive pulmonary toilet is essential in preventing pulmonary complications. Protocols regarding suctioning and tracheostomy care must be closely followed. Nursing coordinates efforts with respiratory therapy or physical therapy in providing chest physiotherapy. Turning and repositioning a patient, in addition to early mobilization, also helps prevent complications. Collaborative efforts with rehabilitation therapists with regard to positioning and movement improve pulmonary function and reduce the risk of skin breakdown.

Although skin breakdown is generally not a life-threatening complication, it is a very debilitating one that can require extensive therapy. The use of high-tech beds sometimes provides a false sense of security with respect to the issue of skin integrity. The ICU should have a protocol for assessing and documenting the condition of the patient's skin to identify areas that are at risk of breaking down. When indicated, however, the use of a specialized bed should occur as a collaborative decision.

Documentation and Flowsheets

As with medical interventions, protocols and standards of care must be established and, most important, consistently implemented. Advancing technologies and treatments dictate ongoing updates and revisions. Additionally, care plans for patients outline progressive treatment interventions, using a goal-oriented approach. More recently, multidisciplinary critical pathways prescribe day-to-day activities and interventions along a continuum of care.[50] They maximize quality of care by establishing a prioritized system of efficient, yet comprehensive service provision.

Physiologic measurements and nursing observations must be documented in a consistent, organized manner. The large amount of patient data collected often becomes the basis for choosing treatment programs. Regardless of the specific designs, the documentation format should allow easy retrieval of information and identification of trends to detect subtle, yet potentially significant changes in patient status. The development of computer applications in critical care and in medical record documentation has made this task easier. Table 2–2 lists the components that should be included in the nursing record.

Psychosocial Issues

The early period after a brain injury is a time of crisis for the family. A great deal of support is needed during this period. Because the nurse is often the most available person, the family often looks to the nurse for support and guidance. The nurse also assumes the primary responsibility for ongoing communication with the family. The nurse must understand the family's need for consistent, timely, and often repetitive information.

From a nursing perspective, it is important to be honest with the family with regard to prognosis and long-term outcome. If it is not possible to predict the

Table 2–2 Suggested Data and Observations To Be Documented in the Nursing Record

Nursing Categories	Physiologic Measurements and Observations
Hemodynamics	Blood pressure, pulse, central pressures (Swan-Ganz readings), cardiac output
Respiratory	Rate, ventilator settings (Fio_2, mode of ventilation, PEEP, ventilator breaths/minute, tidal volume), arterial blood gases, O_2 saturation
Temperature	Baseline temperature and alterations over time
Neurologic	Glasgow Coma Scale, intracranial pressure, pupillary reactions, motor function, sensory function
Intake/diet	Intravenous (IV), gastrointestinal, parenteral nutrition, tube feeding, oral feeds, weights
Output	Urine, chest tubes, gastric, bowel, drains, bladder irrigation, ostomies
Skin integrity	Changes in skin integrity, signs of increased pressure, wounds/dressings
Medications	Medications given, responses to medications, IVs, subcutaneous medications
Interventions	Procedures, special beds, turning and positioning, out-of-bed positioning

patient's prognosis, the best response is to say that it is not possible to predict at the present time but that the patient will be monitored and progress will be continuously assessed. Information given to the family should remain consistent across all team members.

Some family members will have difficulty leaving the hospital because of their fear of something happening to the patient or their sense of responsibility to their loved one. The trusting relationship that develops between the nurse and family helps them accept the suggestion to leave the hospital for periods of time to obtain much-needed rest. Providing a telephone number and a specific nurse contact for family members to call periodically can abate anxiety and tension levels for loved ones.

Trauma Nurse Coordinator

The role of the trauma nurse coordinator (TNC) became a "by-product of the trauma center designation process."[56(p673)] While the leadership role falls to the trauma surgeon, the trauma nurse coordinator is responsible for coordination of resources and personnel necessary to care for the traumatically injured patient from entrance into the hospital until discharge. The role of the TNC has expanded and become better defined over the years, due to the growing complexity of trauma care and the experiences of the pioneers who first filled those positions. The Trauma Coordinators' Subcommittee of the American Trauma Society defines a trauma coordinator as a person who promotes optimal trauma care in the context of a regionalized trauma care system through clinical activities, professional and public education, research, quality assurance, and administrative functions.[57]

Clinical activities include primary and secondary assessments, clinical rounds, patient care follow-up, supervision of care plans, and monitoring of trauma care throughout the hospital admission.[58] Involvement in the initial management of the patient, including the resuscitation phase, helps ensure that newly developed protocols are being followed. The TNC becomes a liaison between the trauma service and other departments, as well as with outside agencies and institutions.

Professional and public education on an internal and external basis is an important aspect of this role. The TNC is intimately involved in trauma care education from prevention to rehabilitation. Professional education can incorporate introducing new equipment and protocols to hospital and prehospital staff, as well as teaching continuing education, such as advanced trauma life support or a trauma nurse core curriculum.

In most institutions, the TNC is involved in research, including involvement in clinical trials, hospital and multicentered studies, and trauma registry data. The trauma surgeon and TNC ensure that the registry is designed to meet the specific needs of the institution and the patients it serves.

Quality improvement (QI) is probably the most vital role undertaken by this team member, including primary responsibility for the design, implementation, and tracking of quality assurance indicators for trauma care. Components of a trauma QI program are multidisciplinary and include the trauma registry, chart audits, mortality and morbidity conferences, clinical care reviews, and medical and nursing care audits. QI projects undertaken by other departments but directly related to the care of the trauma patient should also be incorporated into the trauma QI program. A successful QI program allows the TNC to guide the institution in improving patient outcome.

The scope and definition of this position continue to evolve. Larger institutions may support more than one TNC or subdivide responsibilities between positions. Some institutions have expanded the function of this position into three different, yet related nursing positions: TNC, trauma director, and trauma clinical nurse specialist.[59] This expansion resulted in improved quality care, reduced patient complications and lengths of stay, and increased patient and employee satisfaction.

The TNC role requires that the individual have a broad knowledge of health care delivery and a strong academic and clinical background.[57] Within this role, the TNC promotes consistency of service delivery along the continuum of care to meet the complex and urgent needs of the trauma patient.

Physiatrist

A physiatrist is a medical doctor with training and expertise in physical medicine and rehabilitation. This physician often provides the medical direction for rehabilitation departments. The physiatrist can serve as a valuable acute care team member by offering input toward the neuromedical management of patients with brain injuries. In the acute stage, the physiatrist intervenes to prevent complications that could add to patients' disability later in recovery. The physiatrist occupies the unique position of being the member of the acute physician team most specifically dedicated to functional outcome.

In view of maximizing function, physical medicine and rehabilitation physicians can offer insights into the selection of an efficacious pharmacologic regime. Although drug-induced sedation for some patients with brain injuries may be medically necessary, it must be recognized that the "sedative side-effects can be magnified in the injured brain and that even small changes in arousal can impact on the patient's responsiveness."[60(p1035)] A physiatrist knowledgeable in neuropharmacology can provide input regarding potential replacement drugs that are less sedating to the patient.

The physiatrist can also provide input to the medical team on a myriad of other neuromedical complications, including management of spasticity, contractures, skin integrity, peripheral nerve injuries, and bowel-bladder incontinence. This physician coordinates with the rehabilitation treatment team on employed modalities, splinting, casting, positioning, and the possible use of nerve or motor point blocks.

The knowledge base of the physiatrist can be used to assist in outcome prediction. Part of the role of the physiatrist is to evaluate the postacute rehabilitation needs of the patient and, in coordination with other team members, facilitate an early and timely transfer to a rehabilitation facility. The physiatrist can provide education and support to the family, including anticipated complications and behavioral issues in the recovery process. By obtaining education, the family is better able to make the transition from the acute medical hospital to a rehabilitation environment. The involvement of the physiatrist and rehabilitation team in the early stages of recovery encourages the family, as well as the acute medical team, to maintain a focus on maximizing functional outcome on both a short- and a long-term basis.

Social Worker

A crisis is a turning point in a person's life such that nothing thereafter will be exactly as before. During medical emergencies, families often experience a greater sense of isolation because they are away from familiar resources; this may lead to heightened anxiety, which in turn can result in rapid decompensation and regression.

The social worker's role is to assist the family in dealing with the crisis successfully and to provide guidance, advice, and education. Crisis is time limited. Ideally, the social worker should meet the family members on their arrival at the hospital. The family most needs support and guidance in the first critical hours and days after injury. Thus, the social worker must take action quickly while maintaining composure, a calm approach to issues, and accuracy in assessment.

While in the ED, the social worker, in coordination with the nurse, becomes the liaison between the physician and family. Initial cursory assessments are performed simultaneously with intervention. The social worker must identify the family dynamics, the strengths and weaknesses of family members' coping skills, and the family's level of understanding of the situation. The social worker must be prepared for—and must respect—a variety of family coping patterns and defenses. The social worker must also have knowledge of typical medical/surgical procedures and related terminology. He or she should be present for all family interactions with the physician or other staff to reinforce and clarify the diagnosis, plans for treatment, and the condition of the patient.

Much of the initial focus, in the ED and during the first day in the ICU, is on survival. After this initial period of stabilization, the issues of potential outcome arise. The goals of intervention at this time include helping the family clarify the problem; offering specific, technically accurate information; directing the family toward individual and institutional resources; helping develop explicit awareness and acceptance of feelings associated with the trauma; and offering explicit emotional support or arranging for its provision by friends and extended family. A major component of family crisis intervention involves preserving and encouraging growth in the social network. A dramatic reduction in the family's scope of social activity, with resulting isolation and a sense of abandonment, is common after brain injury.[61] Intervention helps ease this phenomenon for the family and, later on, the patient.

A brief family history at this time is useful for two reasons. From it, the social worker can ascertain more accurately how the family has dealt with stress and conflict in the past. Also, it allows the family to be engaged in an active task, thus helping to alleviate feelings of helplessness.[62] The rapport that is built begins to facilitate the trust that is vital between the family and social worker.

A multitude of other related questions arise that the social worker can address: Can I call for reports on waking and before going to sleep? Whom do I call? Will we be notified of changes in his or her condition? Is visitation limited to certain times and people? How do I tell the children (or elderly parents) about what has happened? Answers to these and other questions must be readily provided to the family. An experienced social worker can anticipate additional questions and provide the necessary information.

The social worker provides support services to two clients: the family and the staff. The treatment team benefits by the presence and intervention of a social service professional in cases in which family relations are unclear or strained. For example, the social worker may ease difficulties encountered in the case of divorced, hostile parents who are both present at the trauma center, or may help sort out spouses and significant others. "Trauma nurses have an extremely pressurized job, because they have primary responsibility for patient care. The social worker can assist the nursing staff by identifying and diffusing the extraneous variables that interfere with nurses' primary caretaker role."[63(p312)]

The social worker may also be responsible for more concrete issues, such as financial concerns. In some trauma centers, additional social workers or discharge planners may be involved. They provide the family with the information necessary to make financial and legal decisions, including guardianship or conservatorship. The social worker, along with other staff, provides information on posttrauma resources, including ongoing rehabilitation.

Within the world of brain injury, the needs of the family in crisis are compounded by the suddenness of the injury, the unresponsiveness of the patient, the helplessness of the family, and the unpredictability of outcome. The social worker provides ongoing support and develops a professional, yet emotional bond with the family. These successful interactions ultimately benefit the family, the patient, the medical staff, and the institution. Additional information on the interaction between the social worker or crisis counselor and the family is given in Chapter 14.

TEAM EFFECTIVENESS

Ideally, an interdisciplinary team approach should be used in a trauma center. This approach requires effort from all team members and must be creatively organized to function well within the design of the trauma center. Interdisciplinary team members not only bear responsibility for their areas of expertise but also share responsibility for the goals of the team. The overall program involves the team's identification of problem areas and establishment of treatment plans based upon those areas. Problem areas involving critical care management of brain injuries frequently involve multiple disciplines. One example is the problem of maintaining adequate nutrition, which includes the progression from parenteral feeding to tube feeding to oral eating. Issues identified by the team may include

- what volume of intake is necessary to meet minimum requirements
- what the optimal means of intake is
- what the potential complications are (eg, swallowing disorders, aspiration pneumonia)
- what preventative measures can be taken to reduce complications or improve the level of function (eg, respiratory treatments, medication, suctioning)
- what progression of interventions should be implemented to maximize recovery

These issues involve different interventions at different times in the recovery process. A variety of professionals should be involved, including the trauma surgeon, surgical intensivist, dietitian, respiratory therapist, and speech/language pathologist or occupational therapist. Certain team members—specifically, the attending physician and dietitian—assume overall responsibility, with all team members participating in the treatment of this problem area.

There are no highly regarded paradigms or standards that one can follow; therefore, team structure and function within critical care units will vary. Successful programs, however, do share commonalities in their structure and function. The essential components leading to success are outlined in Exhibit 2–5.

Both formal and informal communication is important to the team. Most hospitals use daily ICU rounds for updating the condition of all patients and for planning. Medical personnel, including a critical care intensivist, residents, and nurses, participate. Additional staff may participate to provide updated patient information. However, a mechanism should exist (at least once weekly) for *all* team members to meet and discuss issues relative to trauma patients. Such a forum facilitates and encourages members to look at the patient as a whole person, rather than to focus on individual parts. Trauma rounds allow for information dissemination, problem solving, and planning. These meetings facilitate proactive behavior designed to identify and reduce or avoid anticipated problems. A proactive stance also facilitates initiation of early discharge planning. Team members leave each meeting with a consensus on the patients' status, allowing consistent information to be communicated to family members. Successful team communication, including the delineation of what information should be transmitted by what method and to whom, can make the difference between efficiency and redundancy.

The reality in many hospitals, however, is that communication is becoming increasingly more difficult because of decreasing lengths of stay and reduced staffing. Although technology is not a substitute for human interaction, computerized

Exhibit 2–5 Essential Structural and Functional Components of an Integrated TBI Team in the ICU

---

1. Team approach with multiple disciplines working in concert
2. Ongoing communication
3. Establishment and enforcement of protocols and procedures
4. Timelines of interventions
5. Established methods of delivery of care
6. Early, aggressive rehabilitation
7. Staff education
8. Family efforts, including crisis intervention and provision of consistent information and education
9. Aggressive, timely transfer to a rehabilitation facility

---

communication is being used more frequently to assist with interdisciplinary contact.

Staff education is vital in the trauma center. Trauma rounds are one mechanism for ongoing education. Certain programmatic requirements for Level I and II trauma centers are educational, including the trauma registry, audits, quality improvement programs, and research. Changing technology and staff rotations within teaching facilities make ongoing education a necessity. In many centers, health care personnel are required to obtain yearly continuing medical education or continuing education units in the areas of injury or critical care.

Education is also facilitated by the ongoing update of established protocols for management of severe brain injury. Team participation in initiation or modification of protocols facilitates improved carryover and support of procedures. This type of documentation provides the basis for consistent quality of care.

Good documentation, including protocols and patient-specific charting, also improves team performance by reducing wasted time, expediting planning, and avoiding reduplication of services and procedures. Emphasis is placed on documentation of patient status and changes. Other information that is vital to the team but is frequently not documented is (1) the results of team planning or family meetings, (2) family responses to the trauma, (3) significant cultural or ethnic customs that may affect medical treatment or intervention, (4) the identification of a family member/significant other responsible for medical/legal decisions, (5) potential discharge plans and status, and (6) upcoming surgeries, procedures, or precautions. This information can affect interventions with the patient and family and facilitate improved care. Unfortunately, increases in productivity expectations can often result in elimination of tasks considered to be of lower priority, such as documentation. However, with organization and planning, documentation can be completed in a quick, concise, easily retrievable, and streamlined manner. With increasing constraints on lengths of stay, expeditious and comprehensive provision of information to all team members is vital.

SUMMARY

Despite changing economic and professional issues, team approaches can improve the delivery of services to individuals with brain injury. A comprehensive ICU team should include a traumatologist, a critical care intensivist, a neurosurgeon, a nurse, a pharmacist, a physiatrist, physical and occupational therapists, a speech/language pathologist, a respiratory therapist, a dietitian, a trauma nurse coordinator, a social worker, a case manager/discharge planner, and the family. Components of an effective team, with regard to brain injury, include ongoing communication, use of established protocols and procedures, timely interventions, early aggressive rehabilitation, and support and involvement of the family in patient care and planning.

Successful teamwork, although not easy to achieve, benefits all team members, and, more important, patients and their families. Patients and families find it is easier to communicate with a cohesive team than with numerous practitioners who work in isolation. Effective teamwork brings together diverse knowledge and skills and results in quicker decision making. Finding ways to communicate effectively, plan cooperatively, and intervene collaboratively can make the difference between costly, fragmented services and cost-efficient, goal-oriented progress.[64]

REFERENCES

1. Melvin JL. Status report on interdisciplinary medical education. *Arch Phys Med Rehabil.* 1989;70:273–276.
2. Rothberg JS. The rehabilitation team: future direction. *Arch Phys Med Rehabil.* 1981;62:407–410.
3. Therriault VM. The trauma team: a nurse's perspective. *J Emerg Nurs.* 1975;1:27–28.
4. Steiner ID. A study of group performance. *Behav Sci.* 1966;11:273–283.
5. Hallam J, Stammers RB. The distribution of task demands in the multiman-machine system. *Proc Int Conf Man-Machine Sys.* 1982;212:68–72.
6. Lanzetta JT, Roby TB. Group performance as a function of work distribution patterns and task load. *Sociometry.* 1956;19:95–101.
7. Hallam J, Stammers RB. The effects of task characteristics on the organization of the team. *Proc Hum Fac Soc.* 1981;18:546–549.
8. Driscoll PA, Vincent CA. Organizing an efficient trauma team. *Injury.* 1992;23:107–110.
9. Purtilo RB. Ethical issues in teamwork: the context of rehabilitation. *Arch Phys Med Rehabil.* 1988;69:318–322.
10. Dean BZ, Geiringer SR. Physiatric therapeutics. The rehabilitation team/behavioral management. *Arch Phys Med Rehabil.* 1990;71:S275–S277.

11. Preston KM. A team approach to rehabilitation. *Home Health Nurse.* 1990;8:17–23.

12. Keith RA. The comprehensive treatment team in rehabilitation. *Arch Phys Med Rehabil.* 1991;72:269–274.

13. O'Toole MT. The interdisciplinary team: research and education. *Holist Nurs Pract.* 1992;6: 76–83.

14. Strasser DC, Falconer JA, Martin-Saltzmann D. The rehabilitation team: staff perceptions of the hospital environment, the interdisciplinary team environment, and interprofessional relations. *Arch Phys Med Rehabil.* 1994;75:177–182.

15. Kant I. In: Beck LW, ed. *Critique of Practical Reason and Other Writings in Moral Philosophy.* Chicago, Ill: University of Chicago Press; 1949:347.

16. Purtilo RB, Meier RH III. Team challenges: regulatory constraints and patient empowerment. *Am J Phys Med Rehabil.* 1993;72:327–330.

17. Baggs JG, Ryan SA, Phelps CE, Richeson JF, et al. The association between interdisciplinary collaboration and patient outcomes in a medical intensive care unit. *Heart Lung.* 1992;21:18–24.

18. King GE, Lemon JC, Martin JW. Multidisciplinary teamwork in the treatment and rehabilitation of the head and neck cancer patient. *Texas Dent J.* 1992;109:9–12.

19. Martens L, Cameron T, Simonsen M. Effects of a multidisciplinary management program on neurologically impaired patients with dysphagia. *Dysphagia.* 1990;5:147–151.

20. Wells JD, Nicosia S. The effects of multidisciplinary team care for acute spinal cord injury patients. *J Am Paraplegia Soc.* 1993;16:23–29.

21. Deane SA, Gaundry PL, Pearson I, Ledwidge DG, et al. Implementation of a trauma team. *Aust NZ J Surg.* 1989;59:373–378.

22. Spencer JD. Why do our hospitals not make more use of the concept of a trauma team? *Br Med J.* 1985;290:136–138.

23. Fisher GG, Opper FH. An interdisciplinary nutrition support team improves quality of care in a teaching hospital. *J Am Diet Assoc.* 1996;96:176–178.

24. Jones JS, Tidwell B, Travis J, Spencer T, et al. Nutritional support of the hospitalized patient: a team approach. *J Miss State Med Assoc.* 1995;36:91–99.

25. Regenstein M. Nutrition support teams: alive, well, and still growing. *Nutr Clin Pract.* 1992;7:296–301.

26. Hamaoui E. Assessing the nutrition support team. *JPEN.* 1987;11:412–421.

27. Oxford Parenteral Nutrition Team. Total parenteral nutrition: value of a standard feeding regimen. *Br Med J.* 1983;286:1323–1327.

28. Blackburn GL, Bothe A Jr, Lahey MA. Organization and administration of a nutrition support service. *Surg Clin North Am.* 1981;61:709–719.

29. Gales BJ, Gales MJ. Nutritional support teams: a review of comparative trials. *Ann Pharmacother.* 1994;28:227–235.

30. Faubion WC, Wesley JR, Khalidi N, Silva J. Total parenteral nutrition catheter sepsis: impact of the team approach. *JPEN.* 1986;10:642–645.

31. Traeger SM, Williams GB, Milliren G, Young DS, et al. Total parenteral nutrition by a nutrition support team: improved quality of care. *JPEN.* 1986;10:408–412.

32. Nehme AE. Nutritional support of the hospitalized patient: the team concept. *JAMA.* 1980; 243:1906–1908.

33. Dalton MJ, Schepers G, Gee JP, Alberts CC, et al. Consultative total parenteral nutrition teams: the effect on the incidence of total parenteral nutrition-related complications. *JPEN.* 1984;8:145–152.

34. Hickey MM, Munyer TO, Salem RB, Yost RL. Parenteral nutrition utilization: evaluation of an educational protocol and consult service. *JPEN*. 1979;3:433–437.

35. Hassell JT, Games AD, Shaffer B, Harkins LE. Nutrition support team management of enterally fed patients in a community hospital is cost-beneficial. *J Am Diet Assoc*. 1994;94:993–998.

36. Balet A, Cardona D. Importance of a nutritional support team to promote cost containment. *Ann Pharmacother*. 1992;26:265. Letter.

37. O'Brien DD, Hodges RE, Day AT, Waxman KS, et al. Recommendations of nutrition support team promote cost containment. *JPEN*. 1986;10:300–302.

38. Weinsier RL, Heimburger DC, Samples CM, Dimick AR, et al. Cost containment: a contribution of aggressive nutritional support in burn patients. *J Burn Care Rehabil*. 1985;6:436–441.

39. Friedman MH, Higa AM, Davis AJ. A unique team approach to optimal nutritional support with minimal cost. *Nutr Supp Serv*. 1983;3:27–28.

40. Shildt RA, Rose M, Stollman L, Bell B. Organization of the nutritional support service at a medical center: one year's experience. *Milit Med*. 1982;147:55–58.

41. Mutchie KD, Smith KA, Mackay MW, Marsh C, et al. Pharmacist monitoring of parenteral nutrition: clinical and cost effectiveness. *Am J Hosp Pharm*. 1979;36:785–787.

42. Cataldi-Betcher EL, Seltzer MH, Slocum BA, Jones KW. Complications occurring during enteral nutrition support: a prospective study. *JPEN*. 1983;7:546–552.

43. MacDonald HL, Anderson JR, McClean Ross AH, Gove LF, et al. Parenteral nutrition: the team approach. *J R Coll Surg Edinburgh*. 1981;26:173–177.

44. Cohen IL, Bari N, Strosberg MA, Weinberg PF, et al. Reduction of duration and cost of mechanical ventilation in an intensive care unit by use of a ventilatory management team. *Crit Care Med*. 1991;19:1278–1284.

45. Bone RC, Balk RA. Noninvasive respiratory care unit: a cost effective solution for the future. *Chest*. 1988;93:390–394.

46. Hall JB, Wood LDH. Liberation of the patient from mechanical ventilation. *JAMA*. 1987; 257:1621–1628.

47. O'Donohue WJ Jr, Giovannoni RM, Goldberg AI, Keens TG, et al. Long-term mechanical ventilation: guidelines for management in the home and at alternate community sites. Report of the Ad Hoc Committee, Respiratory Care Section, American College of Chest Physicians. *Chest*. 1986; 90(suppl):1S–37S.

48. Petty TL. IMV vs IMC. *Chest*. 1975;67:630–631.

49. Mackay LE, Bernstein BA, Chapman PE, Morgan AS, et al. Early intervention program in severe head injury: long term benefits of a formalized program. *Arch Phys Med Rehabil*. 1992;73:635–641.

50. Cardona VD, Von Rueden KT. Nursing practice through the cycles of trauma. In: Cardona VD, Hurn PD, Bastnagel Mason PJ, Scanlon AM, et al., eds. *Trauma Nursing: From Resuscitation through Rehabilitation*. 2nd ed. Philadelphia, Pa: WB Saunders Co; 1994:62–88.

51. Mitchell PH. Central nervous system I: closed head injuries. In: Cardona VD, Hurn PD, Bastnagel Mason PJ, Scanlon AM, et al., eds. *Trauma Nursing: From Resuscitation through Rehabilitation*. 2nd ed. Philadelphia, Pa: WB Saunders Co; 1994:383–434.

52. Teasdale G, Jennett B. Assessment of coma and impaired consciousness: a practical scale. *Lancet*. 1974;2:81–84.

53. Marshall L, Barba D, Toole BM, Bowers SA. The oval pupil: clinical significance and relationship to intracranial hypertension. *J Neurosurg*. 1983;58:566–568.

54. Hudson-Civetta JA. Allocating nursing care. In: Civetta JM, Taylor RW, Kirby RR. eds. *Critical Care*. 2nd ed. Philadelphia, Pa: JB Lippincott Co; 1992:83–99.

55. Carpenter R. Infections and head injury: a potentially lethal combination. *Crit Care Nurs Q*. 1987;10:1–11.

56. McArdle M, Murrin P. Role of the trauma nurse coordinator. *Nurs Clin North Am*. 1986;21:673–675.

57. Flint CB. The role of the trauma coordinator: a position paper. *J Trauma*. 1988;28:1673–1675.

58. Beachley M, Snow S, Trimble P. Developing trauma care systems: the trauma nurse coordinator. *J Nurs Adm*. 1988;18:34–42.

59. DeKeyser FG, Paratore A, Camp L. Trauma nurse coordinator: three unique roles. *Nurs Manage*. 1993;24:56A–H.

60. Bontke CF, Boake C. Principles of brain injury rehabilitation. In: Braddom RL, ed. *Physical Medicine and Rehabilitation*. Philadelphia, Pa: WB Saunders Co; 1996:1027–1051.

61. Cope DN, Wolfson B. Crisis intervention with the family in the trauma setting. *J Head Trauma Rehabil*. 1994;9:67–81.

62. Moonilal JM. Trauma centers: a new dimension for hospital social work. *Soc Work Health Care*. 1982;7:15–25.

63. Silverman E. The social worker's role in shock-trauma units. *Soc Work*. 1986;31:311–313.

64. Halper AS. Teams and teamwork: health care settings. *ASHA*. June–July 1993;35:34–48.

CHAPTER 3

Basic Knowledge of the Brain and the Clinical Ramifications Post Injury

OVERVIEW OF NEUROANATOMY

From an anatomic and physiologic standpoint, the brain is the most complex, perplexing, and intriguing organ within the human body. The sense of consciousness begins and ends with the brain. The 17th-century French philosopher Rene Descartes declared, "Cogito, ergo sum" (I think, therefore I am).[1] Descartes was basically asserting that what the conscious brain is most sure of is the self. The state of consciousness is a concept of self and of how that self interacts with the outside world. The brain, which is the seat of consciousness, learns, thinks, remembers, and processes. Yet it is an extremely fragile organ that is highly sensitive to even a minor insult. Injury can result in diminishment or negation of the conscious state. Traumatic brain injury (TBI) is a common cause of disabling and destroying of conscious thought and interaction. The common mechanisms leading to a traumatic insult to the brain are vehicular injuries, falls, assaults, and penetrating trauma. To ascertain the consequences of these injuries, it is important that health care providers possess a working knowledge of basic neuroanatomy, neurophysiology, and neuropathophysiology.

Cellular Anatomy

The central nervous system (CNS) is composed of neurons, neuroglia, meningeal cells, and specialized blood vessels. *Neurons,* or nerve cells, conduct nerve impulses and give nervous tissue most of its functional characteristics. A CNS neuron is generally made up of three parts: the cell body, the dendrites, and the axon. The *cell body* is the part of the neuron that contains the nucleus, nucleolus, endoplasmic reticulum, polysome, mitochondria, and Golgi bodies (Figure 3–1). Neurons can be classified according to their functions or according to the number

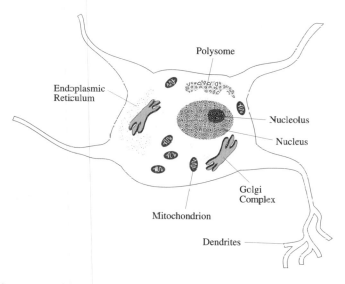

Figure 3–1 Intracellular structures of the neuron.

of processes extending from the cell body. Some neurons have a sensory function and relay information to the CNS from the periphery of the body. The olfactory membrane, inner ear, and retina have these sensory neurons. Motor or effector neurons carry impulses to the periphery to produce movement. There are probably 100 billion neurons in the entire nervous system. The *dendrites* are multiple branching outgrowths from the cell body that serve as receptor areas for the neuron (Figure 3–1). Most signals that are to be transmitted by the neuron enter by way of dendrites, although some enter also by the surface of the cell body. The dendrites of each neuron usually receive signals from thousands of *synapses* or points of contact between neurons or between a neuron or a muscle fiber. The *axon* is the portion of the neuron that is usually called *nerve fiber* (Figure 3–2). Nerve fibers are of two functional types: *afferent fibers*, which transmit sensory information into the brain, and *efferent fibers*, which transmit motor signals back from the CNS to the periphery, especially to the skeletal muscles. Each neuron has one axon leaving the cell body. An axon is usually longer than a dendrite and originates from an axon hillock (Figure 3–2).

A *myelin sheath*, composed of lipids and proteins, surrounds most long axons. The sheath is made of a spiral of plasma membrane from specialized glial cells (*oligodendroglia*), giving the axon a white and glistening appearance; thus the name *white matter* for the great bundles of nerve fibers in the brain that lead to or from the nerve cells (*gray matter*), so called because the great numbers of neu-

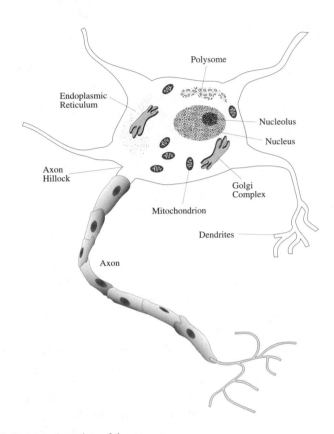

Polysome

Endoplasmic
Reticulum

Nucleolus

Nucleus

Axon
Hillock

Golgi
Complex

Mitochondrion

Dendrites

Axon

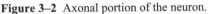

Figure 3–2 Axonal portion of the neuron.

ronal cell bodies all together give it a grayish hue. Injury to the gray matter is significant because it can result in cell loss and because there is no new cell replacement. Neurons differ from other cells in their lack of mitotic ability. Without mitosis, neurons cannot reproduce.

Myelin is what enables an axon to conduct impulses quickly and efficiently. Unmyelinated fibers conduct impulses quite slowly. Within the peripheral nervous system, the Schwann cells or neurilemmal cells perform the same function as the oligodendroglia.

Nerve impulses have the ability to achieve high velocity by what is called *saltatory conduction*. In saltatory conduction, the impulses jump from node to node. Myelin sheaths are interrupted by areas of constriction called *nodes of Ranvier*. At about every 1 to 2 mm, impulses can jump from node to node.

Cells can communicate both chemically and electrically. At the end of a dendrite is a *bouton*, a presynaptic membrane or presynaptic terminal. The part of the cell receiving the impulse is covered by a postsynaptic membrane. The area separating the two membranes is the *synaptic cleft*. In the boutons, vesicles called *synaptic vesicles* contain chemical transmitter substances. Nerve impulses release transmitters into the synaptic cleft to combine with specific molecular binding sites on a receptor and either excite or inhibit the postsynaptic neuron (Figure 3–3). These chemical reactions can change the postsynaptic cell's membrane permeability, affecting its concentration of cations, sodium, and potassium.

The electrical transport of nerve impulses is also related to cellular membrane permeability. In a state of rest, the cell is very permeable to potassium. However, when it is in an excited state, it becomes highly permeable to sodium. The reverse of permeability creates a nerve impulse or action potential that is propagated along the membrane by local circuits of electrical current.

The second group of cell types is the *neuroglia*, better known as *glial cells*. Neuroglia cells provide structural support and important metabolic functions. They make up the major non-neuronal elements of the CNS. Basically, the CNS is composed almost entirely of neurons and neuroglia cells packed tightly together.

Most glial cells are *astrocytes* (or *astroglia*) (Figure 3–4). Their shape is star-like, with numerous processes extending from the cell body. Some of these pro-

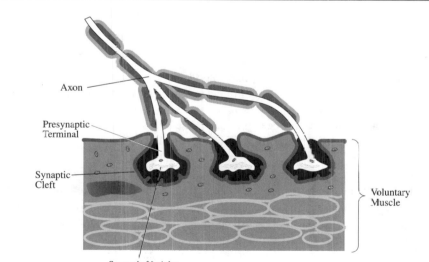

Axon

Presynaptic Terminal

Synaptic Cleft

Voluntary Muscle

Synaptic Vesicles

Figure 3–3 Structures involved in transmitter release into the synaptic cleft, affecting voluntary muscle response.

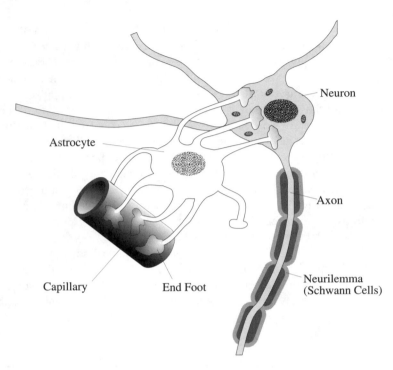

Figure 3–4 Star-shaped astrocyte with processes attached to the surface of a capillary blood vessel.

cesses attach to the surface of capillary blood vessels. Many enzymes that have been isolated from astrocytes suggest their involvement in transport mechanisms between blood and brain.

When brain injury occurs due to trauma or disease, the astrocytes can have both a beneficial and a deleterious effect. These glial cells mobilize and proliferate at the site of injury. They act as scavengers and aid in the healing process by phago-cytosing (ingesting and destroying) cellular debris and toxic products left by in-jured degenerating neurons. However, the proliferation of astrocytes can also re-sult in the development of obstructive scar tissue that fills in spaces resulting from trauma or disease. This scar tissue can block the course of regenerating axons and prevent the formation of new synaptic connections.

Oligodendroglia, discussed earlier, have a significant role in forming myelin sheaths. These cells react to injury by swelling. Another type of glial cell that is abundant in the gray matter is *microglia*. These cells, like astrocyes, are activated when trauma or disease has occurred: they proliferate rapidly and migrate toward the injury. Astrocytes and oligodendroglial cells originate from the same neuroectoderm as neurons. Microglia are mesodermal and are similar to large lymphocytes.

Gross Anatomy of the Brain

The human brain is a thinking, sensing, and controlling system of the body. It receives thousands of pieces of information and then integrates this information into a bodily response. It weighs approximately 1,400 g and generally constitutes about 2% of the total body weight. The brain is that portion of the nervous system that is located in the cranial cavity. Within this cranial vault surrounding the brain are three tissues of membrane, or *meninges*. These provide a layer of nourishing and protective covering for the CNS. The outermost layer enveloping the brain is the *dura mater*, which means "hard mother." It is a tough fibrous layer that protects the entire brain and its contents. The skull's inner *periosteum*, or layer of connective tissue that closely invests the bone, is more adherent to the meningeal dura than to the bone itself; consequently, it is often considered to be the outer layer of the dura. The inner, or *meningeal*, layer of the dura forms folds into the brain itself, as in the *falx cerebri* and *falx cerebelli*. In certain areas, spaces called *dural venous sinuses* form between layers of dura and are filled with venous blood. The epidural space is between the periosteal and meningeal layers of the dura. The subdural space is between the dura and the *arachnoid mater,* a delicate transparent membrane that covers the entire brain and spinal cord. The third or inner layer is the *pia mater,* which is a delicate membrane closely adherent to the surface of the brain. It contains blood vessels meshed in its membranes (Figure 3–5) and cannot be dissected from the brain tissue. The space between the arachnoid mater and the pia mater is called the *subarachnoid space,* and through it flows the spinal fluid.

The brain is divided into five parts: (1) the cerebrum or *(telencephalon)*; (2) the diencephalon; (3) the limbic system; (4) the brainstem, including the mesencephalon, the pons, and the medulla oblongata; and (5) the cerebellum. According to another classification scheme, the telencephalon and the diencephalon together constitute the *prosencephalon,* or *forebrain,* which is the large portion of the brain filling the anterior and superior three fourths of the cranial cavity. The *mesencephalon*, a minute portion of the brain located at the base of the forebrain, is also called the *midbrain*. It is the only connecting link between the forebrain and all the lower portions of the brain and spinal cord. And the pons, medulla, and cerebellum, which all lie in the posterior fossa of the cranial vault, together constitute what is called the *rhombencephalon,* or *hindbrain*.

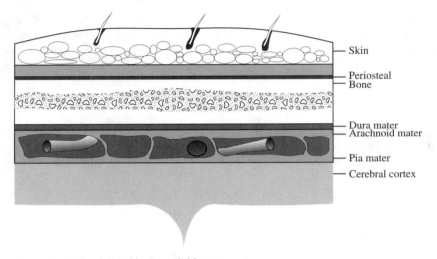

Figure 3–5 Cranial and intracranial layers.

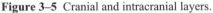

Cerebrum

The cerebrum, which is divided into left and right hemispheres, makes up the largest part of the brain, accounting for 80% of the weight. Its surface layer of gray matter, the cerebral cortex, functions chiefly to coordinate and analyze sensory and motor information. The two cerebral hemispheres are partially separated by the deep longitudinal cerebral fissure. The division of the cerebral hemispheres is complete in the frontal and occipital regions, but centrally, the fissure extends only to the corpus callosum. The corpus callosum is the major interhemispheric pathway; it consists of bundles of nerve fibers that connect the cortex on one side with the corresponding area on the other side. It has four parts: (1) rostrum, (2) genu rostrum, (3) body, and (4) splenium (Figure 3–6). The genu's fibers connect the rostral frontal lobes. The body's fibers connect the remaining parts of the two frontal lobes and the two parietal lobes. The splenium's fibers connect the two temporal and two occipital lobes. A second, minor interhemispheric pathway is the anterior commissure, located several centimeters below the anterior third of the corpus callosum. Unlike the corpus callosum, which has approximately 20 million fibers, the anterior commissure is a much smaller bundle that contains only approximately 1 million fibers. It connects mainly the anterior and medial portions of the two temporal lobes.

The cerebral hemispheres have an abundance of folds. These folds substantially increase the surface area and the volume of the cerebral cortex. The grooves or

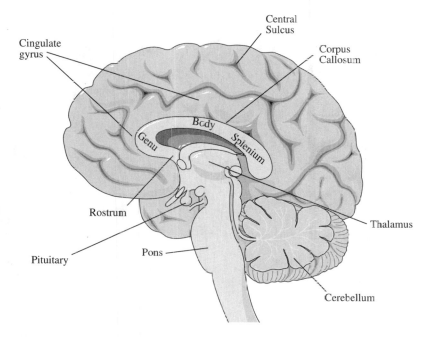

Figure 3–6 The corpus callosum and its four divisions.

clefts of the outer surface of the cerebral cortex are known as *sulci*. The elevated rigid portions of the brain lying between the sulci are called *convolutions* or *gyri*. The deep grooves between lobes and hemispheres are sometimes referred to as *fissures*.

Divisions of the Cerebrum

The cerebral hemisphere is subdivided by several sulci into four major lobes: frontal, parietal, occipital, and temporal (Figure 3–7). The frontal lobe is the largest of the lobes, making up about one third of the hemispheric surface. The convexity of the frontal lobe has four principal gyri. The *precentral gyrus* passes anterior and parallel to the central sulcus, or fissure of Rolando (Figure 3–8). It is the primary motor cortex, containing neurons whose axons give rise to cortical spinal and cortical bulbar tracks. The second and third gyri are the *superior* and *middle frontal gyri*, located to the front of the precentral gyrus. These two gyri are involved with the body and eye movements. The fourth, the *inferior frontal gyrus*, includes, on the left side, Broca's area, an important speech-producing area of the brain. Orbital sulci and gyri give rise to pathways important to expression of emo-

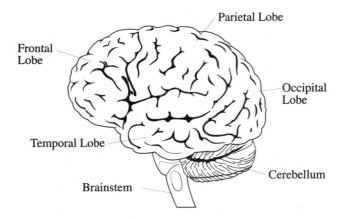

Figure 3–7 Four major lobes of the cerebrum.

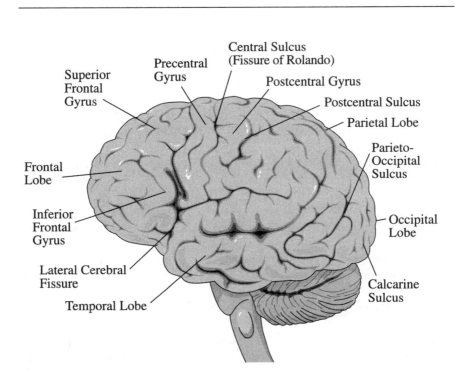

Figure 3–8 Divisions of the frontal, parietal, and occipital lobes.

tion. The most commonly injured portions of the brain are the inferior frontal and temporal lobes. Injuries to the frontal lobe can result in behavioral problems, compromised judgment, difficulties in abstraction, a lack of emotional response, and short-term memory loss.

The parietal lobe is bounded by the central sulcus anteriorly and the parieto-occipital sulcus posteriorly and is bounded laterally by the level of the lateral cerebral (or *Sylvian*) fissure (Figure 3–8). The postcentral sulcus is one of the two major sulci in the parietal lobe and is located behind and parallel to the central sulcus (or fissure of Rolando). The postcentral gyrus is concerned with the somesthesis, or the sense of touch; kinesthesis, or the sense of position of the extremities; vibratory sense; and other fine tactile discriminatory processes. The parietal lobe and inferior parietal lobe are important in the synthetic aspects of multiple sensory experiences brought to consciousness, including body awareness and spatial orientation. On the left, the reception and organization of language functions are centered in the supramarginal gyri and angular gyri, which are subdivisions of the inferior parietal lobe. Injuries to the parietal lobe carry the potential of disrupting all of the above functions.

The occipital lobe is a pyramidal-shaped posterior lobe situated behind the parietal occipital sulcus (Figure 3–8). The walls of the calcarine sulcus are the primary visual cortex. The lateral occipital sulcus divides the occipital lobe into a superior gyrus and an inferior gyrus. The precuneus is situated between the calcarine sulcus and the parietal occipital sulcus. These areas process visual information.

The temporal lobe has been referred to as the *psychic cortex*. When it is stimulated, memory is aroused. The temporal lobe lies inferior to the lateral cerebral fissure (Figure 3–8) and extends back to the level of the parieto-occipital fissure. The transverse temporal gyrus constitutes a primary auditory cortex. It occupies the posterior part of the superior temporal surface. Injuries to the temporal lobe can compromise visual learning skills and emotion, lessen short-term memory, and create difficulties in intellect. Dominant hemispheric damage to this lobe creates problems of speech comprehension and interpretation. Bilateral loss of the inferior temporal lobes abolishes the ability to learn. Furthermore, persons with temporal lobe lesions are at high risk of seizure disorder

A fifth, minor lobe that is deep within the lateral cerebral fissure is sometimes classified as part of the limbic system. This is the oval-shaped *insula*, or central lobe, which has been associated with intra-abdominal visceral motility. If the temporal and frontal lobes are separated, the insula can be exposed. Posteriorly, this fissure separates portions of the parietal and temporal lobes. The *central sulcus* surrounds the insula and separates it from the adjacent frontal, parietal, and temporal lobes. The *cingulate sulcus* begins below the anterior end of the corpus callosum, runs parallel to the corpus callosum, and finally curves up a short distance behind the upper end of the central sulcus. It outlines the *cingulate gyrus*, part of the limbic system, which contains an accessory motor area and is activated when movement is intended.

Deep within the brain matter of the cerebrum are the basal ganglia (Figure 3–9). Their functions are extrapyramidal motor activity, including facilitation and inhibition of primary motor activity. The three most important nuclei of the basal ganglia are the *caudate nucleus,* the *putamen*, and the *globus pallidus*. An additional part of the basal ganglia whose function is not well known is called the *claustrum*. All that is known is that the claustrum establishes connections with the frontal, parietal, and temporal lobes.

The caudate nucleus forms a lateral wall of the anterior horn of the lateral ventricle; the putamen, located just beneath the insular cortex, is the largest and most lateral part of the basal ganglia and is mostly composed of small to medium-sized nerve cells; and the globus pallidus, which is smaller, is located between the internal capsule and the putamen. The principal function of the basal ganglia is to control motor tone and posture, whereas the cerebral cortex is necessary for performance of more precise movements of arms, hands, fingers, and feet. The high degree of coordination of different muscle groups of the body during most motor functions involves certain complex circulatory nerve fibers that are interconnected and is achieved by the cerebral cortex and basal ganglion in the cerebrum, which both interact with the cerebellum.

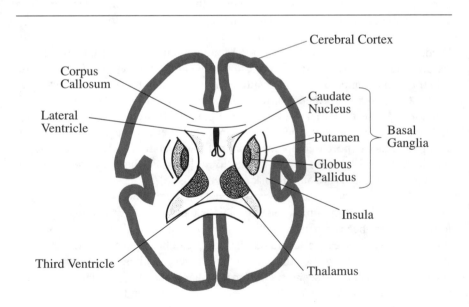

Figure 3–9 The nuclei of the basal ganglia: caudate nucleus, putamen, and globus pallidus.

Organization of the Cerebral Cortex

Over time there have been various attempts to localize functions in the cerebral cortex. The most widely used classification of anatomy is that devised by Brodmann (1909), who studied the cortical structure in horizontal sections stained according to Nissl. He described 47 such areas, shown in Figures 3–10 and 3–11. Discussions of motor and sensory areas of the cortex below will refer to these areas by number.

Unfortunately, Brodmann's areas correspond only fairly well with function as defined by a variety of studies. Broca, Pierre Marie, and Wernicke studied functional losses and correlated them with lesions found at autopsy. They defined the broad areas of speech function in the left hemisphere. Hughlings Jackson studied the progression of focal-onset seizures and then used autopsy correlation. He was most influential in defining both motor and sensory functions around the central sulcus. Foerster and then Penfield used electrical stimulation of the exposed brain in awake patients mainly to define which functions were arrested. This is still a widely used technique to find which areas to avoid during surgery. Movement and sensation are sometimes elicited. Occasionally, stimulation of the temporal lobe

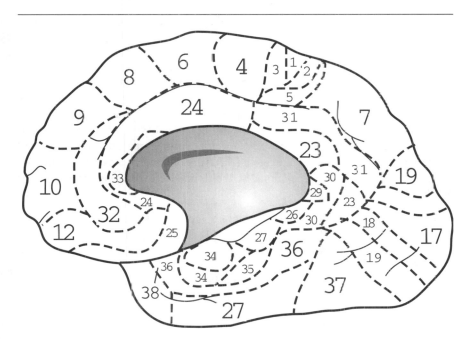

Figure 3–10 Interior of the cerebral cortex as designated by Brodmann (concave surface).

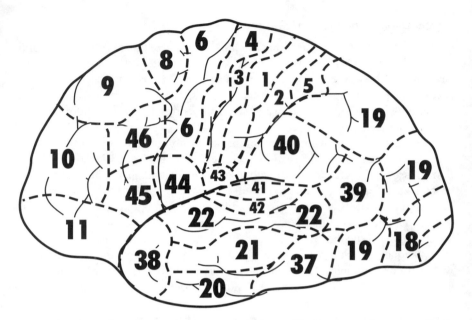

Figure 3–11 Interior of the cerebral cortex as designated by Brodmann (convex surface).

causes the patient to relive past episodes of his or her life. Lassen, starting in the 1960s, confirmed an old observation of Harvey Cushing's that use of a part of the brain increases its blood flow and metabolism. Using radioactive xenon, he confirmed or amended much of the work previously completed and added data on new areas, such as the depths of the lateral cerebral fissure and the interhemispheric fissure. Extensions of this work using positron emission tomography and functional magnetic resonance imaging (MRI) are ongoing and extend our knowledge of cortical function. Functionally, the defined areas of the cortex may be subdivided as follows:

1. *motor areas*, which include primary motor areas, premotor areas, and supplementary motor area
2. *sensory areas*, which include primary and secondary sensory areas and association areas
3. *psychologic areas*, which include the "psychical' areas of the temporal lobe and the prefrontal cortex (shown in Figure 3–12)

Motor Areas of the Cortex

It has been recognized for a long time that stimulation of the precentral gyrus, which corresponds to Brodmann's areas 4 and 6, causes movement of the extremities (Figure 3–12).

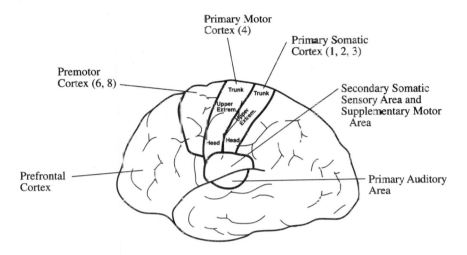

Figure 3–12 Primary motor cortex areas of the brain. Numbers are those of Brodmann's areas.

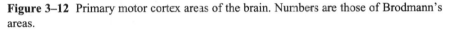

Area 4: Primary Motor Cortex. Area 4 is located along the anterior wall of the central sulcus and the adjacent parts of the precentral gyrus and extends over the anterior part of the precentral gyrus (Figure 3–12). The cortex of area 4 is characterized by an abundance of pyramidal (cone-shaped) cells and the so-called giant cells of Betz, which number about 34,000 per hemisphere. These Betz cells have thick axons but constitute only 3% of the total number of corticospinal fibers.

Stimulation of area 4 causes movement of muscles in the contralateral limbs, mainly the flexor muscles. In a somatotopic pattern called the *homunculus* (Figure 3–13), each part of the body has a well-defined site of representation. The parts that are more frequently used—the face, the hand, and the upper extremities—occupy a much larger area than do the trunk and lower extremities.

Areas 6 and 8: Premotor Cortex and Supplementary Motor Area. Areas 6 and 8 are located rostral to area 4 and extend over the anterior part of the precentral gyrus and the upper part of the superior frontal gyrus (Figure 3–12). Area 4 and area 6 show similarities of structure, but area 6 lacks the giant cells of Betz. Stimulation of area 6 causes rotation of the head and trunk to the contralateral side and flexion and extension of the extremities (primarily the axial and proximal muscle groups), all of which are more complex movements than those that occur with stimulation of area 4 only. The supplementary motor area plays a significant role in the programming of patterns and sequence of movements.

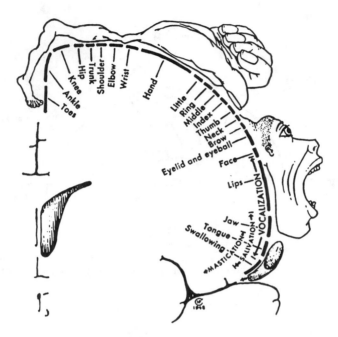

Figure 3–13 Motor homunculus, showing the representation of the various parts of the body in the motor cortex. The face, hand, and foot areas are most widely represented. *Source:* Reprinted with the permission of Simon & Schuster from THE CEREBRAL COR-TEX OF MAN by Wilder Penfield and Theodore Rasmussen. Copyright © 1950 by Macmillan Publishing Company, Renewed 1978 by Theodore Rasmussen.

Cortical Lesions of Areas 4 and 6. When a lesion is confined to area 4, flaccid paresis of the contralateral extremity will follow. The distal muscles of the extremity will be more severely paralyzed than the proximal muscles. Subsequent to a lesion of both area 4 and area 6, there will be more severe paralysis, which is associated with spasticity and increased myotatic (stretching or extending) reflexes. The last two symptoms probably result from the involvement of many corticoreticulospinal fibers that arise from area 6.

Somatosensory Areas of the Cortex

Areas 1, 2, and 3: Somatosensory Cortex. The primary somatosensory area is made up of three narrow strips of the postcentral gyrus, areas 1, 2, and 3 of Brodmann (Figure 3–12). These extend from the depth of the central sulcus over the entire postcentral gyrus. The afferent fibers originate from the thalamus and convey stimuli from the opposite side of the body. The area shows an exact somatotopic localization (homunculus), with the lower extremities at the peak and the face and teeth in the inferior part (Figure 3–13). The sensory cortex enriches perception of delicate discriminatory qualities: for example, the ability to recognize spatial relations and minor differences of intensity. It is also associated with the characterization of pain and temperature, which have only a minor representation in the cortex.

Cortical Lesions of Areas 1, 2. and 3. Lesions of the postcentral gyrus reduce the mechanical discriminatory capacities in both the perception of tactile stimuli and the ability to determine the position of the limbs in space. There is only slight disturbance of pain and temperature sensibility. In the sequence of recovery, the sense of pain is the first to return, and kinesthesia is the last.

Areas 17, 18, and 19: The Visual Cortex. The visual cortex (see Figure 3–10) will be discussed again in Chapter 4's treatment of the cranial nerves. Brodmann's area 17 is located in the posterior part of the cortex on either side of the calcarine sulcus, and is known as the *area striata*. It is regarded as the primary optical area. The fibers of the geniculocalcarine tract terminate, for the most part, on the granular cells of layer IV. The surrounding areas 18 and 19 are essential for eye movements, the interpretation of optic impressions, and the integration of these impressions into other information.

Areas 41, 42, and 22: The Auditory Cortex. The auditory area (Brodmann's areas 41 and 42) lies in the cortex of the superior temporal gyrus and in the depth of the lateral cerebral fissure (see Figures 3–11 and 3–12). The afferent projection fibers originate from the medial geniculate body or directly from the inferior colliculus. The primary auditory cortex (area 41) responds to broad bands of the audible spectrum and is essential for the location of the source of the sound and for changes in frequency. Secondary areas 42 and 22 have a higher threshold of response to sound intensity.

Areas 22, 39, 44, and 45: The Language Neural Circuit. The function of speech production is organized according to a complex model. Neural impulses that originate in the sensory cortical association areas of vision, sound, or general sensation converge on Wernicke's speech area, located in the posterior portion of area 22 (Figure 3–11). In this area, the words to be spoken originate, are generated, and are then transmitted to Broca's speech area, located anterior to area 22 in areas 44 and 45 of the inferior frontal gyrus. In Broca's area, a detailed coordinated program for vocalization is formulated, and the information is passed to the motor cortex (areas 4 and 6), where the motor pathways for the production of the spoken language are activated.

Psychologic Areas of the Cortex

Extensive areas, mainly in the frontal cortex (Brodmann's areas 9, 10, 11, and 45) and the temporal lobes (areas 23, 21, and 22), do not respond to sensory stimulation (see Figures 3–10 and 3–11). These are the areas of anatomic substrate of the higher psychologic functions. They are connected both among themselves and to the thalamus and parietal lobes.

Bilateral lesions of the prefrontal cortex cause defects of intelligence and personality and are manifested through an inability of patients to concentrate and to think in abstract terms. Personality changes may occur, and a patient may lose the power of self-criticism, initiative, stability, and a sense of social correctness. Behavioral testing shows an inability to change the first chosen course of action. Surgical interruption of the fibers from the prefrontal cortex has the effect of dulling the appreciation of pain and may be performed on patients who have severe intractable pain. Areas 39 and 40 of the parietal lobe, which connect with the prefrontal cortex, are necessary for the integration of the entire exteroceptive and proprioceptive input necessary for the recognition of one's own body parts and their position in space. This is usually referred to as recognition of body schema. Lesions in the nondominant, usually right parietal lobe, lead to disturbances of body schema, while those in the left parietal lobe in the same area result in problems with language, mainly aphasia.

The Concept of Cerebral Dominance

It is well recognized that humans have dominant extremities, especially in the upper extremities. The majority of humans are right hand dominant. Since the right hand is controlled by the left hemisphere for motor activity, the left hemisphere plays a leading role. The speech center is in the left hemisphere in over 90% of people. For 40% of left-hand–dominant persons, some speech is found in the right hemisphere. Because both the control of the right hand and the control of language are in the left side, this hemisphere is usually referred to as the *dominant hemisphere*.

Numerous clinical studies have shown the functional inequality of the right and left hemispheres. The left hemisphere functions analytically and is recognized as the center for the execution of mathematical calculations. It is suggested that conscious awareness may be localized in the left hemisphere.

The dominance of the left hemisphere does not mean that the right hemisphere is not important. Recognizing abstract forms and spatial relations through artistic expression is the responsibility of the right hemisphere. However, the left hemisphere, figuratively speaking, allows for right hemisphere expression.

Ventricles

Cerebral spinal fluid (CSF) is contained within interconnective cavities called ventricles. There are four ventricles: two paired lateral ventricles and the third and fourth ventricles (Figure 3–14).

The two lateral ventricles, left and right, are "C"-shaped cavities contained within the cerebral hemispheres. Each of the lateral ventricles is connected with

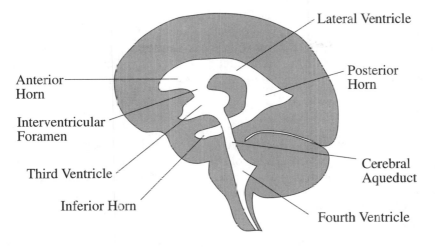

Figure 3–14 Interconnective cavities called ventricles, containing cerebrospinal fluid.

the third ventricle via the interventricular foramen (or foramen of Monro). The lateral ventricles are composed of the following four parts: (1) the anterior horn, located in the frontal lobe; (2) the body, located in the parietal lobe; (3) the inferior or temporal horn, located in the temporal lobe; and (4) the posterior horn, located in the occipital lobe.

CSF is produced by the choroid plexus (special secretory structures that secrete CSF) of the lateral, third, and fourth ventricles. This fluid production is a vascular process of the pia mater projecting into the ventricular cavity. The choroid plexus has a semipermeable filter between arterial blood and the cerebral spinal fluid. The production of CSF does consume energy. The arteries to the plexus are the anterior carotid artery (a branch of the internal carotid artery) and the posterior carotid artery (a branch of the posterior cerebral artery). The volume of CSF varies from 80 to 150 mL, including fluid from both the ventricles and the arachnoid space. The choroid plexus effectively replaces the CSF several times per day.

The third ventricle is a narrow ventricle chamber between the two lateral ventricles. Its roof is formed by a thin layer of ependyma. The lower lateral wall in the floor of the ventricle is formed by the hypothalamus and the subthalamus. There are three openings that communicate with the third ventricle: the two interventricular foramina and the cerebral aqueduct. There are two choroid plexi that enter in the roof of the third ventricle. The fourth ventricle is a cavity overlying the pons and medulla. The cerebral aqueduct connects the third and fourth ventricles. The fourth ventricle contains several tufts of choroid plexus.

The conduits for the passage of CSF and the subarachnoid space that surrounds and protects the brain and spinal cord are the foramen of Magendie and the two lateral foramen of Luschka. Normally CSF is reabsorbed in the bloodstream through arachnoid villi that empty into the venous sinuses of the dura mater and along the dorsal roots of the spinal nerves.

Diencephalon

The diencephalon is sometimes called the "between-brain" because it is surrounded by two cerebral hemispheres of telencephalon. Together, the diencephalon and the telencephalon make up the forebrain. The diencephalon is the forebrain's central core, a mass of gray matter surrounded by the two cerebral hemispheres of the telencephalon. The most important structures of the diencephalon are the thalamus and the hypothalamus.

Thalamus

In each cerebral hemisphere there is a thalamus (Figure 3–9). Basically, the thalamus is a major traffic relay station for receiving sensory and other signals and directing them to appropriate points in the cerebral cortex, where they undergo further analysis, and in deep areas of the cerebrum. It has been called the "gateway to the cerebral cortex" for this reason. The thalamus makes up about four fifths of the diencephalon and is a major source of afferent fibers to the cortex. It receives information from ascending pathways of the auditory, visual, and somatosensory systems. The thalamus comprises 30 separate discrete nuclei, subdivided into five groups: anterior, middle, dorsal medial, lateral, and posterior. The *anterior nuclei* receive fibers from the mammillary bodies and project to the cingulate cortex of the cerebrum. The *middle nuclei* receive fibers conveying sensory information from the reticular formation of the brainstem and have connections with the hypothalamus and the dorsal medial thalamic nuclei. The *dorsal medial nuclei* of the medial group contribute to aspects of emotion, such as a sense of well-being, euphoria, or depression. Memory may also be an important role of the dorsal medial thalamic nuclei. The *lateral nuclei* make essential contributions to the initiation of movement, the control of muscle tone, and the regulation of cortical reflexes. The *posterior nuclei* relay somatic impulses to connections with the parietal and temporal lobes: the lateral geniculate subgroup relays visual input to the calcarine cortex, and the medial geniculate subgroup sends auditory input to the temporal lobes.

Hypothalamus

The hypothalamus is the integrative and control center for the autonomic nervous system (Figure 3–15). Its actions are automatic. No other region of the brain

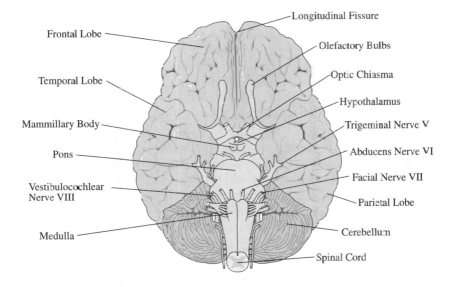

Figure 3–15 The hypothalamus, integrative/control center for the autonomic nervous system.

has so many different and vital functions. It is part of the diencephalon lying below the thalamus on either side of the third ventricle. Separating the hypothalamus from the overlying thalamus is a shallow groove called the *hypothalamic sulcus.* The hypothalamus receives fiber bundles mainly from higher corticoid centers such as visual and auditory. It controls personality, goal-seeking behavior, temperature control, sleep, sexual drive, water metabolism, hunger, secretions of hormones, and emotions, and it maintains a balance between the sympathetic and parasympathetic divisions of the autonomic nervous system.

The essential hypothalamic nuclei have several functions. The *preoptic nucleus,* anteriorly located, is concerned with body temperature control and causes a decrease in both heart rate and arterial pressure. The *medial nucleus* gives a sense of satiety. The *superoptic nucleus,* anteriorly and inferiorly located, controls renal excretion of water. If the electrolyte concentration increases in bodily fluids, the neurons of this area become stimulated. Stimulation causes the production of vasopressin, an antidiuretic hormone from the posterior pituitary gland, which then causes massive reabsorption of water.

Both the lateral and the posterior hypothalamus, in contradistinction to the preoptic area, cause an increase in heart rate and arterial pressure. The lateral hypothalamus is also a thirst and hunger center.

The *paraventricular nucleus* lies within the superoptic region close to the third ventricle in the lateral wall of the hypothalamus. Stimulation of the nucleus causes neuronal cells to secrete the hormone oxytocin, which causes increased contractility of the uterus. The nucleus also causes contractility of milk epithelial cells around the alveoli of the breast, resulting in alveoli emptying milk through the nipples.

The cells of the hypothalamus can in part influence the secretion of various hormones of the anterior lobe of the pituitary gland, which is attached to the hypothalamus. Neurosecretory cells, specialized neurons in the hypothalamus that are very sensitive to the blood concentrations of various anterior lobe hormones, synthesize and secrete hypothalamic releasing and inhibitory hormones that control the secretion of the anterior pituitary hormones. These neurons send nerve fibers into the median eminence and the tuber cinereum, an extension of the hypothalamic tissue that extends into the pituitary stalk. The neurosecretion is carried by portal veins to the anterior lobe of the pituitary, where cells are stimulated to produce various hormones. The function of the hypothalamic releasing and inhibitory hormones is to control the secretions of the anterior pituitary hormone. The most important hypothalamic releasing and inhibitory hormones are thyrotropin-releasing hormone, corticotropin-releasing hormone, growth hormone–releasing hormone, gonadotropin-releasing hormone, and prolactin inhibitory factor. The *thyrotropin-releasing hormone* controls the rate of secretion of thyrotropin in the pituitary gland. This stimulates the thyroid, which controls most chemical reactions of the body. *Corticotropin-releasing hormone* causes the release of adrenocorticotropin. Adrenocorticotropin acts primarily on the adrenal cortex, stimulating the secretion of cortical steroids, which in turn affects metabolism of glucose, proteins, and fats. *Growth hormone–releasing hormone* results in the release of growth hormone and growth hormone inhibitory hormone (*somatostatin*), which inhibits the release of growth hormone. *Gonadotropin-releasing hormone* causes the release of two gonadotropin hormones, luteinizing hormone–releasing hormone and follicle-stimulating hormone. Luteinizing hormone–releasing hormone controls growth of the gonads, as well as the reproductive activities. Follicle-stimulating hormone promotes the growth of ovarian follicles and spermatogenesis. *Prolactin inhibitory factor* results in the inhibition of prolactin secretions. Prolactin stimulates and sustains lactation during the postpartum period. Prolactin secretion is spontaneous. For this reason, hyperprolactinemia is an important sign of hypothalamic dysfunction.

Limbic System

Limbic means "border," and the limbic system borders the structure of the cerebrum and the diencephalon that mainly surrounds the hypothalamus. The major function of the limbic system is to control emotions and behavior. The *amygdala* is located deep inside each anterior temporal lobe. It is thought to control the appropriate behavior of a person for a given social situation. The two amygdalae are connected by the anterior commissure. The *hippocampus* is located on each side and on the medial-most border of the temporal lobe. It is a primitive portion of the cerebral cortex whose function is to interpret for the brain the importance of most sensory experiences. The more important experiences are stored as memories. The *mammillary bodies* lie behind the hypothalamus, functioning in close association with the thalamus, hypothalamus, and brainstem. They help control behavioral functions such as wakefulness, sense of well-being, and feeding reflexes such as swallowing. They receive a large input from the hippocampus by the fornix. The *septum pellucidum* lies anterior to the thalamus, hypothalamus, and basal ganglia. The adjacent cortex causes behavioral changes such as rage. Medial to the cerebrum and part of the deeper limbic system are the *cingulate gyrus*, the *cingulum*, the *insula,* and the *parahippocampal gyrus*. These structures influence conscious and nonconscious behavior.

Brainstem

The brainstem connects the forebrain with the spinal cord. There are three regions of the brainstem: the mesencephalon, the pons, and the medulla oblongata, better known as the medulla (Figure 3–15). Numerous important fiber tracts of the brainstem move upward and downward, transmitting sensory signals from the spinal cord to the thalamus and motor signals from the cerebral cortex to the spinal cord. The brainstem has many important centers that control respiration, arterial pressure, and equilibrium. It also has connecting links superiorly between the cerebellum and the cerebrum and inferiorly between the cerebellum and the spinal cord.

Mesencephalon

The mesencephalon is the smallest of the major subdivisions of the brainstem. It is located between the pons and the diencephalon. It contains sensory and motor pathways and nuclei of two cranial nerves, the oculomotor and the trochlear. The mesencephalon is divided into (1) an anterior section containing the two cerebral peduncles and midbrain tegmentum and (2) the midbrain tectum, a posterior structure. The dividing line between the tegmentum and the tectum is the cerebral aqueduct, which connects the third ventricle in the diencephalon with the fourth ventricle in the lower brainstem.

Each cerebral peduncle has two separate areas: the cortical spinal and cortical pontine fibers. The conduction of motor signals from the cortex to the spinal cord and pons is through the cortical spinal and cortical pontine fibers.

The tegmentum is made up of substantia nigra cranial nerve nuclei, smaller fiber tracts, and reticular gray matter. The neurons of the substantia nigra function as part of the basal ganglion system to control nonconscious muscle activities. An important fiber tract within the tegmentum for transmitting sensory signals from the body to the thalamus is the medial lemniscus. Another tract, the medial longitudinal fasciculus, connects several eye movement nuclei of the brainstem with each other and with the diencephalon. The red nucleus functions with the basal ganglion and cerebellum to coordinate muscle movements; it also helps relay information from the cerebellum to the thalamus and cerebrum. The nucleus of the third and fourth cranial nerves control most of the muscles for eye movements. The periaqueduct gray is a diffuse collection of nuclei that plays a major role in the analysis of reactions to pain. The reticular formation is widely dispersed in the brainstem. Various nerve cells within it are involved in motion of the body as a whole and, most important, in controlling the brain's overall level of activity. Activation of the reticular gray matter is essential to consciousness.

The tectum consists of four small nodule bodies: two superior colliculi, which deal with eye movements and trunk movements and respond to visual signals such as flashes of light; and two inferior colliculi, which serve as relay stations for auditory signals from the ears to the cerebrum and which cause the body to respond to sound coming from multiple directions. At the level of the inferior colliculi are the superior cerebellar peduncles. These two large bundles of nerves are major trunk lines between the cerebellum and the remainder of the brain.

Pons

The *pons*, meaning "bridge," lies between the mesencephalon and the medulla. It is a large mass with two distinct parts: ventral and dorsal. The ventral part provides extensive connections between the two cerebellar hemispheres and the cortical spinal fibers and cortical pontine fibers. These connections allow for efficiency of motor activities. The dorsal part has functions that are both sensory and motor such as vasomotor and respiratory centers, which are shared with the rest of the brainstem. It contains three structures that continue down from the tegmentum of the mesencephalon: the medial lemniscus, the medial longitudinal fasciculus, and the reticular formation. The dorsal portion contains several cranial nerve nuclei: (1) the abducens nerve, which controls eye movement; (2) the facial nerve, which allows for facial expression; (3) the trigeminal nerve, which controls the muscle of mastication and sensation of the face; and (4) the vestibulocochlear nerve, which transmits sensory signals from the ear and from the vestibular apparatus.

Medulla Oblongata

The medulla oblongata, or *myelencephalon*, is a pyramidal-shaped structure between the spinal cord and the pons (Figure 3–15). It lies below the inferior floor of the fourth ventricle. On the anterior surface of the medulla are two protrusions called *pyramids*. They carry corticospinal fibers, which pass from the cerebral cortex through the cerebral peduncle of the midbrain and through the ventral pons. Eventually, these fibers go to all aspects of the spinal cord, carrying signals dedicated to control of movement. Inferiorly, the fibers of the pyramids cross opposite sides before arriving at the spinal cord. This crossover is commonly called *decussation of the pyramids* and allows the left cerebral cortex to control muscle contractions in the right half of the body and the right cortex to control muscle contractions in the left half of the body.

Lateral to each pyramid is a structure called an *olive*. The olive relays signals to the cerebellum and also receives input from the basal ganglion, spinal cord, and the motor cortex. Efferent signals go to the contralateral cerebellum and then to the inferior cerebellar peduncle.

The medulla contains many of the same components as the mesencephalon and pons, such as the medial lemniscus, which receives sensory signals from the spinal cord and the cerebrum. In the posterior and inferior medulla are the gracile and the cuneate nuclei, which receive sensory signals from the dorsal columns of the spinal cord. These fibers decussate to form the medial lemniscus. Due to the crossover, the left side of the brain is excited from the right side of the body, and the right side of the brain from the left side of the body.

Several cranial nuclei are present in the medulla: numbers 9, 10, 11, and 12 (Figure 3–16). (Cranial nerves are discussed in Chapter 4.) Additionally, a large portion of the posterior and lateral medulla is made up of reticular formation. The reticular formation of the medulla and pons contains specialty centers. The vasomotor center transmits signals to the heart and blood vessels. These work in concert to increase blood pressure. The respiratory center is an automatic and rhythmic center that causes respiratory contractions needed for expiration and inspiration. Another specialized center involved with higher brain function is the hypothalamus, which relays messages to the spinal cord to control body temperature, sweating, stimulation of digestive secretions, and excretion of urine. In close proximity to the dorsal medullary reticular formation on each side of the midline is the dorsal motor nucleus of the vagus. This nucleus relays signals to the vagus nerve controlling gastric secretion, gastroperistalsis, control of internal functions, and control of heart rate.

Cerebellum

The cerebellum is the largest part of the hindbrain (Figures 3–7 and 3–15). It is located in the posterior fossa of the skull behind the pons and medulla. Its primary function is to allow the different muscle groups to accomplish complex movements, especially when those movements occur rapidly. It is essentially a control center for the coordination of voluntary muscle activity, equilibrium, and muscle

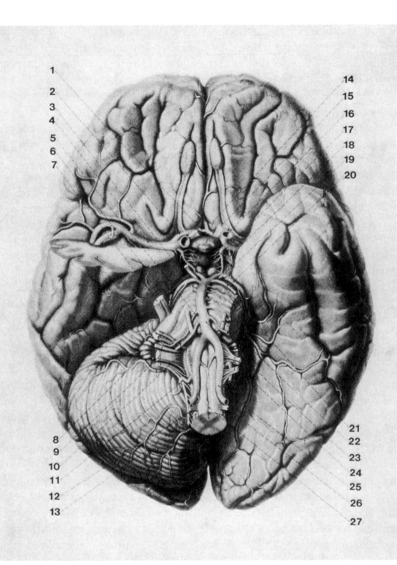

Figure 3–16 Arteries and cranial nerves of the base of the brain. *Source:* Reprinted from J.D. Fix, *Atlas of the Human Brain and Spinal Cord,* pp. 2–3, © 1987, Aspen Publishers, Inc.

Figure 3-16 continued

1. Anterior communicating artery	12. Accessory nerve
2. Anterior cerebral artery	15. Optic nerve
3. Transverse pontine arteries	16. Internal carotid artery
4. Middle cerebral artery	17. Posterior communicating artery
5. Labyrinthine artery	18. Anterior choroidal artery
6. Trochlear nerve	19. Oculomotor nerve
7. Trigeminal nerve	20. Posterior cerebral artery
8. Facial, intermediate, and vestibulocochlear nerves	21. Superior cerebellar artery
	22. Abducent nerve
9. Vagal group (glossopharyngeal, vagal, and accessory nerves)	23. Basilar artery
	24. Hypoglossal nerve
10. Anterior inferior cerebellar artery (AICA)	25. Vertebral artery
	26. First cervical nerve (ventral root)
11. Posterior inferior cerebellar artery (PICA)	27. Ventral spinal artery

tone. The cerebellum does not initiate movement; thus, cerebellar injury does not result in paralysis.

Each cerebellar hemisphere has connections to the brainstem through three bundles of nerve fibers: (1) the superior cerebellar peduncle, connecting the cerebellum to the mesencephalon; (2) the middle cerebellar peduncle, making connections to the pons; and (3) the inferior cerebellar peduncle, which connects with the medulla. Transmissions are made to and from the cerebellum via these three peduncles.

The cerebellum is made up of the vermis and the hemispheres. The *vermis* functions to coordinate subconscious postural body movements. This is done in an association with the brainstem and spinal cord. There are two cerebellar hemispheres, located on the two sides of the cerebellum. These hemispheres function in concert with the cerebrum to coordinate voluntary movements of the extremities. All parts affect speech and swallowing.

The internal structure of the cerebellum is made up of the cerebellar cortex, consisting of several billion nerve cells; the subcortical white matter, made up of nerve fibers; and the deep nuclei. The deep nuclei are located in the center of the cerebellar white matter. The most prominent nucleus is the dentate nucleus. The other three are the fastigial, the emboliform, and the globose nuclei. These deep nuclei give rise to nerve fibers that transmit signals from the cerebellum to other parts of the nervous system. The cerebellar cortex acts as a computer receiving input from the cerebral cortex, the basal ganglia, the spinal cord, and the peripheral muscles, integrating all of these inputs to assist in the coordination of muscle movements.

BLOOD SUPPLY

Approximately 800 mL of blood are needed to flow through the brain each minute to sustain this ever-active organ. The brain consumes about 20% of the oxygen used by the body; it does not store either oxygen or glucose, and it derives its energy almost exclusively from the metabolism of the glucose delivered by the blood.

Blood is supplied to the brain by two arterial systems: the internal carotid arterial system and the vertebral arterial system. Blood is removed from the brain by the jugular venous system and to a lesser extent by the vertebral venous system.

Arterial Blood Supply

Internal Carotid Arterial System

Both the right and left internal carotid arteries enter the cranial cavity through their respective cavernous sinuses. Each divides into two terminal branches:

1. The *anterior cerebral artery* proceeds medially above the optic nerve as far as the longitudinal cerebral fissure. Here the two vessels communicate through the anterior communicating artery, then follow the margin of the corpus callosum on the medial aspect of the hemisphere. They terminate as the pericallosal and callosomarginal arteries at the parieto-occipital fissure (Figure 3–16). The anterior cerebral artery supplies blood to the corpus callosum, the septum pellucidum part of the caudate nucleus and hypothalamus, and the medial cerebral hemispheres.

2. The *middle cerebral artery* curves between the temporal pole and the inferior frontal lobe of the hemisphere to the lateral cerebral fissure, where it divides into several branches that supply blood to the lateral portions of the orbital gyri and to the frontal, parietal, and temporal lobes (Figure 3–16). The peripheral branches anastomose with those of the anterior and posterior cerebral arteries. An important branch, the anterior choroidal artery, enters the sulcus between the temporal lobe and the brainstem, proceeds to the choroid fissure, and supplies the choroid plexus of the lateral ventricle. Other branches (*striate arteries*) penetrate the cerebrum to supply the basal ganglia, the internal capsule, and most of the diencephalon.

The ophthalmic artery is an important branch of the internal carotid artery arising at the "S" bend of the latter. It supplies blood to the eye.

Vertebral Arterial System

The two vertebral arteries enter the cranium through the foramen magnum on the anterolateral aspect of the medulla. At the level of the pontomedullary junction, they join to form the basilar artery, which proceeds rostrally as far as the midbrain level, where it bifurcates to form the left and right posterior cerebral arteries (Figure 3–16).

The vertebral arterial system, through its various branches, supplies blood to the brainstem, the cerebellum, and a large part of the occipital lobe.

Three groups of branches arise from the main stem of the artery. The *paramedian arteries* supply the medial aspect of the medulla and brainstem. One of these descends to the midline and unites with its contralateral artery to form the anterior spinal artery, which supplies the anterior two thirds of the cord as far as the conus terminalis. The *short circumferential arteries* include short pontine branches of the basilar artery supplying the posterolateral and posterior aspect of the brainstem and cerebellum. The *long circumferential arteries*, one on each side, include (1) the posterior spinal artery, supplying the posterior third of the spinal cord; (2) the posterior interior cerebellar artery from the vertebral artery, which supplies the undersurface of the cerebellum; (3) the anterior inferior cerebellar artery, arising from the midsection of the basilar artery and the inferior peduncle of the cerebellum; and (4) the superior cerebellar artery arising from the proximal end of the basilar artery and supplying the superior aspect of the cerebellum and the superior cerebellar peduncle.

Circle of Willis

The two arterial systems just discussed are interconnected at the base of the brain and may form an effective collateral circulation should one of the major arteries become occluded. There is, however, little exchange of blood between these communicating systems. The arterial ring is formed posteriorly by the bilateral posterior communicating arteries, which arise off the internal carotid arteries and join the posterior cerebral arteries (Figure 3–16). The anterior portion of the circle is completed by the anterior communicating arteries, which arise from the anterior cerebral arteries of each side.

Venous Drainage

The veins of the brain form a separate plexus and drain into the venous sinuses of the dura mater and the brain but do not accompany the arteries, as elsewhere in the body. The veins of the cerebrum are short, stocky branches that join the dural sinuses at acute angles. The dural sinuses are valveless channels that are located between the folds of the dura mater. The blood from the upper, lateral, and medial aspects of the cortex drains into the superior sagittal sinus as far as the occipital region, where it drains into the confluence of sinuses between the falx cerebrum and cerebellar tentorium. From this confluence arise the right and left transverse sinuses, which extend laterally in a broad, well-defined groove of the occipital bone. At the level of the vein of Abbe, these become the sigmoid sinus, which passes through the jugular foramen of the skull to continue as the internal jugular vein on each side.

Blood from the deeper parts of the brain drains into the paired internal cerebral veins, which join in the region of the pineal body to form the great vein of Galen. Successively, blood flows posteriorly in the midline through the tentorium as the straight sinus, then into the confluence of sinuses and thence to the internal jugular vein.

There are connections between the veins superficial to the skull and the dural sinuses by means of emissary veins. These veins act as pressure valves if intracranial pressure (ICP) is raised but can also be routes for the spread of infection into the brain.

THE PHYSIOLOGY/PATHOPHYSIOLOGY OF BRAIN INJURY AND ITS MANAGEMENT AND TREATMENT

Brain injury can be classified as primary or secondary. Secondary injuries may occur within seconds or days of the primary insult. Clinical entities such as global anoxia, profound hypotension, metabolic derangement, and infection are common sequelae to secondary brain injury. The primary goal of treatment of persons with brain injury is to prevent secondary insults.[2] The primary injury that occurs at the time of the initiating event will create some degree of irreversible damage. However, some brain tissue injury will be reversible if treated optimally. Neurosurgical and intensive neurotrauma interventions attempt to minimize the secondary insults of brain ischemia leading to cellular damage by evacuating mass lesions, maintaining adequate cerebral perfusion pressure, and correcting derangements of ICP.

Physiology of the Brain

Under normal physiologic circumstances, cerebral blood flow (CBF) is dependent upon cerebral vascular resistance (CVR). CVR depends upon the following:

1. cerebral metabolic rate of oxygen consumption ($CMRo_2$)
2. partial pressure of arterial carbon dioxide ($Paco_2$)
3. partial pressure of arterial oxygen (Pao_2)
4. blood pressure

When conditions are stable, CBF is between 50 and 65 mL/100 g/mm.[3]

The average adult brain weighs between 1,200 and 1,400 g and consumes 40 mL of oxygen per minute, or 15% of the oxygen used by the entire body. As blood traverses the cerebral circulation, 35% of the arterial oxygen content is extracted. This results in a 65% venous saturation in the internal jugular bulb (Table 3–1).

To maintain cellular integrity, the brain consumes 45% of its oxygen supply. The rest is used for electrophysiologic work. In addition, the temperature of the brain has a great deal to do with the maintenance of cellular integrity. A decrease or increase in temperature results in an alteration of $CMRo_2$. This can be either protective (at low temperatures) or destructive (at high temperatures). Hyperthermia should be aggressively prevented because for each degree centigrade increase in temperature, cerebral metabolism increases by 7% to 10%. This will result in increased metabolic demand, which the brain may not be able to meet. Elevated temperatures will also increase the production of CO_2, with a resulting increase in ICP.

When the brain stimulates motor or sensory activity or initiates complex energy-requiring processes, there is greater consumption of oxygen and substrates. An extreme of generalized brain activation is seizure and hyperthermia, resulting in a marked increase in $CMRo_2$. This results in an increased CBF to maintain proper oxygenation.[4] CBF and $CMRo_2$ are integrally linked: with an increase in CBF there is a rise in $CMRo_2$, and as CBF decreases there is a fall in $CMRo_2$.

Imbalance between oxygen supply and demand may occur as a consequence of cerebral oxygen delivery (CDo_2), increased $CMRo_2$, and impaired tissue oxygen uptake. Cerebral oxygen delivery is dependent upon CBF and arterial oxygen saturation (Sao_2). Sao_2 is reciprocally related to CBF. A decrease in hemoglobin concentration is associated with an increase in CBF and a decrease in CDo_2. In comparison to other organs, the brain is very sensitive to ischemia due to its high resting energy requirements and lack of oxygen stores.[3]

Alterations in CBF can be seen with changes in CVR. CVR is extremely sensitive to changes in $PaCo_2$. A decrease in $PaCo_2$ results in a decrease in CBF. This decrease in CBF is due to an increase in CVR. Hypercapnea (elevated $PaCo_2$)

Table 3–1 Normal Values for Cerebral Oxygen Delivery and Consumption

Cerebral blood flow (CBF)	50 mL/100 g/min
Systemic arterial oxygen content (Cao_2)	20 mL/100 mL
Jugular venous oxygen content ($Cjvo_2$)	13 mL/100 mL
Jugular venous oxygen saturation ($Sjvo_2$)	65%
Cerebral oxygen delivery ($CDo_2 - CBF \times Cao_2$)	10 mL/100 g/min
Cerebral metabolic rate of oxygen consumption	
($CMRo_2 = CBF \times [Cao_2 - Cjvo_2]$)	3.5 mL/100 g/min

causes a decrease in CVR, whereas hypocarbia (decreased Pa_{CO_2}) results in an increase in CVR.[5]

CBF is dependent on the inverse relationship of cerebral perfusion pressure (CPP) and CVR. CPP is a factor of the mean arterial pressure (MAP) minus ICP, as per the following formulas:

$$CPP = MAP - ICP$$
$$CBF = \frac{CPP}{CVR}$$

This physiologic control is called *myogenic autoregulation*. It is generally accepted that the lower limit of autoregulation is an MAP of 60 mm Hg and that the upper limit of autoregulation is 150 mm Hg, whereby flow is active. Mean arterial pressures beyond these parameters result in passive CBF.[6]

At the cellular level, when oxygen demand and delivery are adequate during a nerve action potential, sodium (Na^+) flows into the cell by rapid passive diffusion, and there is an exchange of Na^+ and potassium (K^+). During a recovery phase, Na^+ is actively pumped out of the cell, and K^+ is reaccumulated inside the two cations' respective extracellular-to-intracellular gradients. This is accomplished by the membrane-associated "sodium pump" (Na^+, K^+, $-ATPase$). The energy required for the "sodium pump" is provided by the hydrolysis of adenosine triphosphate (ATP) to adenosine diphosphate and inorganic phosphate (Pi).[7]

Calcium (Ca^{++}) ion transport into the cell is through three mechanisms: (1) depolarization-dependent entry activated by an increase in extracellular K^+ or an increase in intracellular Na^+, (2) changes in membrane fluidity, and (3) agonists such as norepinephrine, acetylcholine, 5-hydroxytryptamine, or excitatory amino acid neurotransmitters (glutamate or aspartate) binding to membrane receptors to open calcium channels.[8] Calcium flows across the cell membrane into the cell, and there is a release of Ca^{++} from mitochondria and other spontaneous processes. Active transport of Ca^{++} from the cell and the sequestering of Ca^{++} by the mitochondria require energy from ATP to maintain the integrity of the cell.[9]

The normal pH of the brain is about 7.0. Hydrogen ion (H^+) transport is by passive entry into the cell. Neutralization of intracellular H+ is by chemical buffering and mitochondria-induced transfer of acid or alkali between cytosol and intracellular organelles. Basically, the maintenance of normal intracellular pH requires transport of acid from the cell.[10] This is accomplished by an influx of Na^+ and an efflux of chloride ions. ATPase and Na^+ down its electrochemical gradient are the energy sources required for acid extrusion.

Pathophysiology

Dynamics

An increase in ICP may cause diffuse ischemia due to a reduction in CPP. This ischemic insult can cause mismatching of oxygen supply to oxygen demand. The metabolic needs of the brain become inadequate due to poor CD_{O_2}.

At a cellular level, oxygen deprivation rapidly causes a depletion of high-energy substrates, anaerobic glycolysis, and failure of ATP production. The exhaustion of energy stores leads to failure of the Na^+, K^+, ATPase–dependent ion pump, resulting in massive influx of Na^+, efflux of K^+, and membrane depolarization.[11] This increase in extracellular K^+ stimulates influx of Na^+ and Cl^-, accompanied by H_2O, into glial cells. Another consequence of increased extracellular K^+ is the massive influx of Ca^{++} into the cell.[10] The intracellular accumulation of Ca^{++} leads to the activation of proteases and phospholipases, with the release of free fatty acids, particularly arachidonic acid.[12] The metabolism of arachidonic acid, through the cyclo-oxygenase pathway, produces prostaglandins and the release of destructive free oxygen radicals.[13,14] Free oxygen radicals contain an unpaired electron in the outer orbit ring.[15,16] They are produced during oxidative phosphorylation in the mitochondrial cytochrome oxidase enzyme system in which the production of ATP is linked to the reduction of molecular oxygen to water.[16] The free radicals are tightly bound within the mitochondrial membrane and pose no threat to the cell. When there is decreased perfusion or oxygenation, free radical production is limited due to the decrease in oxygen. However, during the process of reperfusion or reoxygenation, there is greater presence of oxygen, causing a release of free oxygen radicals. These free oxygen radicals attach membrane phospholipids in a reaction that is probably catalyzed by iron.[14] Local inflammatory response is accentuated with the production of not only free oxygen radicals but also proteases, cytokines, and eicosanoids. Additionally, there is a release of excitatory neurotransmitters, such as glutamate and aspartame, which can worsen ionic disequilibrium, particularly of Ca^{++}, by binding to N-methyl-D-aspartate (NMDA) receptors, which control Ca^{++} channels.[17] These excitatory amino acids contribute to neuronal damage in a variety of disorders, such as epilepsy and neurodegenerative diseases[18,19] and have been implicated in the pathogenesis of TBI. When they bind to the NMDA receptors, creating an open receptor–associated ion channel, Na^+ and Ca^{++} are allowed to enter the neuron. The accumulation of Na^+ results in increases in osmotic swelling and eventual cell death. The intracellular accumulation of Ca^{++} is a primary factor in the destruction of the mitochondrial membrane. Mitochondrial sequestration of Ca^{++} is severely limited. All of this causes an additional cascade of events leading to neuronal damage or death.[14]

Treatment

The normal defense against free radical damage is that antioxidative substances and cell enzymes scavenge free radicals.[20] Glutathione peroxidase acts on H_2O_2, and superoxide dismutase is directed against superoxide radical (O_2^-). Vitamin E and beta carotene control lipid peroxidation by free radicals.[21] Current investigators are evaluating the value of administering protective enzymes or free radical scavengers, such as sodium dismutase and tirilazad, following brain injury.[17,22] There has been evidence to suggest that these new agents may be able to ameliorate the pathology caused by the free radicals. However, recent investigations failed to demonstrate clinical or statistical reference.

There is also experimental evidence suggesting that it may be therapeutical to block or gate the calcium ion channel. The cation magnesium is one blocking agent. Following brain injury, there is diminution of intracellular and total magnesium concentration. In the last few years, there have been investigations of agents that readily cross the blood-brain barrier. Diclozipine (MK-801), phencyclidine hydrochloride, ketamine, and dextrophan are all noncompetitive NMDA-receptor antagonists.[23] The administration of MK-801 has been shown to improve brain metabolism status and to reverse the post–acute injury decline of magnesium concentrations.[24–26]

A very well-studied calcium entry blocker is nimodipine. Nimodipine is a dihydropyridine derivative.[27] Not only is it a calcium channel blocker, but there are several studies demonstrating its ability to attenuate cerebral vasospasm.[28,29] In patients with stroke, nimodipine produces markedly increased CBF.[30] Patients with subarachnoid hemorrhage (SAH) have clearly been shown to benefit from the administration of nimodipine. Reports have shown significant improvements in functional outcomes and a decrease in mortality. The mechanism is not as clear. What is postulated is its ability to improve CBF and its prevention of Ca^{++} entry, and its retardation of the formation of free radicals and free fatty acids. Most recently, the potentials of nimodipine have been looked at in the TBI model. From the European literature, the results have been mixed.[31] However, a favorable effect was shown in patients who exhibited traumatic SAH.

CBF is affected by Ca^{++} flux.[32] Posttraumatic vasospasm, caused by Ca^{++}, may be prevented by blocking calcium influx. The European trial and a preliminary investigation by coauthor Anthony S. Morgan suggest a trend toward improvements.[33] The major difference between the European trial and the coauthor's investigation is that in the latter, higher dosages of nimodipine were given for a longer period of time via the gastrointestinal route. The results of this treatment are still pending.

Intracranial Hypertension

Pathology

It is generally agreed that abnormal elevation in ICP is a basic pathologic process in TBI.[34–36] In the supine position, the normal ICP is less than 10 mm Hg. Pressures greater than 15 mm Hg are considered pathologic. The observation that alterations in pressure inside the cranium can affect survival following brain injury dates back thousands of years. In the 18th century, Monro attempted to establish a relationship between intracranial volume and pressure.[37] At that time, he did not factor in cerebrospinal fluid as a cranial component. In the following century, Monro's theory was embraced by Kellie. The Monro-Kellie doctrine holds that due to the inelastic nature of the cranium, even small variations in the contents of this space produce changes in ICP.[38] Burrows in the mid 19th-century gave further clarification of the Monro-Kellie hypothesis by identifying three components of the intracranium as brain, blood, and CSF.

Methods of measuring ICP date back to the 1930s. However, it was not until 1960 that Lundberg published his article on continuous ventricular monitoring.[39] His report outlined the pathophysiology and clinical significance of the "Lundberg waves," classified as A (percussion wave), B (tidal wave), and C (diacrotic wave). A waves are seen with increased cerebral blood volume due to cerebral vasodilatation. Intracranial hypertension compromises venous outflow, thereby causing cerebral vasodilatation. B waves are the most frequent type of ICP waveforms seen. The B waves are ICP reflections of respiration. They are pathologic in that they are reflective of decreased intracranial compliance and increased ICP. Like A waves, B waves are related to changes in intracranial blood volume. Like B waves, but not pathognomonic of increased ICP, are C waves. C waves are caused by increased transmission of arterial pulse waves into the intracranial vasculature due to decreased intracranial compliance.[39,40]

An increasing ICP suggests exhaustion of the compensatory ability of the cranium to absorb further volume increases. Studies have shown that ICPs consistently greater than 20 mm Hg are associated with a greater than 50% to 60% mortality rate, compared to a 15% to 30% mortality rate in patients with ICPs lower than 20 mm Hg.[41–46] Not unexpectedly, raised ICP refractory to treatment carries the highest mortality.[46,47]

Elevations of ICP are indicative of volume changes intracranially—that is, cerebral edema. The total intracranial volume in adults is approximately 2,000 cc: 10% is CSF, 10% blood volume, and 80% parenchymal tissue. Because the brain is basically noncompressible, an increase in intracranial volume initially decreases the production CSF or the volume of cerebral blood.

An increased ICP can compromise CBF. As CBF decreases, there is a progressive decline in CPP below the stable level of 50 mm Hg (the desired level is 70 mm HG). The combination of dysfunctional autoregulation and increased ICP predisposes to cerebral ischemia. In persons with severe brain injury, when autoregulation is comprised and ICP is high, there is a 90% incidence of death.[48]

A corollary to ICP dynamics is the pressure-volume index (PVI). PVI is a reflection of intracranial compliance.[49] Mathematically, PVI can be explained by the following:

$$PVI = V/\log P_1/P_2$$

where V is the volume of fluid added or removed, P_1 is the baseline ICP, and P_2 is the ICP post injection (withdrawal or addition of fluid).

PVI is an indicator of changes in ICP; the lower the PVI value, the less compliant the brain.

ICP is a static measurement that reflects a dynamic process. As compliance lessens, there is a significant risk of refractory intracranial hypertension.

Management and Treatment

The mainstay of treatment of severe brain injury is keeping ICP below 20 mm Hg. To do this, it is of primary concern to address alterations in those homeostatic parameters that can exacerbate ICP. Maintaining normotension, normal arterial oxygenation, and normothermia is of profound importance. Hypotension has been shown to double the mortality rate and significantly increase morbidity following severe brain injury. Hypoperfusion will result in severe ischemic cerebral damage. Hypoxia can significantly impair the recovery process of the person with brain injury. The overall morbidity associated with hypoxia can be overwhelming to the recovering brain-injured patient.[2,44,50,51] Normal arterial oxygenation is essential if the brain-injured patient is to survive. The maintenance of normothermia is quite often difficult in the ICU setting. These patients tend to be hyperdynamic, and their ICU course can be made more complicated due to infections. The basic supportive measures of restoring and maintaining an adequate blood pressure, normal arterial oxygenation, and normothermia can assist in preventing and treating intracranial hypertension. It should be noted that any derangement of homeostasis can cause an increase in ICP.

Hyperventilation. For over two decades, the mainstay for the treatment of increased ICP has been controlled hyperventilation. Controlled hyperventilation lowers ICP by decreasing the P_{CO_2} (hypocapnea). Hypocapnea causes cerebral vasoconstriction and decreases cerebral blood volume. The effect of P_{CO_2} on vessel diameter occurs both through direct action on vascular smooth muscle and stimulation of peripheral chemoreceptors. Carbon dioxide rapidly equilibrates across the blood-brain barrier and results in an abrupt rise in the pH of the brain extracellular fluid with hyperventilation. The usual range for the P_{CO_2} is 27 to 30 mm Hg. It is felt that further decrease of the P_{CO_2} would theoretically reduce cerebral blood flow enough to cause ischemia.[52]

Recently, the use of controlled hyperventilation has been seriously questioned. Past and present research has clearly demonstrated that CBF, during the first day following injury, is markedly decreased[53-55] and that aggressive hyperventilation can precipitate cerebral ischemia. Patients who have subdural hematomas, diffuse injuries, and hypotension have the lowest CBF. In these patients, CBF may be less than 20 to 30 mL/100 g/min. When arterial jugular-venous oxygen content differences (AVD_{O_2}) are looked at in relation to CBF during the first 24 hours following surgery, there is an inverse relationship. The higher the volume percent over 9, the lower the CBF, leading to cerebral ischemia.[52,56] Therefore, prolonged hyperventilation or excessive hyperventilation can result in a significant increase in $AVDo_2$.[52,57]

In addition, hypocapnia is associated with low jugular venous O_2 (Sjo_2) saturation, and desaturations are most commonly associated with low CBF. The normal Sjo_2 is greater than 50%. Values that are either much less or decreased for a prolonged period of time are associated with poor neurologic recovery.[58,59] In 1991, a prospective, randomized clinical study was conducted that compared patients treated with prophylactic hyperventilation for 5 days to a group kept relatively normocapneic.[60] The groups were followed at three and six months post injury. Patients with motor scores of 4 to 5 who were prophylactically hyperventilated had significantly worse outcomes than those who were kept normocapneic.

The current recommendations are that chronic prophylactic hyperventilation in the absence of increased ICP should be avoided during the first five days post severe brain injury. Additionally, the use of prophylactic hyperventilation during the first 24 hours post severe brain injury with elevated ICP should also be avoided. It is accepted, however, that hyperventilation may be of benefit to patients who have acute neurologic deterioration or intracranial hypertension refractory to sedation, paralysis, CSF drainage, and osmotic diuresis.[61] Currently, there are some centers implementing mild hyperventilation, with PCo_2 kept at 30 mm Hg or above.

Mannitol. Osmotic therapy plays a major role in the treatment of intracranial hypertension. The osmotic agent of choice is mannitol. Mannitol is usually given as a bolus of 0.25 to 1.0 g/kg intravenously over five minutes. Continuous intravenous infusions of mannitol are not recommended, as they negate the immediate hemodynamic benefits of mannitol in patients with marginal autoregulation.[62] Small frequent doses, every 2 to 4 hours, result in fewer side effects related to electrolyte shifts. When mannitol is given, it is imperative that serum osmolality not exceed 315 mOsm/mL. This is done to avoid the complications of systemic acidosis and renal failure. Data have suggested that mannitol's effect is probably not dehydration of brain tissue.[63] Mannitol appears to effect change in the cerebral vasculature by several mechanisms. It has been shown that mannitol increases CPP by augmenting systemic pressure and decreasing ICP.[54-68] An additional measure used to maintain a CPP of 70 mm Hg is to use either dopamine or levophed. Mannitol is also associated with a direct effect on circulatory blood, due to its hemodilution properties and its ability to reduce viscosity.[69,70] This primary effect of lowering viscosity results in increasing CBF and CDo_2.[71] As CBF increases, the autoregulatory mechanisms come into effect, causing vasoconstriction and a decrease in ICP.[71] Studies have demonstrated the superior effect mannitol has on improving CBF and controlling ICP compared to hyperventilation, ventriculostomy drainage, and barbiturates.[72,73]

Diuretics. The use of normo-osmotic diuretics alone or in conjunction with mannitol is somewhat controversial. Furosemide alone is less reliable in reducing ICP[74] and can potentially worsen the dehydration effects of mannitol. Electrolyte problems are commonly seen with the use of furosemide. In fact, combined therapy of mannitol and furosemide causes accentuated electrolyte loss.[75] Despite the potential side effects of combined therapy, there is evidence suggesting that mannitol and furosemide work synergistically in lowering ICP.[76,77]

CSF Drainage. A fairly rapid method of reducing ICP is to extricate CSF from the lateral ventricle, using a ventriculostomy catheter. The indwelling ventricular catheter can be used for both fluid removal and pressure monitoring (see section "Technology" below). Removal of as little as 1 or 2 mL can effect a significant drop in ICP. A recent investigation has demonstrated that this technique is effective in reducing ICP but effects minimal change in CBF.[72]

Head Elevation. It has been a common practice to elevate the head of the bed above the level of the heart in those patients who have sustained intracranial hypertension. However, recent investigations have questioned this wisdom. One study advocated raising the head of the bed 45 or 90 degrees,[78] but other investigations have shown an increase of ICP and a decrease of CPP and cardiac output when the head of the bed was raised to 60 degrees.[79] If patients were positioned horizontally, CPP was at its maximum, although ICP was usually found to be higher at the horizontal position.[80] All of the above analyses did not account for CBF. When CBF is evaluated, the optimal head elevation appears to be 30 degrees. At 30 degrees, there is a significant reduction of ICP with no reduction of CPP or CBF.[81]

Barbiturates. There is a subset of patients who, despite aggressive measures to decrease intracranial hypertension, remain refractory to conventional therapy. In this population, which constitutes between 15% and 25% of patients,[82] mortality is virtually 100%.[35,44,49,52] It is felt by many investigators that these patients are candidates for barbiturate therapy.

Barbituric acid was first synthesized in 1864. Its usage has been numerous in areas of sedation, hyponosis, anesthesia, seizure control, and control of elevations of ICP. High-dose barbiturates' effect on ICP has been known since 1937.[83] However, interest in barbiturate therapy was not generated until the mid-1970s with a report of successful control of elevated ICP in patients with brain injury who failed to respond to hypoventilation, osmotic diuretics, and steroids.[84]

Barbiturates appear to lower ICP and to be cerebral protective by suppressing cerebral metabolic rate, increasing cerebral vascular resistance, and inhibiting free radical–mediated lipid peroxidation.[85-87] In addition to the volume-reducing effects, there is a decrease in oxygen demand of brain tissue. This may allow cells to better tolerate the effects of decreased perfusion pressure. The therapeutic dose regimen is 10 mg/kg over 30 minutes followed by 5 mg/kg/h for the next three hours. Maintenance dose is at 1 to 2 mg/kg/h.[88]

There are significant side effects to barbiturate therapy. The most significant effect is myocardial suppression, leading to hypotension, respiratory depression, and hypothermia. Patients who are in barbiturate coma have depressed brainstem reflexes, which make useful neurologic examination not feasible. Electrolyte imbalance can occur with the use of sodium pentobarbital, causing hypernatremia.

In clinical practice, high-dose barbiturates do not appear to be effective when used as initial therapy. Of the prospective randomized clinical trials, none has demonstrated any benefit for prophylactic use of barbiturates.[73,89] When barbiturates are used for refractory intracranial hypertension (failed conventional therapy), there is some efficacious benefit in a small subset of patients, specifically related to mortality but not to functional recovery.[88,90] It is recommended that hemodynamically stable patients who are refractory to conventional therapy be given a trial of high-dose barbiturates. Further analysis will be necessary to determine if high-dose barbiturates play any role in improving functional recovery.[61]

Hypothermia. Within the last few years, there has been a renewed interest in systemic hypothermia in treating persons with severe brain injury. The history of hypothermia begins with cerebral protection from global ischemia during cardiac surgery. Hypothermic perfusion without pump oxygenation was initially tested on dogs at 20°C in 1950.[91] Years later, clinical trials were attempted at 13°C to 15°C for 45 minutes without an oxygenator.[92] However, due to high operative mortality, this technique was discontinued.[93] In the mid- to late 1970s, successful total circulatory arrest at 10°C to 20°C for up to 50 minutes was used in repair of cardiac anomalies in children less than one year of age.[94-96] Since 1981, circulatory arrest at temperatures of 8°C to 10°C has been used in repair of adult ascending aortic arch aneurysms.[97] The neurosurgical experience with profound hypothermia was quite dismal. From 1964 to 1976, the neurosurgical literature reported on over 100 patients undergoing procedures under profound hypothermia with circulatory arrest using cardiopulmonary bypass to cool and rewarm.[98] Because of patients' suffering from intracranial hemorrhage during rewarming, plus the technical challenge of the procedure, this approach was abandoned.

Moderate hypothermia (surface cooling at 30°C) was investigated both clinically and experimentally from 1955 to 1974. In dogs and primates, systemic hypothermia at 30°C reduced mortality and cerebral edema. The literature between 1958 and 1974 describes treating 121 patients with sustained surface cooling for severe brain injury.[98] Temperatures ranged from 28°C to 34°C. These patients were treated from 2 to 10 days. Mortality figures were between 43% and 72%. Consequences of moderate hypothermia are cardiovascular, metabolic, and neurologic toxicity.

In the last few years, there is some evidence suggesting a therapeutic role for mild to moderate hypothermia. In the animal model, hypothermia appears to exert a cellular-protective effect by preventing toxic levels of extracellular excitatory amino acids.[99] Additionally, investigators have shown that physiologic parameters involved in the development of cerebral edema, such as ionic homeostasis and calcium influx, are temperature sensitive.[90,100] Recent clinical analyses have demonstrated reductions in ICP, CBF, and $CMRo_2$.[101] And from a disability standpoint, there has been a trend toward a better outcome in patients treated by hypothermia compared to those who were normothermic. Current hypothermia investigations are showing the impact of mild hypothermia on uncontrollable intracranial hypertension following severe brain injury. In these studies, mild hypothermia significantly reduced ICP and decreased both CBF and $CMRo_2$. Arterio–jugular venous oxygen difference was decreased, and there was significant improvement in mortality and morbidity rates.[99,102] From the available data, it is fairly clear that further investigations with hypothermia are warranted to determine its clinical application in persons with severe brain injury.

Management of Posttraumatic Seizures. Posttraumatic seizure (PTS) is a manifestation of acute injury response that can complicate management of the person with a severe brain injury. One major consequence is elevated ICP. The incidence of PTS is 10% to 15%, and 50% of these patients have their first onset of seizure within one year post injury.[103,104]

The actual biochemical or cellular cause of PTS remains a mystery. Proposed biochemical effects are contusions or cortical lacerations leading to extravasation of red cells and hemolysis, leading to hemoglobin deposition and subsequent uptake of neutrophils. Through a series of chemical reactions, iron is liberated, yielding free radical intermediates.[105] These free radicals react with methylene groups adjacent to the double bonds of polyunsaturated fatty acids and lipids within cellular membranes, causing hydrogen abstractions and subsequent propagation of peroxidation reactions.[106] This nonenzymatic reaction initiates lipid peroxidation, causing disruption of membranes and subcellular organelles.[107] Lipid peroxidation is believed to be a major cause of posttraumatic cell damage and death.[108] The normal configuration of membrane-bound polyunsaturated fatty acids is lost due to lipid peroxidation.[109] The loss of membrane functional and structural integrity ultimately leads to the destruction of the cell.

Biochemical injury can also alter densities and distribution of ion channels on the neuronal membrane. The alteration of Na^+ and Ca^{++} currents changes thresholds and leads to progressive depolarization. Intracellular destruction may develop, leading to an increase in extracellular K^+ or a reduction of extracellular Ca^{++}.

Glutamate may also be a factor. When the brain is ischemic, there is a release of glutamate (a potent excitatory neurotransmitter). Glutamate activates receptors, causing depolarization of cell membrane.[110] An excess of intracellular calcium activates damaging enzymes, causing cytotoxicity and neuronal death.

Posttraumatic seizures occurring within seven days are classified as early seizures, and those developing later than seven days post injury are described as late seizures.[111,112] Risk factors for incurring a posttraumatic seizure are severity of brain injury and development of one or more seizures.[113] Persons with severe brain injury and neurologic deficits, without dura interruption, have an incidence of posttraumatic epilepsy between 7% and 39%.[113] With disruption of the dura and deficits, there is a 20% to 57% incidence of seizure disorder.[113] Other risk factors are hemiplegia, intracerebral hematomas, penetrating wounds, central parietal injury, and depressed skull fractures.[114]

For years, anticonvulsants have been used in an attempt to prevent PTS. Early retrospective analyses suggested that prophylactic phenytoin was effective.[115] Initial prospective double-blind studies using phenytoin or low-dose phenytoin combined with phenobarbital were unsuccessful in preventing seizures.[116] When carbamazepine was evaluated in a prospective randomized double-blind study, there was a positive benefit of preventing early PTS, but not late PTS.[117]

A fairly current investigation using phenytoin demonstrated quite clearly a significant reduction in early PTS but not late PTS.[118] However, when neurobehavioral effects were examined, it was found that phenytoin impaired performances in neuropsychologic tests at one month post brain injury.[119]

The current recommendation is that phenytoin and carbamazepine are effective in preventing early PTS in those patients who are at high risk for seizures during the first week post brain injury. However, patients who are not at risk should probably not receive early anticonvulsant prophylaxis. This is particularly pertinent in light of the risk of neurobehavioral side effects.

Steroids. Since the 1960s, steroids have been used in the treatment of cerebral edema. Their most significant benefit is their proven effectiveness in patients with brain tumors.[120,121] Unfortunately, the same cannot be said in the area of severe brain injury. Studies that have supported their use either have been retrospective or have failed to apply statistical relevance and were poorly designed. There are numerous well-designed studies that do not support the administration of steroids for brain injuries.[122–126] Potential side effects of steroid usage are immune suppression, gastrointestinal hemorrhage, and metabolic instability.[125] The current recommendation is to avoid the use of steroids for severe brain injury because of their lack of efficacy and their potential complications.

Technology

ICP Monitoring. ICP technology has been continually evolving (Figure 3–17). However, the ventricular catheter remains the monitoring device to which all others are compared. The ventriculostomy catheter is generally inserted in the midpupillary line on the right side, just anterior to the coronal suture. It is inserted at a depth of about 7 cm, entering the frontal horn of the lateral ventricle. The device is then tunneled under the scalp and attached via a fluid-filled tube to an external pressure transducer. Advantages include the ability to drain CSF (therefore, it has therapeutic value) and the ability to monitor ICP at low cost and with relative ease of insertion. However, ease of insertion may be compromised by compression of ventricles as a result of interstitial edema or space-occupying lesions, and infection is a potential risk factor.

The subarachnoid bolt or screw is often used in clinical practice to measure ICP in the subarachnoid space.[127] The bolt is twist-drilled through the dura. Therapeu-

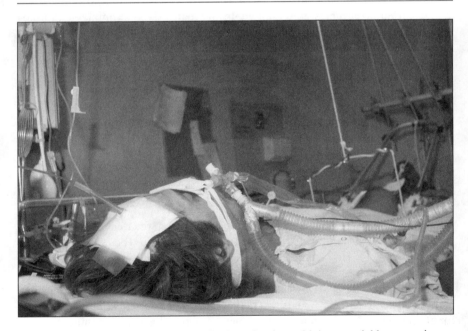

Figure 3–17 Intracranial pressure monitoring of patient with intracranial hypertension.

tic removal of CSF is feasible, and there is a low infection rate and decreased bleeding with this device.[128] The main advantage of these bolts is that they do not require cannulation of the lateral ventricle. This becomes important when the lateral ventricles are compressed. However, when there is extensive cerebral swelling, the bolt may be compromised, resulting in erroneous readings. In addition, artifacts can be seen with head positioning or tube movement.

In recent years, fiber-optic monitoring devices have been developed: specifically, the Camino system (Camino Laboratories, San Diego, Calif).[129] The fiber-optic catheter can be placed in the lateral ventricle or the subdural or extradural space. The compactness of the Camino device facilitates continuous monitoring. The device permits detection in swings in ICP caused by changes in position, ventilation, and stimulation. Patients who require computed tomography (CT) scans and surgical procedures can have their ICP continuously monitored.

Transcranial Doppler Ultrasonography. Transcranial Doppler (TCD) ultrasonography (TCD) is an indirect, noninvasive method for estimating changes in CBF. TCD was first described in the early 1980s.[130] Since its development, it has become a convenient bedside tool for ascertaining intracranial dynamics.

Sonography, or sound waves, measures blood velocity in the major intracranial vessels through thin bone windows within the skull. Piezoelectric crystals emit ultrasonic signals transmitted to the bloodstream. On the basis of the Doppler principle, frequency is shifted as a result of red blood cell movement. With changes in the frequency of the ultrasound before and after it is reflected by red blood cell movement, one can calculate the velocity of blood. Parameters that are provided are flow velocities, pulsatility amplitude between systolic and diastolic flow velocities, and shape of the Doppler profile.[131] The narrowing of a vessel, as in stenosis, vasospasm, or hyperemia, will result in an increase in velocity.[132] An ICP rising to the level of the diastolic arterial pressure will cause an absence of diastolic flow velocity. As ICP increases, flow velocity reappears, but flow is reversed. At this point, there is little chance of survival for the person who has sustained a severe brain injury.

The advantages of this procedure are its easy accessibility for the cortically impaired patient and its low cost. The major disadvantage is that it requires technical skill to provide reproducible results. Additionally, there are problems with interpretation of data. Patients who are agitated and unable to maintain adequate positioning can potentially alter the readings of the data. However, TCD can provide valuable information about CPP in patients with elevated ICP, will detect vasospasm, and can be useful in making a determination of brain death.

Continuous Jugular Venous Oximetry. Laboratory and clinical investigations have shown that in the severely brain injured, abnormalities of CBF in response to alterations in perfusion pressure, blood gas analysis, and metabolic demand occur after the primary injury.[133–135] The injured brain continues to be susceptible to transient episodes of hypoxia and ischemia. Therapeutic changes in $PaCo_2$ or Pao_2 can result in significant changes in CBF. In conjunction with monitoring ICP, arterial pressure, and arterial oxygen content (Sao_2), the use of continuous fiber-optic oximetry of jugular venous oxygen saturation ($Sjvo_2$) can assist in assessing the relationship between perfusion pressure and CBF.[136] Assuredly, awareness of the impact of therapeutic intervention on CBF becomes crucial. However, the data generated from $Sjvo_2$ are dependent on the conditions that hemoglobin concentration and $CMRo_2$ remain relatively constant, that dissolved oxygen can be ignored, and that differences between Sao_2 and $Sjvo_2$ will reflect CBF by the Fick principle.

Normal jugular bulb oxygen saturation ($Sjbo_2$) is 62% to 70%.[137] Values below 50% to 55% are considered to be oligemic. Those greater than 75% to 80% are often considered hyperemic. Basically, the amount of oxygen extracted by the brain is reflected in the difference between Sao_2 content and $Sjbo_2$. When the brain's requirement is not met by the oxygen received, it will extract more oxygen, resulting in a lower $Sjbo_2$. If the brain exceeds its oxygen requirements, then the $Sjbo_2$ will be higher. A low $Sjbo_2$ is usually associated with decreased CBF. However, anemia, hypoxia, acidosis, fever, and PTS can also lower $Sjbo_2$.[138]

The fiber-optic catheter used for jugular venous oximetry is a number 4 French. It is inserted retrogradely into the jugular vein approximately 10 cm. The size of the catheter allows for easy insertion, and monitoring is performed easily without interfering with routine clinical care.

A disadvantage of the catheter is its susceptibility to angulation, resulting in unsatisfactory light-intensity signals. It is commonly necessary to withdraw the catheter or reposition the head and neck. Several calibrations are needed for readjustments. A principal difficulty with the technique is the inability to verify $CMRo_2$. This is particularly true when patients need suctioning, potentially causing a decrease in $CMRo_2$. In contradistinction, patients who are agitated or coughing many times have an increase in $CMRo_2$. Other limitations are that $Sjbo_2$ is based on global oxygen metabolic measurements, although there may be situations of heterogeneous CBF patterns.[139] Additionally, if a patient suffers a cerebral infarct, the jugular bulb catheter may register an unreliable elevated value due to localized lack of oxygen extraction.

When circumstances are optimal, continuous jugular venous oximetry can be useful. But if this technology is to become reliable, improvements need to be made on catheter design and efforts made to adjust for some of its limitations as it relates to $CMRo_2$ and localization of ischemic areas resulting in heterogeneous CBF patterns.

Bedside Cerebral Blood Flow Monitoring. Autoregulation within the brain attempts to provide adequate CBF to meet fluctuations in delivery and demand for oxygen by cerebral tissues. Injury to the brain can result in autoregulation's being less then optimal.[52] A relatively new technology for assessing regional cortical CBF, based on a heat diffusion principle, uses a heat source and detector placed on the cerebral cortex.[140]

There are currently two methods under evaluation for continuous bedside monitoring of CBF, a heat diffusion and laser flowmetry (early stages of investigations). In the heat diffusion method, a Silastic catheter is placed under the dura and directly on a gyrus of the cerebral cortex.[140] The catheter exits the dura, bone, and scalp and is connected to a monitor or computer. There are two gold discs embedded at the distal end of the thermal diffusion catheter resting in the cerebral cortex. One disc is for heat source, and the other measures temperature.

The difference in temperature between the two discs reflects the ratio at which heat is dissipated, thereby reflecting cerebral tissue perfusion. The greater the difference in temperature between heated and nonheated discs, the lower the CBF, and the smaller the temperature gradient, the higher the CBF.

The major advantage of the heat diffusion method is recording minute-to-minute changes in CBF. Differences in regional CBF can be related to the patient's clinical condition. Disadvantages with the CBF catheter are the risk of infection; loss of contact of the catheter to the cerebral cortex, resulting in inaccurate readings; erroneous CBF readings due to the collection of fluid or blood between the catheter and cerebral cortex; and a discouragingly high cost ($80,000).

As the technology of continuous bedside CBF monitoring improves and its cost is less prohibitive, it is expected to prove to be a valuable adjunct to the care of the patient with a severe brain injury.

Hematomas

Subdural hematomas (SDHs) form when cortical veins bridging the arachnoid membrane and the dura are torn. There are three types of SDHs: acute, subacute, and chronic. An *acute* SDH is a manifestation of the rapidity of the venous collection and the compromise to underlying structures associated with neurologic dysfunction. It occurs within 24 hours of injury. The diagnosis is definitively made with CT scanning (Figure 3–18). There is a 15% incidence for acute SDH. It is associated with a high mortality rate, but if the injury is treated with surgical evacuation within 4 hours, mortality can drop from 90% to 30%.[141,142] Patients with acute SDH have a poor functional prognosis. *Subacute* SDH presents symptoms within two weeks after injury. It is associated with insidious lethargy, confusion, hemiparesis, or hemispheric deficits. Surgical intervention usually results in improvement. *Chronic* SDH usually presents weeks to months following the initial trauma. The mechanism is commonly a result of a mild brain injury. Persons at greatest risk are those who are elderly or those who are alcoholic. The clinical manifestations are papilledema and progressive mental status change; focal signs (hemiparesis, aphasia) may or may not be present. Diagnosis is made by CT. Patients should have drainage or evacuation.[143,144]

Epidural hematoma (EDH) occurs when there is a rupture of the middle meningeal artery, with progressive accumulation of blood in the space between the dura and the skull (Figure 3–19). The incidence is about 5%. EDH can also arise from injured venous channels in the bone at a point of fracture or from a lacerated major dural venous sinus. The clinical features at presentation are oculo-motor nerve, subcortical, and brainstem dysfunction. One inconsistent finding may be a "lucid interval," in which a brief period of unconsciousness is followed by a conscious state with minimal symptoms. As the hematoma enlarges, the patient may develop the classic triad of coma, fixed and dilated pupils, and decerebrate posturing, indicating a transtentorial herniation. The diagnosis is made by clinical presentation and CT scanning. Patients who are symptomatic or have a fairly large hematoma should be surgically treated.[143,144]

Intracerebral hematoma is direct bleeding into the parenchyma of the brain (Figure 3–20). The incidence is 2% or less. Patients can have rapid deterioration or

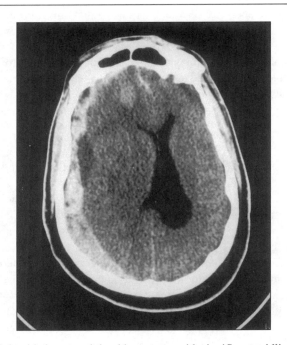

Figure 3–18 Right-sided acute subdural hematoma with significant midline shift.

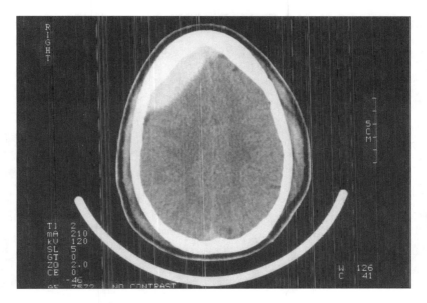

Figure 3–19 Right-sided epidural hematoma.

present conscious, yet hemiplegic. ICHs are most often located in the frontal and temporal regions. Those that are larger than 2 cm and are associated with a midline shift and neurologic deterioration should be evacuated.

Depressed skull fractures are breaks of the outer layer of one or more fractured segments lying below the level of the inner table of the surrounding intact skull (Figure 3–21). There is an association of intracranial hematomas with an incidence of more than 5%, most of which are intracerebral.[145] Twenty-five percent of persons with depressed skull fractures will be unconscious, and another 25% will have posttraumatic amnesia of less than one hour.[145]

Patients with compound depressed skull fractures who are symptomatic and who may or may not have an associated hematoma will require surgical intervention. Early surgical intervention entails the elevation and restoration of the fracture site, repair of the dural laceration, and evacuation of contused necrotic brain or hematomas. The objective is to prevent infection and to lessen the morbidity of neurologic deficits and posttraumatic epilepsy.[145]

Other Pathology

A contusion is a bruise of brain tissue; it is usually hemorrhagic. It contains both red blood cells and degenerated tissue. Whereas a hematoma is clotted blood that

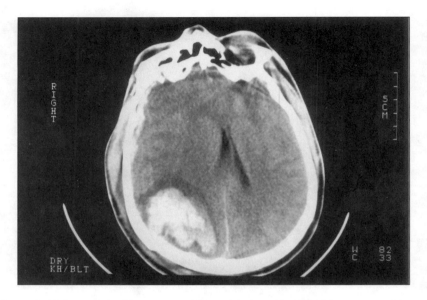

Figure 3–20 Intracerebral hematoma with a residual small subdural hematoma with cerebral edema and compression of the ventricles.

acts as a mass capable of displacing surrounding brain, a contusion is caused by the movement of the brain over the rough edges of bone at the base of the skull. Common sites for contusions are the base of the frontal and temporal lobes of the brain.

Traumatic subarachnoid bleeding occurs with very severe brain injury. The SAH extends over cerebral convexities. The origin of SAH has been associated with the traumatic shearing of microvessels coursing within the subarachnoid space. A sequela of SAH is the potential initiation of vasospasm.[146] SAH can compromise CBF due to vasospastic properties (catecholamine-laden blood).[147] SAH also carries the risk of functionally obstructing CSF absorption by plugging of arachnoid villi. Over time, this would potentiate the development of intracranial hypertension.

From the last decade to the present, there has been a great deal of emphasis placed upon traumatically induced axonal injury. Current thinking has ascribed a selective vulnerability of axons to traumatic brain injury. There are some investigators who feel that diffuse axonal injury (DAI) is the hallmark of traumatic brain injury.[148,149] Diffuse coronal injury is associated with disruptions

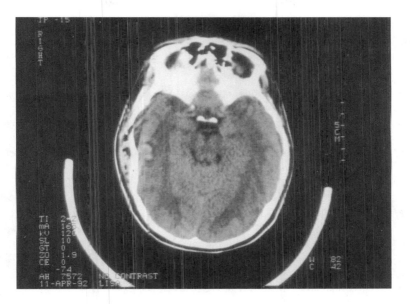

Figure 3–21 Depressed skull fracture with associated small epidural hematoma.

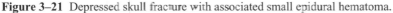

throughout both cerebral hemispheres. This may explain the sequelae of prolonged coma and high mortality for persons with severe brain injury. Diagnostically, DAI can be challenging. Despite a severe shearing injury, the brain may appear normal, particularly with the use of CT scanning. In these situations, MRI might prove beneficial. Experimental and clinical investigations are needed to increase our understanding of DAI from a pathologic and clinical standpoint.

SUMMARY

If we are to make an impact on the process of functional recovery, it is basic that clinicians possess a working knowledge of neuroanatomy, neurophysiology, and the current thinking on the pathophysiology of brain injury. Equally important, it is imperative that treatment measures be consistent with current thinking. As our understanding of the brain and its response to injury continues to increase, there will come new awareness. With new awareness comes hope for improved experimental and finally clinical intervention.

REFERENCES

1. Descartes. *Discourse on Method and Meditations,* translated by LJ LaFleur. Indianapolis: Bobbs-Merrill; 1960:41.

2. Chestnut RM, Marshall LF, Klauber MR, Blunt BA, et al. The role of secondary brain injury in determining outcome for severe head injury. *J Trauma.* 1993;34:216–222.

3. Prough DS, Rogers AT. Physiology and pharmacology of cerebral blood flow and metabolism. *Crit Care Clin.* 1989;5:713–728.

4. Roland PE, Friberg L. Localization of cortical areas activated by thinking. *J Neurophysiol.* 1985;53:1219–1243.

5. Grubb RL Jr, Raichle ME, Eichling JO, Ter-Pogossian MM. The effects of changes in $PaCO_2$ on cerebral blood volume, blood flow, and vascular mean transit time. *Stroke.* 1974;5:630–639.

6. Strandgaard S, Paulson OB. Cerebral autoregulation. *Stroke.* 1984;15:413–416.

7. Albers RW, Siegel GJ, Stahl WL. Membrane transport. In: Albers RW, Agnanoff BW, Siegel GJ, Molinoff PB, eds. *Basic Neurochemistry.* Boston, Mass: Little, Brown, and Co; 1981:107–109.

8. Siesjo BK. Historical overview: calcium, ischemia, and death of brain cells. *Ann NY Acad Sci.* 1988;522:638–661.

9. Fiskum G. Mitochondrial damage during cerebral ischemia. *Ann Emerg Med.* 1985;14:810–815.

10. Roos A, Boron WF. Intracellular pH. *Phys Rev.* 1981;61:296–434.

11. Astrup J. Energy-requiring cell functions in the ischemic brain: their critical supply and possible inhibition in protective therapy. *J Neurosurg.* 1982;56:482–497.

12. Raichl ME. The pathophysiology of brain ischemia. *Ann Neurol.* 1983;13:2–10.

13. White BC, Aust SD, Arfos KE, Aronson LD. Brain injury by ischemic anoxia: hypothesis extension—a tale of two ions? *Ann Emerg Med.* 1984;13:862–867.

14. White BC, Wiegerstein JG, Wineger CD. Brain ischemic anoxia: mechanism of injury. *JAMA.* 1984;251:1586–1590.

15. Southern PA, Powis G. Free radicals in medicine. I. Chemical nature and biologic reactions. *Mayo Clin Proc.* 1988;63:381–389.

16. Fisher AB. Intracellular production of oxygen-derived free radicals. In: Halliwell B, ed. *Oxygen Radicals and Tissue Injury.* Bethesda, Md: Federation of American Societies for Experimental Biology; 1988:34–51.

17. Cotman C, Inversen L. Excitatory amino acids in the brain: focus on NMDA receptors. *Trends Neurosci.* 1987;10:263–265.

18. Meldrum B. Excitatory amino acid antagonists as potential therapeutic agents. In: Jenner P, ed. *Neurotoxins and Their Pharmacological Implications.* New York, NY: Raven Press; 1987.

19. Meldrum B. Possible therapeutic applications of antagonists of excitatory amino acid transmitters. *Clin Sci.* 1985;68:113–122.

20. Siesjo BK. Brain death in ischemia and aging: are free radicals involved? *Monogr Neural Sci.* 1984;11:1–7.

21. Muizelaar JP, Marmarou A, Young HF, Choi S, et al. Improving outcome of severe head injury with oxygen radical scavenger polyethylene glycol conjugated superoxide dismutase: a phase II trial. *J Neurosurg.* 1993;78:375–382.

22. McIntosh TK, Thomas M, Smith D, Banbury M. The novel 21-aminosteroid U74006 attenuates cerebral edema and improves survival after brain injury in the rat. *J Neurotrauma.* 1992;9:33–46.

23. McIntosh TK, Morgan AS. New trends: neurodiagnostics and therapeutics. *Trauma Q.* 1992;8:58–73.

24. McIntosh TK, Soares H, Hayes R, Simon R. The NMDA receptor antagonist MK-801 in the treatment of experimental brain injury in the rat. In: Cavaliero J, Lehman J, eds. *Frontiers in Excitatory Amino Acid Research*. New York, NY: Alan R Liss; 1988.

25. McIntosh TK, Vink R, Soares H, Hayes R, et al. Effects of the N-methyl-D-aspartate receptor blocker MK-801 on neurologic function after experimental brain injury. *J Neurotrauma.* 1989;6:247–259.

26. McIntosh TK, Vink R, Soares H, Hayes R, et al. Effect of noncompetitive blockade of NMDA receptors in the neurochemical sequelae of experimental brain injury. *J Neurochem.* 1990; 55:1170–1179.

27. Barrett GH, Bose B, Little JR, Jones SC, et al. Effects of nimodipine in acute focal cerebral ischemia. *Stroke.* 1986;17:884–890.

28. Allen GS, Ann HS, Preziosi TJ, Battye R, et al. Cerebral arterial spasm: a controlled trial of nimodipine in patients with subarachnoid hemorrhage. *N Engl J Med.* 1983;308:619–624.

29. Petruk KC, West M, Mohr G, Weir BK, et al. Nimodipine treatment in poor-grade aneurysm patients: results of a multicenter double-blind placebo-controlled trial. *J Neurosurg.* 1988; 68:505–517.

30. Gelmers HJ, Gorter K, deWeendt CJ, Wiezer HJ. A controlled trial of nimodipine in acute ischemic stroke. *N Engl J Med.* 1988;318:203–207.

31. Teasdale G, Bailey I, Bell A, Gray J, et al. The effects of nimodipine on outcome after head injury: a prospective randomised control trial. The British/Finnish Co-operative Head Injury Trial Group. *Acta Neurochir.* 1990;51:315–316.

32. Kostron H, Twerdy K, Stampfl C, Mohsenipour I, et al. Treatment of cerebral vasospasm with calcium channel blocker nimodipine: a preliminary report. *Neurol Res.* 1984;6 29–32.

33. A multicenter trial of the efficacy of nimodipine in outcome after severe head injury: the European Study Group on Nimodipine in Severe Head Injury. *J Neurosurg.* 1994;80:797–804.

34. Miller JD, Becker DP, Ward JD, Sullivan HG, et al. Significance of intracranial hypertension in severe head injury. *J Neurosurg.* 1977;47:503–516.

35. Narayan RK, Kishare PR, Becker DP, Ward JD, et al. Intracranial pressure: to monitor or not to monitor. A review of our experience with severe head injury. *J Neurosurg.* 1982;56:650–659.

36. Marshall LF, Barba D, Toole BM, Bowers SA. The oval pupil: clinical significance and relationship to intracranial hypertension. *J Neurosurg.* 1983;58:566–568.

37. Monro A. *Observations on the Structure and Function of the Nervous System*. Edinburgh, Scotland: Creed and Johnson; 1783.

38. Kellie G. An account of the appearances observed in the dissection of two of the three individuals presumed to have perished in the storm of the 3rd, and whose bodies were discovered in the vicinity of Leith on the morning of the 4th November 1921, with some reflections on the pathology of the brain. *Trans Med-Chir Soc Edinburgh.* 1824;1:84.

39. Lundberg N. Continuous recording and control of ventricular fluid pressure in neurosurgical practice. *Acta Psychiatr Scand.* 1960;36(suppl):1–193.

40. Rosner MJ, Becker DP. Origin and evolution of plateau wave: experimental observations and a theoretical model. *J Neurosurg.* 1984;60:312–324.

41. Morgan AS. Traumatic brain injury: improving functional recovery. *J Nat Med Assoc.* 1989;81:1133–1137.

42. Palter MD, Dobkin E, Morgan AS, Previost S. Intensive care management of severe head injury. *J Head Trauma Rehabil.* 1994;9:20–31.

43. Saul TG, Ducker TB. Effects of intracranial pressure monitoring and aggressive treatment in mortality in severe head injury. *J Neurosurg.* 1982;56:498–503.

44. Miller JD, Butterworth JF, Gudeman SK, Faulkner JE, et al. Further experience in the management of head injury. *J Neurosurg.* 1981;54:289–299.

45. Marshall LF, Smith RW, Shapiro HM. The outcome with aggressive treatment in severe head injury. Part I: the significance of intracranial pressure monitoring. *J Neurosurg.* 1979;50:20–25.

46. Alberico AM, Ward JD, Choi SC, et al. Outcome after severe head injury. *J Neurosurg.* 1987;67:648–656.

47. Loughlead MG. Brain resuscitation and protection. *Med J Aust.* 1988;148:458–466.

48. Graham DI, Adams JH, Doyle D. Ischemia brain damage in fatal non-missile head injuries. *J Neurol Sci.* 1978;39:213–234.

49. Maset AL, Marmarou A, Work JD, et al. Pressure-volume index in head injury. *J Neurosurg.* 1987;67:832–840.

50. Miller JD, Becker DP. Secondary insults to the injured brain. *J R Coll Surg (Edinburgh).* 1982;27:292–298.

51. Miller JD, Sweet RC, Narayan RK, Becker DP. Early insults to the injured brain. *JAMA.* 1978;240:439–442.

52. Obrist WD, Langfitt TW, Jaggi JL, Cruz J, et al. Cerebral blood flow and metabolism in comatose patients with acute head injury. *J Neurosurg.* 1984;61:241–253.

53. Bouma GJ, Muizelaar JP, Stringer WA, Choi SC, et al. Ultra early evaluation of regional cerebral blood flow in severely head injured patients using xenon enhanced computed tomography. *J Neurosurg.* 1992;77:360–368.

54. Bouma GJ, Muizelaar JP, Choi SC, Newlon PG, et al. Cerebral circulation and metabolism after severe traumatic brain injury: the elusive role of ischemia. *J Neurosurg.* 1991;75:685–693.

55. Fiesihi C, Batlistine N, Beduschi A, Boselli, et al. Regional cerebral blood flow and intraventricular pressure in acute head injuries. *J Neurol Neurosurg Psychiatry.* 1974;37:1378–1388.

56. Gotoh F, Meyer JS, Takagi Y. Cerebral effects of hyperventilation in man. *Arch Neurol.* 1965;12:410–423.

57. Nordstrom CH, Messeter K, Sundbang G, et al. Cerebral blood flow, vasoreactivity, and oxygen consumption during barbiturate therapy in severe traumatic brain lesions. *J Neurosurg.* 1988; 68:424–431.

58. Cruz J. On-line monitoring of global cerebral hypoxia in acute brain injury: relationship to intracranial hypertension. *J Neurosurg.* 1993;79:228–233.

59. Sheinberg M, Kante MJ, Robertson CS, Contant CF, et al. Continuous monitoring of jugular venous oxygen saturation in head-injured patients. *J Neurosurg.* 1991;76:212–217.

60. Muizelaar JP, Marmarou A, Ward JD, Kontos MA, et al. Adverse effects of prolonged hyperventilation in patients with severe head injury: a randomized clinical trial. *J Neurosurg.* 1991; 75:731–739.

61. Bullock R, Chestnut RM, Clifton G, Ghajar J, et al. Guidelines for the Management of Severe Head Injury. *J Neurotrauma.* 1996;13:639–734.

62. Marshall LF, Smith RW, Rauscher LA, et al. Mannitol dose requirements in brain-injured patients. *J Neurosurg.* 1978;48:169–172.

63. Nath F, Galbraith S. The effect of mannitol on cerebral white matter water content. *J Neurosurg.* 1986;65:41–43.

64. Procaccio F, Menasce G, Sacchi L, et al. Effects of thiopentone and mannitol on cerebral perfusion pressure and EEG in head injured patients with intracranial hypertension. *Agressologie.* 1991;32:381–385.

65. Shalmon E, Reichenthal E, Kasp T. Transient effects of mannitol on cerebral blood flow following brain injury. *Acta Neurochir (Wien).* 1990;51(suppl):116–117.

66. Zornow MH, Oh YS, Scheller M-S. A comparison of the cerebral and haemodynamic effects of mannitol and hypertonic saline in an animal model of brain injury. *Acta Neurochir (Wien).* 1990;51(suppl):324–325.

67. Mendalow AD, Teasdale GM, Russell T, Flood J, et al. Effect of mannitol on cerebral blood flow and cerebral perfusion pressure in human injury. *J Neurosurg.* 1985;63:43–48.

68. Wise BL, Chater ML. The value of hypertonic mannitol solution in decreasing brain mass and lowering cerebrospinal fluid pressure. *J Neurosurg.* 1962;19:1033–1041.

69. Muizelaar JP, Wei EP, Kontos HA, Becker DP. Mannitol causes compensatory cerebral vasoconstriction and vasodilation in response to blood viscosity changes. *J Neurosurg.* 1983;59:822–828.

70. Burke AM, Quest DO, Chien S, Cerri C. The effects of mannitol on blood viscosity. *J Neurosurg.* 1981;55:550–553.

71. Muizelaar JP, Lutz HA III, Becker DP. Effects of mannitol on ICP and CBF and correlation with pressure autoregulation in severely head injured patients. *J Neurosurg.* 1984;61:700–706.

72. Fortune JB, Feustel PJ, Graca L, Hasselbarth J, et al. Effect of hyperventilation, mannitol, and ventriculostomy drainage on cerebral blood flow after head injury. *J Trauma.* 1995;39:1091–1099.

73. Schwartz ML, Tater CH, Rowed DW. The University of Toronto Head Injury Treatment Study: a prospective randomized comparison of pentobarbital and mannitol. *Can J Neurol Sci.* 1984;11:434–440.

74. Levin A. Treatment of increased intracranial pressure: a comparison of different hyperosmotic agents and the use of thiopental. Presented at Annual Meeting of the American Association of Neurological Surgeons; May 1978; New Orleans, La.

75. Wilkinson HA, Rosenfeld S. Furosemide and mannitol in the treatment of acute experimental intracranial hypertension. *Neurosurgery.* 1983;12:405–410.

76. Schettini A, Stakurski B, Young HF. Osmotic and osmotic-loop diuresis in brain surgery: effects in plasma and CSF electrolytes and ion excretion. *J Neurosurg.* 1982;56:679–684.

77. Tarnheim PA, MiLaurin RL, Saweya R. Effect of furosemide on experimental traumatic cerebral edema. *Neurosurgery.* 1979;4:48–51.

78. Kenning JA, Toutant SM, Saunders RL. Upright patient positioning in the management of intracranial hypertension. *Surg Neurol.* 1981;15:148–152.

79. Durwood OJ, Amacher AL, DelMaestro RF, et al. Cerebral and cardiovascular responses to changes in head elevation in patients with intracranial hypertension. *J Neurosurg.* 1988;69:15–23.

80. Rosner MJ, Coley IB. Cerebral perfusion pressure, intracranial pressure and head elevation. *J Neurosurg.* 1986;65:636–641.

81. Feldman Z, Kanter MJ, Robertson CS, Contant CF, et al. Effect of head elevation on intracranial pressure, cerebral perfusion pressure, and cerebral blood flow in head-injured patients. *J Neurosurg.* 1992;76:207–211.

82. Becker DP, Miller JD, Ward JD, Young HF, et al. Outcome from severe head injury with early diagnosis and intensive management. *J Neurosurg.* 1977;47:491–502.

83. Horsley JS. The intracranial pressure during barbital narcosis. *Lancet*. 1937;1:141–143.

84. Shapiro HM, Wyte SR, Loeser J. Barbiturate-augmented hypothermia for reduction of persistent intracranial hypertension. *J Neurosurg*. 1974;40:90–100.

85. Demopoulos HB, Flamm ES, Pietronigro DD, et al. The free radical pathology and microcirculation in the major central nervous system. *Acta Physiol Scand*. 1980;492(suppl):91–119.

86. Kassell NF, Hitchon PW, Gerk MK, et al. Alterations in cerebral blood flow, oxygen metabolism, and electrical activity produced by high-dose theopental. *Neurosurgery*. 1980;7:593–603.

87. Pierce EC, Lambertsen CJ, Deutsch S, Chase PE, et al. Cerebral circulation and metabolism during theopental anesthesia and hyperventilation in man. *J Clin Invest*. 1962;41:1664–1671.

88. Eisenberg H, Frankowski R, Contant C, et al. High dose barbiturate control of elevated intracranial pressure in patients with severe head injury. *J Neurosurg*. 1988;69:15–23.

89. Ward JD, Becker DP, Miller JD, et al. Failure of prophylactic barbiturate coma in the treatment of severe head injury. *J Neurosurg*. 1985;62:383–388.

90. Marshall LF, Smith RW, Shapiro HM. The outcome with aggressive treatment in severe head injuries. Part 2. Acute and chronic barbiturate administration in the management of head injury. *J Neurosurg*. 1979;50:26–30.

91. Bigelow WG, Callaghan JC, Hopps VA. General hypothermia for experimental intracardiac surgery: use of artificial pacemaker for cardiac standstill and cardiac rewarming in general hypothermia. *Ann Surg*. 1950;132:531–543.

92. Drew CE, Anderson IM. Profound hypothermia in cardiac surgery: report of three cases. *Lancet*. 1959;1:748–750.

93. Mohri H, Merendino KA. Hypothermia with or without a pump oxygenator. In: Gibbon JH, Sabiston DC, Spencer FC, eds. *Surgery of the Chest*. Philadelphia, Pa: WB Saunders Co; 1969:643–673.

94. Smith DL, Wilson JM, Ebert PA. Cardiac surgery in infants up to one year old. *Cardiovasc Med*. 1978;18:925–940.

95. Castaneda AR, Lamberti J, Sade RM, Williams RG, et al. Open heart surgery during the first three months of life. *J Thorac Cardiovasc Surg*. 1974;5:719–731.

96. Rittenhouse EA, Mohri H, Dillard DH, Merendino KA. Deep hypothermia in cardiovascular surgery. *Ann Thorac Surg*. 1974;17:63–98.

97. Crawford ES, Saleh SA. Transverse aortic arch aneurysm: improved results of treatment employing new modifications of aortic reconstruction and hypothermic cerebral circulatory arrest. *Ann Surg*. 1981;196:180–188.

98. Clifton GL, Allen S, Berry J, Koch SM. Systemic hypothermia in treatment of brain injury. *J Neurotrauma*. 1992;2:487–495.

99. Shiozaki T, Sugimoto H, Taneda M, Yoshida H, et al. Effect of mild hypothermia on uncontrollable intracranial hypertension after severe head injury. *J Neurosurg*. 1993;79:363–368.

100. Williams WM, Lee ST, DelCerro M, et al. Effect of 2450 MHz microwave energy on the blood-brain barrier to hydrophilic molecules. D. Brain temperature and blood-brain barrier permeability to hydrophilic traces. *Brain Res*. 1984;319:191–212.

101. Marion DW, Obrist WD, Carlier PM, Penrod LE, et al. The use of moderate therapeutic hypothermia for patients with severe head injuries: a preliminary report. *J Neurosurg*. 1993;79:354–362.

102. Marion DW, Penrod LE, Kelsey SF, Obrist LD, et al. Treatment of Traumatic Brain Injury with Moderate Hypothermia. *N Engl J Med*. 1997;336:540–546.

103. Hauser WA. Prevention of post-traumatic epilepsy. *N Engl J Med*. 1990;323:540–541.

104. Willmore AE, Blumer D. Posttraumatic epilepsy. *Neurol Clin North Am.* 1992.10:869–878.

105. Aisen P. Some physicochemical aspects of iron metabolism. *Ciba Found Sym.* 1976;51:1–17.

106. Fong KL, McCay BP, Poyer JL, et al. Evidence of superoxide-dependent reduction of Fe3+ and its role in enzyme-generated hydroxyl radical formation. *Chem Biol Interact.* 1976;15:77–89.

107. Triggs WJ, Willmore LJ. In vivo lipid peroxidation in rat brain following intracranial Fe2+ injection. *J Neurochem* 1984;42:976–980.

108. Payan H, Toga M, Berard-Bad er M. The pathology of post-traumatic epilepsies. *Epilepsia.* 1970;11:81–94.

109. Hall ED. The role of oxygen radicals in traumatic injury: clinical implications. *J Emerg Med.* 1993;11:31–36.

110. Faden AI, Demediuk P, Panter SS, et al. The role of excitatory amino acids and NMDA receptors in traumatic brain injury. *Science.* 1989;244:798–800.

111. Yablon SA. Posttraumatic seizures *Arch Phys Med Rehabil.* 1993;74:983–1001.

112. Temkin NR, Dikmen SS, Winn HR. Posttraumatic seizures. *Neurosurg Clin North Am.* 1991;2:425–435.

113. Caveness WF. Epilepsy, a product of trauma in our time. *Epilepsia.* 1976;17:207–215.

114. Feeny DM, Walker AE. The prediction of posttraumatic epilepsy. *Arch Neurol.* 1979;36:8–12.

115. Wohns RN, Wyler AR. Prophylactic phenytoin in severe head injuries. *J Neurosurg.* 1979;51:507–509.

116. Young B, Rapp RP, Norton JA, et al. Failure of prophylactically administered phenytoin to prevent late posttraumatic seizures. *J Neurosurg.* 1983;58:236–241.

117. Glotzner FL, Haubitz I, Miltner F, et al. Anfalls prophylaxe mit carbamazepin nach schweren schadelhighverletzungen. *Neurochir.* 1983;26:66–79.

118. Temkin NR, Dikmen SS, Wilensky AJ, et al. A randomized, double-blind study of phenytoin for the prevention of post-traumatic seizure. *N Engl J Med.* 1990;323:497–502.

119. Dikmen SS, Temkin NR, Miller B, et al. Neurobehavioral effects of phenytoin prophylaxis of posttraumatic seizures. *JAMA.* 1991;265:1271–1277.

120. Renaudin J, Fewer D, Wilson CB, Boldrey EB, et al. Dose dependency of Decadron in patients with partially excised brain tumors. *J Neurosurg.* 1973;39:302–305.

121. French LA, Galicich JH. The use of steroids for control of cerebral edema. *Clin Neurosurg.* 1964;10:212–223.

122. Dearden NM, Gibson JS, McDowall DG, et al. Effect of high-dose dexamethasone on outcome from severe head injury. *J Neurosurg.* 1986;64:31–88.

123. Giannotta SL, Weiss MH, Apuzzo ML, Martin E. High dose glucocorticoids in the management of severe head injury. *Neurosurgery.* 1984;15:497–501.

124. Braakman R, Schouten HJ, Blaauw-Van Dishoeck M, Minderhoud JM. Megadose steroids in severe head injury. *J Neurosurg.* 1983;58:326–330.

125. Saul TG, Ducker TB Salzman M, Carro E. Steroids in severe head injury: a prospective randomized clinical trial. *J Neurosurg.* 1981;54:596–600.

126. Guidemann S, Miller J, Becker D. Failure of high dose steroid therapy to influence intracranial pressure in patients with severe head injury. *J Neurosurg.* 1979;51:301–306.

127. Vries JK, Becker DP, Young HF. A subarachnoid screw for monitoring intracranial pressure: technical note. *J Neurosurg.* 1973;39:416–419.

128. Barnett GH, Chapma PH. Insertion and care of intracranial pressure monitoring devices. In: Ropper AH, Kennedy SF, eds. *Neurological and Neurosurgical Intensive Care.* Gaithersburg, Md: Aspen Publishers, Inc; 1988:43.

129. Bray RS, Chodraff RG, Narayan RK, et al. A new fiberoptic monitoring device: development of the ventricular bolt. *ICP.* 1989;7:45–47.

130. Aaslid R, Markwalder TM, Nones H. Non-invasive transcranial Doppler ultrasound recording of flow velocity in basal cerebral arteries. *J Neurosurg.* 1982;57:769–774.

131. Hassler W, Steinmetz H, Gawlowski J. Transcranial Doppler ultrasonography in raised intracranial pressure and in intracranial circulatory arrest. *J Neurosurg.* 1988;68:745–751.

132. Williams MA, Razumovsky AY, Diringer M, Hanley DF. Transcranial Doppler ultrasonography in the intensive care unit. In: Babikan VG, Wechsler LR, eds. *Transcranial Doppler Ultrasonography.* St Louis, Mo: CV Mosby; 1993:175–189.

133. Muizelaar JP, Ward JD, Marmarou A, et al. Cerebral blood flow and metabolism in severely head-injured children. Part 2: autoregulation. *J Neurosurg.* 1989;71:72–76.

134. Cold GE, Christensen MS, Schmidt K. Effect of two levels of induced hypocapnia on cerebral autoregulation in the acute phase of head injury coma. *Acta Anaesthesiol Scand.* 1981;25:379–401.

135. Lewelt W, Jenkins LW, Miller JD. Autoregulation of cerebral blood flow after experimental fluid percussion injury of the brain. *J Neurosurg.* 1980;53:500–511.

136. Cruz J, Miner ME, Allen SJ, et al. Continuous monitoring of cerebral oxygenation in acute brain injury: assessment of cerebral hemodynamic reserve. *Neurosurgery.* 1991;25:743–749.

137. Gibbs EL, Lennox WG, Nims LF, Gibbs FA. Arterial and cerebral venous blood: arterial-venous differences in man. *J Biol Chem.* 1942;144:325–332.

138. Robertson CS, Narayan RK, Gokaslan ZL, et al. Cerebral arteriovenous oxygen differences as an estimate of cerebral blood flow in comatose patients. *J Neurosurg.* 1989;70:222–230.

139. Fortune JB, Feustel PJ, Weigle CG, Popp AJ. Continuous measurement of jugular venous oxygen saturation in response to transient elevations of blood pressure in head-injured patients. *J Neurosurg.* 1994;80:461–468.

140. Dickman CA, Carter P, Baldwin HZ, Harrington T, et al. Continuous regional cerebral blood flow monitoring in acute craniocerebral trauma. *Neurosurgery.* 1991;28:467–470.

141. Seelig JM, Becker DP, Miller JD, et al. Traumatic acute subdural hematoma: major mortality reduction in comatose patients treated within four hours. *N Engl J Med.* 1981;304:1511–1518.

142. Bowers SA, Marshall LF. Outline of 200 cases of severe head injury tested in San Diego County: a prospective analysis. *Neurosurgery.* 1980;6:237–242.

143. Crokard A, Hayward R, Hoff JT, eds. *Neurosurgery: The Scientific Basis of Clinical Practice.* 2nd ed. Oxford, England: Blackwell Scientific Publications; 1992:993.

144. Cooper PR, ed. *Head Injury.* 2nd ed. Baltimore, Md: Williams & Wilkins; 1987.

145. Gudeman SK, Young HP, Miller JD, Ward JD, et al. Indications for operative treatment and operative techniques in closed head injury. In: Becker DP, Gudeman SK, eds. *Textbook of Head Injury.* Philadelphia, Pa: WB Saunders Co; 1989:138–181.

146. Millikan CH. Cerebral vasospasm and ruptured intracranial aneurysm. *Arch Neurol.* 1975; 32:433–439.

147. Pickard JD, Boisuert DP, Graham DI, Fitch W. Late effects of subarachnoid hemorrhage on the response of the primate cerebral circulation to drug-induced changes in arterial blood pressure. *J Neurol Neurosurg Psychiatry.* 1979;42:899–903.

148. Gennarelli JA, Thibault LE, Adams JH, et al. Diffuse axonal injury and traumatic coma in the primate. *Ann Neurol.* 1982;12:564–574.

149. Jane JA, Rimel RW, Pobereskin LH, et al. Outcome and pathology of head injury. In: Grossman GR, Gildenberg PL, eds. *Head Injury: Basic and Clinical Aspects.* New York, NY: Raven Press; 1982:15–29.

CHAPTER 4

Cranial Nerve, Maxillofacial, and Blunt Carotid Injuries

Cranial nerve and maxillofacial injuries result in major functional deficits for patients with severe brain injuries. The correct diagnosis and prompt treatment of these injuries is essential for the best outcome of these patients. A thorough understanding of the anatomy of the cranial nerves, their physiology, and the most frequent mechanisms of injury is of utmost importance for the appropriate diagnosis and treatment. This chapter will describe the anatomy and physiology of the cranial nerves in detail. The different signs and symptoms of the injuries to the cranial nerves will be reviewed, with an outline of the important features for correct diagnosis and management. The anatomical features of maxillofacial injury in relation to severe brain injury will be discussed. The latter part of this chapter will discuss blunt injury to the carotid artery and its relationship to suspected brain injury. The importance of a prompt and accurate diagnosis will be emphasized.

ANATOMY AND PHYSIOLOGY OF THE CRANIAL NERVES

There have been various attempts to classify the cranial nerves according to function. Some anatomists suggest eliminating three of them from the classification, namely, the olfactory (I), the optic (II), and the spinal accessory (XI) nerves, because the first two are extensions of brain cells and the third is an amalgamation of the upper three nerves of the spinal cord.[1]

For purposes of this review, the nerves will be taken in sequence. An exception will be the sixth, the abducens, which will be discussed with the oculomotor and trochlear nerves before the fifth nerve, the trigeminal (Figure 4–1). The general visceral efferent and afferent components as they apply to certain cranial nerves and reflexes associated with them will be discussed in the appropriate section dealing with that nerve.[2]

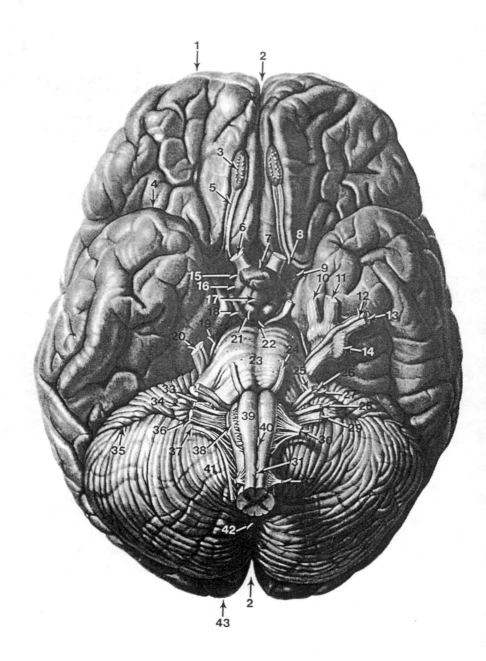

Figure 4–1 Base of the brain with the cranial nerves. *Source:* Reprinted from J.D. Fix, *Atlas of the Human Brain and Spinal Cord,* p. 4, © 1987, Aspen Publishers, Inc.

Figure 4–1 continued

Key:

1. Frontal pole
2. Longitudinal cerebral fissure
3. Olfactory bulb
4. Temporal pole
5. Olfactory tract
6. Optic nerve
7. Hypophysis
8. Olfactory trigone
9. Anterior perforated substance
10. Ophthalmic branch of trigeminal nerve
11. Maxillary branch of trigeminal nerve
12. Motor root of trigeminal nerve
13. Mandibular branch of trigeminal nerve
14. Trigeminal ganglion
15. Optic chiasm
16. Optic tract
17. Tuber cinereum
18. Oculomotor nerve
19. Trochlear nerve
20. Sensory root of trigeminal nerve
21. Mammillary body
22. Interpeduncular fossa
23. Pons (basilar sulcus)
24. Abducens nerve
25. Facial nerve
26. Intermediate branch of facial nerve
27. Vestibulocochlear nerve
28. Glossopharyngeal nerve
29. Vagus nerve
30. Hypoglossal nerve
31. Pyramidal descussation
32. Ventral root of first cervical nerve
33. Choroid plexus of fourth ventricle
34. Flocculus
35. Horizontal fissure
36. Cranial root of accessory nerve
37. Spinal root of accessory nerve
38. Olive
39. Pyramid
40. Ventral median fissure
41. Tonsil
42. Vermis of cerebellum
43. Occipital pole

Table 4–1 summarizes the names, components, and functions of the cranial nerves.

I—Olfactory Nerve (Figure 4–2)

Major Function

The olfactory nerves, with their sensory organs situated in the upper part of each nasal cavity, are the transmitters and interpreters of odors, either noxious or pleasant. Thus, an odor that provokes an appetite will induce reflex salivation, and a foul odor will induce nausea and even vomiting. Emotions play a large part in these reactions in that odors may be pleasant or offensive.

Major Subdivisions and Pathways

From the site of reception of olfactory stimuli to the site of their interpretation in the brain, the subdivisions of the olfactory nerve are the olfactory mucosa in the

Table 4–1 The Cranial Nerves: Components and Major Functions

Name	Components	Major Functions
I. Olfactory Nerve	Special visceral afferent	Smell
II. Optic Nerve	Special somatic afferent	Vision
III. Oculomotor Nerve	General somatic efferent	Movement of eyes
	General visceral efferent	Miosis: contraction of ciliary muscle (accommodation)
IV. Trochlear Nerve	General somatic efferent	Movement of eyes
	General somatic afferent	Proprioception from eye muscles
V. Trigeminal Nerve	Special visceral efferent	Movement of muscles of mastication and of stapedium muscle
	General somatic afferent	Sensation from anterior half of head and face and from meninges
VI. Abducens Nerve	General somatic efferent	Movement of eyes
VII. Facial Nerve	Special visceral efferent	Movement of facial muscles of expression, tension on ossicles of the ear
	General visceral efferent	Salivation and production of tears
	Special visceral afferent	Taste (anterior two thirds of tongue)
	General visceral afferent	Secretion of saliva, tears, vasodilation
VIII. Vestibulocochlear Nerve	Special somatic afferent	Hearing and equilibrium sensors
IX. Glossopharyngeal Nerve	Special visceral efferent	Movement of muscles of pharynx
	General visceral efferent	Salivation
	Special visceral afferent	Taste (posterior third of tongue)
	General visceral afferent	Sensibility (posterior third of tongue and pharynx)
	General somatic afferent	Sensibility (middle ear and Eustachian tube)
X. Vagus Nerve and Cranial Root of XI	General visceral efferent (parasympathetic)	Motor to viscera of chest and abdominal cavity
	Special visceral efferent	Motor to viscera of chest and abdominal cavity

Table 4–1 continued

Name	Components	Major Functions
	General visceral afferent	Sensibility of abdominal cavity
	General somatic afferent	Sensibility of auditory canal and dura
XI. Spinal Accessory Nerve (Spinal Root)	General somatic efferent	Sternocleidomastoid and trapezius muscles
XII. Hypoglossal Nerve	General somatic efferent	Movement of tongue muscles

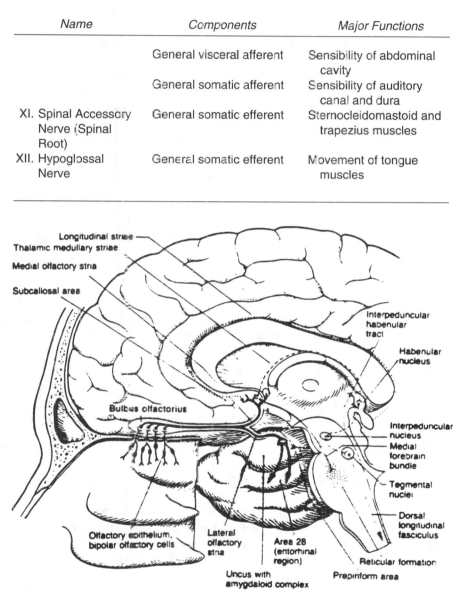

Figure 4–2 The olfactory nerve (tract) and its cortical terminals. *Source:* Reprinted with permission from P. Duus, *Topical Diagnosis in Neurology, Anatomy, Physiology, Signs, Symptoms,* 2nd revised edition, © 1989, Thieme Medical Publishers, Inc.

nasal cavity, the fila olfactoria, the olfactory bulbs, the olfactory tract, the "paleo-cortex" in the temporal lobe uncus, and the subcallosal area in the medial aspect of the occipital lobe.

The olfactory mucosa covers an area of 2 cm² in the upper part of each nasal cavity and extends toward the superior nasal concha and the nasal septum. The highly specialized olfactory epithelium consists of sensory cells, supporting cells, and Bowman's glands. The latter produce the serous fluid in which aromatic substances go into solution. The sensory cells are bipolar neurons, and their peripheral processes terminate at the surface of the epithelium in the form of short olfactory hairs. The central processes are unmyelinated delicate fibers that join to form the fila olfactoria. These fila olfactoria pass through the foramina in the cribriform plate of the ethmoid bone and connect with the olfactory bulb on their respective sides.

The olfactory bulbs are protruding portions of the telencephalon that form the second set of neurons. The axons of the olfactory bulbs form the olfactory tracts, which proceed posteriorly and laterally in the olfactory sulci to the gyri recti. At the level of the anterior perforated substance, they form the olfactory trigone, from which each divides into the medial and lateral striae.

Cortical and Other Connections

The fibers of the medial striae connect with those of the other side and pass through the area beneath the rostrum of the corpus callosum. Those of the lateral striae continue posteriolaterally to the amygdala and thence to the parahippo-campal gyrus of the cortex (Brodmann's area 28).

II—Optic Nerve (Figure 4–3)

Major Functions

The optic nerves form part of the visual system. This latter consists of a peripheral apparatus of reception and integration, namely, the retina; an afferent fiber system (the optic nerve, chiasm, optic tract), and a central area of reception for the retinal impulses at the level of the lateral geniculate body on the posterolateral side of the thalamus. From there, the fibers of the optic tract diverge and synapse in three different areas. Of the three main routes that the retinal impulses travel, two connect the retina with the cerebral cortex, and the third is a subcortical route. The first route, the retino-geniculo-calcarine route, is involved in discriminatory sensory functions such as spatial analysis of the environment, interpretation of shapes, visual acuity, and color vision. About 80% of the optic fibers that synapse in the lateral geniculate body belong to this system. The second route, the retino-tecto-thalamo-cortical system, is in charge of motor aspects of visual

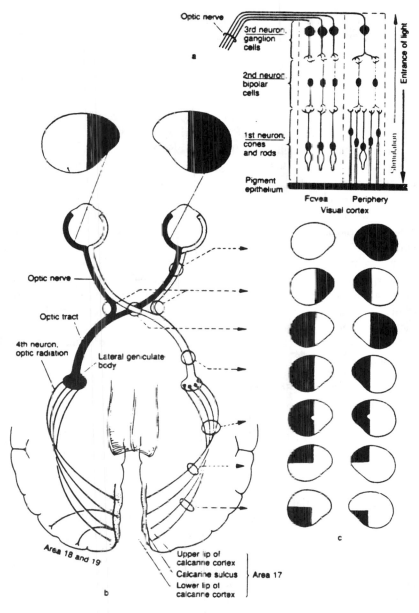

Figure 4–3 The optic nerve and optic pathway. a. Microscopic structure of retina. b. Visual pathway interrupted by lesions. c. Corresponding defects of visual fields. *Source:* Reprinted with permission from P. Duus. *Topical Diagnosis in Neurology, Anatomy, Physiology, Signs, Symptoms,* 2nd revised edition, p. 82, © 1989, Thieme Medical Publishers, Inc.

function, such as tracking movements of the eye to follow the chosen object even when it moves. The third visual route, the retino-mesencephalic system, is involved mainly in the production of subcortical optical reflexes, such as the light reflex.

Major Subdivisions and Pathways

The retina, which is essentially an extension of the forebrain, is the receptor of visual impulses. A full description of the retina is beyond the scope of this review. In summary, it is a complicated 10-layer system, of which 3 layers of neurons are of special interest because they carry the visual impulses. Beginning from the external layer and moving in toward the optic nerve is the first layer of neurons, called the *cones and rods*; the second layer of neurons, the *bipolar cells*; and the third layer, the *ganglion cells*. Approximately 1 million axons emerge from these ganglion cells and run in the retinal fiber layer to the head or papilla of the optic nerve (Figure 4–3). From here, the optic nerves pass posteriorly through the lamina cribrosa of the sclera of the eye as far as the chiasm. On arrival at the chiasm, the nerve fibers that originate in the nasal half of the retina cross through the chiasm to the opposite side. The fibers that originate in the temporal side of the retina continue ipsilaterally. Behind the chiasm, they join the crossed fibers from the contralateral eye to form the optic tracts. Each tract proceeds posteriorly to terminate in the lateral geniculate body, which is attached to the posteriolateral aspect of the thalamus.

Cortical and Other Connections

The lateral geniculate body is the final destination for the majority of the optic fibers. Each fiber synapses with about six cells in this body. New fibers from the principal cells of the lateral geniculate body extend along the wall of the lateral ventricle as the optic radiation to the calcarine fissure (Brodmann's area 17; see Figure 3–10) of the occipital lobe, where they synapse (Figure 4–4).

Brodmann's area 17 is surrounded by areas 18 and 19 (see Figure 3–10), which extend from the medial aspect of the occipital lobe over its convexity. These areas are related to area 17 and are called association areas for visual imprints (fields of optical memories). Electrical stimulation of areas 18 and 19 produces an optical aura such as flashing lights, color, simple forms, and lines. Visual impressions, which arrive at area 17, probably become conscious experiences in the adjacent association areas, where they can be compared with former experiences and interpreted. Destruction of areas 18 and 19 results in an inability to recognize objects by their forms, sizes, and outlines or to be aware of their significance (optical agnosia, alexia). This can become more apparent if the optical commissural fibers of the splenium of the corpus callosum, which interconnects both visual areas, is interrupted.[2]

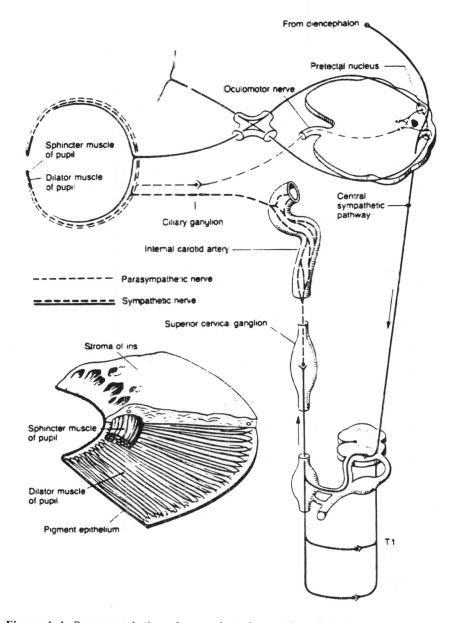

Figure 4–4 Parasympathetic and sympathetic innervation of the inner eye muscles. *Source*: Reprinted with permission from P. Duss, *Topical Diagnosis in Neurology, Anatomy, Physiology, Signs, Symptoms,* 2nd revised edition, p. 100, © 1989, Thieme Medical Publishers, Inc.

III—Oculomotor Nerve (Figure 4–1)

The fibers of the oculomotor nerves are mainly somatic efferent. These nerves also carry general visceral fibers from the parasympathetic system that act on the sphincter muscles of the pupils.

The branches of the nerve innervate the following external ocular muscles: the superior levator palpebrae muscle; the superior, inferior, and medial recti muscles; and the inferior oblique muscle on the ipsilateral side. Contraction of these muscles causes the eyes to look upward and outward; to turn inward (nasally); and to look downward and outward—that is, to the temporal side. The parasympathetic fibers accompany the branches for the inferior oblique muscles and, by innervating the sphincter muscles of the pupil and the ciliary muscle, cause the pupil to contract and the convexity of the lens to increase for accommodation.

Major Subdivisions and Pathways

The oculomotor nerves have nuclei located at the level of the superior colliculus in the alar plate of the midbrain and ventral to the gray matter of the cerebral peduncles. The axons from the nucleus in the superior colliculus pass proximally through the red nucleus and exit on the medial side of the cerebral peduncle. They continue on course on each side between the superior cerebellar and the posterior cerebral arteries to the posterior clinoid process, where they enter the sinus cavernosum. At this level, they divide into inferior and superior branches that reach the orbit via the orbital fissure.

Cortical and Other Connections

The oculomotor nuclei connect with three nuclei in their immediate vicinity; with the pontine oculomotor center; and with the hypoglossal nucleus propositus. The pontine oculomotor center projects to the abducens nucleus, thus controlling horizontal eye movements. Homolateral and heterolateral fibers from the cerebral cortex converge on the nucleus, as do fibers from the vestibular nuclei. Afferent fibers from the ophthalmic branch of the trigeminal nerve ensure proprioceptive innervation of the eye muscles. Parasympathetic axons originate from the Edinger-Westphal nuclei, situated rostral and dorsal to the somatomotor nucleus.

IV—Trochlear Nerve (Figure 4–1)

Major Functions

Trochlear nerves are purely somatomotor to the external ocular muscles. Each innervates the ipsilateral superior oblique muscles. Contraction of these muscles causes the eyes to look downward and inward with slight abduction.

Major Subdivisions and Pathways

The nuclei of the trochlear nerves are located in the caudal end of the mesencephalon near the inferior colliculi, distal to those of the oculomotor nerves. The efferent fibers leave the brain dorsal to the aqueduct and, having crossed over to the opposite side, extend laterally and cranially through the sinus cavernosum and reach the orbit via the superior orbital fissure.

VI—Abducens Nerve (Figure 4–1)

Abducens nerves are also purely somatomotor to the external ocular muscles. They innervate the lateral rectus muscles, which cause the eyes to turn to the lateral side.

Major Subdivisions and Pathways

The nuclei of the abducens nerves are situated in the wall of the fourth ventricle; fibers of the seventh nerve are between them and the ventricle. Efferent fibers of the abducens nerves emerge from the brain at the pontomedullary junction proximal to the pyramids. They proceed rostrally through the subarachnoid space on either side of the internal carotid artery, penetrate the dura, and join the oculomotor nerve and the trochlear nerve in the cavernous sinus. From there, they proceed to the lateral rectus muscles of each eye.

Cortical and Other Connections

The cortical and vestibular connections are similar to those described for the oculomotor and trochlear nerves.

Autonomic Innervation and Reflexes of the Eye (Figure 4–4)

Any discussion of the nerves of oculomotion would be incomplete without considering the effects of the parasympathetic and sympathetic systems on the eye.

Major Functions

For objects to be sharply visualized, light rays emitted from these objects must fall on the fovea centralis of both retinas. There is therefore need for conjugate eye movements. Movements in the horizontal plane follow simultaneous contraction of the lateral rectus muscles of one eye and the medial rectus muscle of the other eye. Movement in the vertical plane is more complicated. To appreciate binocular vision at a short distance, the two visual axes must be aimed at the same point so that a single image is perceived. This is accomplished by the two eyes' converging to make the two visual axes meet at the fixation point. The dilator muscle of the pupil, which runs in a ray fashion from the inner to the outer circumference of the eye, and in which the pigment of the pupil is present, is controlled by the sympathetic nervous system. The second muscle of the pupil, the sphincter, is circumferentially placed around its inner margin and is controlled by the parasympathetic system. The light reflexes are mediated through the parasympathetic system. The pupil reacts to incident light by contraction, not only of the eye to which the light is focused, but to the other eye as well (the consensual light reflex). The accommodation reflex is also mediated through the parasympathetic system. It comes into action when objects within 6 m of the eye are to be sharply depicted on the retina. The curvature of the lens has to increase to allow this to occur, and this movement is effected by contraction of the ciliary muscle.

Major Subdivisions and Pathways

The pathway of the sympathetic system is summarized as follows. Afferent impulses from the hypothalamus proceed through the central sympathetic tract of the midbrain, where they cross and continue into the cervical cord to a ciliospinal center located in the lateral horn of the gray matter at the level of C-8 or T-1. The afferent fibers enter the nuclei at this level, and, from there, efferent preganglionic fibers proceed via the sympathetic trunk to the superior cervical ganglion, where they synapse. Postganglionic fibers accompany the internal carotid artery to the ciliary ganglion and hence to the orbit via the short ciliary nerves. The pathway of the parasympathetic system has already been covered under the discussion of the oculomotor nerve.

Cortical and Subcortical Connections

Coordination of the eye movements is accomplished mostly through the medial longitudinal fasciculus adjacent to the lateral nucleus of the oculomotor nerve. Fibers from the vestibular nuclei come via this pathway. Both the light and the accommodation reflexes are regarded as subcortical reflexes.

V—Trigeminal Nerve (Figure 4–5)

Major Functions

The trigeminal nerve is a mixed nerve containing both special motor and general somatic afferent fibers. The motor fibers innervate the muscles of mastication, namely, the masseter, the pterygoids, and the temporalis muscles; the tensor tympani; the mylohyoid; and the anterior belly of the digastric muscles. The sensory and larger portion carries afferent fibers for pain, touch, pressure, and temperature from an extensive area of the face, nose, and mouth.

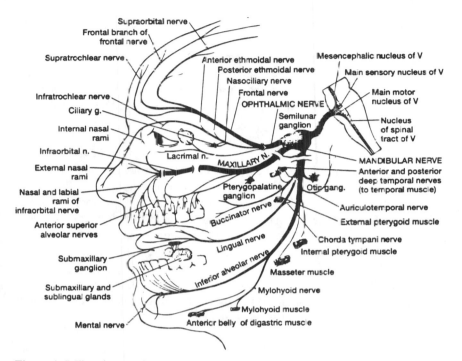

Figure 4–5 The trigeminal nerve and its branches. Source: Reprinted with permission from S.G. Waxman and J. deGroot. *Correlative Neuroanatomy,* 22nd edition, p. 116, © 1995, Appleton & Lange.

Major Subdivisions and Pathways

The trigeminal nerve, in its peripheral portion, divides into three principal branches:

1. the *ophthalmic nerve,* which is purely sensory and innervates the forehead, eyes, and nose
2. the *maxillary nerve,* which is also only sensory and supplies the skin of the maxilla, including the upper teeth, the mucosa of the upper lip, the cheeks, the palate, and the maxillary sinus
3. the *mandibular nerve,* which is the sensory innervation for the tongue; the mandible, including the lower teeth; the lower lip; part of the cheek; and part of the external ear. It is a mixed nerve, and the motor fibers supply the muscles already named.

The sensory fibers from the above-named parts of the face proceed through these branches to the trigeminal ganglion. The central processes enter the pons and terminate either in the principal nucleus (mainly those for touch and pressure from the face) or in the spinal nuclei extending from the cervical cord toward the midbrain (mainly those for pain and temperature). The motor portion of the trigeminal nerve has its nucleus in the pontine tegmentum, which is located just medial to the principal sensory nucleus.

Cortical and Subcortical Connections

These motor nuclei receive their central stimulation through the corticonuclear tract, which originates in the lower portion of the precentral gyrus. Most of the motor impulses come from the contralateral side, but there are some from the ipsilateral side; thus, if there is an interruption at this level, the muscles of mastication may show little weakness. If the nucleus or the peripheral portion of the mandibular branch is damaged, there will be weakness of the chewing muscles on the ipsilateral side.

The sensory nuclear complex receives fibers from the glossopharyngeal and vagus nerves, from the first four cervical spinal cord nerves, and from the primary somatosensory area (Brodmann's area 4; see Figures 3–10 and 3–11). The masticatory nucleus receives afference from the cortex via the corticobulbar fibers. Efferent fibers from the trigeminal complex synapse in the cerebellum, the thalamus, and the reticular formation.

VII—Facial Nerve (Figure 4–6)

Major Functions

The facial nerve is a mixed nerve. It consists of special visceral efferent fibers that form the main bulk of the nerve and a smaller intermediate branch that has general visceral efferent and general and special afferent fibers. The special visceral efferent component innervates the muscles of the facial expression and the platysma, the stylohyoid, the posterior part of the digastric in the neck, and the stapedius in the middle ear. The general visceral efferent fibers, which have vasomotor and salivary secretion actions, innervate the submandibular, sublingual, and lacrimal glands. The general afferent fibers, with their nuclei in the geniculate ganglion, are sensory to part of the external auditory meatus and a small area of skin behind the ear. The special visceral afferent fibers originate from the taste buds on the anterior two thirds of the tongue and convey messages of taste to the gustatory nucleus of the solitary tract.

Major Subdivisions and Pathways

The nucleus of the special visceral efferent component of the nerve is a combination of a few nuclei placed in the ventrolateral aspect of the lower pons near the

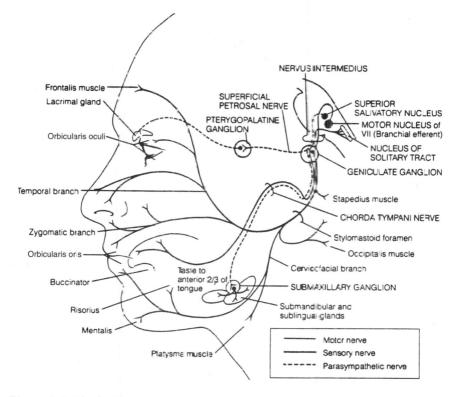

Frontalis muscle

Lacrimal gland

Orbicularis oculi

Temporal branch

Zygomatic branch

Orbicularis oris

Buccinator

Risorius

Mentalis

Platysma muscle

NERVUS INTERMEDIUS

SUPERFICIAL PETROSAL NERVE

PTERYGOPALATINE GANGLION

SUPERIOR SALIVATORY NUCLEUS

MOTOR NUCLEUS of VII (Branchial efferent)

NUCLEUS OF SOLITARY TRACT

GENICULATE GANGLION

Stapedius muscle

CHORDA TYMPANI NERVE

Stylomastoid foramen

Occipitalis muscle

Cervicofacial branch

SUBMAXILLARY GANGLION

Submandibular and sublingual glands

Taste to anterior 2/3 of tongue

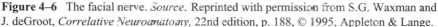

——— Motor nerve
——— Sensory nerve
- - - - Parasympathetic nerve

Figure 4–6 The facial nerve. *Source.* Reprinted with permission from S.G. Waxman and J. deGroot, *Correlative Neuroanatomy,* 22nd edition, p. 188, © 1995, Appleton & Lange.

medulla oblongata. These nuclei are in close proximity to those of the abducens nerve. The axons, having curved around the abducens nerve, emerge from the brain at the inferior margin of the pons. The nerve then enters the internal auditory meatus and extends through the facial canal of the petrous bone. It leaves the skull through the stylomastoid foramen, from which the motor fibers spread out to innervate the muscles as described above.

The general visceral efferent fibers, which form part of the intermediate nerve, have their origin in the superior salivatory nucleus. These efferent fibers pass through the chorda tympani and the greater petrosal nerve to the submandibular, sublingual, and lacrimal glands to ensure increased secretion of these glands.

The general afferent fibers, on their way to the geniculate ganglion, join auricular branches of the vagus nerve. The postganglionic fibers join those of the special afferent fibers from the taste buds. These latter first join the lingual nerve, a branch of the trigeminal nerve, and pass from it through the chorda tympani to the intermediate nerve. From there, having passed through the geniculate ganglion, the preganglionic fibers ascend to the nucleus of the solitary tract in the medulla oblongata. In this nucleus, they are joined by taste fibers from the posterior third of the tongue that are transmitted through the glossopharyngeal nerve and by sensory fibers from the epiglottis that are transmitted through the vagus nerve. They all have their relay station in the nucleus of the solitary tract, from which they cross and go to the contralateral thalamus.

Cortical and Subcortical Connections

Having passed through the thalamus, the general sensory and special afferent fibers proceed to the posterior central convolution of the cortex near the insula (Brodmann's areas 3, 1, and 2; see Figures 3–10 and 3–11).

There are three nerves involved in the appreciation of the sense of taste: the seventh, as discussed here; the fifth (trigeminal), with which it is connected through the lingual nerve; and the ninth (glossopharyngeal), which carries gustatory fibers from the posterior third of the tongue. As a result, it is rare to get complete loss of taste with injury.

Cortical control of the facial muscles is interesting in that the supranuclear control of the forehead musculature is located in both cerebral hemispheres, whereas that for the remaining musculature is located in the contralateral precentral gyrus. This explains how in a high-level pons or cortical lesion, the musculature in the forehead on the contralateral side will not be involved, whereas in a local or postnuclear lesion of the facial nerve, the forehead muscle on the ipsilateral side will be paralyzed.

The motor nucleus receives afferent fibers from the spinal tract nucleus, the superior colliculus, the reticular formation, and the cerebral cortex. Because of these connections, the motor nucleus is part of several reflex arcs. One of the most important is the corneal reflex, in which sensory stimuli originating in the mucus membrane of the eye are carried via the ophthalmic branch of the trigeminal nerve to its principal sensory nucleus. From there, interconnector neurons pass to the motor nucleus of the facial nerve. Efferent impulses arise from here and pass through the nerve to the orbicularis oculi muscles, causing reflex closure of the eyes. A lesion unilateral of the trigeminal nerve will cause the eyes to close when the contralateral eye is irritated, whereas there will be no reflex closure of the eyes if the facial nerve is involved. There will continue to be sensitivity in the cornea if the lesion is only of the facial nerve.

Another reflex is the blink reflex, which is stimulated when a bright light is shone in the eye. Impulses pass along through the tecto bulbo tract to the motor nucleus, causing the eyelids to close. A similar response occurs in the acoustic palpabreal or cochlear palpabreal reflex when observed blinking of the eyelids occurs in response to a loud, sharp noise. The acoustic reflex is produced with contraction of the stapedius muscle supplied by the seventh nerve in response to auditory stimuli transmitted to the middle ear through the vestibulocochlear nerve, as described in the following section.

VIII—Vestibulocochlear Nerve (Figure 4–7)

Major Functions

The vestibulocochlear nerve has two components: a vestibular one that controls equilibrium and a cochlear one that controls the sense of hearing. The peripheral receptors of the nerve are localized in complex, communicating, fluid-filled epithelial tubes situated in the bony labyrinth of the petrous bone. Those of the vesti-

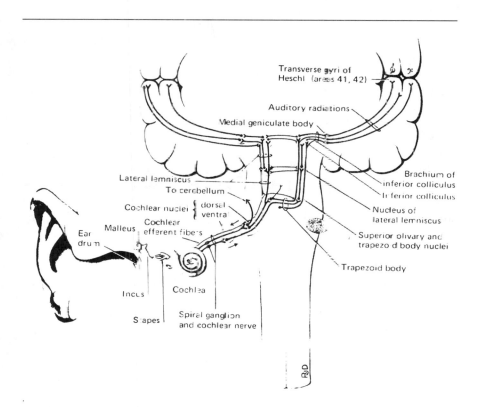

Figure 4–7 Diagram of the auditory pathways. *Source*: Reprinted with permission from C.R. Noback, M.L. Stromingr, and R.J. Demarest, *The Human Nervous System: Introduction and Reviews,* p. 257. © 1991, Williams & Wilkins.

bular component are localized in the semicircular canals. The receptors of the cochlear component are localized in the organ of Corti in the cochlea.

Major Subdivisions and Pathways

Hearing is appreciated when sound waves entering the ear are transformed into mechanical movements of the auditory ossicle of the middle ear. In turn, these movements are transformed into pressure waves of the perilymph, which sends messages through the cochlea to the round window of the inner ear. The pressure waves cause vibration of the basilar membrane, which causes stimulation of the hair cells of the organ of Corti, and these sensory receptors are transformed into electrical action potentials. The special sensory cells of the organ of Corti are connected to the spiral ganglion situated in the spiral canal of this same organ. Central axons from this ganglion form the cochlear nerve, which is joined by the vestibular nerve in the internal acoustic meatus.

The vestibular system is complex and consists of the labyrinth, the vestibular nerve, and the central vestibular pathways. The labyrinth, situated in the petrous bone, consists of the utricle, the saccule, and three semicircular canals. This labyrinth is a membranous organ that is separated from the bony labyrinth by a thin space filled with perilymph. The organ itself is filled with endolymph. The receptor organs are the "hair" cells. They protrude into the endolymphatic space and are situated in the saccule, the utricle, and the ampullae of the semicircular canals. These "hair" cells respond to changes in orientation or movement of the body by sending electrical impulses to vestibular afferents that pass to their cell bodies in the vestibular (Scarpa's) ganglion, found in the internal auditory meatus. Central fibers from these form the vestibular nerve, which unites with the cochlear nerve as they pass through the internal acoustic meatus to enter the brainstem at the pontomedullary junction (Figure 4–1). They join the vestibular nuclei near the floor of the lateral ventricle.

Cortical and Subcortical Connections

Immediately after entering the brainstem, the fibers of the cochlear nerve divide into an ascending branch, which synapses in the ventral cochlear nucleus, and a descending branch, which synapses in the dorsal nuclei. The fibers project ipsilaterally and heterolaterally through a complicated system to the superior olivary nucleus, the lateral lemniscus in the tegmentum to the inferior colliculus, and the medial geniculate body of the thalamus via the geniculotemporal tract to the upper temporal gyrus (Brodmann's areas 41 and 42; see Figure 3–11). Each cochlea is represented bilaterally in the acoustic cortex.

Efferent fibers, which exert a regulatory influence on incoming acoustic information, descend from all the acoustic nuclei. The best known of these is the olivocochlear tract, which accompanies the vestibular nerve as far as the labyrinth, then parts from it via the vestibulocochlear anastomosis and terminates on the hair cells.

From the vestibular nuclei, secondary neurons go to various parts of the cerebellum, and efferent stimuli return from these endings in the cerebellum through the vestibular nerves to the hair cells of the labyrinth. Here they exert a regulatory, predominantly inhibitory influence. Efferent stimuli also come directly to the vestibular nuclear complex and to spinal motor neurons, where they exert their influence on muscle tone and balance. The central connections of the vestibular system are not fully understood. For more details, the reader is referred to a treatise on neuroanatomy. It is more recently held that the vestibular sensations occupy an area in the parietal lobe adjacent to the portion of the postcentral gyrus where the head is represented.[3]

IX—Glossopharyngeal Nerve (Figure 4–8)

Major Functions

The special visceral efferent fibers through the pharyngeal branches supply the superior pharyngeal constrictor and stylopharyngeal muscles. These are important muscles in the pharyngeal phase of deglutition, especially of liquid ingestion. The general visceral efferent fibers through the tympanic nerve supply parasympathetic impulses to the parotid gland. These regulate salivary flow.

The special visceral efferent fibers convey impulses from the taste buds on the posterior third of the tongue. They also communicate through the carotid nerve with the vagus nerve and the sympathetic branches influencing the control of blood pressure in the carotid sinus.

The general visceral afferent fibers convey visceral sensation from the parotid gland, the carotid sinus, the mucous membrane of the pharynx, the middle ear, and the posterior third of the tongue. The general somatic afferent fibers convey cutaneous sensation from a small area behind the ear.

Major Subdivisions and Pathways

The special visceral efferent fibers of the glossopharyngeal nerve originate from the nucleus ambiguus, situated between the spinal nucleus of the trigeminal nerve and the inferior olive. The general visceral efferent fibers originate in the inferior salivatory nucleus. The nerve passes through the jugular foramen to the superior and inferior ganglia, which contain the cell bodies of the afferent components of the nerve. Having received communications from the sympathetic system and the vagus, the nerve proceeds as the tympanic nerve to enter the tympanic plexus on the promontory of the medial wall of the middle ear. From there, sensory fibers are distributed through the lesser petrosal nerve to the mucous mem-

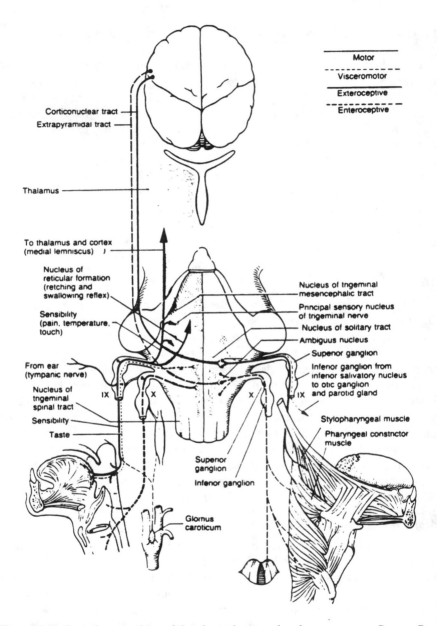

Figure 4–8 Central connections of the glossopharyngeal and vagus nerves. *Source:* Reprinted with permission from P. Duus, *Topical Diagnosis in Neurology, Anatomy, Physiology, Signs, Symptoms,* 2nd revised edition, p. 122, © 1989, Thieme Medical Publishers, Inc.

branes of the pharynx and middle ear. The lesser petrosal nerve ends in the otic ganglion, from which postganglionic fibers are distributed via the auricotemporal branch of the trigeminal nerve to the parotid gland.

Cortical and Subcortical Connections

The connections of the glossopharyngeal, trigeminal, and vagus nerves have been referred to above. The glossopharyngeal nerve is also closely related to the intermediate branch of the facial nerve, as already discussed. From the nuclei of origin, the nerve has efferent and afferent connections with the motor and sensory cortex and the thalamus.

X—Vagus Nerve (Figure 4–8)

The complex vagus nerve has many parts, of which two principal ones are recognized: a branchial component that is involved in the innervation of branchial arch derivatives and a parasympathetic or visceral component that innervates as far as the descending colon, including respiratory, cardiac, and digestive organs and blood vessels. The branchial component terminates in the inferior laryngeal nerve, and all branches caudal to this are parasympathetic or sensory fibers for the viscera.

Major Functions

Special visceral efferent fibers that originate in the nucleus ambiguus near the nucleus of the glossopharyngeal nerve innervate the voluntary muscle of the larynx, pharynx, palate, and upper two thirds of the esophagus. These fibers include fibers from the cranial portion of the eleventh (accessory) nerve.

General visceral efferent fibers that arise in the dorsal nucleus of the vagus nerve supply preganglion parasympathetic impulses to involuntary muscles and glands of the heart, esophagus, stomach, trachea, bronchi, intestines, and other abdominal viscera.

Special visceral afferent fibers convey taste from the epiglottis and palate. General visceral afferent fibers convey visceral sensation from the carotid body, base of the tongue, pharynx, larynx, trachea, bronchi, lungs, heart, esophagus, stomach, and intestines. General somatic afferent fibers convey cutaneous sensation from the external ear, external acoustic meatus, and dura mater of the posterior cranial fossa.

Major Subdivisions and Pathways

The vagus nerve emerges with the glossopharyngeal nerve in the groove dorsal to the inferior olive. It leaves the skull through the jugular foramen in the same dural sheath as the accessory nerve. In this foramen, it forms the superior ganglion containing the nuclei for the general somatic afferent fibers. On exiting, it forms the inferior ganglion containing the nuclei for the visceral afferent components. Caudal from the inferior ganglion, the nerve descends along the line of the internal carotid artery and the common carotid artery and enters the mediastinum via the superior thoracic aperture. The nerve on the right side passes over the subclavian artery; that on the left, over the arch of the aorta and behind the root of the lungs. Both come into contact with the esophagus; the right nerve descends posterior to it and the left descends anterior to it. They form a plexus around the esophagus, and the terminal branches enter the abdominal cavity through the esophageal hiatus of the diaphragm.

Cortical and Subcortical Connections

The connections with the trigeminal and glossopharyngeal nerves are affected through the nucleus ambiguus. This nucleus also receives impulses from the cortex through the corticobulbar fibers. The nucleus ambiguus is important for affecting reflexes such as swallowing, coughing, and vomiting.

XI—Accessory Nerve (Figure 4–9)

Major Functions

The accessory nerve has two portions: the cranial, which was discussed with the vagus nerve; and the spinal, which is generally understood when the nerve is named. The spinal division of the accessory nerve is the somatic motor nerve to the ipsilateral sternocleidomastoid and trapezius muscles. It also carries sensory fibers, mainly proprioceptive, impulses centrally from these muscles.

Major Subdivisions and Pathways

The spinal division of the accessory nerve originates in the ventrolateral anterior horns of C2-5. The axons of this division ascend in the lateral funiculus before they leave the cord, near the dentate ligament. They pass rostrally through the foramen magnum into the cranium and unite with the cranial portion of the nerve. Subsequently, the nerve leaves the cranium through the jugular foramen. The cranial accessory nerve parts company and joins the vagus nerve to become the recurrent laryngeal nerve, supplying the intrinsic laryngeal muscles. The spinal accessory nerve descends in the neck until it reaches the two muscles it innervates.

Cortical and Subcortical Connections

Since this is a spinal motor nerve arising from the anterior horn cells at C-6 and upward, it will have the same cortical connections as have any of these nerves via

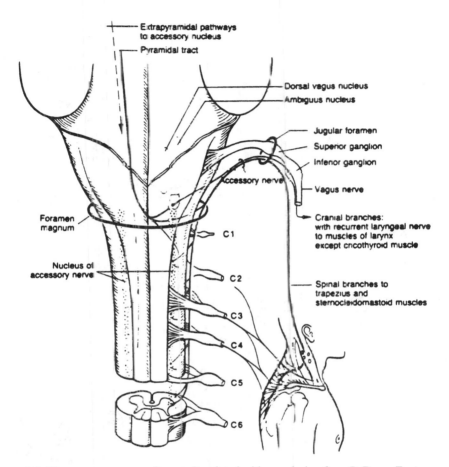

Figure 4–9 The accessory nerve. *Source*: Reprinted with permission from P. Duus, *Topical Diagnosis in Neurology, Anatomy, Physiology, Signs, Symptoms,* 2nd revised edition, p. 126, © 1989, Thieme Medical Publishers, Inc.

the pyramidal tracts to the motor cortex (Brodmann's areas 4 and 6; Figures 3–10 and 3–11).

XII—Hypoglossal Nerve (Figure 4–10)

The hypoglossal nerve is a somatic motor nerve only. It innervates both intrinsic and extrinsic muscles of the tongue. The latter are the genioglossus, hyoglossus, and styloglossus muscles.

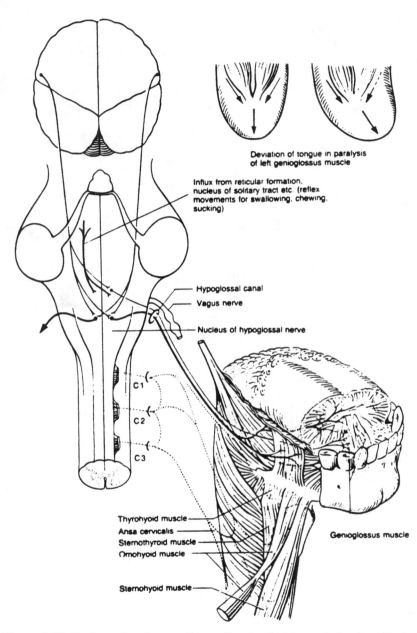

Deviation of tongue in paralysis
of left genioglossus muscle

Influx from reticular formation,
nucleus of solitary tract etc. (reflex
movements for swallowing, chewing,
sucking)

Hypoglossal canal

Vagus nerve

Nucleus of hypoglossal nerve

C 1

C 2

C 3

Thyrohyoid muscle

Ansa cervicalis

Sternothyroid muscle

Omohyoid muscle

Sternohyoid muscle

Genioglossus muscle

Figure 4–10 The hypoglossal nerve. *Source:* Reprinted with permission from *Topical Diagnosis in Neurology, Anatomy, Physiology, Signs, Symptoms,* 2nd revised edition, p. 129, © 1989, Thieme Medical Publishers, Inc.

Major Subdivisions and Pathways

The nucleus of the hypoglossal nerve is located in the lower medulla oblongata near the midline and deep to the floor of the fourth ventricle. Each nucleus is made up of several groups of motor neurons that innervate individual tongue muscles. The axons emerge from the brainstem between the pyramid and the inferior olive (Figure 4–1). The nerve leaves the cranium through its own canal near the margin of the foramen magnum. In the neck, the nerve passes between the internal jugular vein and the internal carotid artery and joins fibers of the three upper cervical segments to innervate the muscles of the hyoid bone and the muscles of the tongue, namely, the styloglossus, hyoglossus, and genioglossus.

Cortical and Subcortical Connections

Corticobulbar fibers from the sensory cortex synapse in the nucleus of the hypoglossal nerve. Other fibers come from the reticular formation, the trigeminal nuclei, and the solitary nucleus. It is via these fibers that reflex movements such as sucking and swallowing are executed.

DIAGNOSIS AND MANAGEMENT OF CRANIAL NERVE INJURIES

The exact incidence of damage to the cranial nerves secondary to brain injury varies according to the mechanism and severity of the injury. It will also depend on the patient selection and length of follow-up. There is general agreement that the olfactory and facial nerves and audiovestibular function are damaged most often by blunt brain injury.[4] Trauma to the optic nerve and each of the ocular motor nerves is intermediate in frequency, whereas the trigeminal nerve trunk and the lower cranial nerves are rarely injured. Cranial nerve findings can predict the type of brain injury. It is uncertain how often, how soon, and how well patients recover from traumatic cranial neuropathies. Follow-ups are notoriously poor in these patients. Changes in return of function vary with the nerve involved: the facial nerve usually recovers, the ocular motor nerves return to normal about 40% of the time,[5] and the first two cranial nerves show significant improvement in less than one third of cases.[4] Lesions of the audiovestibular nerve are usually permanent.

The different signs and symptoms of the injuries to the different cranial nerves described above will be presented. Emphasis on aggressive treatment and rehabilitation will afford patients the best possible outcome.

I—Olfactory Nerve

The function of the olfactory nerve is neglected by many during the evaluation of a patient with brain injury. This neglect in testing the sense of smell transfers to the patient the burden of detecting a loss of taste and smell. Anosmia occurs more commonly with occipital than with frontal injuries.[4] Most studies agree that the olfactory nerve is the cranial nerve most often damaged by blunt brain injury. Its incidence ranges from 5% up to 30% with severe brain injuries or anterior fractures.[4-7] Recovery occurs in more than one third of cases, usually during the first three months. Some patients, however, are reported to show improvement as late as five years after injury.[4] Trivial injuries can cause permanent loss of smell, but the incidence of anosmia parallels the severity of brain injury. Anosmia has been postulated to occur when the fila olfactoria have been traumatically severed at the cribriform plate and the regenerating axon has failed to reach the olfactory bulb.[7] It is unlikely that either medical therapy or additional time will allow healing.

II—Optic Nerve

About one fourth of civilian optic nerve injury is due to penetrating injury.[4] Gunshot wounds are the usual cause and usually are associated with the preference for aiming a handgun at the temple when attempting suicide. This frequently results in one or both optic nerves being destroyed.[8] Indirect optic nerve injury results from injury to the ipsilateral outer eyebrow with astonishing regularity.[4] Forces exerted there are transmitted directly to the optic nerve canal, the usual site of traumatic optic neuropathy.[9] Occasionally, temporal-parietal blows will damage the optic nerve, but occipital trauma rarely produces optic neuropathy. The optic nerves, like the olfactory and trochlear nerves, can be damaged by trivial blows, but most traumatic optic neuropathies are associated with severe brain injury.[4]

The most common result of optic nerve injury is complete blindness in one eye, but any degree of impairment of visual acuity may occur.[10,11] About 10% of patients will show signs of bilateral optic nerve or chiasmal damage.[12] Many chiasmal lesions are asymmetric, with unilateral severe optic neuropathy associated with contralateral temporal hemianopsia.

Clinical evaluation of the conscious brain-injured patient consists of prompt testing of visual acuity and fields and use of the swinging-flashlight test to search for an afferent pupillary defect. In the unresponsive brain-injured patient, evaluation depends on afferent pupillary function, and the frequent association of efferent pupillary damage may make this a difficult task. Fundoscopy is necessary to rule out vitreous or retinal hemorrhage as the cause of visual loss. Radiographic and laboratory testing are of limited value in the presence of immediate visual loss. Fractures through the optic canal can be demonstrated in half of such patients, but this finding is of limited practical concern. Sheath hemorrhages of the optic nerve may be seen with other intracranial bleeding without interfering with the vision, and their presence after brain injury is expected.[13]

Prompt treatment is imperative in cases of delayed visual loss. Otherwise, no therapy has been shown to be of definite benefit. The optic nerve and the spinal cord are both central nervous system tracts contained within bone canals, and effective therapy for one should benefit the other. Recent evidence that immediate, high-dose steroid therapy results in improved outcome after spinal cord injuries[14] is a strong recommendation for its prompt use in nearly all cases of traumatic optic neuropathy. Surgery is unlikely to benefit the majority of traumatized optic nerves and remains controversial in the literature.[11,15] Indirect optic nerve injury usually produces immediate visual loss, and recovery may occur in more than one third of patients. Delayed visual loss is potentially reversible, and it is presumably due to edema or ischemia within the canal or compression from an evolving orbital subperiosteal hematoma.

Nerves of Oculomotion

The nerves of oculomotion are discussed together due to their related function regarding the control of the movement of the eyes, as explained before. Lesions of these nerves may occur in isolation or in association with these and other cranial nerves. Blunt trauma is the mechanism responsible for most of the injuries. The incidence of lesions to these nerves is unclear, but it is considered that these lesions are not as frequent as with the other cranial nerves.[4] It has been reported that the third and sixth nerves are each injured more often than the fourth, but injuries in the latter nerve tend to be more frequently irreversible.[4] In one large series, the incidence of injury to these nerves due to cranial injuries was reported to be responsible for up to 25% of all cases of paralysis.[4]

III—Oculomotor Nerve

Paralysis of the oculomotor nerve is a well-recognized syndrome characterized by palpebral ptosis; inability to rotate the involved eye upward, downward, and inward, with outward and slightly downward deviation of the eyeball; and a dilated, nonreactive pupil.[16] To assess the traumatic nature of primary third-nerve palsy, the following criteria are required: (1) the presence of a fixed, dilated pupil and involvement of the muscles innervated by the third cranial nerve from the very onset of the injury; (2) the absence of a relevant intracranial space–occupying lesion; (3) the disappearance of all evidence of central nervous system damage but persistent third-nerve palsy; and (4) no evidence of direct orbital injury, traumatic mydriasis, or blindness.[16,17] The principal temptation is overdiagnosis of oculomotor nerve paresis in the face of concomitant orbital trauma. The possibility of recovery depends on the exact anatomic lesion and not on the ophthalmologic findings in the acute phase of the palsy. The recovery of this nerve has ranged from 0% to close to 75%.[16]

IV—Trochlear Nerve

Palsies of the trochlear nerve are rarely diagnosed early. As lethargy improves, the patient complains of vertical diplopia on looking downward. Examination shows one eye to be slightly higher, especially on gaze down and in. The most common mistake in diagnosing a trochlear nerve palsy is overlooking lesser paresis of the opposite fourth nerve. The recovery of deficits in this nerve depends on the severity of cranial injuries, and a wide range of deficits have been reported in the literature, with the worst prognosis being for bilateral palsy.[18]

VI—Abducens Nerve

Minor degrees of lateral rectus limitation are ambiguous after brain injury, and patient cooperation is necessary to establish a diagnosis of sixth-nerve palsy. However, the discovery of a sixth-nerve palsy in a person with severe brain injury is usually a delayed finding. Although bilateral third-nerve palsies are rare, bilateral fourth- and sixth-nerve pareses are common and may even be confused with each other in a stuporous patient who exhibits esotropia (strabismus in which there is a manifest deviation of the visual axis of an eye toward that of the other eye, resulting in diplopia) on downward gaze.[4]

Careful examination of the patient with brain injury is of paramount importance to make the correct diagnosis of injury to these nerves. Cooperation of the patient, when possible, is of utmost importance in a patient with diplopia. Computed tomography (CT) should be done on all severe brain injuries. It may be useful to elucidate whether a third-nerve palsy was immediate due to direct injury or delayed due to tentorial herniation; it may also reveal a preexisting intracranial pathology affecting one of these nerves. In the same manner, CT and magnetic resonance imaging (MRI) are useful in sorting out the cause of delayed diplopia.

Initial treatment of diplopia consists of patching the involved eye for comfort. As mentioned before, recovery may occur spontaneously depending on the degree of the brain injury. Surgery of the extraocular muscles is usually delayed 9 to 12 months or until diplopia has been stable for 6 months.[4] Surgery aims to eliminate diplopia in the forward and the downward reading positions[19] and can be very helpful for persisting trochlear palsies, less so for abducens pareses, and sometimes of benefit with third-nerve damage.

V—Trigeminal Nerve

Branches of the trigeminal cranial nerve are frequently injured by facial laceration and fractures.[4] One of the most common causes of maxillary nerve injury is an orbital floor blowout fracture.[20] The gasserian ganglion and the trigeminal trunk are rarely involved in closed brain injuries. When an injury to this nerve occurs, it is usually associated with other cranial nerves, especially VI and VII.[4] The symptoms are usually the loss of sensation and numbness of the area of the trigeminal nerve. No treatment is indicated.

VII—Facial Nerve

Because of its long, tortuous course through the temporal bone, the facial nerve is especially vulnerable to penetrating or blunt cranial trauma. The result of these injuries is the paralysis of facial expression. The majority of these injuries are caused by penetrating trauma,[4,21] and the reported incidence of facial nerve paralysis is approximately 20%[21] of all cranial nerve injuries. Blunt trauma to the facial nerve can be caused by objects entering the middle ear and exposing the horizontal segment of the facial nerve.[4] However, injury to this nerve is associated most frequently with basal skull fractures involving the temporal bone. Temporal bone fractures usually are classified as longitudinal or transverse with respect to the long axis of the temporal bone. Seventy percent to 80% of temporal bone fractures are longitudinal, and 10% to 30% are transverse.[22,23] Most cases of facial paralysis secondary to temporal bone fracture are caused by longitudinal fractures, with an incidence of 10% to 20% of these fractures.[23,24] Facial palsy is associated with 40% to 50% of transverse temporal bone fractures, but this type of fracture is less frequent than the longitudinal.

The tympanic and mastoid segments are the areas frequently involved in a facial nerve injury secondary to gunshot wounds. Middle-ear disruption and conductive hearing loss are the usual symptoms.[23]

Diagnostic Tests

Topographic Testing. Knowledge of the three major branches of the facial nerve within the temporal bone allows one to localize the site of the lesion within the fallopian canal.[25] Injuries of the vertical mastoid segment result in loss of taste on the ipsilateral anterior two thirds of the tongue. Lesions involving the horizontal segment within the middle ear produce loss of both the stapedius reflex and ipsilateral taste. The former is manifested by hypersensitivity to loud sounds. Finally, a lesion of the most proximal labyrinthine segment of the facial nerve results in impaired ipsilateral lacrimation in addition to the loss of the stapedius reflex and ipsilateral taste. Lesions within the internal auditory canal commonly involve both the seventh and eighth cranial nerves, so facial nerve symptoms are combined with hearing loss and vertigo.[4,25]

Electrical Stimulation. The Hilger stimulator is the most commonly used device for percutaneous electrical stimulation of the facial nerve. Absence of response on the involved side immediately after an injury may be evidence of a complete interruption of this nerve. The nerve may continue to stimulate for up to four days because the distal segment remains intact.[4] After a four-day waiting period, repeat percutaneous stimulation should provide a good estimate of the level of facial nerve function. If the involved side stimulates as well as the normal side, the prognosis is excellent for return of function. Absence of stimulation on the involved side after four days is an indicator of poor prognosis, and surgical evaluation may be indicated.

Imaging Studies. High-resolution CT with bone windows is the radiologic procedure of choice for evaluating injury to the temporal bone and skull base.[26] This test will reveal the involvement of any fracture or hematoma, suggesting the possible location of the nerve injury. The combination of this test and the above methods will increase the accuracy of the diagnosis of facial nerve injuries.

Treatment

In clean facial lacerations with immediate onset of facial paralysis, repair should be undertaken as soon as the patient's condition permits.[23] If repair cannot be accomplished within three days due to contamination, then three weeks becomes the theoretical optimal time for repair of extracranial nerve injury because of the dynamics of axonal regeneration, although this idea is not accepted universally.[23] As suggested earlier, if there is only partial paresis and the facial nerve stimulates after four days, the prognosis is good and the need for surgical intervention is unlikely.[4] The most clear-cut indication for surgery is a temporal bone fracture (especially transverse) with immediate onset of facial paralysis and electrical evidence of degeneration (on a nerve electrical stimulation test). This lesion is usually associated with severe loss of auditory and vestibular function as well.[4,23] The surgical approach for repair of the facial nerve depends on residual auditory function. If functional hearing remains in the involved ear, the nerve is explored and repaired by a transmastoid and middle-fossa approach. If hearing has been lost, repair is accomplished by a translabyrinthine approach.[4,23] Grafting of the facial nerve is a frequent technique used for injuries to this nerve and should be done as early as possible,[27] but repair even months after trauma can be successful if medically necessary.

Prophylactic eye care using artificial tears should be instituted in all patients with facial paralysis, regardless of whether they have adequate or inadequate tear production.[28] Further, the patient's eye should be taped closed with paper tape. Partial or complete tarsorrhaphy is often required in patients with permanent facial paralysis. A simple marginal lid adhesion tarsorrhaphy can easily be reversed if facial nerve function returns.[4]

With prolonged facial paralysis, electrical stimulation of the denervated muscles can help maintain tone and prevent contractures.[4] The muscles can also be massaged to relieve spasms and avoid contractures. As nerve function recovers, exercises can be performed in front of a mirror to aid in recovery of muscle function.[4]

VIII—Vestibulocochlear Nerve

Sensorineural hearing loss and vertigo, characteristic of inner-ear concussion, frequently accompany a longitudinal temporal bone fracture, but the bony labyrinth is rarely fractured.[4] Damage to the eighth cranial nerve is infrequent. Transverse fractures of the temporal bone are commonly associated with damage to both the seventh and the eighth cranial nerves. Because the tympanic membrane remains intact, bleeding is usually confined to the middle ear, where it can be seen through the intact membrane. Auditory and vestibular symptoms frequently follow cranial injury that does not result in temporal bone fracture. The absence of associated brainstem symptoms and signs and the usual rapid improvement in symptoms following this labyrinthine concussion support a peripheral localization of the lesion.[4] Sudden deafness following an insult to the cranium without associated vestibular symptoms is often partially or completely reversible.

The most common neurologic sequela of brain injury is benign positional vertigo. The conscious patient develops sudden brief attacks of vertigo and nystagmus precipitated by changes of head position such as turning over in bed, getting in and out of bed, bending over and straightening up, and reaching for an object on a high shelf.[29] The attacks of vertigo last for less than a minute, but the patient is then left with a more nonspecific dizziness along with nausea and imbalance. The mechanism of posttraumatic positional vertigo is thought to result from dislodgment of calcium carbonate crystals from the macula of the utricle, causing the crystals to become attached to the cupula of the posterior semicircular canal.[4] The prognosis is good: most spontaneous remissions occur within three months, and almost all patients have remissions within two years of the cranial injury. Subsequent recurrences are not infrequent.

The first step in evaluating a patient who develops dizziness or hearing loss immediately after a cranial injury is a careful examination of the external auditory canal and tympanic membrane. Laceration of the tympanic membrane with blood in the external auditory canal is common with a longitudinal fracture of the temporal bone, whereas hemotympanum is often seen with a transverse fracture.[4] Audiometric examination can help document the magnitude of hearing loss and site of the lesion. As in the case of the facial nerve, the radiologic procedure of choice for evaluating injury to the temporal bone and skull base is CT.

There is no specific treatment for sensorineural hearing loss owing to temporal bone injury unless there is evidence of a perilymph fistula. Damage to the vestibular apparatus results in acute symptoms with gradual improvement as central compensation occurs. Symptomatic treatment of vertigo is helpful initially, and the conscious patient is encouraged to begin vestibular exercises as soon as possible to accelerate the compensation process.[4] Posttraumatic positional vertigo, like other varieties of benign positional vertigo, responds to positional exercises.[30]

Vagal System: Glossopharyngeal (IX), Vagus (X), Spinal Accessory (XI), and Hypoglossal (XII) Nerves

The lower cranial nerves will be discussed together because lesions to these nerves secondary to injury are rare. When injury occurs, the primary dysfunction is alterations in swallowing, speech, and airway protection.[31] The styloid process, under cover of the tympanic plate of the temporal bone, defines a space opposite the first cervical vertebra. The ninth, tenth, eleventh, and twelth cranial nerves pass through this gap, about 1 cm wide, and these are vulnerable to injury that affects the styloid process.[32] A compression neuropathy of the cranial nerves passing through this space may result in dysphagia.[33] Injury to the lower cranial nerves is rare and occurs more frequently with penetrating injury. Penetrating wounds to the neck may cause damage to the vagus or the hypoglossal nerve, producing dysphagia. Lesion to the spinal accessory nerve is not associated with dysphagia. Loss of trapezius function causes a severe shoulder disability, but loss of innervation to the sternocleidomastoid is rarely noticeable.[23]

The preferred assessment for patients with dysphagia associated with head and neck injury includes examination for a foreign body obstruction or anatomic lesion. The gag reflex should be examined, and any symmetry of palatal motion should be noted.[32] Indirect laryngoscopy of vocal cord function is appropriate. Endoscopy can be important in assessing nasal pharyngeal closure. Video fluoroscopy, however, may be necessary for diagnosis of those injuries that can cause pain and aspiration.[34] For patients with swallowing disorders associated with cranial injury, a speech/language pathologist is beneficial in teaching patients to become successful oral feeders. More than three months of therapy may be required. Surgical management of lesions to these nerves is usually unsuccessful or not indicated. Teaching dysphagic patients to swallow is the most important therapy, and rapid participation by the speech/language pathologist will allow these patients to regain the possibility of eating in a prompt manner.

MAXILLOFACIAL INJURIES

Maxillofacial injuries are common in this country. In the United States, the annual incidence of maxillofacial injuries requiring hospital treatment sustained by vehicle occupants involved in road traffic collisions has been estimated as 139 per 100,000 population. Stated differently, approximately 54% to 70% of motor vehicle injuries involve facial trauma.[35] It is common at all ages, but the causes are related directly to age, sex, and alcohol consumption.[36] A large review of maxillo-facial injuries found that the most common cause of soft tissue injury was falls, whereas for maxillofacial fractures, the most common cause was interpersonal violence. Falls accounted for most of the injuries in children and the elderly, whereas interpersonal violence was mainly responsible for injuries occurring in patients aged 15 to 50 years.

Maxillofacial injury is frequently found in patients suffering from severe brain injury. The incidence of closed head injury with facial fractures has been reported to be from around 17% up to 50%.[37–39] and a significant number are considered severe.[37]

The face is divided into three regions: the upper region, including the frontal bones and sinuses; the middle region, including the orbits, nasal bones, zygoma, and maxilla; and the lower region, consisting of the mandible.[40] Soft tissue injury of the face is common and may vary from a minor abrasion to destruction of most of the face.[41] Although extremely distracting during resuscitation and stabilization of the patient, most soft tissue injury is not life threatening and should be dealt with after the airway, respiratory, cardiovascular, and neurologic systems are evaluated and stabilized. Bleeding is one of the most dangerous findings associated with these types of injuries, and its prompt control is important during the initial phases of the management of these patients. The cheek is the area of the face lacerated most frequently. Deep structures of concern include the facial nerve, parotid gland, and parotid duct.[41]

Facial fractures can be life threatening when the airway is compromised. The reported incidence of these fractures varies in the literature.[41–43] Fractures of the midface are the most common, including the zygoma, orbital floor, nasal bones, and maxilla. In a classic paper, Le Fort describes specific types of facial fractures of the maxilla along lines of bone weakness.[44,45] These fractures are rarely encountered in clinical practice. The mandible is frequently fractured in trauma to the face. It is important to point out that fractures of the mandible and maxilla, Le Fort II and III, are frequently associated with obstruction of the airway. Also, severe fractures of the maxilla and the orbit are more often associated with brain injury (Figures 4–11 and 4–12).

MANAGEMENT OF MAXILLOFACIAL INJURIES

General Management

The initial management of the patient with severe brain injury and maxillofacial injury follows the guidelines established by the American College of Surgeons in the Advanced Trauma Life Support Program. Establishment of an adequate airway is the first priority.[45] Asphyxia due to upper-airway obstruction is a major

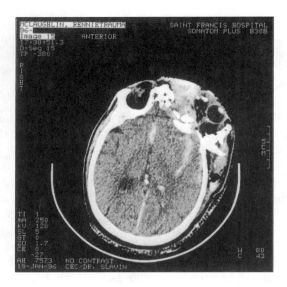

Figure 4–11 CT scan of a patient with extracranial injury with orbital fracture and optic nerve injury.

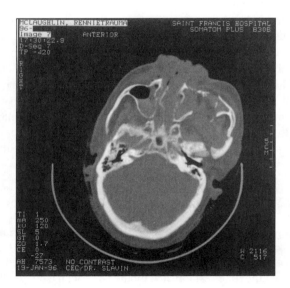

Figure 4–12   Same patient as in Figure 4–11, but with additional maxillary sinus and zygomatic fracture.

cause of death from facial injuries.[40] The airway may be compromised by mechanical obstruction from several sources. Fractures of the mandible and maxilla can cause compromise by posterior displacement of bony fragments or attached soft tissue into the pharynx. Airway management of the patient with maxillofacial injuries must be performed in a manner that will not compromise the integrity of the cervical spine. Multiple studies have shown a 10% to 20% association of cervical spine injury in the multiply traumatized patient with maxillofacial injury.[47,48] Endotracheal intubation is the usual and preferred method for securing an airway. It should be performed using the oral route. If intubation is unsuccessful or inadvisable secondary to the nature of the injury present, establishment of a surgical airway (cricothyroidotomy) in the neck is necessary without hesitation.

Breathing and circulation are the next priority. Significant bleeding associated with severe facial injuries is generally controlled with pressure or packing. If these measures fail to control bleeding, ligation of the internal maxillary or carotid artery may be required. Control of bleeding may be accomplished via surgery or angiographic embolization.

A quick neurologic evaluation includes examination of the pupils and assessment of the mental status of the patient. Movement of the extremities is noted. A patient with significant facial injuries should undergo a CT of the brain after the secondary assessment (detailed examination from head to toes) is completed in most cases if no other life-threatening injury is identified. This should proceed despite a normal initial neurologic examination.

Exposure of the patient is completed and a secondary survey from head to toes is carried out after the primary survey is completed. Palpation of all facial bones should be performed, feeling for step-off or tenderness suggestive of bony disruption, or soft tissue crepitus suggestive of sinus fracture. Examination of the mandible includes examination of the temporomandibular joint with the jaw in both open and closed positions. Finally, the examiner should examine for maxillary fracture: one hand is placed on the frontal bone to stabilize the head, while the examiner attempts to rock the maxilla by firmly grasping and exerting pressure on the upper alveolar ridge. Extraocular movement and facial muscle movement are assessed. Cerebrospinal fluid leak is associated in fractures of the cribriform plate or nasal bones. A high index of suspicion for associated intracranial injury is of utmost importance in this situation.

Radiologic Evaluation

Establishing the fracture configuration of craniofacial trauma in three dimensions is essential to the primary successful management of midface and upper-face injuries.[49] CT has replaced plain facial films because of a better definition of the type of bony injuries. MRI has been used recently in the diagnosis of craniofacial injury, but it has not shown a major advantage over CT scan. Axial CT views of the cranium and face significantly enhance the surgeon's ability to locate sites of fracture and contribute to the preliminary diagnosis of craniofacial injuries. Scanning of the facial bones should be completed at the same time that the cranium is imaged if the patient's general condition does not preclude a more extended CT scan examination. When orbital volume changes are suspected or naso-orbital-ethmoid fractures are diagnosed, coronal CT scans can be used to facilitate three-dimensional representation or reconstruction of the fractures, provided that the neck is stable and the patient is cooperative.

Specific Management

As previously mentioned, the initial goals in the management of maxillofacial trauma are to establish and maintain a patent airway and to correct any insult to the respiratory, cardiovascular, or neurologic system. The secondary goals are (1) to reestablish the integrity of the facial bones and their relationship to each other, thus restoring appearance and facial structure and function; (2) to reestablish normal ocular movement; (3) to reestablish previous dental occlusion; (4) to ensure closure that maximizes healing and minimizes scarring; (5) to prevent wound infections; and (6) to provide psychologic support to the patient.[41]

It has been clearly established that most of the secondary goals mentioned above can be achieved with good anatomic reduction of most of the fractures. Knowing the fracture configuration of the craniofacial injury by the appropriate radiologic test is of utmost importance. The development of techniques for repair of these injuries using open reduction and internal fixation of many of the maxillofacial fractures has been a tremendous advance in reestablishing a distorted anatomy. The different techniques and special treatment of the diverse fractures of the maxillofacial area are beyond the scope of this chapter. However, a few important aspects are important to emphasize in the management of maxillofacial trauma when it is related to severe brain injury.

Timing of the Repair

The old tenet of waiting several days after maxillofacial fractures to allow facial edema to subside has been challenged by several authors in recent years. It is accepted that early fixation should be done when possible to achieve better results and faster recovery.[37,50–54] There are several advantages of early fixation. First, early fixation allows easier manipulation and better alignment of fracture fragments.[55] Second, a multiply injured patient may develop complications that are unrelated to his or her craniofacial injuries such as pneumonia, acute respiratory distress syndrome, or sepsis. These complications often prevent or increase the risk of a subsequent trip to the operating room.[50] Third, there is some evidence that early fixation may reduce infection and hospital stay.[54] One of the problems of early repair is its definition. In the literature, early repair of maxillofacial injuries has been reported from the day of admission up to two weeks after the injury.[56] Most plastic surgeons in a recent survey agreed that a facial fracture should be repaired within two weeks. However, there is evidence that there is no need to wait the traditional 7 to 10 days for resolution of edema, and it may be advantageous for the patient to receive definitive treatment as soon as possible or after stabilization of life-threatening injuries.

Another controversial issue regarding the management of craniofacial injuries is the optimal timing in the presence of severe intracranial injury. We have mentioned the frequent association of brain injury with maxillofacial trauma. The traditional philosophy has been to delay definite treatment of these injuries until stabilization of a severe brain injury. The reasons for this are not clear but are related to the risk of raising the intracranial pressure.[54,57] A recent study found no difference of outcome in patients treated early despite severe brain injury.[54] The general recommendation, until more convincing evidence arises, is delayed treatment in the patient with severe brain injury showing a Glasgow Coma Scale score less than 8, intracranial hemorrhage with midline shift, basal cistern effacement, or an intracranial pressure greater than 15 mm Hg. Definitive treatment should be delayed until there is no evidence of neurologic deterioration. However, all attempts to accomplish this treatment within two weeks of the injury should be made.

The last aspect of treatment to consider in a patient with maxillofacial injury is the use of angiography. Angiography is important in the patient who has uncontrollable bleeding associated with maxillofacial injury. Embolization may be proved lifesaving when used in these patients.[57] Angiography should be used when vascular injury is suspected, especially in gunshot wounds to the maxillofacial area.[58–60]

BLUNT INJURY TO THE CAROTID ARTERY

Blunt injury to the internal carotid artery is an uncommon clinical entity, accounting for less than 3% of all carotid injuries.[61] This type of injury can be associated with severe brain injury, but in several cases its diagnosis is delayed when the alteration of mental status is attributed to a possible intracranial injury and when the carotid injury is not suspected initially. Early diagnosis and prompt treatment are imperative to prevent the severe permanent neurologic complications that can result from the thrombosis and embolism that occur with blunt carotid injuries.[61,62]

Understanding the pathophysiology of this injury requires a knowledge of the anatomic relationship of the carotid artery to its surrounding structures. The common carotid artery ascends in the neck medial to the internal jugular vein and normally has no branches.[63] The bifurcation is usually located at the level of the superior border of the thyroid cartilage. Variations in the levels at which the carotid bifurcates are more often above this position than below. The common carotid is in close relationship to the internal jugular vein and the vagus nerve. The location of the injuries to the carotid artery that are potentially related to neurologic sequelae are at the level of the carotid artery, near the bifurcation, and at different levels of the internal carotid artery. We have to remember that more than 90% of the cranial blood flow is provided by the carotid arteries via the internal carotid. Bilateral lesions will produce ischemia of the brain tissue if not recognized early. Unilateral injuries may not cause neurologic symptoms due to flow provided by the contralateral side via the circle of Willis, but this type of communication provides adequate flow to the contralateral side in only 20% of normal individuals.[64] The lack of contralateral blood flow in the majority of patients makes recognition of unilateral carotid injuries equally important to prevent adverse complications.

The internal carotid artery ascends in the neck ventral to the longissimus capitis muscle and the transverse process of the upper cervical vertebrae. With severe hyperextension and contralateral rotation of the head, the carotid artery is stretched over the bony lateral articular process of the atlas and axis. In the majority of these cases, the initial defect of the artery is an intimal tear that can lead to the formation of a thrombus. Propagation of this thrombus either proximally or distally could totally occlude the common carotid artery, the internal carotid artery, or its branches, leading to severe neurologic sequelae or death. The treatment of this condition is anticoagulation therapy, starting with heparin IV and continuing with oral anticoagulation for three to six months.

The diagnosis of carotid injury requires a high index of suspicion. Patients who sustain severe hyperextension of the neck, such as motorcycle accident victims and persons ejected from cars, are at a high risk to have carotid injury. If there is alteration in the mental status or if the patient is unconscious and a CT scan of the brain is normal, carotid injury should be suspected. Despite the awareness of this injury, the diagnosis of most carotid injuries is delayed several hours or, more commonly, days after the injury. The procedure considered as a gold standard is the angiography. Recently, Doppler ultrasonography has been proposed to be as accurate as the angiography, with the advantage of being less invasive. However, angiography is still recommended in patients in whom carotid injury is highly suspected, with ultrasonography reserved as a screening method.

Angiography is recommended in patients with carotid injuries because of the type of lesions that can occur besides the intimal tear and thrombosis of the artery. Pseudoaneurysms may occur if there is disruption of the media and the adventitia.[61–64] The treatment of this condition is resection, with reconstruction of the artery if possible. In cases where the pseudoaneurysm is intracranial, balloon catheter occlusion of the internal carotid artery orifice of the pseudoaneurysm and ligation of the proximal cervical carotid artery is the treatment of choice. Carotid cavernous fistula results when the integrity of the cavernous portion of the carotid artery has been disrupted, creating an abnormal communication between the high-pressure arterial system and the low-pressure venous system. The signs of this condition are an audible bruit, pulsation of the orbit, chemosis (excessive edema of the conjunctiva), diplopia, visual disturbance, headaches, and exophthalmos.[61] The use of a detachable latex balloon to occlude the fistula while the carotid blood flow is maintained is the recommended treatment.

In summary, blunt carotid injury is an uncommon entity, with higher incidence in those victims for whom the mechanism of the accident involves hyperextension of the neck. The diagnosis of this entity requires a high index of suspicion. Any patient with unexplained neurologic abnormality or deterioration, especially with a normal CT scan of the brain, should raise the possibility of embolic and/or ischemic events secondary to carotid artery injury and should prompt four-vessel cranial arteriography. The most common injury is an intimal tear of the carotid, and the recommended treatment is anticoagulation. The use of intra-arterial devices and surgery may be necessary to treat pseudoaneurysms or carotid cavernous fistulas.

REFERENCES

1. Martinez-Martinez PFA. *Neuroanatomy, Development, and Structure of the Central Nervous System.* Philadelphia, Pa: WB Saunders Co; 1982:164.

2. Duus P. *Topical Diagnosis in Neurology: Anatomy, Physiology, Signs, Symptoms.* New York, NY: Thieme Medical Publishers Inc; 1989:85.

3. Nolte J. *The Human Brain: An Introduction to Its Functional Anatomy.* 3rd ed. St. Louis, Mo: Mosby Year Book; 1993:208.

4. Keane JR, Baloh RW. Posttraumatic cranial neuropathies. *Neurol Clin.* 1992;10:849–867.

5. Rush JA, Younge BR. Paralysis of cranial nerves III, IV and VI: cause and prognosis in 1000 cases. *Arch Ophthalmol.* 1981;99:76–79.

6. Zusho H. Posttraumatic anosmia. *Arch Otolaryngol.* 1982;108:90–92.

7. Jafek BW, Eller PM, Esses BA, Moran DT. Post-traumatic anosmia: ultrastructural correlates. *Arch Neurol.* 1989;46:300–304.

8. Keane JR. Blindness from self-inflicted gunshot wounds. *J Clin Neuro Ophthalmol.* 1986;6:247–249.

9. Gross CE, DeKock JR, Panje WR, Hershkowitz N, et al. Evidence for orbit deformation that may contribute to monocular blindness following minor frontal head trauma. *J Neurosurg.* 1981; 55:963–966.

10. Kline LB, Morawetz RB, Swaid SN. Indirect injury of the optic nerve. *Neurosurgery.* 1984;14:756–764.

11. Lessell S. Indirect optic nerve trauma. *Arch Ophthalmol.* 1989;107:382–386.

12. Savino PJ, Glaser JS, Schatz NJ. Traumatic chiasmal syndrome. *Neurology.* 1980;30:963–970.

13. Keane JR. Retinal hemorrhage: its significance in 100 patients with acute encephalopathy of unknown cause. *Arch Neurol.* 1979;36:691–694.

14. Bracken MB, Shepard MJ, Collins WF, Holford TR, et al. A randomized, controlled trial of methylprednisolone or nalozone in the treatment of acute spinal-cord injury. *N Engl J Med.* 1990;322:1405–1411.

15. Fujitani T, Inoue K, Takahashi T, Ikushima K, et al. Indirect traumatic optic neuropathy: visual outcome of operative and non-operative cases. *Jpn J Ophthalmol.* 1986;30:125–134.

16. Kruger M, Noel P, Ectors P. Bilateral primary traumatic oculomotor nerve palsy. *J Trauma.* 1986;26:1151.

17. Solomons NB, Solomon DJ, De Villiers JC. Direct traumatic third nerve palsy. *S Afr Med J.* 1980;58:109–111.

18. Keane JR. Fourth nerve palsy: historical review and study of 215 patients. *Neurology.* 1993;43:2439–2443.

19. Sabates NR, Gonce MA, Farris BK. Neuro-ophthalmological findings in closed head trauma. *J Clin Neuro Ophthalmol.* 1991;11:273–277.

20. Greenwald HS Jr, Keeney AH, Shannon GM. A review of 128 patients with orbital fractures. *Am J Ophthalmol.* 1974;78:655–664.

21. Williams MJ. Blunt trauma leading to facial nerve paralysis. *J Emerg.* 1991;9(suppl 1):27–28.

22. Cannon CR, Jahrsdoerfer RA. Temporal bone fractures. *Arch Otolaryngol.* 1983;109:285–288.

23. Adkins WY, Osguthorpe JD. Management of trauma of the facial nerve. *Otolaryngol Clin North Am.* 1991;24:587–611.

24. Hasso AN, Ledington JA. Traumatic injuries of the temporal bone. *Otolaryngol Clin North Am.* 1988;21:295–316.

25. Dobie RA. Electrical and topognostic tests of the facial nerve. In: Cummings CW, ed. *Otolaryngology: Head and Neck Surgery.* Vol 4. St Louis, Mo: CV Mosby; 1986:2821.

26. Kinney SE. Trauma. In: Cummings CW, ed. *Otolaryngology: Head and Neck Surgery.* Vol 4. St Louis, Mo: CV Mosby; 1986:3033.

27. Barrs DM. Facial nerve trauma: optimal timing for repair. *Laryngoscope.* 1991;101:835–848.

28. Smith MF, Goode RL. Eye protection in the paralyzed face. *Laryngoscope.* 1979;89:435–442.

29. Baloh RW, Honrubia V, Jacobson K. Benign positional vertigo: clinical and oculographic features in 240 cases. *Neurology.* 1987;37:371–378.

30. Brandt T, Daroff RB. Physical therapy for benign paroxysmal positional vertigo. *Arch Otolaryngol.* 1980;106:484–485.

31. Netterville JL, Civantos FJ. Rehabilitation of cranial nerve deficits after neurotologic skull base surgery. *Laryngoscope.* 1993;103(suppl 60):45–54.

32. Smoot EC III, Konrad HR. Dysphagia associated with head and neck trauma: report of a case. *J Oral Maxillofac Surg.* 1989;47:190–194.

33. Haidar Z, Kalamchi S. Painful dysphagia due to fracture of the styloid process. *Oral Surg Oral Med Oral Path.* 1980;49:5–6.

34. Lazarus C, Logemann JA. Swallowing disorders in closed head trauma patients. *Arch Phys Med Rehabil.* 1987;68:79–84.

35. Karlson TA. The incidence of hospital-treated facial injuries from vehicles. *J Trauma.* 1982;22:303–310.

36. Hussain K, Wijetunge DB, Grubnic S. Jackson CT. A comprehensive analysis of craniofacial trauma. *J Trauma.* 1994;36:34–47.

37. Haug RH, Savage JD, Likavec MJ, Conforti PJ. A review of 100 closed head injuries associated with facial fractures *J Oral Maxillofac Surg.* 1992;50:218–221.

38. Derdyn C, Persing JA, Broaddus WC, Delashaw JB. Craniofacial trauma: an assessment of risk related to timing of surgery. *J Plastic Reconstr Surg.* 1990;86:238–245.

39. Sinclair D, Scwartz M, Gruss J, McLellan B. A retrospective review of the relationship between facial fractures, head injuries, and cervical spine injuries. *J Emerg Med.* 1988;6:109–112.

40. Shepperd SM, Lippe MS. Maxillofacial trauma: evaluation and management by the emergency physician. *Emerg Med Clin North Am.* 1987;5:371–392.

41. Lower J. Maxillofacial trauma. *Nurs Clin North Am.* 1986;21:611–628

42. Scherer M, Sullivan WG, Smith DJ Jr, Phillips LG. An analysis of 1,423 facial fractures in 788 patients at an urban trauma center. *J Trauma.* 1989;29:388–390.

43. Marciani RD. Management of midface fractures: fifty years later. *J Oral Maxillofac Surg.* 1993;51:960–968.

44. Le Fort R. Experimental study of fractures of the upper jaw: parts I and II. *Plast Reconstr Surg.* 1972;50:497–506.

45. Le Fort R. Experimental study of fractures of the upper jaw: part III. *Plast Reconstr Surg.* 1972;50:600–607.

46. American College of Surgeons. *Resources for Optimal Care of the Injured Patient.* Chicago, Ill: American College of Surgeons; 1993.

47. Bertolami CN, Kaban LB. Chin trauma: a clue to associated mandibular and cervical spine injury. *Oral Surg Oral Med Oral Pathol.* 1982;53:122–126.

48. Lewis V, Manson PN, Morgan RF, Cerullo RJ. Facial injuries associated with cervical fractures: recognition, patterns and management *J Trauma.* 1985;25:90–93.

49. Marciani RD, Gonty AA. Principles of management of complex craniofacial trauma. *J Oral Maxillofac Surg.* 1993 51:535–542.

50. Brandt KE, Burruss GL, Hickerson WL, et al. The management of mid-face fractures with intracranial injury. *J Trauma.* 1991;31:15–19.

51. Conforti PJ, Haug RH, Likavec M. Management of closed head injury in the patient with maxillofacial trauma. *J Oral Maxillofac Surg.* 1993;51:298–303.

52. Piotrowski WP. The primary treatment of frontobasal and midfacial fractures in patients with head injuries. *J Oral Maxillofac Surg.* 1992;50:1264–1268.

53. Heine RD, Catone GA, Bavitz JB, et al. Naso-orbital ethmoid injury: report of a case and review of the literature. *Oral Surg Oral Med Oral Pathol.* 1990;69:542.

54. Chang C, Chen Y, Noordhoff MS, et al. Maxillary involvement in central craniofacial fractures with associated head injuries. *J Trauma* 1994;37:807.

55. Gruss JS, Phillips JH. Complex facial trauma: the evolving role of rigid fixation and immediate bone graft reconstruction. *Clin Plast Surg.* 1989;16 93.

56. Thaller SR, Kawamoto HK. Care of maxillofacial injuries: survey of plastic surgeons. *Plast Reconstr Surg.* 1992;90:568.

57. Wenig BL. Management of panfacial fractures. *Otolaryngol Clin North Am.* 1991;24:93.

58. Ardekian L, Samet N, Shoshani Y, et al. Life-threatening bleeding following maxillofacial trauma. *J Craniomaxillofac Surg.* 1993;21:336.

59. Cohen MA, Boyes-Varley G. Penetrating injuries to the maxillofacial region. *J Oral Maxillofac Surg.* 1986;44:197.

60. Thorne CH. Gunshot wounds to the face: current concepts. *Clin Plast Surg.* 1992;19:223.

61. Welling RE, Saul TG, Tew JM, Tomsick TA, et al. Management of blunt injury to the internal carotid artery. *J Trauma.* 1987;27:1221–1226.

62. Fabian TC, George SM, Croce MA, Mangiante EC, et al. Carotid artery trauma: management based on mechanism of injury. *J Trauma.* 1990;30:953–963.

63. Wind GG, Valentine RJ. Carotid arteries. In: Wind GG, Valentine RJ, eds. *Anatomic Exposures in Vascular Surgery.* Baltimore, Md: Williams & Wilkins; 1991:490.

64. Fry RE, Fry WJ. Extracranial carotid artery injuries. *Surgery.* 1980;88:581–586.

CHAPTER 5

Implications of Patient Data and Use of Technology

Health care providers working with patients with severe brain injury must have a thorough understanding of brain injury and its management, secondary insults to the brain, deterioration and stabilization, factors that may affect intervention, and the equipment used for treating and monitoring the patient. The patient with severe brain injury commonly has injuries to multiple systems; therefore, many specialists are consulted to care for this patient. Extensive workup, multiple procedures, and various equipment may be necessary to stabilize and monitor the patient with a brain injury. Secondary trauma, such as hypoxia or hypotension, may have been sustained at the scene of the accident, en route to the hospital, or after arrival at the hospital. The health care providers must also understand the impact of injuries and functional alterations in other systems on the brain and the patient.

IMPLICATIONS OF PATIENT DATA

Information in the chart of a trauma patient should be well documented, allowing team members a complete understanding of the patient's condition. Information regarding the systems that sustained injury, what the injuries were, and how much secondary, as well as initial trauma, the brain has sustained is important in treating this patient population, not only in the intensive care unit (ICU), but during the entire hospitalization, and in making recommendations for posthospital discharge and rehabilitation needs. The team must know the patient's history and medical condition from the time of the injury until critical care intervention begins in the ICU, and then throughout the patient's ICU course.

The medical record contains demographic information, evaluations done by the emergency medical service (EMS) providers and the emergency department (ED), consults, history and physical notes, admission notes, physician progress notes, laboratory and test results, and surgical, X-ray, and other procedural reports. Within this documentation, pertinent information includes

- mechanism of injury
- patient status
  1. initial evaluations in the field and in the ED
  2. identification and treatment of life-threatening injuries
  3. identification and treatment of complications
  4. identification and treatment of non–life-threatening injuries
- past medical history

Within the first 24 hours, life-threatening injuries should have been assessed and treatment initiated. Identification and treatment of other injuries and complications should occur as early as 48 hours after admission. As complications arise, equipment and medications may vary. Lesser injuries may be discovered during assessment by the intensivist or during routine nursing care or rehabilitation sessions.

Documentation of all information from the accident until the time that the physician, nurse, therapist, or other team member enters the patient's room is necessary for the caregivers to understand the extent of injury to the brain and to other systems that may affect the brain. When patients are transferred from outlying hospitals, thorough documentation should be present in the chart regarding the initial responder's findings and treatment, the initial ED's findings and treatment, and information during transport to the receiving hospital. Additionally, all events that occurred in the ED, radiology department, surgical suite, and ICU must be documented for a complete profile of the patient. Initial information regarding the patient's status during resuscitation is necessary to have an understanding of the extent of the injuries the patient sustained. For example, a patient that becomes responsive with fluid resuscitation may not have sustained a severe brain injury and may instead have been hypovolemic.

It is therefore imperative to do a thorough chart review, reviewing information from the scene of the accident, the trauma room, the operating room, and the ICU. The chart review may be time consuming, but it should always be completed before assessing the patient to obtain a clear picture of the patient's condition.

Mechanism of Injury

The reader begins the chart review by discerning the mechanism of injury. The ambulance "run sheet" has valuable information on this subject. The patient may have been injured by a fall; involved in a motor vehicle, pedestrian, motorcycle, bicycle, all-terrain vehicle, roller-skating or rollerblading accident; assaulted with an object; or involved in a fight. The mechanism of injury has a direct impact on the degree and severity of injuries sustained. The use of restraints alters the potential injuries that a driver or passenger can receive. Air bags in combination with proper use of seat belts create the potential for different injuries than those sustained by an air bag alone. The professional, when reading the description of the collision in the chart, should be aware of the types of injuries the patient may have sustained, including any intrusion into the interior compartment, and the use of safety equipment.

Motor Vehicle Collisions

Frontal Collision. Studies have determined that use of seat belts and air bags saves lives,[1-3] especially in frontal collisions. Lap belt use prevents driver or passenger ejection. Abdominal and chest injuries, as well as head and brain injuries, may still occur to the driver as a result of steering wheel impact, but the severity of the injury is reduced. Additional injuries from lap belt use include lumbar spine fractures (Chance fracture) and intestinal injuries, referred to as the "seat belt syndrome.[3-6]

Three-point restraints (lap belt and shoulder restraint) have decreased life-threatening injuries and lifelong disability.[3-7] The development of the automatic shoulder belt in recent years creates new problems when individuals do not wear the corresponding lap belt. Use of the shoulder restraint alone creates the potential for rib, sternal, and clavicle fractures; chest trauma; intra-abdominal injuries; and cervical spine fractures.[3] Injuries that may be sustained when the occupant is wearing a shoulder and lap restraint include rib fracture, chest contusions, abrasions, and cervical strains.[3-7]

In collisions in which the engine or the frame of the car intrudes into the passenger compartment, more extensive injuries occur. Frontal collisions with intrusion into the interior compartment decrease the effectiveness of restraints as parts of the interior of the vehicle, such as the steering wheel or dash, strike the person. Intrathoracic injuries, including pneumothorax, hemothorax, and diaphragmatic tears and intra-abdominal injuries (eg. spleen, liver injuries), may occur. Lower-extremity injuries also occur frequently in frontal collisions, regardless of the type of restraint used.[8] Intrusion into the interior compartment is not necessary for these fractures to occur. When the engine is forced into the occupant area, however, more severe lower-extremity injuries, including fractures, dislocations, and open wounds, do occur.[9]

Air bags are effective in frontal collisions if no further impact on the vehicle occurs. Injuries that may be identified in persons not restrained but protected by air bag deployment are cervical or thoracic fractures and possibly right atrial tear. These injuries are considered to be the result of the body's flexing on impact and then the air bag's inflating. Air bag inflation has been measured at between 98 and

211 mph.[10] The person's height dictates how close to the air bag compartment he or she sits. Persons 5 foot 3 inches or shorter are more susceptible to severe injuries from the deployment of the air bag because of their close proximity to the steering wheel for visibility and control access. Subdural hematomas, cerebral edema, cardiac rupture, cardiac perforation, fractures of the upper extremities, and ocular trauma may result from contact with the air bag module (cover over the air bag).[11] Additionally, eye injuries may be sustained from the inflation of the air bag, whether additional restraints are used or not.[10,11] In multiple-impact collisions, the air bag is ineffective after its initial deployment. The person not restrained will have multiple injuries in this collision.

Rollover Collisions. Three-point restraints provide the greatest protection in rollover collisions. The support lessens the impact on objects within the passenger compartment. With shoulder restraints alone, there is an increased likelihood that the person may slip under the restraint or be caught at the neck or chin, sustaining severe cervical spine and neck injuries. Lap belts alone allow the upper body and head to flex and extend, creating the potential for further chest, neck, facial, and brain injuries to occur. The air bag offers no restraint of the person in rollover collisions.

Lateral Collisions. No restraint prevents severe injuries in lateral collisions. Severe brain injury can frequently occur with three-point restraint usage as a result of the head's striking the side of the car. Additionally, there is a higher incidence of pelvic injuries when intrusion into the occupant compartment occurs. Thoracic and abdominal injuries, including pneumothorax, hemothorax, and liver and spleen lacerations, occur more frequently with lateral collisions, especially when there is intrusion.[9]

Motorcycle Collisions

Use or nonuse of a helmet makes a difference in the injuries a person may sustain in a motorcycle collision. Severe brain injury is reduced with the use of helmets.[12,13] Craniofacial trauma is more common in nonhelmeted motorcyclists, with facial fractures three times more likely to occur in persons not wearing a helmet.[12] Orbit fractures are the most common facial fracture seen in motorcycle collisions.[14] Le Fort fractures are more common in persons not wearing helmets. Trunk injuries are also common in helmeted motorcyclists.[14] Cranial, brain, and neck injuries (including spinal cord injuries) are five to nine times more likely in nonhelmeted motorcyclists. Patients with rib fractures must also be suspect for liver, spleen, aorta, heart, and lung injuries. Spleen and liver injuries commonly occur together because of their close proximity.[14]

Injuries sustained in all-terrain vehicle collisions can be similar to those of motorcyclists, due to the speed possible at the time of the collision. The nonuse of helmets affects the severity of brain and facial injuries sustained by this group of riders as well.

Bicycle Injuries

Severe brain injury secondary to bicycling has been dramatically reduced with the use of helmets. In children, bicycling is the leading cause of recreational injuries.[15] Unhelmeted bicyclists sustain 39% to 86% more brain injuries than helmeted bicyclists.[15-19] Bicycle collisions with motor vehicles have a significantly higher rate of brain injury occurrence than collisions with other objects or falls from the bicycle.[18] Helmet use reduces the facial injuries sustained when a bicycle collides with a motor vehicle.[17,19] Injuries including those of the neck, extremities, and pelvic girdle still occur with persons wearing helmets.[19] Extremity and pelvic girdle injuries are the other most common injuries in bicycle collisions.[19] Fractures of the upper extremity are more common than fractures of the lower extremity, and neck fractures are the most common non–head/brain injury.[15]

Other Mechanisms of Injury

Pedestrian injuries vary according to the mechanism of injury. A low-velocity impact, such as pedestrian versus bicycle, may result in less severe injuries than a high-velocity impact, such as pedestrian versus motor vehicle. The risk of being thrown is also reduced in these situations. The higher the speed and force of impact, the greater the amount and severity of injury. With falls, the distance that the person fell should be identified, as well as the type of surface on which the person landed, the position he or she was in when found, and any objects the person may have hit or have been hit by.

Patient Status

"In-Field" Information

The EMS "run sheet" has valuable information regarding the person's initial status, including vital signs and neurologic signs; the timing of interventions; and any initial medical care completed (Exhibit 5–1). Prolonged extrication may indicate that medical interventions required for the patient's stabilization were delayed. The longer the time spent before arrival at the trauma center, the greater the chance for poor outcomes and severe disability in this population. The brain can tolerate ischemic blood flow for only a limited time before irreversible infarction occurs.[20] The concept of the "golden hour" reinforces the timely intervention and management of airway, breathing, and circulation. Likewise, it has been found that evacuating subdural hematomas within four hours significantly reduces the mortality and morbidity rate[21] with these patients.

Exhibit 5–1 An EMS "Run Sheet"

Ambulance "Run Sheet"

Name:		Dispatch:	Arrival:
Address:		Depart scene:	Arrive Hospital:

Complaint:

Mechanism of Injury:

Eye Opening	Verbal Response	Motor Response	Pupils	Vital Signs		
Spontaneous	Oriented	Follow commands	Equal	BP	BP	BP
Voice	Confused	Push away pain	Reactive	P	P	P
Pain	Inappropriate	Withdrawal	Non-reactive	R	R	R
None	Sounds only	Flex inappropriate	Dilated			
	None	Rigid extension	Constricted			
		None	Sluggish			

Skin:	Normal	Pale	Cyanotic	Diaphoretic	Hot	Cool	Jaundice
Chest sounds:	Clear	Rhonchi	Stridor	Rales	Wheezes	Decreased	Absent
Abdomen:	Normal	Obese	Rigid	Distended	Tender		

Procedures: Airway:

Cervical
  Collar:
Backboard:
Splints:

Oral
Nasal
Oxygen
Mouth to Mouth
Intubated: Oral
Nasal

CPR:

Collapsed time:
CPR Inititated:
CPR Stopped:

Medications/Response:

Physical Assessment:

Although agitation and confusion can be signs of brain injury, the reviewer should not automatically assume that the person sustained a brain injury when statements regarding such behavior are made in the report. A large percentage of persons involved in a trauma can be hypotensive or have elevated levels of alcohol or drugs in their systems that may explain their confusion or agitation. It is estimated that at least 70% of patients involved in automobile collisions have alcohol on board, and of these, 50% are above the legal blood alcohol level limit.[22] Studies of motorcycle collisions report lower alcohol percentages, ranging from 12% for helmeted riders to 37.9% for nonhelmeted drivers.[12,13]

The EMS report should be reviewed for mention of blood pressure (BP), pulse, respiratory status, and, if used, cardiopulmonary resuscitation (CPR). An elevated blood pressure and a decreased pulse may be indicative of brain ischemia. A decrease in respirations or labored breathing may be indicative of brain hypoxia or ischemia. With cardiopulmonary arrest, the length or suspected length of time the person was in arrest before CPR was initiated is important. Cardiopulmonary arrest will cause both hypoxia to the brain and ischemia. The longer the period of arrest, the greater the hypoxia. Hypoxia and ischemia are the major causes of secondary brain insults in the trauma patient.

A witnessed seizure necessitates clarification of the presence of premorbid epilepsy, alcohol-related seizure history, or new onset. Prophylactic antiseizure medication, if ordered, may decrease the level of alertness and cognition.[23] A report of the patient found "seizing" should alert the reader to the possibility of further insult to the brain. The length of the seizure and the potential for prolonged reduction in oxygen saturation may result in secondary insult to the brain from hypoxia or anoxia. Medications used to stop seizure activity may affect the patient's early responses.

A chart review should identify whether the patient was intubated at the scene and, if so, whether intubation was traumatic (ie, took several attempts to succeed or failed with several attempts). This information may be relevant to various team members, including the speech/language pathologist, in addressing pharyngeal and laryngeal function as it relates to speech and swallowing skills.

Changes in Glasgow Coma Scale (GCS)[24] score should be noted. A lowering of scores from in-field to hospital records may indicate a progressive brain insult. Dramatic improvements in scores may result from some medical interventions (eg, fluid resuscitation). In these circumstances, the initial GCS score may not be indicative of the actual severity of the brain injury.

Emergency Department, Procedures, and Intensive Care Information

The ED report can also provide valuable information to team members regarding the nature and extent of injuries. Results of computed tomography (CT) scans, radiography studies (X-rays), magnetic resonance imaging (MRI) tests, and other procedures should be reviewed; as well as information on airway, breathing, circulation (the ABCs), neurologic status, other injuries, and any treatment provided (Exhibit 5–2).

Airway. Injuries to the trachea may result from direct trauma. Injury or swelling of the vocal cords, the trachea, the esophagus, or the pharynx may also occur from traumatic intubation. These injuries can have an impact on extubation of the patient. The use of intubation versus tracheostomy or cricothyroidotomy ventilation affects nursing care as well as rehabilitation. Maxillofacial fractures, lacerations in the oral cavity, palate injuries, and injuries to the tongue may affect feeding and speech.

Breathing. Record review should include the patient's respiratory status, including lung expansion or any difficulties with breathing. Chest X-rays should be reviewed for possible fractures of the ribs, sternum, and scapula, since these fractures may affect breathing or clearing of secretions because of discomfort. Laboratory reports for blood gases and pH must be reviewed. Respiratory acidosis leads to poor tissue perfusion, which may result in hypoxia to the brain. Respiratory alkalosis may cause an increase in intracranial pressure (ICP) by increasing cerebral blood flow and cerebral vasodilation.[25]

Pneumothorax, pneumomediastinum, or hemothorax usually requires insertion of chest tubes. Multiple rib fractures may result in a flail chest. Lung contusions may also be present. A patient with a diaphragmatic tear will require surgery emergently to repair the injury. Chest tubes or fractures may cause discomfort to the agitated patient or may cause difficulty in mobilizing the patient later, when he or she is medically stable. The patient with thoracic injuries may require a longer period of intubation and ventilation, which increases the potential for complications such as atelectasis, pneumonia, acute respiratory distress syndrome (ARDS), empyema, and sepsis. The therapist responsible for chest physical therapy must review this information thoroughly, as timely pulmonary toilet intervention is crucial for this patient population. Pain management may be necessary to mobilize these patients, but the use of pain medications may suppress coughing and increase accumulation of secretions, which can lead to further complications. Pain control allows good pulmonary toilet and helps prevent some complications. The amount of shoulder movement that can be tolerated during physical or occupational therapy may be restricted until the pain is under control.

Circulation. Major blood loss (hypovolemia) will cause secondary insults to the brain through ischemia or hypoxia. Assessment procedures such as peritoneal lavage and CT scan reports should be noted. Procedures used to control bleeding should also be noted.

Exhibit 5–2 An Emergency Department/Trauma Center Report

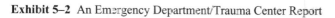

Trauma Center/Emergency Department

Name: _____   Date: _____
Address: _____   Time of Accident: _____
_____   Time admitted to ER: _____

Mechanism of Injury

AUTO	Pedestrian	Assault
Driver	Motorcycle	Fall
Passenger	ATV	Crush
Seatbelt	Bicycle	GSW
Car seat	HELMET	Stabbing
		Other:

Extrication Time: _____

Description of incident:

Prehospital Treatment

EMT
Paramedic
Ambulance
Air transport
Transfer from other hospital

Observation/Interventions:

Vital Signs:
R-Respirations
BP-Blood Pressure
P-Pulse
T-Temperature

Pupils:
R-Brisk   S-Sluggish
E-Equal   R-Reactive
N-Nonreactive
Size: 2, 3, 4, 5, 6, 7, 8,
9 mm

X-rays:

C-spine
Thoracic Spine
Lumbar Spine
Pelvis
CXR
Other X-rays:

Time	R	BP	P	T

Time	Left	Right

CT Scan: _____
Angiography: _____
Peritoneal Lavage: _____
Wounds: _____

continues

Exhibit 5–2 continued

Lab Work:

| Blood Work: |
| ABG: |
| Trauma Blood: |
| Urinalysis: |

Abnormalities:

| Neuro |
| Neck |
| Spine |
| Chest |
| Abdomen |
| Pelvis |
| Extremities |

Glasgow Coma Score

Eye Opening	
To Verbal Stimulus	3
Spontaneous	4
To Pain	2
None	1
Verbal	
Oriented	5
Disoriented	4
Inappropriate	3
Incomprehensible	2
None	1
Motor	
Obeys Commands	6
Localizes Pain	5
Flexion Withdrawal	4
Flexion Abnormal	3
Extension	2
None	1
Total	

Fluids:

| |
| |
| |
| |

Transfusions:

| |
| |
| |

Medications:

| |
| |
| |
| |
| |

Airway:

| Patent |
| Oral |
| Nasal |
| ET   Size |
| Other |
| Suction |

Breathing:

| Spontaneous |
| Normal |
| Retractive |
| Assisted |
| Oxygen |
| Lung Sounds: |
| right |
| left |
| Chest Tubes: |
| right |
| left |
| Other |

Trauma Score:

GCS Score:	
14–15	5
11–13	4
8–10	3
5–7	2
3–4	1
Respiratory Rate	
10–24	4
25–35	3
>35	2
<10	1
0	0
Respiratory Effort	
Normal	1
Shallow/Retractive	0
Systolic Blood Pressure	
>90	4
70–90	3
50–69	2
<50	1
0	0

continues

Exhibit 5–2 continued

Skin:		Pulses:	Trauma Score (con't.)	
Normal		Carotid	Capillary Refill Time	
Pale		Radial	Normal (<2 sec)	2
Cyanotic			Delayed	1
Warm		Femoral	None	0
Cold			Total Trauma Score	
Dry				
Diaphoretic				
External Bleeding:				
Site:				

Treatment/Procedures:

Discharge To:	Condition:	Signatures:
ICU	Stable	
OR	Unstable	
Floor	Guarded	
Morgue	Serious	
Home	Critical	
Other:	Dead	
	DOA	

If gross blood was found during the peritoneal lavage, the reader should review the chart to see if laparotomy was performed and what injuries were found and repaired. Retroperitoneal hematomas are not usually explored, but if a pelvic injury is present (especially if an "open-book" pelvic ring injury is found), an external fixator may be applied to help stop the bleeding and stabilize the pelvis. The external fixator may limit full range of motion of the hips and may limit sitting completely upright.

Neurologic compromise to an extremity may occur if bleeding causes pressure on the brachial or lumbosacral plexus. A compartment syndrome may develop in the arm or leg if expanding hematomas are present and if compartment releases were not performed before neurologic compromise occurred. In complex fractures of the upper or lower extremity, where the vascular supply was interrupted, external fixators may be applied to align the fracture so that surgery can be performed to revascularize the area.[26]

The team should also note if coagulopathy, during or after surgery, is documented. Disseminated intravascular coagulopathy (DIC) may occur in the patient with severe blood loss as a result of the fluid resuscitation necessary to stabilize the patient.[27] Patients who develop DIC may develop increased bleeding in the brain, which may become life threatening.

Aortic tears must be emergently repaired. Hypoxic episodes to the spinal cord may occur secondary to the aortic clamping necessary to enable repair and may masquerade as spinal cord injury. Paresis or paralysis secondary to aortic clamping may recover partially or completely over time, depending on how long blood supply to the spinal cord was compromised. ED records may note movement of all four extremities before surgery but no movement in the lower extremities after surgery.

Neurologic Assessment. Team members must be aware of the presence of epidural, subdural, or intracerebral hematomas; subarachnoid hemorrhage; or midline shifting of the brain. They must also find out whether evacuation of hematomas was performed. Small hematomas may not be evacuated emergently; rather, they may be monitored with further CT scans and frequent neurologic evaluations. If the hematoma causes midline shift, injury may occur to the area of the brain opposite the bleed as a result of compression against the skull. Hemiparesis or hemiplegia may occur on the same side as the hematoma or on the opposite side. Brain injuries can be diffuse. CT scans may report edema of the brain, contusions, intracerebral hemorrhages, or blood in the ventricles or other areas of the brain. Contusions and intracerebral hemorrhages may cause edema and neurologic deterioration. The team must review CT scan results to gain a clear understanding regarding the degree of neurologic injuries.

Edema causes increased ICP and, if not controlled, may lead to herniation.[28] Three different areas of herniation may occur, depending on the structure under which the brain is forced. If the brain is forced under the falx cerebri (cingulate or subfalcine herniation), this may decrease the patient's level of consciousness and possibly occlude the anterior cerebral arteries.[29] Tentorial herniations include central herniation and transtentorial herniation. Portions of the temporal lobes, midbrain, and diencephalon are forced downward through the tentorium. Signs of a tentorial herniation may include hemiparesis progressing to decorticate or decerebrate rigidity. The patient is in coma and will have a dilated, nonreactive pupil on the side of the compression. With increased herniation, both pupils may become dilated and nonreactive, and alterations in breathing will occur.[30] The third location for herniation is the foramen magnum. The brainstem is forced downward, resulting in alterations in vital signs, including respiratory pattern, blood pressure, and pulse. Hypertension with elevation of systolic and decrease in diastolic pressure, bradycardia, and slowed respirations (Cushing's triad) are signs of impending foraminal herniation.[31] Respiratory pattern changes deteriorate from Cheyne-Stokes in the early stage to ataxic in the late stage of herniation, until apnea occurs.[25] The patient may be noted to exhibit decerebrate posturing, later becoming flaccid.

CT scan results of the brain can be negative or normal by report. A negative report does not rule out the presence of brain injury. Diffuse axonal injuries may not be apparent on CT scan unless a significant amount of bleeding or edema has occurred. The patient may be in deep coma and unresponsive to painful stimuli yet may have a normal CT scan.[32] In these cases, the clinical presentation may be more indicative of the brain injury.

Basilar skull fractures, often not seen on X-ray or CT scan, are frequently diagnosed secondary to clinical manifestations. An ecchymotic area behind the ear (Battle's sign), blood behind the tympanic membrane (hemotympanum), cerebrospinal fluid (CSF) and blood draining from the ear (otorrhea) or nose (rhinorrhea), and bilateral ecchymosis around the eyes (raccoon's eyes) are all signs of a basilar skull fracture. Ecchymosis occurring only in the area of the orbicularis oculi muscles, bilaterally, is considered raccoon's eyes, whereas ecchymosis beyond this area or unilaterally is usually a sign of nasal injuries or direct trauma to the eye area. A hemotympanum or otorrhea may decrease hearing. Audiologic consultation may be considered after CSF leakage has ceased.

Spinal Injuries. Motor vehicle collisions are the most common cause of spinal cord injuries.[33] These injuries may or may not produce neurologic changes. X-rays, CT scans, MRIs, neurosurgical, and orthopaedic consults should be reviewed, as well as reports pertaining to the patient's ability to move the extremities.

A patient whose cervical spine has not been cleared for injury should continue to wear a firm cervical collar. Team members should not move the neck until the cervical evaluation is completed and injuries have been either ruled out or reported stable for movement. Thoracic and lumbar spine injuries may also be identified as stable or unstable by the neurosurgeon and the orthopaedic surgeon. Cervical or lumbar spine injuries may prevent full range of motion of the upper or lower extremities. Range of motion may be performed on patients with stable injuries, who do not have an altered level of consciousness, since movement may be performed to patient tolerance. But in patients with severe brain injury who may have a delayed response to pain or discomfort or may not respond to painful stimulus, full range of motion cannot be performed safely.

Neurologic changes secondary to a spinal injury should be documented in EMS, ED, and hospital records. A patient with spinal fracture or changes in the alignment of the spine may demonstrate no neurologic deficits, some changes, or paralysis. The level and stability of the injury and the neurologic status will all affect interventions. If the spinal cord injury is considered a complete injury, or a complete transection, the level of intact sensation and movement should be documented. Patients with incomplete spinal cord injuries should be thoroughly evaluated for intact sensation and movement below the level of the injury. This information aids in monitoring recovery during therapy or deterioration in the patient's condition.

Surgical stabilization procedures should be reviewed. If the injuries were not stabilized, the immobilization or traction device being used must be noted. Skeletal traction versus a halo vest may restrict movement of the patient. When Crutchfield, Gardner, or other types of tongs are being used with patients with severe brain injury, a rotating bed or a turning frame that supports and maintains correct body alignment should be used. Such a bed or frame may also be used for a patient with thoracic or lumbar vertebrae instability or fractures until the patient is stable enough for spinal surgery. The rotating bed makes access to the patient and range of motion difficult. Alignment is a critical issue until surgical stability occurs.

Orthopaedic Injuries. X-rays, CT scans, MRI reports, and consults from other physicians must be reviewed. Many patients sustaining severe brain injury also have other injuries; therefore, a thorough review of all X-rays should be included in the chart review. Life-threatening injuries may be the only ones evaluated and treated initially. The team may discover minor injuries while evaluating or treating the patient, or it may have to deal with known injuries that cannot be addressed until the patient stabilizes.

If acetabular or femur fractures are addressed with skeletal traction, movement of the hip may be restricted. Knee flexion and extension may also be restricted due to location of the skeletal pin. Ankle motion is not affected. When agitation is present, chemical paralysis or sedation may be needed until stabilization occurs, reducing the potential for further soft tissue injury or fracture malalignment.

Unstabilized upper-extremity fractures are usually splinted, preventing range of motion. External fixators may be used, especially if the fracture is open and wound care is required. Agitated patients may harm themselves or others with the external fixator device and may require sedation if padding of the device or calming of the patient is not possible.

The team must be aware of all fractures present and whether open or closed reductions were performed. Intramedullary rods (or nails) are now commonly used for stabilization of long bone fractures and allow early mobilization of the extremity and the patient.[34] Documentation of weight-bearing status is vital information for many team members. Patients with concomitant brain injury may have impaired cognition affecting their ability to understand or retain information regarding weight-bearing ability. Direct contact with the orthopaedist will help identify any precautions that must be taken during range of motion or other activities.

Facial fractures frequently are not stabilized surgically on admission. The oromaxillofacial surgeon usually waits until the patient is stable or until swelling decreases. Oral movement should not be encouraged until the mandible or maxilla has been stabilized or until the physician approves movement. Temporomandibular joint disorders may also be present and should be documented. Fractures of the orbit may cause muscle entrapment, preventing certain eye movements or causing injury to the eye itself. Muscle entrapment must not be confused with dysconjugate eye movement. Eye injuries must not be confused with brain or cranial nerve injuries affecting the eyes. Eye injuries restricting opening of the eyes must be noted and avoided in treatment.

An outline of the human body is beneficial during the chart review (Figure 5–1). The team is able to mark the location of fractures, casts, external fixators, or traction. If traction was applied, the type of traction should be noted. Weight-bearing status or other restrictions can also be noted on the diagram. The team can mark lacerations, abrasions, wounds, and burns anatomically on the chart. Surgeries, chest tube placement, and A-line or other line placement can also be included in the diagram. The team may note identified brain injuries on the chart. The diagram should be reviewed by all members of the team, and additions should be made, if necessary, during the hospital course. Use of this diagram benefits all team members, as there is an awareness of all the injuries present. New team members can use the diagram as a quick system for reviewing the injuries sustained by the patient with severe brain injury.

Alcohol or Drug Usage. Alcohol usage is common in motor vehicle collisions.[35] ED blood work usually includes blood alcohol concentration level and the presence of illicit drugs. The reader should note an alcohol level over the legal limit, which may be recorded as greater than 0.10 mg% or greater than 100. The presence and/or history of drug or alcohol use suggests the potential for withdrawal, including delirium tremens and withdrawal seizures. Confusion and agitation may be indicative of drug withdrawal. The use of heroin and other strong drugs reduces a patient's response to sedating and pain-controlling medications.

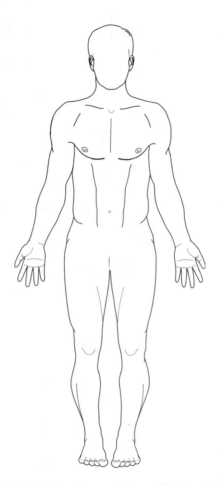

Figure 5–1 Outline of the body for documentation of injuries, procedures, and weight-bearing status.

Management may require heavy medication for patients who develop drug or alcohol withdrawal, further impairing their cognitive status.

Medications. Medications may affect patient assessment and treatment. Medications should be reviewed when changes in patient status are noted. Pain medications, such as morphine, will dull the patient's reaction to painful stimulation. Medications may also affect the size and responsiveness of the pupils. Therefore, when changes are noted in the pupils, medication effects must be distinguished from changing neurologic status. The patient's response to commands may also be slowed. Paralytic agents, pain medications, seizure medications, sedatives, and medications given to control the effects of withdrawal from alcohol or drugs will alter the patient's performance. The team must understand that difficulty in arousal, lethargy, and delayed or sluggish responses may be the result of medication rather than brain injury.

Past Medical History

Past medical history may affect the patient's evaluation, treatment, or hospital course. It is important that an accurate history be obtained from the family or the patient's physician as quickly as possible. A history of chronic obstructive pulmonary disease, asthma, bronchitis, or other respiratory problems or a history of smoking may directly affect the length of ventilatory support needed. A person with diabetes may have peripheral neuropathies that will affect the assessment, since response to painful stimulus to the finger or toe may be decreased or absent. A history of deep-vein thromboses or peripheral vascular disease increases the risk for vascular complications during the acute stay due to the immobility of the patient during the critical phase. Cardiac monitoring may show irregularities that were present premorbidly with patients who have a history of cardiac problems. Additionally, the cardiovascular system may not tolerate the stresses of pneumonia or ARDS.

Preexisting visual or hearing problems should be identified, including the use of hearing aids, glasses or contact lenses, specific visual impairments, or the presence of unequal pupils prior to the accident. Preexisting hearing problems may affect the team's ability to interact with the patient. An audiologist may need to evaluate the patient's hearing and may be of assistance in procuring equipment that will assist the patient during his or her early rehabilitation or later stages of recuperation.

Identification of preexisting neurologic conditions is imperative. A previous history of a cerebral vascular accident, peripheral nerve injury, multiple sclerosis, or other neurologic illness or disease, such as cerebral palsy, dementia, or mental retardation, will directly affect the patient's evaluation, care, and rehabilitation. Persons who have sustained brain injury are more susceptible to subsequent brain injury. The team must be aware of the possibility of cumulative trauma to the brain, which may exacerbate deficits. Premorbid educational problems, learning disabilities, or behavioral or psychologic problems should also be noted. These problems must be taken into consideration during assessment and treatment.

It is of utmost importance that the team review the patient's status daily during this critical time. The patient's medical and neurologic status may fluctuate for several days to weeks, depending on the brain injury, other associated injuries, or infections that may develop. The team must have knowledge of the equipment used in the ICU, what limitations this equipment places on therapy, what changes in the vital signs and neurologic signs mean, and what effect other injuries have on the treatment of the patient.

USE OF TECHNOLOGY

The purpose of equipment used in the ICU is to monitor, evaluate, treat, and maintain a patient's physical and neurologic systems. The specific pieces of equipment will vary according to the patient's needs. Initially, BP, heart rate and rhythm, respiratory rate, and frequently ICP are monitored. A ventilator is used as part of the treatment for the acute brain injury. Intravenous (IV) lines are in place for fluid resuscitation. Urinary catheters are used for bladder decompression and output monitoring. Nasogastric tubes are used for gastric decompression. Equipment may be added over time to evaluate or treat complications. If complications arise, some equipment use may be prolonged: for example, prolonged ventilator use may be necessary if the patient develops persistent respiratory insufficiency. Normative values for some of the monitored functions are shown in Table 5–1.

Some equipment in the ICU may affect intervention with this unstable patient population (Table 5–2). Rehabilitation needs of the patient should be considered by the team (physician, nurse, and rehabilitation personnel) when they are contemplating insertion of arterial, central venous pressure (CVP), and Swan-Ganz lines, and other equipment such as special beds. A mutual understanding of the special beds available, why a particular bed is recommended, and a bed's effect on tone and/or agitation is necessary, facilitating a joint educated decision regarding the best bed for a particular patient. The use of splinting devices to position the hands or feet must also be a team decision, or adverse effects may occur. Care must be taken to avoid automatic use of "off-the-shelf splints" with patients who have increased tone or posturing because many splints used for support will stimulate increased tone in patients with severe brain injury. A splint to maintain the

Table 5–1 Normative Values for Some Monitored Functions

Monitored Function	Normal Range
Mean arterial pressure	50–170 mm Hg
Cerebral perfusion pressure	50–130 mm Hg
Intracranial pressure	0–15 mm Hg (or torr)
Cardiac output	3.0–7.0 L/min
Cardiac index	2.5–4.5 L/min/m^2

Table 5–2 Common Equipment Used in the ICU, Its Purpose, and the Precautions Necessary When It Is in Use

Equipment	Purpose	Precautions
Cardiac monitor	Records heart rate, cardiac rhythm	If electrode comes off, replace it or ask nurse to replace it. **CAUTION:** if heart rate alters dramatically or cardiac rhythm changes, **stop treatment.**
Arterial line (A-line)	Records blood pressure, mean arterial pressure; used for frequent blood draws for blood gases	Limited movement where present—usually wrist or groin. **If it comes out, call nurse immediately and apply direct pressure.**
Central venous pressure line (CVP)	Assesses blood volume; used for hyperalimentation, rapid fluid resuscitation	If in subclavian vein, usually no restriction. If in jugular vein, **do not do full range of motion to neck.**
Swan-Ganz catheter	Records pulmonary artery pressure, pulmonary capillary wedge pressure, right arterial pressure, CVP, and cardiac output	If in subclavian vein, usually no restriction. If in jugular vein, **do not do full range of motion to neck.**
Intracranial pressure (ICP) monitor	Monitors intracranial pressure	**Do not turn head. CAUTION: if remains elevated (over 20 mm Hg), do not treat except to position to decrease posturing, which may decrease the ICP.**

continues

Table 5–2 continued

Equipment	Purpose	Precautions
Ventilators	Used to breathe for patient, assist in breathing; rate of breathing set	Alarms will sound if rate of breathing or resistance to breath alters from parameter set. **Allow patient to rest.** Alarm will sound if tubing detaches: reconnect tubing or ask nurse to reconnect. Must be sure tubes are not pulled. Will cause coughing, choking, and discomfort to patient, **which may cause increased ICP.**
Ventilator tubes	Nasal intubation, oral intubation, tracheo-stomy	
Nasogastric (NG) tube	Removes secretions from stomach; then used for feeding	Patient must not be allowed to pull on it. If tube starts coming out, feeding may go into lungs. **Get nurse to stop feeding before continuing with treatment.**
Dobhoff tube Gastrostomy tube Jejunostomy tube	Provides nourishment	Patient must not be allowed to pull on it. If the Dobhoff tube starts coming out, feeding may go into lungs. **Get nurse to stop feeding immediately.**
Chest tubes	Remove air, fluids, and blood from chest and assist in reinflating lungs following hemothorax or pneumothorax	Crimping tube or elevating it above level of chest may cause clotting within the tube, thus preventing drainage of fluids and air and preventing reinflation of the lungs. **CAUTION:**

continues

Table 5–2 continued

Equipment	Purpose	Precautions
		drainage system is on floor, near bed. Care must be taken not to kick it while working around the bed. Patient can be turned and sat up with chest tubes present.
Pulse oximeter	Records oxygen saturation	Electrode is frequently on finger or toe. If it falls off, replace. May put on another extremity until range of motion or exercise of that extremity is done.
Temperature probe	Monitors patient's temperature	May cause discomfort during movement of the legs. **Discomfort may increase the ICP; stop treatment until it normalizes.**
Urinary catheter	Collects patient's urine from the bladder	May cause discomfort during movement of the leg if pulled on. **If ICP increases, stop treatment until it normalizes.**
Fecal collection bag	Collects patient's fecal waste; used when diarrhea present frequently to prevent skin irritation	May cause discomfort during movement of the legs. **If ICP increases, stop treatment until it normalizes.**
Cooling Blanket	Used to reduce or increase patient's temperature to a normal level	May cause shivering and discomfort, **which may cause increased ICP. May need to delay treatment until temperature normal.**

foot in dorsiflexion may stimulate the positive supporting reaction. This reaction causes increased extension and plantarflexion, worsening tone in a patient with decorticate or decerebrate posturing. Input from the physical or occupational therapist, combined with staff education, will optimize treatment.

The therapist must be aware of limitations secondary to the equipment in use. The monitor can provide input regarding those interventions that aggravate the patient or facilitate negative reactions (eg, increased BP or increased heart rate). Decreased ICP can be noted when the patient is positioned to decrease posturing. Conversely, ICP can be increased when discomfort is caused during range of motion.

The cardiac monitor simultaneously displays vital signs and information regarding brain perfusion. The ICP may also be displayed on this or a separate one. Other equipment used with this patient population includes the ventilator, chest tubes, different types of lines and tubes inserted or attached to the patient, special types of beds, and temperature monitoring and regulating devices (Figure 5–2).

Ventilatory Support

Ventilators are used to maximize oxygen intake and exchange and support breathing for the patient. Mild hyperventilation ($Pco_2>30$ mm Hg) helps manage

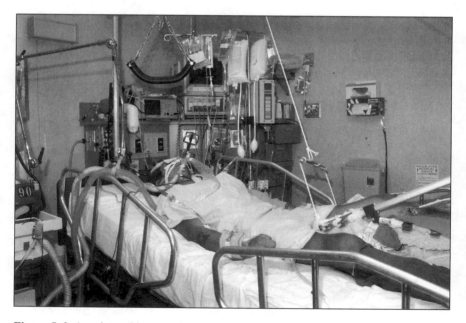

Figure 5–2 A patient with severe brain injury, attached to and surrounded by equipment in the intensive care unit.

intracranial hypertension. Arterial carbon dioxide reduction reduces cerebral blood flow, thus assisting in maintenance of a safe range of ICP.[36] Frequent blood gases are completed to ensure that carbon dioxide and oxygen remain in the desired range. Ventilators set to control the patient's respiratory rate and volume (control mode ventilation) are used when no effort in breathing is desired or initiated by the patient.[37]

Orotracheal or nasotracheal intubation is the more common initial approach for ventilatory support. The vocal cords may be injured during intubation, especially with nasotracheal insertion, since visualization of the vocal cords is not possible.[38] If ventilator support is needed over time, a tracheostomy will be performed. Care must be taken when moving the patient or the patient's head or arm on the side of the ventilator so as not to pull the ventilator tubing. Tension on this tubing may cause irritation, discomfort, agitation, or uncoupling of the tubing from the orotracheal, nasotracheal, or tracheostomy attachment. Pulling on the orotracheal or nasotracheal tube may also cause irritation or stretching of the vocal cords. Coughing or choking may occur and will cause the alarm to sound. Patients may develop increased ICP from increased thoracic pressure associated with the coughing or choking.[39]

Respiratory rate and breathing pattern should be observed before treatment and then throughout the treatment session. Treatment should stop if fluctuations occur, with attempts to quiet the patient and return the rates to normal levels. Therapy may need to be coordinated with weaning schedules. Continuous positive airway pressure mode is frequently used for weaning. The patient breathes spontaneously, but the baseline airway pressure is kept elevated for better alveolar ventilation. This patient may fatigue from the effort of breathing or if additional activity requirements are placed on him or her.

Hemodynamic Monitors

The monitor used with patients in the ICU displays the vital signs of the patient, including the heart rate and rhythm, BP, MAP, respiratory rate and pattern, and oxygen saturation. Information on the monitor must be noted before, during, and on completion of treatment while the patient is considered unstable. Alterations in vital signs between visits or during intervention may indicate improvement or deterioration in the patient. Increases or irregularities in the heart rate or rhythm; fluctuations in the BP, especially affecting MAP; changes in the respiratory rate; and decreases in the oxygen saturation level are all signs to stop treatment, either momentarily until the vital signs return to acceptable levels or completely if the vital signs remain erratic.

Electrocardiogram

The electrocardiogram (ECG) monitors the heart rate and rhythm. The pattern on the monitor varies according to the electrode placement and what part of the

ECG is selected for monitoring. The heart rate is also displayed on the monitor. Notation as to whether the heart rate is regular and within the normal range should be made. Arrhythmias should be documented if noted. Monitoring the display during interaction is important. If irregularities not previously documented are observed, the patient's nurse should be contacted.

Tachycardia is frequently seen following trauma.[40] If the heart rate becomes too high, medication may be administered to lower it. The team must be careful treating this patient, since the heart rate may not adjust to the demands placed upon it. Bradycardia may be normal in some individuals, especially athletes. A suddenly occurring bradycardia may be indicative of lower brainstem dysfunction secondary to brain herniation or excessive medication used to treat tachycardia. Bradycardia, apnea, and an increased BP are signs of Cushing's triad (symptoms of transforaminal herniation), necessitating evaluation and treatment to correct the cause of the bradycardia; therefore, all other interventions should be deferred. Arrhythmias may occur secondary to injury to the chest (cardiac contusion) or secondary to the release of catecholamine from the injury to the brain.[41] An occasional premature atrial contraction (PAC) or premature ventricular contraction (PVC) is acceptable, but repetitive or frequent PACs or PVCs require that the cardiac status be evaluated and treated.

Arterial Line

The arterial line (A-line) is used for monitoring the systemic arterial BP, calculating the MAP, or calculating the mean systemic arterial pressure (MSAP) and may also be used for frequent arterial blood sampling to monitor blood gases.[25,42] The therapist should observe the BP and the MAP before and during treatment.

Hypotension and hypertension cause the MAP to decrease or increase and must be monitored carefully in this patient population. The MAP frequently displayed on the monitor is calculated using the following equation: MAP or MSAP = $1/3$(systolic − diastolic) + diastolic.[25] The normal MAP range is 50 mm Hg to 170 mm Hg. Throughout this range, there is autoregulation of blood flow in the normal brain.[25] This autoregulation protects the brain from changes in the arterial pressure and also changes in the ICP. With brain injury, the desired range is 60 mm Hg to 150 mm Hg.

The radial artery is the more common site used (radial A-line) for measuring MAP, but the groin may also be used (femoral A-line). Range of motion of the joint where the A-line is located may be limited. With a femoral A-line, full hip flexion, abduction, and rotations may cause dampening of the waveform, irritation of the artery, or loosening of the A-line. A radial A-line using a short catheter limits movement at the wrist. Consideration of the limitations on range of motion is important in patients with severe brain injury. Patients with decorticate or decerebrate posturing or with extensor tone in the lower extremities will not be able to receive adequate range of motion to the lower extremity where a femoral A-line is placed. Contractures may develop quickly if range of motion is not maintained. Radial A-line placement may be more difficult in patients with decorticate posturing than in those with decerebrate posturing secondary to wrist position. Splinting of the wrist may be necessary to prevent deformity and maintain line function.

Central Venous Pressure Line

The CVP line is used for monitoring venous pressure and assessing blood volume. Central venous catheterization (CVC) may also be used for hyperalimentation, vasopressor administration, rapid fluid resuscitation, and passage of a Swan-Ganz catheter.[42]

The peripheral vessels may be difficult to access in a patient with considerable blood loss; therefore, a subclavian or a femoral central venous catheter may be placed. This access is also used to provide nutritional support until gastric feedings can be instituted. A hypermetabolic state is present in patients who have sustained trauma and brain injury specifically.[43] Early parenteral feeding facilitates replenishment of the nutrients needed for healing.

Maintaining fluid balance in the patient with a severe brain injury is extremely important. Too much fluid can increase the ICP. Dehydration will cause hypotension and decreased cardiac output, resulting in decreased cerebral perfusion and ischemia to the brain. CVP monitoring is used to monitor the intravascular fluid volume and to evaluate responses to the fluid resuscitation.[41]

The CVP catheter is frequently placed in the subclavian vein, using either a supraclavicular or an infraclavicular approach. The line is normally sutured in place and will not move when the patient is moved or during range of motion. If the line is not sutured in place, range of motion of the shoulder should be limited to approximately 90 degrees of flexion or abduction to prevent movement of the catheter or discomfort to the patient.

The CVP catheter may be inserted into the internal or external jugular vein, especially if pulmonary injuries are present. This placement limits full range of motion of the neck because of discomfort or irritation of the vein from movement of the catheter.[25] This discomfort may result in increased posturing, restlessness, or agitation.

The femoral vein is another site for CVP line placement and will prevent full range of motion of the hip in flexion, abduction, and both internal and external rotation. As with A-line placement, contractures may quickly develop when posturing is present or in patients with high tone when adequate range of motion cannot be provided to the hip.

Intravenous Lines

Intravenous lines are placed for administering medications or fluids. Fluids may be administered for nutrition or as part of fluid resuscitation. Medications to control the heart rate or BP may be administered through this route. Pain medications, sedation, antibiotics, and seizure medication may also be given. All team members should have a general knowledge of medications and their effect on vital signs, patient stability, and sensorium. An educated clinician is better able to distinguish an emergent alarm from an intravenous medication pump (I-Med pump). Cardiac, BP, and seizure medication disruptions are more urgent then fluid resuscitation alarms.

Neurologic Monitoring

An ICP monitor is used to assess ICP and the effect of treatments aimed at reducing the ICP level. The display of the pressure may be on the monitor with the vital signs or on a separate monitor specific to recording the ICP.

Normal ICP is between 0 and 15 mm Hg (or torr).[25] Pressures of 20 mm Hg or more over a sustained period can result in cerebral hypertension, which results in decreased cerebral perfusion, neuronal cell death, brain compression, and herniation.[44] Hematomas, contusions, midline shifts, and edema of the brain are contributors to an increased ICP.

Increased blood flow to the brain causes an increase in blood volume in the brain. Blood flow to the brain relates to cerebral perfusion and ICP. The formula for calculating cerebral perfusion pressure (CPP) is CPP = MSAP − ICP. The cerebral perfusion pressure must be between 50 and 130 mm Hg. A CPP of 50 mm Hg or less results in ischemia. A CPP of 130 mm Hg or more results in an increased ICP, due to increased blood flow to the brain.[25] Brain death occurs when the MAP and ICP are equal.

A decrease in flow out of the brain also causes cerebral hypertension and can occur if the neck is not maintained in a neutral position. Rotation or flexion of the neck can cause compression of the internal jugular vein,[45-53] which is the main outflow route for blood in the brain. If the ICP is elevated and the patient's head is not in a neutral position, the head must be realigned by the team member.

External Drains

A nasogastric (NG) tube may be placed through the nostril or the mouth. The initial purpose of a nasogastric tube is to decompress the stomach, remove secretions as they develop, and introduce medications. Following major trauma, ileus can occur. The NG tube removes the gastric secretions that cannot be passed easily due to ileus.

Chest tubes are inserted into the chest wall to correct a pneumothorax or hemothorax. The patient may have difficulty being extubated because of pulmonary injury. The physical or respiratory therapist who does postural drainage must monitor secretions and provide appropriate pulmonary toilet if needed. Chest tubes are attached to an underwater seal and a suction drainage system. The tubing from the chest to the container should not be crimped, since the drainage of blood, fluid, or air may be stopped. The chest tube(s) should be kept below the level of the chest. If blood is draining through the tube, it may clot and block the tube, preventing further fluids or air from draining through.[37] The system must remain intact for proper drainage and to prevent infections from occurring. Internal and external rotation range of motion of the shoulders should be done to prevent capsulitis. Patients may be turned or sat up with chest tubes in place.

Urinary catheters are used to decompress the bladder and monitor urinary output. Suprapubic catheters, rather than indwelling urinary catheters, may be placed in trauma patients with bladder or uretheral injuries. Patients in the ICU may have an external catheter in place for a period of time. An alert patient can communicate discomfort from the catheter. In the comatose patient, discomfort may be displayed through fluctuations in vital signs, increases in ICP, or restlessness and agitation.

A fecal collection bag provides a method of removing waste and protecting the skin from breakdown as a result of irritation produced by prolonged exposure to liquid fecal material. Diarrhea may occur when feedings are started. The clinicians/therapists must safeguard the patient from discomfort caused at the system attachment during movement of the patient. Discomfort may increase ICP, change vital signs, or increase agitation.

Orthopaedic Equipment

Traction

Traction may be used for unstable spinal injuries or orthopaedic injuries, especially acetabular or femur fractures. Fractures not stabilized on admission require either an orthotic device or traction. Alignment must be maintained until stabilization can be performed. Agitated or restless patients with unstable fractures should not be treated unless satisfactory immobilization is in place. If calming the agitated patient is not possible and the alignment of the fracture is in jeopardy, sedation may be necessary to prevent further injury. Posturing may result in malalignment through increased muscle tone. Positioning of the posturing patient may help maintain proper alignment of unstabilized fractures. However, sedation or chemical paralysis may need to be considered.

External Fixators

External fixators may be used to maintain the alignment of a fracture until reduction can be performed or to reduce a fracture or separation. Open wounds at fracture sites are more easily managed with an external fixator in place. Internal fixation may not be indicated with open wounds because of potential development of infections at the site of surgery. Agitated patients may take external fixators apart or hit them on bed rails, causing malalignment, weakness, or damage to the fixator device. Sedation of the agitated patient may be necessary.

Special Beds

Alternating air flow beds, whether standard or rotating, firm rotating beds, turning frames, and special mattresses may be used with critically ill or injured patients. The team members must understand their purposes and potential effects on the patient with a severe brain injury (Table 5–3). When routine turning of the patient is not possible because of injuries or elevated ICP, special beds may be necessary until turning the patient side to side and mobilizing the patient are possible.

Critically ill patients who cannot be mobilized will develop pressure ulcers if pressure cannot be relieved at bony prominences, such as the sacrum, coccyx, and heels. Atelectasis and pneumonia develop secondary to immobility of the body and lack of position changes of the trunk. The cardiovascular system decreases its ability to react to changes when the patient remains immobile. There is also an increased risk for vein thromboses and pulmonary emboli. Urinary tract infections and urinary tract calculi may develop from the inactivity.[54,55] Foam, egg crate, and air mattresses or air beds reduce the risk of pressure sores. Rotating beds reduce the risk of pressure sores and cardiovascular, urinary, and pulmonary complications.

Air flow beds prevent skin breakdown in patients maintained in a supine position because weight is more evenly distributed, thus preventing ischemia. The air flow bed, in distributing the weight of the patient evenly, may decrease the amount of stimulation the comatose patient receives. Without early therapeutical intervention, this patient will have increased sensory deprivation. Additional time with stimulation may be necessary to arouse the patient. Posturing and tone are known to increase when the body senses lack of support. Decerebrate or decorticate posturing may cause an increase in the ICP. Therefore, increased support is necessary for the shoulders, neck, and the knees to counteract the effects of the bed. The patient should be mobilized as soon as possible when this type of bed is used. Sitting the patient in a chair for a period of time each day will help to counteract the decreased sensory input resulting from the air flow bed.

Rotating air flow beds allow the left and right sides of the bed to alternately inflate and deflate, thereby rotating the patient. In addition to maintaining skin integrity, these beds help prevent pulmonary complications in inactive supine patients. Rotating air flow beds do stimulate the comatose patient by the constant

Table 5–3 Specialty Beds and Mattresses Used in the ICU, Their Purposes, and Interventions That May Be Necessary with Each Type of Bed

Type of Bed/Mattress	Purpose	Therapy Intervention
Alternating air flow beds: multiple segments, each pressurized according to the patient's needs and weight	To prevent skin breakdown	Need to add support to patients who are posturing.
Rotating air flow beds	To prevent skin breakdown and respiratory complications	Need to add support to patients who are posturing; need to evaluate neck position to maintain in neutral; need to evaluate if posturing increases on rotation. Agitation may increase with rotation.
Firm rotating beds with head, trunk, and extremity support	To maintain alignment of the head, trunk, and extremities while preventing respiratory and circulatory complications, especially for patients with spinal injuries in traction	Need to evaluate support to ensure that friction does not occur during rotation, causing skin breakdown, and to ensure that proper alignment is maintained.
Turning frames	To prevent skin breakdown and maintain alignment of head and trunk while preventing respiratory and circulatory complications	Need to evaluate trunk alignment to ensure that movement is not occurring on turning of patient. Need to monitor ICP during turning, as patient may not tolerate this movement early post injury.

continues

Table 5–3 continued

Type of Bed/Mattress	Purpose	Therapy Intervention
Air mattresses, water mattresses, quilted mattresses, and egg crate/foam mattresses	To prevent skin breakdown	Need to ensure that integrity of the skin remains unjeopardized. Also need to ensure that adequate support to decrease posturing is maintained.

rotation. Increased decerebrate or decorticate posturing may occur as a result of this rotation. Additionally, this patient must be observed for neutral head alignment. Neutral head alignment must be maintained to prevent increased ICP and decreased perfusion of the brain during the first few days after injury.[45–53] Rotation may stimulate the head to turn to one side if there is an imbalance of tone in the neck. Decerebrate and decorticate posturing, as well as the head's not being in a neutral position, will cause increased ICP. It is imperative not to cause secondary insults to the brain during the first 48 to 72 hours while edema, cerebral perfusion, and ICP are not yet under control. The patient must be monitored for posturing and head position. Teams must design optimal interventions based on patient priorities. Constant rotation may contribute to internal agitation in patients at Rancho Los Amigos Scale of Cognitive Functioning[56] level IV. The perception of support and then removal of support during inflation and deflation may initiate this internal agitation.

Firm-surface rotating beds with supports for proper body alignment are used, especially with spine injuries, when proper alignment must be maintained before surgical stability. These beds maintain neck alignment, relieve pressure over bony prominences, reduce pooling of pulmonary secretions, and stimulate the cardiovascular system. When the body feels support, posturing and increased tone are easier to manage. ICP may rise if the patient has a unilateral space–occupying mass. This increase in ICP may occur when the patient is rotated to the side where the mass is located or is brought to the neutral position.[55] Positioning to support the shoulders and back of the knees should be completed. Regular evaluation is necessary to ensure that adequate support is maintained during rotation so that skin shearing does not occur. The patient with cervical traction should be checked for alignment, which can shift from the constant rotation. Treating a patient in constant rotation is difficult. Because the bed is firm, it cannot be stopped frequently or for long periods of time, since skin integrity might be jeopardized. The bed, however, is stopped periodically for skin care. Therapy sessions may be coordinated during those times.

Turning frames allow pressure relief, full skin inspection, and good pulmonary toilet. Postural drainage for the lower lobes is more effective with a turning frame than with a rotating air flow or firm-surface rotating bed, since neither rotates to 90 degrees and neither allows the use of the prone position. Proper alignment may be maintained in any position. Tone may be decreased with changes from supine to side-lying to prone. The upper extremities can be positioned to reduce the risk of contractures developing. With severe brain injury, these positions may not be possible during the first days because of increased ICP. This must be the primary concern during this critical period.

Special mattress pads are designed to distribute the weight of the patient equally. These include air, water, soft foam, and quilted pads added to the mattress that have effects similar to those of air beds. The team should evaluate these patients in a similar manner to patients on air beds.

Nutritional Support

Once peristalsis returns, the NG tube may be used to provide nutrition until the patient is able to eat or until a different source of feeding is in place. A Dobhoff tube is a smaller and more flexible tube that is also placed through either the nostril or the mouth to the stomach. This tube is more comfortable for the patient and replaces the NG tube once feeding the patient is safe. Patients with severe brain injury frequently have early placement of either a gastrostomy tube or a jejunostomy tube. These sources for feeding the patient involve less risk of aspiration or of the feeding tube's displacing and feedings entering the lungs. The patient must be prevented from pulling on these tubes. If a Dobhoff or NG tube is dislodged, feedings may mistakenly enter the patient's lungs. If a gastrostomy or jejunostomy tube is dislodged, replacement may be difficult, or surgical intervention to replace it may be necessary.

THE UNSTABLE PATIENT

Equipment Used with the Unstable Patient

Patients with severe brain injury are subject to many complications, including atelectasis, pneumonia, urinary tract infections, ARDS, systemic infections, and thromboses. The ventilator is typically used from 48 to 72 hours. If the patient cannot be weaned, ventilatory support must be continued. Aspiration pneumonia is the most frequent cause of lung infection in the intubated trauma patient with brain injury requiring prolonged intubation. Lung injuries are also frequent in this patient population.

Swan-Ganz Catheterization

A Swan-Ganz catheter is used for monitoring myocardial function and hemodynamic status. Measurement of pulmonary artery pressure, pulmonary capillary wedge pressure, right ventricular pressure, right atrial pressure, CVP, and cardiac output is performed with the Swan–Ganz catheter,[57] a triple-lumen catheter. In addition to cardiac monitoring, one line may be used for pulmonary artery blood sampling and one for CVP monitoring and central venous blood sampling.

Monitoring of cardiac function and ventricular output is essential in patients who have sustained trauma because of the potential for compromise of cardiovascular status. Hypovolemia, frequent with trauma, stresses the cardiac system. Fluid resuscitation must be monitored closely so that it does not compromise cardiac performance.

Venous blood sampling through the Swan-Ganz is used to analyze venous oxygen saturation and tension for tissue oxygenation assessment. The adequacy of oxygen transportation and oxygen consumption, as well as the respiratory ability to oxygenate the blood, is monitored. This analysis determines circulatory sufficiency, tissue extraction of the oxygen, and the balance between delivery and consumption of the oxygen.

In sepsis, the cardiac index increases. Cardiac output is elevated by an increase in heart rate and a reduced afterload (secondary to a decrease in systemic vascular resistance) and is referred to as a *hyperdynamic cardiovascular state*. Oxygen consumption also increases. The cardiac workload may be similar during running or exercising vigorously. The heart, unable to maintain this workload for long periods of time (necessary with sepsis), decreases function, creating a low output.[57]

The approach for Swan-Ganz catheterization is through the subclavian vein or either the right external or internal jugular vein. When the subclavian vein is used, either a supraclavicular or infraclavicular approach may be used. Pneumothorax, secondary to puncturing the lung during the procedure, is a possible complication of Swan-Ganz catheter placement. The Swan-Ganz catheter, if sutured in place, allows range of motion of the shoulder. If the Swan-Ganz catheter is placed in the neck, full range of motion of the neck should be avoided because of discomfort or movement of the tip of the catheter. As with the arterial line and the CVP monitoring catheter, the Swan-Ganz catheter requires calibration. A fluid-filled pressure bag will be seen hanging from an IV pole, and a transducer will be attached to a manifold on an IV pole.

Jet Ventilators

Jet ventilation is a type of high-frequency ventilation.[37] It may be necessary when lung compliance is poor because of pulmonary contusions, ARDS, and sepsis. The patient is usually chemically paralyzed, since the machine may be set at

100-plus respirations per minute under high pressure. These patients are usually extremely critical; therefore, aggressive therapy should not be pursued. Splints may be applied to maintain the wrists, hands, and ankles in a neutral position. Gentle, passive range of motion should be done two to three times a week to maintain joint integrity, and positioning should be done to maintain alignment. Patients chemically paralyzed may or may not be given pain medication; therefore, the patient may feel pain but will be unable to demonstrate it. Joints should not be forced through range of motion, and stretching should be avoided.

Cooling Blankets

Cooling blankets are used to help rapidly reduce an elevated temperature. An elevated temperature results in an increase in the patient's metabolism. In an unstable patient with severe brain injury, the brain has increased metabolic needs for healing. Therefore, the temperature must be decreased rapidly to allow the metabolic needs of the brain to be met. Stimulation and movement of the patient, as well as the motor movements from shivering, place increased metabolic demands on the brain and potentially increase the ICP if the demands cannot be met. Treatment sessions may need to be deferred until the temperature decreases.

If the stabilized patient develops an elevated temperature, treatment may occur without jeopardizing the metabolic needs of the brain. The patient, however, may not be as responsive.

Neurologic Status

When deterioration in the patient's neurologic condition has occurred since admission or over the last 24 hours, the team should discuss whether treatment should be delayed until the neurologic condition stabilizes. The patient's nurse or ICU physician knows the patient's present condition and should be consulted before any treatment is started to ensure that no deterioration has occurred within the last few hours.

A patient who previously followed commands or purposefully moved all four extremities but who changes to randomly moving, not moving one side, posturing, or displaying no movement should not be treated until he or she is fully assessed by the physician. A patient previously exhibiting decorticate posturing and now flaccid or exhibiting decerebrate posturing or a patient who had one or both pupils responsive to light and now has pupils that are changed in size or fixed and dilated has deteriorated and needs a complete medical evaluation with possible intervention.

Unilateral or bilateral pupillary dilation may be signs of a downward shift of one or both sides of the brain above the tentorium, causing a transtentorial herniation. This situation usually results from an expanding hematoma. The neurosurgeon must evaluate the patient and either evacuate the hematoma or clear the patient for intervention by the team. The neurosurgeon may also request that the patient be maintained in a nonstimulating environment, possibly including paralysis. The members of the rehabilitation team should not treat this patient until stabilization has occurred.

Further herniation and compression downward of the brain can result in herniation through the foramen magnum of the brainstem. This condition is terminal if control of the brain swelling or of the pressure causing the shift is not possible. The patient should be monitored until neurologic stability is achieved.

An expanding hematoma (epidural, subdural, subarachnoid) may cause shifting of the brain to one side or downward and requires surgical evacuation emergently. Signs may include unilateral dilation of a pupil that is unresponsive to light, a decrease in alertness from that previously noted, and weakness of one side of the body or hemiplegia. A CT scan may note shift of the midline structures to the left or right or a downward shift of the brain, and an expansion in the size of the hematoma may be reported. The CT scan may also note disappearance of the ventricles.

An elevated ICP (over 20 mm Hg) for an extended period of time results in increased mortality or morbidity. This patient should not be aggressively treated, except for positioning to inhibit posturing. Inhibition of decerebrate or decorticate posturing may help decrease the ICP.[53] The head must be maintained in a neutral position. If multiple procedures were just performed on the patient, rest should be provided because multiple procedures in a short period of time will elevate the ICP. Frequently, with rest, the ICP will lower.[53]

Medications have an impact on motor and cognitive function. Deterioration in physical and mental status necessitates that medications be reviewed. Paralytic agents, if given, may be responsible for what appears to be neurologic deterioration. When patients become more alert, they may need to be medicated to reduce agitation, to stabilize vital signs, or to keep them from fighting the ventilator.

The team must know if medications were given that would affect perception of pain and movement. Some medications may cause dysconjugate gaze. Some medications alter the manner in which vital signs react to stimulation. Medications that regulate heart rate and BP may prevent the heart from responding to exertion. This lack of response prevents oxygen and nutrients from being transported to areas where they are needed. If oxygen and nutrients are not able to supply the needs of the brain, secondary brain injuries may occur. These insults are hypoxic or ischemic. Treatment sessions may need to be scheduled before administration of medication to maximize patient performance.

Brain Death

An important issue affecting therapy intervention is significant deterioration with impending determination of brain death. It is appropriate at those times for the rehabilitation team to refrain from any intervention. The nurse or physician can provide input to the therapist regarding cessation of all rehabilitation services. These services can be reinstated if the medical situation and stability of the patient improve.

SUMMARY

Team members must perform a thorough chart review, including reports from the scene of the accident, transport, the ED, and the ICU, for this complicated patient population in order to understand the extent of the injuries incurred and the stability of the patient.

Knowledge of the mechanism of initial injury alerts the team to the potential severity of the brain injury and the interventions and technologies needed to treat, monitor, and help prevent further brain injury from occurring. The team must be knowledgeable concerning primary and secondary brain injury and the mechanisms involved in each. Knowledge of the other systems of the body is necessary to understand the effects of other injuries on the brain and on treatment of the patient. Surgical procedures not performed on admission because of instability of the patient must be known, since they affect interventions by the team. Past medical history, alcohol or drug usage, and medications must be known, since these may affect the treatment.

Team members must understand the technology being used and the purpose it serves in the treatment and monitoring of the patient. They must also be aware of what restrictions the technology may place on treatment They must know which equipment has the potential to cause problems that may affect outcome and which interventions are necessary to prevent problems. The impact of complications and the additional technology needed when complications arise must also be known.

Awareness of the patient's neurologic status, including stability and deterioration, is mandatory. All team members must know what interventions may affect the neurologic status. They must also know what are appropriate interventions, and when the interventions are appropriate, in order to help the patient achieve his or her maximum potential.

REFERENCES

1. Viano DC. Restraint effectiveness, availability and use in fatal crashes: implications to injury control. *J Trauma*. 1995;38:538–546.

2. Zador PL, Ciccone MA. Automobile driver fatalities in frontal impacts: air bags compared with manual belts. *Am J Public Health*. 1993;83:661–665.

3. Hendey GW, Votey SR. Injuries in restrained motor vehicle accident victims. *Ann Emerg Med*. 1994;24:77–84.

4. Shalaby-Rana E, Eichelberger M, Kerzner B, Kapur S. Intestinal stricture due to lap-belt injury. *AJR*. 1992;158:63–64.

5. Grace DM, Fenton JA, Duncanson ME. Devastating lap-belt injury: a plea for effective rear-seat restraints. *Can Med Assoc J*. 1994;151:331–333.

6. O'Neill MJ. Delayed-onset paraplegia from improper seat belt use. *Ann Emerg Med*. 1994;23:1123–1126.

7. Redelmeier DA, Blair PJ. Survivors of motor vehicle trauma: an analysis of seat belt use and health care utilization. *J Gen Intern Med*. 1993;8:199–203.

8. Burgess AR, Dischinger PC, O'Quinn TD, Schmidhauser CB. Lower extremity injuries in drivers of airbag-equipped automobiles: clinical and crash reconstruction correlations. *J Trauma*. 1995;38:509–516.

9. Siegel JH, Mason-Gonzalez S, Dischinger P, Cushing B, et al. Safety belt restraints and compartment intrusions in frontal and lateral motor vehicle crashes: mechanisms of injuries, complications, and acute care costs. *J Trauma*. 1993;5:736–759.

10. Blacksin MF. Patterns of fracture after air bag deployment. *J Trauma*. 1993;35:840–843.

11. Smock WS, Nichols GR II. Airbag module cover injuries. *J Trauma*. 1995;38:489–493.

12. Johnson RM, McCarthy MC, Miller SF, Peoples JB. Craniofacial trauma in injured motorcyclists: the impact of helmet usage. *J Trauma*. 1995;38:876–878.

13. Wagle VG, Perkins BS, Vallera A. Is helmet use beneficial to motorcyclists? *J Trauma*. 1993; 34:120–122.

14. Sarkar S, Peek C, Kraus JF. Fatal injuries in motorcycle riders according to helmet use. *J Trauma*. 1995;38:242–245.

15. Li G, Baker SP, Fowler C, DiScala C. Factors related to the presence of head injury in bicycle-related pediatric trauma patients. *J Trauma*. 1995;38:871–875.

16. Thomas S, Acton C, Nixon J, Battistutta D, et al. Effectiveness of bicycle helmets in preventing head injury in children: case-control study. *Br Med J*. 1994;308:173–176.

17. Bjornstig U, Ostrom M, Eriksson A, Sonntag-Ostrom E. Head and face injuries in bicyclists, with special reference to possible effects of helmet use. *J Trauma*. 1992;33:887–893.

18. Maimaris C, Summers CL, Browning C, Palmer CR. Injury patterns in cyclists attending an accident and emergency department: a comparison of helmet wearers and non-wearers. *Br Med J*. 1994;308:1537–1540.

19. McDermott FT, Lane JC, Brazenor GA, Debney EA. The effectiveness of bicyclist helmets: a study of 1710 casualties. *J Trauma*. 1993;34:834–845.

20. Becker DP. Common themes in head injury. In: Becker DP, Gudeman SK, eds. *Textbook of Head Injury*. Philadelphia, Pa: WB Saunders Co; 1989:1–22.

21. Morgan AS. The trauma center as a continuum of care for persons with severe brain injury. *J Head Trauma Rehabil*. 1994;9:1–10.

22. Rimel RW, Jane JA. Characteristics of the head-injured patient. In: Rosenthal M, Griffith ER, Bond MR, Miller JD, eds. *Rehabilitation of the Head Injured Adult*. Philadelphia, Pa: FA Davis Co; 1983:9–21.

23. Yablon SA. Posttraumatic seizures. *Arch Phys Med Rehabil*. 1993;74:983–1001.

24. Teasdale G, Jennett B. Assessment of coma and impaired consciousness: a practical scale. *Lancet*. 1974;2:81–84.

25. Mitchell PH. Central nervous system I: closed head injuries. In: Cardona VD, Hurn PD, Mason PJ, Scanlon AM, et al, eds. *Trauma Nursing from Resuscitation through Rehabilitation*. 2nd ed. Philadelphia, Pa: WB Saunders Co; 1994:383–434.

26. Powell JN, Chapman P. The impact of early orthopedic management on patients with traumatic brain injury. *J Head Trauma Rehabil.* 1994;9:57–66.

27. Ansell JE. Acquired bleeding disorders. In: Rippe JM, Irwin RS, Alpert JS, Fink MP, eds. *Intensive Care Medicine.* 2nd ed. Boston, Mass: Little, Brown and Co; 1991:1013–1023.

28. Miller JD. Early evaluation and management. In: Rosenthal M, Griffith ER, Bond MR, Miller JD, eds. *Rehabilitation of the Head Injured Adult.* Philadelphia, Pa: FA Davis Co; 1983:37–58.

29. Miller JD, Pentland B, Berrol S. Early evaluation and management. In: Rosenthal M, Griffith ER, Bond MR, Miller JD, eds. *Rehabilitation of the Adult and Child with Traumatic Brain Injury.* 2nd ed. Philadelphia, Pa: FA Davis Co; 1990:21–51.

30. Cowley RS, Swanson B, Chapman P, Kitik BA, et al. The role of rehabilitation in the intensive care unit. *J Head Trauma Rehabil.* 1994;9:32–42.

31. Pang D. Pathophysiologic correlates of neurobehavioral syndromes following closed head injury. In: Ylvisaker M, ed. *Head Injury Rehabilitation: Children and Adolescents.* San Diego, Calif: College-Hill Press; 1985:3–70.

32. Butterworth JF, Prough DS. Head trauma. In: Rippe JM, Irwin RS, Alpert JS, Fink MP, eds. *Intensive Care Medicine.* 2nd ed. Boston: Little, Brown and Co; 1991:1459–1478.

33. Walleck CA. Central nervous system II: spinal cord injury. In: Cardona VD, Hurn PD, Mason PJ, Scanlon AM, et al, eds. *Trauma Nursing from Resuscitation through Rehabilitation.* 2nd ed. Philadelphia, Pa: WB Saunders Co; 1994:434–465.

34. Gibson JM. Multiple injuries: the management of the patient with a fractured femur and a head injury. *J Bone Joint Surg Am.* 1960;42:425–431.

35. Weigelt JA, Klein JD. Mechanism of injury. In: Cardona VD, Hurn PD, Mason PJ, Scanlon AM, et al, eds. *Trauma Nursing from Resuscitation through Rehabilitation.* 2nd ed. Philadelphia, Pa: WB Saunders Co; 1994:91–113.

36. Sherman DW. Managing an acute head injury. *Nursing.* April 1990;20:47–51.

37. Hurn PD, Hartsock RL. Thoracic injuries. In: Cardona VD, Hurn PD, Mason PJ, Scanlon AM, et al, eds. *Trauma Nursing from Resuscitation through Rehabilitation.* 2nd ed. Philadelphia, Pa: WB Saunders Co; 1994:466–511.

38. Kaur S, Heard SO, Welch GW. Airway management and endotracheal intubation. In: Rippe JM, Irwin RS, Alpert JS, Fink MP, eds. *Intensive Care Medicine.* 2nd ed. Boston: Little, Brown and Co; 1991:3–16.

39. Snyder M. Relation of nursing activities to increases in intracranial pressure. *J Adv Nurs.* 1983;8:273–279.

40. Manzi DB, Weaver PA. *Head Injury: The Acute Care Phase.* Thorofare, NJ: Charles B Slack Inc; 1987.

41. Horn LJ, Garland DE. Medical and orthopedic complications associated with traumatic brain injury. In: Rosenthal M, Griffith ER, Bond MR, Miller JD, eds. *Rehabilitation of the Adult and Child with Traumatic Brain Injury.* 2nd ed. Philadelphia, Pa: FA Davis Co; 1990:107–126.

42. McQuillan KA. Initial management of traumatic shock. In: Cardona VD, Hurn PD, Mason PJ, Scanlon AM, et al, eds. *Trauma Nursing from Resuscitation through Rehabilitation.* 2nd ed. Philadelphia, Pa: WB Saunders Co; 1994:151–178.

43. Logeman, JA, Pepe J, Mackay LE. Disorders of nutrition and swallowing: intervention strategies in the trauma center. *J Head Trauma Rehabil.* 1994;9:43–56.

44. Palter MD, Dobkin E, Morgan AS, Previost S. Intensive care management of severe head injury. *J Head Trauma Rehabil.* 1994;9:20–31.

45. Mitchell PH, Ozuna J, Lipe HP. Moving the patient in bed: effects on intracranial pressure. *Nurs Res.* 1981;30:212–218.

46. Jess LW. Assessing your patient for increased I.C.P. *Nursing*. 1987;17:34–42.

47. Boortz-Marx R. Factors affecting intracranial pressure: a descriptive study. *J Neurosurg Nurs.* 1985;17:89–94.

48. Mitchell PH. Intracranial hypertension: implications of research for nursing care. *J Neurosurg Nurs.* 1980;12:145–154.

49. Lee ST. Intracranial pressure changes during positioning of patients with severe head injury. *Heart Lung.* 1989;18:411–414.

50. Lipe HP, Mitchell PH. Positioning the patient with intracranial hypertension: how turning and head rotation affect the internal jugular vein. *Heart Lung.* 1980;9:1031–1037.

51. Mitchell PH. Intracranial hypertension: influence of nursing care activities. *Nurs Clin North Am.* 1986;21:563–576.

52. Sherman DW. Managing acute head injury. *Nursing.* 1990;20:46–51.

53. Palmer M, Wyness MA. Positioning and handling: important considerations in the care of the severely head-injured patient. *J Neurosci Nurs.* 1988;20:42–49.

54. Gonzalez-Arias SM, Goldberg ML, Baumgartner R, Hoopes D, et al. Analysis of the effect of kinetic therapy on intracranial pressure in comatose neurosurgical patients. *Neurosurgery.* 1983;13:654–656.

55. Tillett JM, Marmarou A, Agnew JP, Choi SC, et al. Effect of continuous rotational therapy on intracranial pressure in the severely brain-injured patient. *Crit Care Med.* 1993;21:1005–1011.

56. Hagen C, Malkmus D, Burditt C. Intervention strategies for language disorders secondary to head trauma. Presented at American Speech-Language-Hearing Association Convention; short course; November 1979; Atlanta, Ga.

57. Vary TC, Kearney MT. Pathophysiology of traumatic shock and multiple organ system failure. In: Cardona VD, Hurn PD, Mason PJ, Scanlon AM, et al, eds. *Trauma Nursing from Resuscitation through Rehabilitation.* 2nd ed. Philadelphia, Pa: WB Saunders Co; 1994:114–150.

CHAPTER 6

Management of Complicating Associated Injuries

The mechanism of injury for the person with brain injury greatly affects other associated injuries that he or she suffers. These additional injuries will have an effect not only on the patient's immediate care but ultimately on his or her survival and rehabilitation. Details of the mechanism of injury may help direct the caregivers as to the possibility of associated injuries. In the case of motor vehicle accidents, several important considerations are the extent of damage to the vehicle, the patient's location within the vehicle or outside the vehicle if ejected, whether the patient was a pedestrian struck by a vehicle, the speed at which the accident occurred, steering column damage, windshield disruption, and injury or death of other occupants (Figure 6–1). For patients having fallen, the height of the fall and the surface on which the patient landed are important to know. It is estimated that 2% to 20% of patients with traumatic brain injury have at least one other major organ system injury. These may include spinal cord injury, musculoskeletal injuries, thoracic and cardiovascular injuries, abdominal visceral injuries, maxillofacial injuries, and cranial nerve injuries. In this chapter we will discuss injuries in all of these categories, except for maxillofacial and cranial nerve injuries, which have already been discussed in Chapter 4. The presence of these comorbid conditions greatly influences the patient's needs, in terms of both acute medical and surgical interventions and ultimate rehabilitation.

SPINAL CORD INJURY

Spinal cord injury is primarily a disease affecting young adult males. Sixty percent of these injuries occur between the ages of 16 and 30 years, and 82% of patients are male.[1-3] The incidence of spinal cord injury in the United States is approximately 8,000 to 10,000 new cases annually.[1-3] Most of these patients, 40%

215

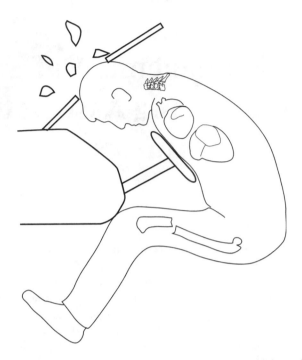

Figure 6–1 As seen with this unrestrained driver in a motor vehicle accident, multiple organs and systems may be affected in the person with a traumatic brain injury; thoracic, abdominal, and long bone fractures are common.

to 50%, present following motor vehicle accidents. Other common causes include falls (20%), especially among the elderly; sports-related injuries (15%), particularly diving accidents; and violent injuries (15%).[1,2]

It stands to reason that, given the mechanism of injury, these patients are at high risk for associated traumatic brain injury. Selecki et al found that a third of patients sustaining a spinal cord injury had a concurrent major head injury as well.[4] Reiss et al found that 60% of patients with cervical spinal cord injuries had other major associated injuries that included skull and facial fractures, cerebral contusions and intracranial hematomas, and other major system injuries such as intrathoracic, intra-abdominal, musculoskeletal, and neurovascular injuries. Only 16% of the patients that they reviewed had an isolated cervical spinal injury.[5]

The frequency of cervical spinal injury found in conjunction with brain injury has been estimated to be up to 10%.[6,7] Although this figure has been questioned by some clinicians as being higher than is normally seen in practice, there does appear to be some association.[8] Hills and Deane reviewed over 8,000 blunt trauma patients and found that those with clinically significant brain injury were at greater risk of having sustained a cervical spine injury than those without brain injury, 4.5% versus 1.1%. The risk appeared to increase with the severity of brain injury, being 6.4% for patients with a Glasgow Coma Scale (GCS) score of 12 or less and 7.3% for patients with a GCS score of 8 or less.[6]

Penetrating injuries to the head, of course, have different implications for spinal cord injury. In a review of patients sustaining gunshot wounds to the head, Kennedy et al found that if the wound was confined to the calvaria, the spine was not at risk for injury. But in those in whom the wound extended beyond the calvaria, 10% sustained an associated cervical spine injury.[9]

Initial Evaluation

Especially in the case of a person with brain injury, for whom a reliable neurologic examination may be difficult to obtain, the caregiver in the acute setting, both prehospital and emergency department, must maintain a high level of suspicion for spinal cord injury. Given the association between brain injury and spinal cord injury, certain principles should be adhered to when initiating care. Of course, any resuscitation of a trauma victim starts with the "ABCs" as outlined by the Advanced Trauma Life Support Program: airway, breathing, and circulation.[10] These are the priorities in initial management, and although proper immobilization of the patient should be strictly carried out, it must not interfere with potential lifesaving maneuvers. It is also important to remember that one must not focus exclusively on obvious injuries or those that have been already diagnosed by a transferring institution. All systems must be evaluated efficaciously, prioritizing first the treatment of those conditions that may be life threatening.

Adequate airway control is one of the first issues to address in the patient with a severe brain injury. The maintenance of adequate gas exchange with sufficient arterial oxygenation and the maintenance of adequate tissue perfusion with the avoidance of hypotension are two major factors critical to survival that may also help minimize the occurrence of secondary brain injury.[2] In addition, protection of the lungs from aspiration can be afforded through proper airway management.

In the patient with brain injury, it is especially important to adhere to cervical spine precautions when securing the airway, given the possibility of concurrent spinal cord injury. In a review of 300 patients with cervical spine injury, Bohlman noted that 23% had a delay in diagnosis because of the effects of either brain injury or alcoholic intoxication. He further observed that 6% of the patients developed their spinal cord injury with neurologic deficit after arrival at the hospital, often because of improper immobilization.[11]

Intubation more often than not becomes necessary in the patient with a clinically significant brain injury. But even without brain injury, the multiply traumatized patient will often have compromised pulmonary mechanics. A high to midcervical spinal cord lesion can result in diaphragmatic dysfunction because of phrenic nerve paralysis. Low cervical or thoracic lesions may lead to intercostal muscle paralysis.[2,3] Associated injuries, including cardiothoracic injuries, such as pneumothorax, hemothorax, pulmonary contusion, cardiac contusion, and major vascular injuries, and intra-abdominal injuries, can all contribute to an impaired respiratory status. All of these factors can lead to the need for mechanical ventilation.

When intubation becomes necessary, it can be safely accomplished with the maintenance of proper spinal precautions. Options as to the route of intubation include blind nasotracheal, fiber-optic, oroendotracheal, and finally surgical airway by cricothyroidotomy if severe maxillofacial trauma coexists and prohibits intubation by conventional means. Nasotracheal intubation in the conscious patient and fiber-optic techniques may help minimize movement of an unstable cervical spine fracture.[2] When the oroendotracheal route is chosen, either because other routes are contraindicated or because of the need for immediate airway control, the caregiver performing the intubation should avoid neck extension by using a chin lift.[2] To do this, one should remove the cervical spine collar, since it can interfere with proper positioning and with laryngoscopy. During this maneuver, it is critical that neck axial in-line stabilization be maintained by an assistant, usually standing below the head of the patient and using both hands to fixate the occiput, the base of neck posteriorly, and the mandible. A second assistant can be responsible for cricoid pressure during the intubation.

It is also important to sedate adequately and perhaps administer a neuromuscular blocking agent when securing the airway in the patient with brain injury and a possible spinal cord lesion. Further neurologic decompensation in the setting of an unstable spine lesion might otherwise occur in a combative patient. Sedation and paralysis might also prevent excessive rises in intracranial pressure during the particularly noxious act of intubation.

Mechanism and Type of Spinal Cord Injury

The two most important mechanisms by which the spinal cord can become injured are direct force vectors and vertebral column fractures and dislocations.[2] Multiple force vectors such as flexion, extension, distraction, compression, axial rotation, and shearing may lead directly to injury through stretching of the spinal cord. This in turn results in both gray and white matter injury over several segments of the spinal cord.[2,12] The spinal cord syndromes can result from this type of injury. These will be reviewed later in this chapter.

The more common mechanism by which the spinal cord becomes injured is direct injury to the vertebral column.[2] The majority of clinically significant vertebral column fractures are located in the lower cervical spine and near the thoracolumbar junction.[1,2,13] A lack of supporting structures may contribute to an increased susceptibility in these regions. For instance, the thoracic vertebral column is offered stability from the ribs and thoracic musculature, both of which are absent in the cervical and lumbar spine regions. In addition, there is a change in the curvature of the spine from a lordotic position in the cervical and lumbar regions to a kyphotic one in the thoracic spine.[13] It is at these junctions that the vertebral column appears to be most at risk from blunt trauma (Figure 6–2). Between 5% and 20% of spinal fractures are multiple, and up to 5% of patients have injuries at multiple noncontiguous levels.[13]

Depending upon the location and mechanism of injury, several descriptive types of bony disruption can occur. Fracture dislocations represent a serious in-

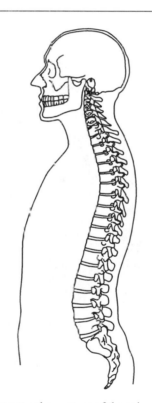

Figure 6–2 Differences in the natural curvature of the spine may contribute to the prevalence of lower cervical and thoracolumbar spinal injuries. Note the lordotic position of the cervical and lumbar spine in relation to the kyphotic thoracic spine.

jury and the most common mechanism by which the cervical spinal cord becomes traumatized. This type of injury results in a neurologic deficit in 75% of patients.[13] Flexion-rotation, shear, and flexion-distraction are the three forces that can produce a fracture dislocation. Conventional radiographs will demonstrate displacement of one vertebral body with respect to the others, and often one will see associated fractures of the bony elements (Figure 6–3).

Compression or wedge fractures are most commonly found in the thoracolumbar spine. Up to 50% of all thoracic and lumbar spine fractures are of this variety.[13] The mechanism of injury is hyperflexion of the spine, with the axis of rotation located in the center of the intervertebral disc. Compression or wedge fractures represent a failure of the anterior elements of the spine, and thus radiographically one will see anterior wedging of the vertebral body, often with a fracture of the anterior-superior bony cortex[14] (Figure 6–4). These fractures do not usually result in a neurologic deficit.[13,14]

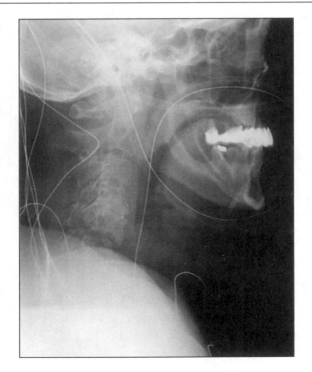

Figure 6–3 After falling down a flight of stairs, a 66-year-old woman presented as a complete C-6 quadriplegic. A plain radiograph of her lateral cervical spine demonstrates a C5–6 fracture dislocation.

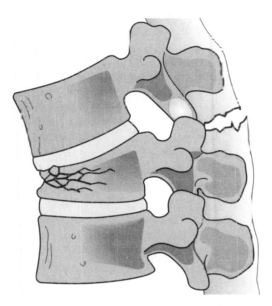

Figure 6–4 Depiction of a compression fracture of the thoracolumbar spine.

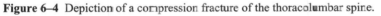

Burst fractures make up roughly 15% to 20% of thoracolumbar spinal injuries. The mechanism of trauma is axial compression during some spinal flexion.[13] The fractures represent a failure of both the anterior and middle elements of the spine, and with the more serious or unstable burst fractures there may also be involvement of the posterior elements.[14,15] Burst fractures are of clinical importance in that there is frequently an associated neurologic deficit.[13,15] Radiographs will reveal a comminuted fracture of the vertebral body, often involving both superior and inferior vertebral end plates, and this may result in posterior retropulsion of bony fragments into the neural canal (Figure 6–5). Computed tomography (CT) is helpful in evaluating extension of the fragments into the neural canal, although this does not necessarily translate into a neurologic deficit. [3]

The lap seat belt–type of fractures, sometimes referred to as Chance fractures, make up about 6% of major thoracolumbar spinal injuries.[13] As the name implies, the injury occurs in a patient involved in a vehicular accident who is wearing a lap belt without a shoulder harness. This causes hyperflexion with distraction of the posterior spinal elements, the axis of rotation being anteriorly located because of the lap seat belt.[13,14] A typical radiograph shows a horizontal fracture through the posterior arch and pedicles extending into the posterior aspect of the vertebral body. One will also usually see an increase in the height of the posterior aspect of the vertebral body (Figure 6–5).[13]

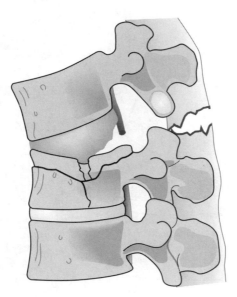

Figure 6–5 Depiction of an unstable burst fracture of the thoracolumbar spine.

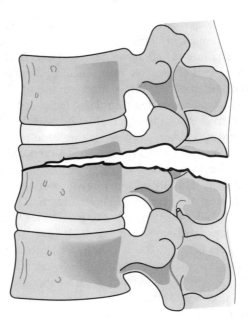

Figure 6–6 Depiction of a Chance fracture of the thoracolumbar spine.

Classification of Spinal Injuries

Once the diagnosis of spinal fracture has been confirmed radiographically, one must determine whether a neurologic deficit coexists. This can be a difficult challenge in the patient with brain injury because of limitations in performing the neurologic examination.

Skeletal Level of Injury

The simplest classification for spinal injuries is the skeletal level of injury, which is defined as the single vertebra or the two adjacent vertebrae with the greatest damage, the latter being referred to as the *motion segment*.[1] As this classification scheme does not take into account neurologic function, it may be all that can be used initially in the unconscious patient with brain injury. It is important to remember that spinal precautions and immobilization should still be maintained in the unconscious patient even if plain radiographs of the spine are normal, since multiple force vectors may have caused injury to the spinal cord itself or to supporting soft tissues and ligaments without an actual bony fracture or subluxation.

Neurologic Level of Injury

A functional-anatomic classification is the next step in the clinical evaluation of a spinal injury in that it takes into account the neurologic level of injury as determined by the neurologic examination.[1] If the patient with brain injury has only a diminished level of consciousness and is able to follow simple commands, one can still determine if a motor or sensory deficit exists with fairly good accuracy. The more severe the brain injury, of course, the less reliable the neurologic examination. However, the examiner can still assess neurologic function by carefully observing the patient for any movement of the extremities, either spontaneously or with stimulus.

The neurologic level of injury is defined as the most caudal segment with good motor and sensory function.[1] A myotome has good motor function if it has a power of at least a grade 3 out of 5. Power grades in descending order of function are as follows[1]:

5: normal power
4: movement through full range of motion against some resistance
3: movement through full range of motion against gravity
2: movement through full range of motion with gravity eliminated
1: trace movement
0: no movement

Key muscles at each spinal cord level have been designated by the American Spinal Injury Association to help determine the motor neurologic level of injury[1]:

C-1 to C-4	diaphragm
C-5	elbow flexion—biceps
C-6	wrist extension
C-7	elbow extension—triceps
C-8	finger flexion, distal phalanx
T-1	hand intrinsics
T-2 to L-1	rely on sensory level
L-2	hip flexion—iliopsoas
L-3	knee extension—quadriceps
L-4	ankle dorsiflexion—tibialis anterior
L-5	great toe extension—extensor halluces longus
S-1	ankle plantar flexion—gastrocnemius
S-2 to S-5	rectal sphincter tone and sensation

Key dermatome areas have also been defined for determining the sensory level (Figure 6–7).

Reflexes are another important part of the neurologic examination. These include deep tendon, abdominal, cremasteric, and plantar reflexes. Rectal sphincter tone and sensation as well as perianal reflexes can be used to assess sacral sparing.[1]

Complete versus Incomplete Spinal Cord Injury

An incomplete spinal cord injury exists if there is any nonreflex neurologic function remaining, either motor or sensory, in the region of the spinal cord below the neurologic level of injury.[1] This does not include the zone of partial preservation, which is the region of the spinal cord immediately below the neurologic level of injury having some remaining sensory or motor function. If the zone of partial preservation is confined to within three consecutive segments caudal to the neurologic level of injury, the lesion is still considered a complete injury.[1]

Functional Classification

The degree of spinal cord impairment can be further classified by the Frankel system, which defines the amount of preservation of function below the neurologic level of injury.[1,16] This can also be useful in following patients as they recover and possibly regain neurologic function. The Frankel classes are defined as follows[1,16]:

> *Frankel A lesion:* complete injury; no preservation of motor or sensory function below the zone of partial preservation
> *Frankel B lesion:* incomplete injury; only preserved sensation below the zone of partial preservation
> *Frankel C lesion:* incomplete injury; preserved but useless voluntary motor function (grade 1 or 2) below the zone of partial preservation

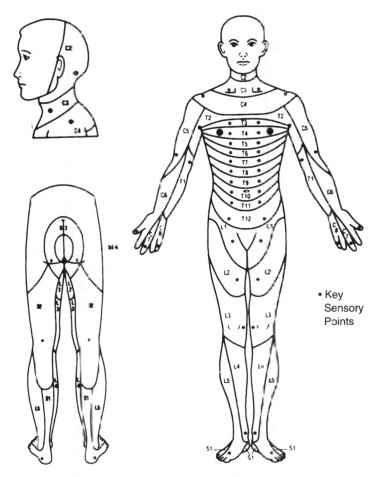

Figure 6–7 Areas to test to determine sensory level of injury. *Source:* Reprinted with permission from J.F. Dituno, *Standards for Neurologic and Functional Classification of Spinal Cord Injury,* p. 10 © 1992, American Spinal Injury Association.

Frankel D lesion: incomplete injury; preserved useful voluntary motor function (at least grade 3) below the zone of partial preservation
Frankel E lesion: return of normal motor and sensory function, though reflexes may be abnormal

All of these classification schemes, including the skeletal level of injury, the neurologic level of injury, and especially the Frankel system taking into account the degree of functional preservation, have important implications when it comes to the eventual rehabilitation and functional recovery of the spinal cord–injured patient.[16] Moreover, the degree of spinal cord injury becomes even more critical in the patient with a coexisting brain injury, since it will be a major determinant in the outcome of such a patient. As complete a neurologic examination as possible must be done early in the acute care setting and then on an ongoing basis in the subacute phase. Fifty percent of patients with spinal fractures resulting in a neurologic deficit present with a Frankel A (complete) lesion, and of these, 94% will remain at this level of spinal cord injury upon discharge from the hospital.[1] Since the spinal cord lesion becomes more incomplete with descending levels of Frankel classification, the prognosis for functional recovery and rehabilitative potential improves greatly.[16]

Spinal Cord Syndromes

As previously mentioned, multiple force vectors can lead to direct injury of the spinal cord, not necessarily with a bony fracture or subluxation of the vertebrae. Even a seemingly minor accident, especially in the elderly, can cause cord injury. The spinal cord injury syndromes result from vector-related forces that translate into specific patterns of neurologic deficit.[1]

Central Cord Syndrome

The central cord syndrome is usually seen with hyperextension injuries of the cervical spine. It commonly occurs in older individuals or in those with congenital or acquired cervical stenosis. As the name implies, the injury results in hemorrhagic necrosis of the central gray matter and the more medially located white matter of the spinal cord. Since the corticospinal and spinothalamic tracts are organized such that the upper body cervical fibers are more medial and the caudal sacral fibers are laterally located, the caudal fibers are relatively spared from disruption. This in turn results in a type of "upside-down quadriplegia," with greater motor weakness in the upper extremities than in the lower extremities.[1]

Brown-Séquard Syndrome

The Brown-Séquard syndrome results from injury to one side of the spinal cord. It may be more often found in penetrating trauma, but it can also follow blunt injury or asymmetric herniation of the nucleus pulposus. The ascending and descending fibers are interrupted, and this results in contralateral sensory deficits in pain and temperature, ipsilateral sensory loss of fine touch and position, and ipsilateral motor weakness. Damage to the nerve roots at the neurologic level of injury can also lead to ipsilateral flaccid weakness and anesthesia in the corresponding muscle groups and dermatome. It is rare to see this classical picture in its pure form; more often the prominent findings will be ipsilateral spastic weakness and contralateral loss of pain and temperature sensation.[1]

Anterior Cord Syndrome

This is a rare syndrome by which the anterior region of the cord supplied by the anterior spinal artery becomes injured. Clinically, this translates into weakness and loss of pain and temperature sensation below the level of injury. Again, this pattern of injury is rare, but it can follow flexion forces, vascular injuries, or acute central herniations of the nucleus pulposus.[1]

Cauda Equina–Conus Medullaris Syndrome

This type of injury results from low-level spine trauma at or below the thoracolumbar junction. The lower–motor neuron dysfunction leads to flaccid motor weakness with anesthesia in the affected dermatomes. Sacral reflexes will also be affected, resulting in flaccid bladder and rectal tone with subsequent incontinence of urine and feces.[1]

Spinal Shock

Special mention should be made of spinal shock. This is seen clinically as total flaccidity with the complete absence of motor and sensory function as well as deep tendon reflexes below the level of injury. Spinal shock is a phenomenon that occurs immediately at the time of the trauma and can last variable periods of time, anywhere from minutes to hours to sometimes weeks after the injury. The length of time appears to be related to the severity of the impact. The exact cause of spinal shock is uncertain, but it is probably multifactorial: the supraspinal facilitatory tracts may be interrupted, ascending inhibitory impulses may be unopposed, and there may be an alteration in the normal extracellular electrolyte milieu, especially that of potassium, at the injury site.[2]

The return of the most primitive spinal single-arc reflexes, such as the bulbocavernosus reflex, signals the end of spinal shock. This may not, however, be a consistent or reliable finding. It appears that the longer the spinal shock lasts, the worse the prognosis for functional recovery. If it extends beyond 24 hours after the injury, the prognosis is very poor.[2]

Secondary Spinal Cord Injury

Another important concept in trauma to the spinal cord is that of secondary injury. Just as the brain can suffer from secondary injury, so can the spinal cord. Many factors can contribute to the progression of the spinal cord injury response.[2] There can be an alteration in central and systemic vasomotor autonomic tone; and with hypertension, hemorrhage and edema can occur in the injured area. Hypotension can also enhance tissue ischemia.[2,17] Shifts in the local metabolism from aerobic to anaerobic because of decreased tissue oxygen tension can result in acid-base and electrolyte disturbances in the region of the spinal cord injury, causing depolarization and possibly neuronal cell death. Increased intracellular calcium can lead to uncoupling of oxidative phosphorylation with decreased levels of adenosine triphosphate.[17,18] Intracellular calcium also will act as a second messenger to activate intracellular proteins such as phospholipases and proteinases, an occurrence that can result in fatal cell membrane destruction.[17–19] The breakdown of cell membranes leads to free fatty acid release. Lipid peroxidation occurs as free radicals attack polyunsaturated fatty acids, forming destructive lipid-free radical intermediates and fatty acid hydroperoxides.[2,17] Free fatty acids, including arachidonic acid, will also be metabolized to thromboxanes, prostaglandins, and leukotrienes. These can promote platelet aggregation and further tissue ischemia.[2,20,21]

Pharmacologic Therapy

The above discussion only touches briefly upon the many factors contributing to secondary injury. However, whether secondary injury actually translates into clinical significance is not clear. The neurologic deficits of most patients do not progress beyond the time of injury.[2] Nonetheless, the theoretical advantage of using high-dose glucocorticoids in the acute management of the spinal cord–injured patient is based upon reducing or minimizing secondary injury.[22] Bracken et al demonstrated in the second National Acute Spinal Cord Injury Study that methylprednisolone given in high doses within 8 hours of injury significantly improved neurologic recovery in spinal cord–injured patients. In this trial, methylprednisolone was administered as an intravenous bolus at a dose of 30 mg/kg followed by a 23-hour maintenance infusion rate of 5.4 mg/kg. The treatment group was compared to a placebo group and a group given high-dose naloxone. At six weeks and at six months, those treated with methylprednisolone showed improvement in both motor and sensory function.[23]

The mechanism of action by which high-dose glucocorticoids have a beneficial effect is not entirely understood. Proposed explanations include the suppression of edema formation, enhancement of spinal cord blood flow, the deceleration of a cascading inflammatory response, the facilitation of spinal cord impulse generation, and, perhaps most important, the inhibition of free radical–mediated membrane lipid peroxidation and cell destruction.[2,22–24] It is this last mechanism by which steroids may have their greatest therapeutic role: through the stabilization of cell membranes by inhibiting free radical reactions associated with the spinal injury, ultimately averting disruption in nervous system activity.[22,23]

Other pharmacologic and treatment interventions have been proposed to help reduce secondary injury in the spinal cord. These include dimethyl sulfoxide (DMSO), naloxone, osmotic diuretics, thyrotropin-releasing hormone (TRH), calcium channel blockers, hypothermia, and hyperbaric oxygen therapy.[2,21,25] None of these has been proven to be of benefit in terms of an improved cxlinical neurologic function, but they are worth mentioning.

Naloxone and TRH are opiate antagonists that might serve to block opiate receptors, there being a significant release in endogenous opioids following spinal cord trauma. This in turn might help augment spinal cord blood flow.[26] DMSO is a diuretic agent that might reduce local edema. In addition, it can act as a vasodilator, an anti-inflammatory agent, and a free radical scavenger.[2,21] Osmotic diuretics such as mannitol may have a similar mechanism of action. Antioxidant and free radical scavengers such as these have been shown to be of benefit in experimental animal models if given prophylactically before the injury. However, they have not confirmed the same desirable outcome if given after the injury.[2,21] In theory, calcium channel blockers might prevent large influxes of calcium into the neural cells, thereby preventing the cascade of events leading to cell destruction.[2,27] Hypothermia can reduce the metabolic demands of injured neural tissues and may also decrease local edema and inflammatory responses. Again, clinical benefit has not been proven for any of these modalities.[2]

Surgical Management of Brain Injury in Association with Spinal Cord Injury

If, following initial evaluation, surgical intervention for the treatment of brain injury becomes necessary, special precautions must be taken to protect the spine in the case of either known or suspected spinal injury. The patient should be carefully logrolled when transferred onto the operating room table. A Mayfield headrest should be used to provide adequate exposure during craniotomy while maintaining neutrality of the head and spinal column. A cervical collar is kept in place during the surgery.[28]

Following the craniotomy, external immobilization with either tong or halo traction is applied in the case of confirmed cervical spine injury. Under some circumstances, depending upon the size and location of the craniotomy, a traction device cannot be applied; in this case, the patient should be kept in a Philadelphia collar and a roto-rest bed postoperatively. Once the scalp flap has healed, a halo brace can be applied. A major limitation of traction and brace devices is the subsequent ability to use head CT scanning as a follow-up diagnostic tool in the brain-injured patient. The scatter artifact caused by the metallic pins can seriously impair the quality of head CT. Nonetheless, the CT scan can often be correctly interpreted in light of other clinical data. In rare situations, temporary removal of the traction device with placement of a cervical collar during CT scanning might be necessary, although such maneuvering can certainly put the spinal cord at risk for further injury.[28]

Definitive therapy of a stable spinal injury might simply consist of a cervical traction device or other spinal orthosis, such as a thoracolumbosacral orthosis brace for thoracic or lumbar spinal injuries. However, in the case of an unstable spinal injury, surgical reduction and fixation might be necessary soon after injury. It is extremely rare that a spinal procedure will be carried out in the same setting as the craniotomy. Ideally, the spinal operation can be delayed until after brain edema has resolved sufficiently, usually 72 hours, so as to minimize the risks of subsequent surgery.[28] After all, any hypotension or blood loss associated with the spinal surgery could contribute to secondary brain injury. If early operative spinal intervention within the first five days following injury is anticipated, an intracranial pressure (ICP) device can be inserted during the craniotomy and used during subsequent operations as a monitor and guide to therapy.

Treatment of Spinal Cord Injury

There are two major goals in the treatment of spinal cord injury: to decompress the neural elements and to stabilize the spine.[2] When a neurologic deficit exists, the surgeon must ensure that further spinal cord injury does not occur because of cord compression caused by a bone fragment, displaced disc, or hematoma. Equally important in the treatment process is to achieve both immediate and long-term stability of the spine. Instability would result in a spine that could not tolerate normal physiologic loads without incurring possible further neurologic deficit, limiting pain, or progressive structural deformity.[29]

Initial stability can often be achieved with simple immobility, using a halo vest or Gardner-Wells tongs in the case of a cervical spine fracture. If a subluxation exists, reduction can be attained with the addition of traction by attaching weights over a pulley apparatus. Cervical traction in the axial direction will often also allow positioning of bone fragments and decompression of the spinal canal. Starting with about 3 to 4 kg of weight on the traction system, serial plain lateral radiographs of the neck are taken, with gradual increases in the weight as necessary until the subluxation is reduced. Distraction of the vertebral bodies is an indication that too much weight is being applied, the maximum weight being between 25 and 35 kg.[29]

In those patients with an incomplete neurologic deficit after initial reduction, a CT-myelography can be helpful in ruling out impingement on the neural canal. When dealing with extrinsic cord compression, early operation within the first day after injury is indicated for a patient with progressive neurologic deterioration despite adequate immobilization.[2] Early operation may also be necessary for those patients who cannot be properly immobilized or adequately reduced using traction. For example, locked facet joints between two subluxed vertebrae can prevent closed reduction, and this may need to be addressed with operative facetectomy.

Traditional views maintain that early operation is not indicated for a complete spinal cord injury with total absence of motor and sensory function below the level of injury, whether or not there is neural compression. The argument has been that in these patients, the damage to the spinal cord has already occurred, most likely at the time of the initial impact, and that efforts to reverse this clinical picture with operative decompression have little to no bearing on the patients' final neurologic functional outcome.[29]

Proponents of conservative management have extended this approach to the spinal cord–injured patient who is neurologically stable but has an incomplete neurologic deficit. Several authors have found that early operation on such patients may in fact be detrimental, with an increased risk of neurologic deterioration or an increased morbidity without the benefit of improved outcome. Marshall et al, in a multicenter retrospective analysis, reported that neurologic deterioration occurred exclusively in patients operated upon within five days of injury.[30] Of the 283 spinal cord injury patients in this study, 14 (4.9%) experienced neurologic deterioration during initial hospital management, and 12 of these were associated with specific events. Four of 134 patients undergoing operative intervention deteriorated. Since each of the three patients with a cervical cord injury who deteriorated was operated on within the first five days and no deterioration was observed in patients operated on beyond five days, the authors concluded that early surgery on the cervical spine may be hazardous.[30] This confirmed earlier data from Heiden et al, who found that early operation in the cervical spinal cord–injured patient increased morbidity.[31] This view would argue for prolonged conservative treatment with immobilization followed by operative decompression and fixation if needed for long-term stability.

More recently, however, these traditional opinions have come into question. What of the systemic risks of prolonged immobilization? What of the delay in getting these patients started on a rehabilitation program? Not only are the monetary costs associated with prolonged hospitalization extremely high, but the physical and psychosocial effects on the patient and his or her family can be extraordinary. Finally, and perhaps most important, does early operation really adversely affect neurologic and functional outcome? To answer these questions, a careful look at some of the more recent literature may be helpful.

In a retrospective review, Levi et al sought to clarify the ideal timing of operative anterior decompression and stabilization in patients with both incomplete and complete cervical cord injury.[32] Of the 50 patients with incomplete neurologic deficits, 10 underwent surgery within 24 hours, and the remaining 40 patients underwent delayed surgery at a mean of 13 days (range 2 to 77 days) past the injury.

These two subgroups were similar in terms of their motor scores and functional grade improvements at discharge compared to admission and in terms of the average length of stay in the acute hospital setting. Although the early-surgery group of patients with incomplete deficits was small (only 10 patients), none had a worsened functional outcome at discharge, and operative morbidity was similar to the delayed-surgery group. A more notable difference was observed in the 53 patients with complete neurologic deficits. In this group, 35 patients underwent early surgery within 24 hours, and 18 underwent delayed surgery again at a mean of 13 days (range 2 to 45 days) following injury. In a comparison of these subgroups, the motor scores and functional grade improvements were similarly small, but the early-surgery group had a significantly shorter acute hospital stay (5 weeks vs 6 weeks) and a significantly less frequent need for chest physiotherapy procedures, which served as a marker for easier patient care and sooner mobilization. The authors concluded that early operation is the preferred treatment for patients with middle to lower cervical spine trauma, since it may facilitate earlier mobilization and rehabilitation and does not increase the complication rate or induce any adverse effects compared to delayed surgery.[32]

In another study, Murphy et al compared the outcome of surgical and nonsurgical management of cervical spinal cord injury.[33] In this retrospective analysis, 102 patients were divided into four groups: patients with cervical instability managed with nonsurgical immobilization (35 patients), patients with cervical instability undergoing surgical fixation within 2 weeks of injury (44 patients), patients with cervical instability undergoing surgical fixation more than 2 weeks after injury (14 patients), and finally patients who were admitted with a stable cervical column but with a spinal cord injury and a neurologic deficit (9 patients). Patients treated with early surgical stabilization (less than 2 weeks from the time of injury) were hospitalized a mean of 21 fewer days than the group managed nonoperatively with external immobilization of the unstable spine and 29 fewer days than the late-surgery group. In addition, the first therapeutic leave of absence from primary rehabilitation was achieved on average 40 days sooner in the early-surgery group compared to the nonsurgical group. Functional outcomes and complications for the surgical and nonsurgical treatment groups were similar. These authors concluded that early operative reduction and internal fixation of the unstable cervical spine not only reduced hospital length of stay but also allowed for earlier achievement of the goals of rehabilitation.[33] Prolonged external stabilization with a halo vest or other bulky orthoses, on the other hand, might significantly hinder certain rehabilitative efforts such as upper-extremity dressing, facial hygiene, wheelchair mobility, and independent transfers.[16] All of these factors can greatly affect total hospital costs as well as the physical and emotional well-being of the patient.

The same reasoning has been considered for other regions of the spine. Krengel et al reported 14 patients with incomplete thoracic-level paraplegia, all of whom were treated by early operative reduction, decompression, and stabilization. Twelve had surgery within 24 hours, and the remaining 2 had surgery at 36 hours and 5 days after injury. Most patients in this series underwent posterior instrumentation and stabilization. Among the 13 surviving patients, 7 were initially classified as Frankel B, and of these, 4 recovered to Frankel E, 2 recovered to Frankel D, and 1 remained Frankel B. Six patients were initially Frankel C, 5 of whom improved to Frankel E and 1 of whom improved to Frankel D. The authors concluded that early surgical reduction, decompression, and stabilization are safe and improve neurologic recovery compared to that of historical controls treated by closed reduction or late operative intervention.[34]

Not all investigators, however, have found that operative intervention correlates with functional recovery. In a review of 22 patients with thoracolumbar fractures associated with spinal cord injury and a neurologic deficit, Lemons et al reported that despite posterior instrumentation, decompression, and fusion, the extent of spinal canal reconstruction failed to correlate with neurologic recovery.[35] They found instead that the greater the initial spinal canal compromise, the more severe the neurologic deficit, both initially and at up to 15 months follow-up. Although the timing of operative intervention was not considered, surgical efforts to restore near-anatomic spinal realignment, as assessed by postoperative axial canal dimensions, did not result in greater neurologic recovery. These authors concluded that the degree of bony and neurologic injury directly reflects the kinetic energy transferred at the time of impact and that ongoing compression and distortion of the neural canal does not significantly contribute to the overall neurologic injury or to the potential for recovery.[35]

The literature is certainly full of controversy regarding the timing of operative intervention and whether surgery positively affects neurologic outcomes. But regardless, it is clear that spinal cord–injured patients require aggressive care and management from the time of injury. With the more recent treatment approaches, it would appear that early definitive surgical intervention may hold significant advantages over the more traditional approaches of prolonged nonsurgical immobilization or late operation. First, it may provide an environment more conducive to fuller neurologic recovery. Experimental studies have suggested that recovery from incomplete cord injury does not occur until mechanical compression is relieved. A decompressed, realigned, stable spine may allow for some neurologic recovery before irreversible changes in white matter occur.[36] Second, early surgical stabilization may facilitate patient mobility and thereby prevent some of the adverse systemic and psychological effects associated with prolonged bed rest. The brain-injured patient may also be less prone to agitation, necessitating excessive sedation, if environmental stimuli and mobility begin early. The net consequence would be less difficult nursing care and reduced hospital costs. Finally, all of this would hopefully translate into an earlier start for rehabilitation and a return to more independent living.

ICU Management of the Patient with Brain and Spinal Cord Injury

The critical care environment plays an important role in the early stages after spinal cord injury. During this phase, an interactive team of caregivers work together to promote the patient's medical and psychologic stability and wellness. Nurses, respiratory therapists, physical and occupational therapists, social workers, trauma surgeons, intensivists, neurosurgeons, orthopaedic surgeons, and physiatrists all have specific areas of expertise. When their services are coordinated and delivered with mutual respect, not only is the patient's acute care optimized, but a successful rehabilitation program is initiated.[3] The value of a multidisciplinary approach holds for any multiply injured trauma patient, though it may have its greatest impact on the patient with brain and spinal cord injury.

In the spinal cord–injured patient, autonomic disturbances can affect a variety of organ systems, and these must be recognized and dealt with appropriately in the acute and subacute phases. In patients with T-6 lesions and higher, there will be a loss of sympathetic tone, since the sympathetic ganglion has been disrupted. This is accompanied by unopposed parasympathetic activity from the vagus nerves.[1,3] Initially, this can lead to neurogenic shock characterized by hypotension and bradycardia. Other symptoms include excessive pulmonary secretions and bronchospasm, a loss of thermoregulation, and gastrointestinal and genitourinary dysfunction.[1,3,37] Depression of the blood pressure and heart rate is usually self-limited, although vasoactive drugs, such as scopolamine patches, dopamine, epinephrine, or norepinephrine, and rarely even a pacemaker may be required.[37] This is especially important in light of maintaining adequate cerebral perfusion in the patient with brain injury.

Gastrointestinal disturbances include gastric distention and an adynamic ileus.[1,3] Although parenteral nutrition may be necessary at first, enteral feedings should be instituted as soon as gastrointestinal function permits. A bowel regimen including stool softeners, enemas, and cathartics will help maintain bowel motility. Acute hemodynamic decompensation can result from noxious somatic or visceral stimulation, the latter being caused by distention of a hollow viscus organ such as the stomach, bowel, or bladder. The underlying stimulus must be quickly removed to restore stability.[1,3] In the case of a distended viscus, effective intervention might include the placement of a nasogastric tube or Foley catheter or the evacuation of an impacted rectum.

Respiratory insufficiency with the need for mechanical ventilation is a common problem in the spinal cord–injured patient. Quadriplegics and high-thoracic paraplegics must rely solely on diaphragmatic contraction for their breathing.[1,16] The paralysis of intercostal and abdominal musculature, along with associated chest and abdominal injuries, will significantly impair normal respiratory mechanics.[16] As previously mentioned, the loss of sympathetic activity with unopposed vagal outflow to the lungs results in bronchospasm and excessive pulmonary secretions.[1,37] In a small number of patients, this can even result in an acute respiratory distress syndrome (ARDS) pattern, sometimes referred to as *neurogenic pulmonary edema*. Careful ventilatory management in this group of patients includes the cautious titration of positive end-expiratory pressure to balance the need for improved oxygenation against the resultant elevation in ICP.[28]

Nurses and respiratory therapists and/or physical therapists must be actively involved in maintaining good pulmonary toilet: careful posturing, frequent suctioning, and chest physiotherapy are all very important maneuvers.[3,16,37] Frequently the patient with brain and spinal cord injury requires a tracheostomy, either because of prolonged mechanical ventilation or simply for maintaining adequate pulmonary toilet if ability to cooperate is impaired. Weaning from the ventilator should be aimed at improving diaphragmatic strength and endurance, and this often requires time and patience. Following removal from the ventilator, good pulmonary toilet must be continued and augmented by incentive spirometry and assisted coughing with abdominal compression.[16] Without these measures, patients may develop diaphragmatic fatigue, atelectasis, or an inability to clear copious bronchial secretions and pneumonia, all of which constitute significant morbidity in this patient population.

Particular attention must also be paid to skin integrity and the avoidance of joint contractures in the intensive care unit (ICU). Initially, the patient must be carefully repositioned every two hours around the clock to prevent skin breakdown.[1,3,37] In the patient with an unstable spine, logrolling techniques can be used to maintain axial alignment. Special rotating beds and flotation beds have been used to avoid sustained pressure on a given area of skin.[37] Special-care beds with compartmentalized air mattresses can be helpful in that they provide a low-pressure surface with continuous alterations in the degree of inflation and pressure in the various segments of the bed. It must be remembered that special beds are only an adjunct to expert nursing care.[37] Eventually, skin tolerance gradually builds up, and turning can be done less frequently. By this time, many patients will have learned techniques for maintenance of their own skin integrity.[1,16] Another essential aspect of care is the prevention of joint contractures, which, if they occur, can significantly impair optimal rehabilitation and mobility. Early range-of-motion exercises should be carried out by experienced therapists.[16,37] The use of intermittent splints will also help maintain joints in a neutral position in between therapy sessions.

Not to be overlooked is the tremendous need for psychologic support for the patient and family members. The psychologic stresses can be compounded by brain injury, the net result being cognitive deficits, behavioral disturbances, and depression.[3,16] In the ICU environment, the nurses become the first line in recognizing these disturbances and, to their credit, offer perhaps the greatest support to the patient following spinal cord injury with or without brain injury. Social workers can help address long-term issues such as discharge planning or placement. Other members of the multidisciplinary team must also be sensitive to the patient's psychosocial needs during this acute phase. This will help pave the road toward a successful transition to a rehabilitation center.

MUSCULOSKELETAL INJURIES

Patients sustaining brain injury following high-energy blunt trauma are at high risk for associated musculoskeletal injuries. Most often, these multiple injuries follow motor vehicle accidents. Of course, the extent and type of musculoskeletal injuries can vary tremendously depending upon the mechanism of trauma. Although fractures of the upper extremity can occur in the multiply injured patient, they are much less common than those of the lower extremity.[38] Further, upper-extremity fractures are more likely to be noncomminuted isolated fractures that are amenable to simple closed reduction and have a high likelihood of proper reunion. Therefore, in this section, the focus will be on two general groups of musculoskeletal injuries that have the most significant impact on both the acute care and long-term rehabilitation of the patient with severe brain injury: pelvic fractures and long bone fractures of the lower extremity.

Pelvic Fractures

The incidence of pelvic fractures among patients sustaining multiple trauma has been estimated to be around 30%. Greater than 60% of pelvic fractures result from motor vehicle accidents, with pedestrians appearing to be at higher risk than vehicle occupants. An additional 30% of pelvic fractures are caused by falls from a height.[39] The mortality rates of pelvic fractures ranges between 6% and 19% but may be as high as 50% when associated with hypotension in the multiply injured patient.[39-41]

Pelvic Anatomy

To fully comprehend the significance of pelvic fractures, one must have a sound understanding of pelvic anatomy (Figure 6–8). The pelvic ring is made up of three bones with strong ligamentous attachments holding them together: two paired innominate bones and a sacrum in the center posteriorly. The innominate bone is further divided into several components: the ileum, ischium, and pubis. The sacrum is firmly suspended from the two innominate bones by the very sturdy posterosuperior sacroiliac ligaments along with several accessory ligaments that reinforce the pelvic ring and floor: the anterior sacroiliac, sacrotuberous, and

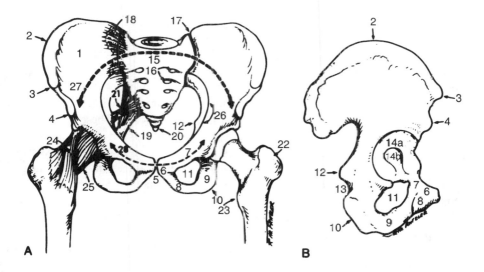

Figure 6–8 Pelvic anatomy. A, Anterior view of pelvis. B, Lateral view of right innominate bone. 1 = iliac fossa, 2 = iliac crest, 3 = anterior superior iliac spine, 4 = anterior inferior iliac spine, 5 = symphysis pubis, 6 = body of pubis, 7 = superior ramus of pubis, 8 = inferior ramus of pubis, 9 = ramus of ischium, 10 = ischial tuberosity, 11 = obturator foramen, 12 = ischial spine, 13 = lesser sciatic notch, 14 = acetabulum (14a = articular surface, 14b = fossa), 15 = sacrum, 16 = anterior sacral foramina, 17 = sacroiliac joint, 18 = anterior sacroiliac ligament, 19 = trochanter of femur, 20 = coccyx, 21 = sacrospinous ligament, 22 = greater trochanter of femur, 23 = lesser trochanter of femur, 24 = iliofemoral ligament, 25 = pubofemoral ligament, 26 = arcuate line, 27 = posterior or femorosacral arch, through which main weight-bearing forces are transmitted, 28 = anterior arch. *Source:* Reprinted with permission from P. Rosen and R. Barkin, eds., *Emergency Medicine: Concepts and Clinical Practice,* 3rd edition, p. 659, © 1992, Mosby-Year Book, Inc.

sacrospinous ligaments. In addition, the iliotransverse ligament connects the posterior ilium to the transverse processes of the fifth lumbar vertebra. At the symphysis pubis, a thick fibrocartilaginous disc supported by the inferior pubic ligament forms the anterior junction between the two innominate bones. The posterior portion of the pelvis carries more importance than the anterior part; not only does it provide stability, but it also serves to bridge the upper body to the lower extremities for important functional purposes such as standing, walking, and sitting.[39,42,43]

Classification of Pelvic Fractures

There have been many different classification schemes of pelvic fractures. Some rely on radiographic appearance to judge stability or lack of stability, others categorize with respect to the degree of the complexity, and still others base the classification on the direction of the injurious forces.

The Key and Conwell classification system rates fractures according to their complexity, determining if there is a break in the pelvic ring and, if so, whether the fractures are single or double.[39] Type I fractures include avulsion fractures, which usually follow sports-related injuries, fractures of a single ramus, isolated fractures of the iliac wing, and fractures of the sacrum or coccyx. These are stable injuries and heal well with bed rest. Type II fractures are those involving a single break in the pelvic ring and occur as a fracture near or a subluxation of the symphysis pubis or sacroiliac joints. There is relative mobility at these regions, which may allow a single break to occur. Fractures of two ipsilateral rami are also defined as type II fractures. In general, type II fractures are considered stable if not displaced and can be managed nonoperatively.[39] A thorough search for a second disruption within the pelvic ring must be made when one suspects a type II fracture, since a single break in a ring is quite unusual. In fact, for this reason, this entire classification scheme has received criticism and is less often used.[44]

Type III fractures occur as double breaks in the pelvic ring, with disruptions at two or more sites. In general, these result from severe forces and are often associated with significant hemorrhage into the retroperitoneal space.[39] Several classically described variants exist. A straddle fracture occurs with fractures to all four ischiopubic rami, or with ipsilateral ischiopubic fractures and diastasis of the symphysis pubis.[39,43] Up to one third of these patients will have associated genitourinary tract injury.[39] Straddle fractures result from lateral compression or from a fall straddling a hard object.[39,43] A Malgaigne fracture represents a severe injury resulting from vertical shear force in which there is disruption of the anterior elements at the level of the symphysis pubis or both ipsilateral ischiopubic rami, as well as disruption of the posterior pelvis involving the ipsilateral sacroiliac joint, ilium, or sacrum.[39,45] The forces involved in the mechanism of injury usually result in multiple associated injuries and a high degree of morbidity and mortality.[39,45] In an open-book fracture, anteroposterior compressive forces exerted against the anterosuperior iliac spines cause separation of the symphysis pubis as well as both sacroiliac joints. A sprung pelvis, also referred to as a dislocated pelvis, is a wide separation of the symphysis pubis and one or both sacroiliac joints. A bucket-handle fracture results from a lateral compression force combined with an upward rotary force. This results in an oblique fracture through the contralateral ischiopubic rami and a disruption around the ipsilateral sacroiliac joint.[39]

Finally, type IV fractures are those involving the acetabulum. These are frequently associated with other breaks in the pelvic ring. They must be managed aggressively, since the slightest uneven surface between the femoral head and acetabulum will cause rapid erosion of the articular cartilage, leading to posttraumatic arthritis.[39]

A separate classification scheme as proposed by Pennal et al and Tile and later refined by Young and Burgess categorizes all pelvic ring fractures on the basis of the direction of injurious forces (Figure 6–9).[46–48] These forces are lateral compression, anteroposterior compression, vertical shear, and combined mechanical injury. Each is further subdivided into three types (types I, II, and III) with increasing severity of the fracture.[44,43] Lateral compression presents as a horizontal fracture through the pubic rami or as an "overlapping" type of fracture. A crush-impacted fracture of the sacrum is frequently seen as well. In anteroposterior compression, one sees a diastasis of the symphysis pubis or vertical fractures through the pubic rami; the more severe types (II and III) also involve disruption of the sacroiliac joints. In vertical shear, as seen with falls from a height, vertically oriented fractures occur through both the anterior and posterior portions of the pelvic ring, with superior displacement of the fractured segment. Finally, combined mechanical injuries result from multiple force vectors.[44,48] This classification scheme may be more useful clinically to the orthopaedic surgeon as he or she decides upon the method of fixation and what corrective forces should be applied. It can also help predict which patients will have significant hemorrhage or other associated injuries. Type III lateral compression fractures, types II and III anteroposterior

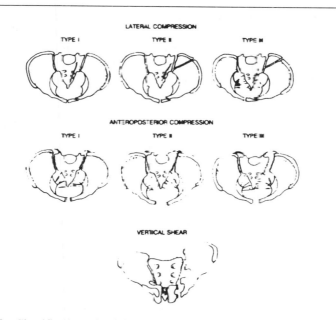

Figure 6–9 Classification of pelvic ring fractures based on the direction of injurious forces. *Source:* Reprinted with permission from J.W.R. Young and C.S. Resnick, *American Journal of Roentgenology,* Vol. 155, p. 1171, © 1990, American Roentgen Ray Society.

compression fractures, types II and III vertical shear fractures, and combined mechanical force injuries all have a high incidence of these comorbid conditions.[44]

Injuries Coexisting with Pelvic Fractures

Given the mechanism of injury, patients with major pelvic fractures are at high risk for other injuries remote from the pelvis, including trauma to the brain, chest, and abdomen, all of which can pose serious threats to survival. The incidence of brain injury in patients with pelvic fractures has been reported to be 26% but exceeds 50% in some series.[49] Injuries to the central nervous system account for many of the deaths in these patients. A small number of patients with pelvic fractures, approximately 6%, will have sustained a ruptured thoracic aorta. Intraabdominal injuries occur in 16% to 26% of patients with pelvic fractures, and in up to 55% of patients with pelvic fractures that are associated with hemodynamic instability.[49–51]

In addition to associated systemic injuries, pelvic fractures also put local structures at risk. Bladder and urethral disruptions occur frequently with damage to the anterior portion of the pelvic ring, as is seen with anteroposterior compression and vertical shear fractures.[49,50] Approximately 7% to 17% of male patients with severe pelvic fractures will have an injury to the posterior urethra. The lower lumbar and sacral nerve roots are at risk for injury, since they are adherent to the anterior surface of the sacrum.[42,49] The pudendal nerves, coursing medially to the ischial rami on their way to the genitalia, can also be damaged. Trauma to the rectum and reproductive organs can be seen as well.[42,49] These associated injuries must be carefully looked for during the evaluation once the patient is adequately resuscitated.[49]

Perhaps the most serious life-threatening sequela of pelvic fractures is that of hemorrhage. High-energy pelvic fractures can result in vascular disruptions with significant hemorrhage into the extraperitoneal space. Small amounts of widening of the pelvic ring, as seen, for example, with a diastasis of the symphysis pubis, can markedly increase the potential space of the pelvis, into which a large volume of retroperitoneal bleeding can occur.[39,42,50] The normal volume in the adult pelvis, about 1.5 L, can increase to as much as 5 L with just a 2-cm diastasis of the pubic symphysis.[50] By far the most common sources of bleeding are from disruption of the rich venous plexus within the pelvis, as well as from bony surfaces at the fracture sites.[42,50] Fortunately, in these cases, the pelvic hematoma will usually tamponade by an intact retroperitoneum, and active bleeding will cease. However, as the severity of the pelvic fracture increases with high-force impacts, resulting in bony and ligamentous disruption, arterial branches may also be injured.[50] The incidence of identifiable arterial bleeding has been estimated to be between 5% and 15%.[50,51] Rarely, a major artery such as the common iliac, external iliac, internal iliac, or femoral artery will be involved.[39,50] More frequently, however, branches of the internal iliac artery such as the superior gluteal artery and internal pudendal artery are the source of bleeding. The superior gluteal artery is particularly at risk with posterior pelvic fractures, since the artery courses around the superior margin of the sciatic notch.[39,50] The internal pudendal artery is in close proximity to the inferior ligaments of the pelvis and pubic rami and therefore is at risk with severe fractures through the pubic rami anteriorly.[50] Other branches of the internal iliac artery, including the lateral sacral, obturator, and vesical arteries, are less frequently involved.[50]

Management of Pelvic Fractures

In the multiply injured patient exhibiting hemodynamic instability, sources of hemorrhage must be quickly found and controlled while the resuscitation is in progress. Bleeding may be occurring intraperitoneally from an abdominal injury or extraperitoneally from an unstable pelvic fracture. Diagnostic peritoneal lavage (DPL) via an open supraumbilical approach can be used to quickly determine if an intra-abdominal injury is contributing to significant hemorrhage.[39,51] It must be kept in mind that the false-positive rate of DPL may be as high as 29% in patients with pelvic fractures. This is because of slight, perhaps inactive bleeding from minor intra-abdominal injuries or, in the case of a large retroperitoneal hematoma from a pelvic fracture, blood seeping intra-abdominally from small tears in the peritoneum or from diapedesis of red blood cells through an intact peritoneum.[50,52] Therefore, only in patients with a grossly positive (frank blood) DPL is there a high likelihood of active bleeding from an intra-abdominal source.[41] These patients should undergo immediate laparotomy. A newer alternative to DPL is ultrasonography to look for evidence of a hemoperitoneum. The use of CT in the evaluation of abdominal and pelvic injuries should be restricted to hemodynamically stable patients.

Once major intra-abdominal injury is ruled out or addressed with a laparotomy, if the patient with a major pelvic fracture remains hemodynamically unstable, extraperitoneal hemorrhage into the pelvic basin must be considered. External fixation of the pelvis is a first step toward stabilizing the bones and restoring the normal volume of the pelvis. It acts as an effective splint to reduce bleeding from the disrupted venous plexus and fractured bony surfaces so that tamponade is more likely to occur (Figure 6–10).[39,51] A pelvic external fixator can be applied quickly in 15 to 20 minutes. Two or three "half pins" are driven into each anterior iliac crest, and an anterior frame then links the two innominate bones.[39] The external fixator does have limitations, however. It cannot be used when significant iliac wing comminution prevents stable application.[39] In addition, anterior fixation by itself is unlikely to control hemorrhage from arterial sources or gain stability in the posterior portion of the pelvis.[50]

Angiographic embolization can therefore be of great benefit to patients with hemodynamic evidence of ongoing hemorrhage. Approximately 10% of patients with pelvic fractures will require embolization.[50,51] But within the different cat-

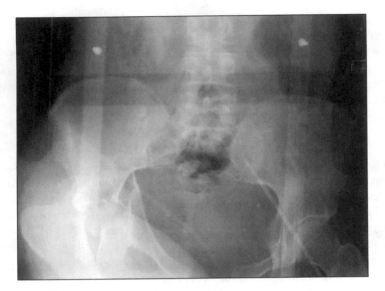

Figure 6–10 A young woman involved in a motor vehicle accident was found to be in shock on arrival in the emergency department. An anterior-posterior radiograph demonstrates a complex severe pelvic fracture that involves superior displacement of the entire right hemipelvis along with destruction of the right acetabulum and femoral head. She underwent external fixation of the pelvis to control extraperitoneal hemorrhage into the pelvic basin.

egories of pelvic fractures based on the injurious forces and the severity of injury, there are marked differences in the incidence of arterial hemorrhage necessitating angiographic embolization. An analysis of a large series of patients by Burgess et al revealed that the majority of patients had lateral compression mechanisms and isolated iliac wing fractures. Only 1.7% of these patients required arterial embolization. On the other hand, a smaller group of patients who had sustained more severe fractures from anteroposterior compression, vertical shear, and combined mechanical injury mechanisms required embolization in 20% of cases.[53]

When angiography identifies injury to the major arteries of the pelvis, such as the common iliac, external iliac, or common femoral arteries, temporary control with balloon occlusion will allow time for immediate preparations for surgical repair and reconstruction. When the internal iliac artery or its branches are found to be the source, careful embolization can stop or slow down bleeding significantly so that clotting will occur without creating large areas of ischemia and necrosis.[50]

Once life-threatening hemorrhage has been successfully treated, management turns to restoration of normal pelvic anatomy and function so that early rehabilitation can take place. It has been shown in the treatment of both long bone fractures and pelvic fractures that early definitive fixation leads to fewer complications and a more timely recovery.[54,55] When Latenser et al reviewed multiply injured patients with unstable pelvic fractures, they found that early internal or external fixation within eight hours of arrival at the emergency department was associated with decreased hospital length of stay, fewer complications and blood transfusions, shorter disability times, a more frequent discharge to home rather than to a rehabilitation facility, and, finally, overall better survival when compared to those patients in whom early fixation was not routinely used.[56]

When choosing an approach to fixation of pelvic fractures, one must address breaks through both the anterior and posterior portions of the pelvic ring. An anterior external fixator can be augmented by internal or external fixation of the posterior elements. But external fixation alone has its limitations: it cannot adequately stabilize all complex fractures, and it further imposes functional restrictions and reduced mobility upon patients.[56] This can in turn lead to increased complications such as deep-vein thrombosis formation, pulmonary embolism, and other adverse pulmonary sequelae such as atelectasis and pneumonia.[54,56] For this reason, operative internal fixation has gained more and more support. Through an ilioanterior approach, the anterior symphysis and rami as well as the posterior sacroiliac regions of the pelvis can be reduced and fixated using reconstructive plates and screws.[57] This is best accomplished early, since reduction maneuvers are technically difficult after the third postinjury day and since after seven days the likelihood of successful reunion diminishes greatly.[56]

Although more accurate reduction can be accomplished with early surgical intervention, the ideal operative timing for severe pelvic fractures must be carefully balanced with the risks of surgery in the patient with brain injury. Excessive blood loss and hypotension may become a problem during operative pelvic fixation. This can lead to impaired tissue perfusion and oxygen delivery to the already compromised brain. The risk of secondary brain injury is especially great within the first 72 hours following traumatic brain injury, when brain edema is at its maximum. For these reasons, the patient with brain injury should be hemodynamically stable for at least 24 hours prior to definitive repair of a pelvic fracture. If early fixation within the first three days is considered the best option in terms of functional outcome, then an ICP monitoring device can be an important adjunct in the perioperative and intraoperative management of the patient with brain injury.

Because of the higher incidence of sepsis, complex open pelvic fractures carry a much higher morbidity and mortality risk than do closed pelvic fractures. Thorough debridement and irrigation of the wounds along with antibiotics play an important role in their management.[42,58] An elective colostomy is a strong consideration for open pelvic fractures in which fecal soilage could lead to ongoing contamination of the perineal wound and pelvis, resulting in the development of systemic sepsis and multiple organ failure.[58,59]

Treatment of associated anorectal trauma is based upon debridement and, if possible, repair of the injury, drainage of the perirectal space, diversion of the fecal stream with a colostomy, and distal washout of the defunctionalized rectum.[59,60] Regarding genitourinary tract injuries, there is some controversy regarding early versus delayed urethroplasty. Delayed urethroplasty may lead to higher stricture rates but fewer problems with impotence and incontinence. Nonetheless, advocates of early repair claim comparably good results.[42] Rupture of the bladder can be managed by primary closure at the time of the initial procedure.

Long Bone Fractures of the Lower Extremities

Lower-extremity fractures are frequently seen in the multiply injured patient. Although by themselves long bone fractures are rarely life threatening, they can be associated with significant morbidity in these seriously injured patients. Further, orthopaedic injuries can greatly influence both the patient's acute and late care. Early fixation of the fracture and mobilization are an important management goal to prevent complications and facilitate overall rehabilitation.[54,55]

In the patient with brain injury and multiple associated injuries, it is critical not to overlook long bone fractures. The mechanism of injury can provide important clues as to the presence of orthopaedic injuries. For example, the unrestrained occupant of a deceleration type of motor vehicle accident will be subject to injuries of the hip, femur, and knee because of impact while the hip and knee are in a flexed position. The ankle and foot, as they press against the brake or clutch, are likewise at risk. A fall from a height can be associated with multiple complex fractures, including those to the calcaneus, talus, tibial plateau, pelvis, or vertebrae.[61]

The patient with brain injury may not be able to indicate local pain at a fracture site. Therefore, one must carefully look for evidence of bony disruption during a detailed secondary survey in the emergency department. Physical examination will almost always reveal deformity and/or swelling at the fracture or dislocation site; the truly occult fracture is quite rare. Shortening, rotation, or angulation of the extremity is usually seen with long bone fractures. Dislocations cause the extremity to be in a characteristic position.

With any orthopaedic injury, the bone will absorb a certain amount of energy before it fails and hence fractures. The normal healthy bones of a young person will be able to withstand much greater forces than the osteoporotic bones of an elderly individual. Therefore, it will take higher-energy impacts to cause disruption of normal bone in the younger population. Once failure occurs, the absorbed energy is released from the bone and to the surrounding tissues. As a result, high-impact injuries will be associated with a greater likelihood of comminution, displacement, and soft tissue injury.[61] Peripheral nerves, vascular structures, muscles, tendons, ligaments, and skin can all be damaged by these types of injuries.

Specific Orthopaedic Injuries

Hip Dislocation. Posterior dislocations of the hip are a common injury among motor vehicle occupants. During deceleration, impact against a flexed knee drives the femoral head posteriorly out of the hip joint. The typical position of the extremity is that of wide abduction and external rotation of the hip. The sciatic or peroneal nerves may be damaged with the dislocation. Closed reduction followed by four to six weeks of skeletal traction is usually curative; however, an associated posterior acetabular fracture can prevent stable reduction. In this instance, open arthrotomy of the hip may be necessary.[61]

Proximal Femur Fractures. Fractures of the proximal femur can be of three types: intracapsular (femoral neck fractures), intertrochanteric, and subtrochanteric. The first two types are common injuries among the elderly following a fall, though extensively comminuted and displaced fractures through the proximal femur can occur as a result of major trauma in younger patients. The lower extremity will be seen as shortened and externally rotated.[61] The major risk with femoral neck fractures is a loss of blood supply to the femoral head, resulting in aseptic necrosis. This occurs in as many as 30% of cases and can be delayed for several years after the trauma. Depending upon the extent of comminution and displacement, if adequate internal fixation of an intracapsular fracture cannot be achieved, excision of the femoral head and hemiarthroplasty with an endoprosthesis may be necessary.[62] There is evidence that emergent fixation of femoral neck fractures within 12 hours of injury in younger patients decreases the incidence of aseptic necrosis.[63] Patients with intertrochanteric fractures, more common among the elderly, and subtrochanteric fractures, found usually in younger patients following major trauma, likewise benefit from urgent internal fixation so as to promote early mobilization and rehabilitation.[6]

Femoral Shaft Fractures. Femoral shaft fractures are usually seen with high-energy trauma and as a result are frequently associated with extensive soft tissue contusion and bleeding. If severe, this can lead to compartment syndrome of the thigh, resulting in muscle necrosis and the threat of limb loss.[64] Early internal fixation with reamed intramedullary nailing (rodding) has been used with great success in achieving proper reunion.[65] This can be done immediately after more life-threatening injuries have been addressed and the patient is hemodynamically stable. Once again, early fixation will allow for rapid mobilization of the patient with progressive weight bearing on the affected extremity.

Injuries Surrounding the Knee. Injuries about the knee include supracondylar femur fractures, fractures of the patella, tibial plateau fractures, and dislocations and ligamentous injuries of the knee. The primary goal in treating these injuries is to quickly restore the joint surface and fixate the bone fragments so as to achieve early mobilization of the joint and the patient. Bone fixation can be accomplished using a variety of methods: intramedullary nails, plates, cancellous screws, and autogenous bone grafts from the iliac crest are some of the reconstructive materials.[61]

Particular attention should be directed toward tibiofemoral (knee) dislocations resulting from high-energy forces to the knee. The popliteal vessels coursing through the popliteal fossa are at risk of damage with posterior disruption of the knee joint. Stretching of the vessels can lead to endothelial intimal tearing with subsequent thrombosis and peripheral ischemia. A vascular injury may not at first be clinically obvious, but if there is a discrepancy in the distal pulses, angiography of the extremity is indicated. Duplex scanning is another option if a vascular injury is suspected on the basis of the mechanism of injury.[66] If a vascular injury is detected, it must be repaired immediately to prevent irreversible distal ischemia. Neuropraxia can also result from stretching of the deep peroneal and tibial nerves.[61]

Ligamentous and meniscal injuries of the knee are usually associated with hemarthrosis, which may require aspiration to relieve pain and to look for fat droplets indicating an intra-articular fracture. Physical examination to detect instability of the joint as well as arthroscopy and magnetic resonance imaging can be used to identify these injuries in a delayed fashion once the multiply injured patient is clinically stable and on the road toward rehabilitation.[61]

Tibial Fractures. High-energy impacts to the leg can result in comminuted open tibial fractures with extensive soft tissue injury. In fact, the tibia is the most common bone in the lower extremity associated with open fractures. These complex injuries present a challenge to the orthopaedic and reconstructive surgeon. External fixators may be needed to stabilize the bone fragments, particularly when there is a highly comminuted fracture of the proximal or distal tibia along with extensive disruption of the surrounding soft tissues.[67,68] Important surgical procedures also include debridement of all necrotic and devitalized tissue, judicious use of antibiotics, repair of major vascular injuries, and soft tissue coverage of exposed bone with eventual delayed closure of open wounds through the use of skin grafting, myocutaneous rotational flaps, or microvascular free flaps.[68,69]

Compartment Syndrome

Compartment syndrome is always a risk following any closed or open fracture of the lower extremity, but especially with fractures of the tibia in which significant crush injury has led to associated muscular or vascular damage.[70] Edema and hemorrhage within the fascial compartments cause the pressure within the compartment to eventually exceed microcirculatory pressures. This in turn leads to ischemia and necrosis of the muscles, nerves, and other soft tissues within the tight compartments.[70,71] If four-compartment fasciotomy of the calf is delayed beyond an irreversible point, not only will limb loss be likely, but dire systemic consequences will result. Restoration of vascular flow at this stage will allow a massive outpouring of free radicals and cytokines into the systemic circulation, leading to an overwhelming systemic inflammatory response as well as acute renal failure from rhabdomyolysis and myoglobinuria.[70,71]

The Mangled Extremity

The so-called mangled extremity, in which combined injuries to the skeletal, vascular, myocutaneous, and nervous structures have occurred, deserves special mention. These are fortunately rare injuries, comprising less than 1% of femoral fractures and 2% to 3% of tibial fractures. Not all of these extremities will be able to be successfully salvaged, in which case amputation becomes necessary.[72,73] Although repair and reconstruction should be aggressively considered, some of the clinical factors that might suggest the need for primary amputation include bone loss of greater than 5 cm, circumferential loss of skin and muscle, irreparable injury to nerves that would result in a loss of motor and sensory function of the foot and ankle, and persistent infection despite multiple debridements.[73,74] After salvage attempts, Poole et al found that the need for amputation was best predicted by severity of injury to the sciatic or tibial nerves and by failure of arterial repair, likely to have been caused by poor microcirculatory outflow in the crushed muscle beds.[74]

Rehabilitation with a well-fitted prosthesis is often a much better option for these patients than having to cope with the chronically disabling problems of neuropathy, pain, fracture nonunion, persistent infection, and vascular insufficiency. Further, persistent attempts to salvage a mangled extremity can result in prolonged hospitalization, narcotic dependency, and delayed rehabilitation, all while expensively draining operating room, nursing, blood bank, and emotional resources.[72,74]

Fat Embolism Syndrome

Another complication of musculoskeletal trauma is that of fat embolism syndrome (FES). Particularly in the patient with coexisting brain injury, FES can complicate both neurologic and overall systemic care. Fat embolism denotes the presence of fat globules in the lung parenchyma and peripheral circulation. There are many clinical situations, both traumatic and nontraumatic, in which fat emboli have been reported. In terms of major trauma with associated musculoskeletal injury, the prevalence of fat embolism is actually quite common, estimated to be greater than 90%.[75] FES, on the other hand, is a very specific clinical entity encompassing a classic triad of organ system involvement that includes pulmonary, neurologic, and cutaneous manifestations.[75] The syndrome occurs in about 1% to 4% of patients with isolated fractures of the tibia or femur and may reach as high as 5% to 10% in patients with bilateral or multiple bone fractures.[75,76] Although it can occur at any age, it is most common among trauma patients in their second or third decade.[75]

There are several mechanisms by which FES is thought to occur. A mechanical theory proposes that fat droplets are released from the marrow of long bone fractures and that these fat droplets then enter torn veins near the fracture site. They are then transported to the pulmonary vascular bed, some being trapped there and others going on to reach the systemic circulation. The result is fat emboli, not only in the pulmonary vascular bed, but also in other locations such as the brain, retina, kidney, or skin.[75]

Certain metabolic and biochemical reactions may propagate or even initiate these events. Mediators released at the site of fractures may affect the solubility of lipids, causing coalescence of normally small chylomicrons (less than 1 μm in diameter) into fat globules 10 to 40 μm in diameter. These larger globules are then capable of occluding capillaries in the pulmonary and other vascular beds.[75,76] In addition, free fatty acids may play a significant role. They may be released from the site of musculoskeletal trauma or mobilized from fat stores in the body as a result of high catecholamine output. Free fatty acids can also be formed during the breakdown of fat in the lung parenchyma from pulmonary lipases. Overall, free fatty acids can produce a very intense and destructive inflammatory response in the lung, leading to endothelial cell damage, capillary leak, and inactivation of lung surfactant, culminating in a pattern of ARDS.[75,76]

The clinical findings primarily include pulmonary, cerebral, and cutaneous manifestations. There is often a latent period from 12 to 72 hours after the trauma before signs and symptoms appear. Pulmonary findings are the most common manifestation and are usually the first to occur. The patient develops tachypnea, dyspnea, and hypoxemia, often accompanied by tachycardia and fever.[75,76] A Pao_2 of less than 60 mm Hg in the setting of an Fio_2 of less than 40% is documented by arterial blood gas. In severe cases, the development of ARDS will be marked by progressive hypoxemia and worsening pulmonary compliance requiring mechanical ventilatory support.

Central nervous system involvement includes variable symptoms ranging from mild disorientation to coma. In between these two extremes, the patient can experience headache, irritability, delirium, stupor, and seizures. Focal neurologic deficits are rare, though hemiparesis and hemiplegia have been reported. These neurologic manifestations occur in up to 80% of afflicted patients.[75] Cerebral edema caused by fat emboli contributes to the neurologic deterioration, and this edema can certainly compound that associated with primary brain injury. Clinical assessment and management of the patient with brain injury may consequently become more complicated and difficult. But in the setting of FES alone, the cerebral edema generally resolves with full neurologic recovery.[75]

Cutaneous manifestations occur in about half of patients, usually by the second or third day following the initial trauma. This will be seen as a petechial rash in nondependent portions of the body such as the chest, axilla, and conjunctiva. Funduscopic examination may also reveal retinal exudates and edema and perivascular or petechial hemorrhages.[75]

Other clinical and laboratory findings may include thrombocytopenia, anemia, hypocalcemia, increased erythrocyte sedimentation rate, raised serum lipid or lipase levels, and the presence of fat globules in the urine, sputum, or blood.[75,76] These findings are nonspecific, however, and may be found in many trauma patients without FES. Still, they can be useful in confirming suspicions in the proper clinical setting.

The treatment of FES may be somewhat preventative in the sense that early definitive fracture management may reduce its incidence. There is evidence that the risk of FES increases when operative fixation is delayed. Early intramedullary nailing of femoral shaft fractures, for example, may decrease the probability of FES.[75,77] Supportive pulmonary and systemic care is also an important aspect of care. Careful fluid management can prevent exacerbation of pulmonary and cerebral edema. Prophylactic corticosteroids may benefit high-risk patients: steroids are thought to stabilize cellular and capillary membranes and to decrease the inflammatory response caused by free fatty acids.[75] Morbidity and mortality of FES is often related to coexisting multiple injuries. In uncomplicated cases resulting from isolated skeletal trauma, patients generally do well with supportive care. However, in the setting of multiple trauma or with the development of coma or severe ARDS, prognosis can significantly worsen.

Timing of Operative Fixation for Long Bone Fractures

Early operative fixation of long bone fractures within 24 hours of injury is in most instances the optimal treatment strategy: it allows for more rapid mobilization of the extremity and the patient while diminishing the risks of FES and prolonged immobilization. However, there may be concern about the hemodynamic stability of the multiply injured patient. If intraoperative hypotension occurs during an orthopaedic procedure in a patient with brain trauma, such instability may contribute to secondary brain injury and negatively influence neurologic outcomes. This clinical scenario once again emphasizes the importance of adequate resuscitation and stabilization of the patient prior to operative fixation of long bone fractures. More life-threatening conditions that can contribute to shock must first be excluded or appropriately managed. Once hemodynamic stability has been ensured, it is safe to proceed with early surgical intervention for orthopaedic injuries (Figures 6–11 and 6–12).

In a retrospective review of 100 consecutive patients with lower-extremity long bone fractures, Marion et al found that there was no significant difference in the incidence of intraoperative hypotension among patients undergoing early internal fixation within 24 hours of injury (29%) and those undergoing delayed internal fixation beyond 24 hours (24%), lending support to the safety of early operative fixation.[78] Early surgery does carry many advantages in terms of rapid mobility and functional outcome, but it must be performed under hemodynamically stable conditions. As with early repair of other injuries, ICP monitoring should be strongly considered for the patient with severe brain injury.

THORACIC AND CARDIOVASCULAR TRAUMA

Thoracic injuries are a frequent occurrence in the multiply injured trauma patient. It is estimated that one half of unrestrained occupants in motor vehicle accidents will have sustained some form of thoracic injury. Blunt trauma from any cause, including traffic accidents and falls, can result in chest injury in up to a third of cases.[79] It is not surprising, therefore, that after blunt trauma, the patient with brain injury is at high risk for associated thoracic injury. Although high-energy impacts may lead to catastrophic thoracic and brain injuries resulting in fatalities at the scene of an accident, those who reach the hospital alive should be salvageable if the thoracic component of their injuries is quickly and appropriately managed. The mortality rate of blunt thoracic trauma is directly related to the occurrence of multisystem injuries. For isolated chest trauma, the mortality rate ranges from 4% to 10%. However, when one other system is injured, it increases to 15%, and when two or more systems are involved, it can be as high as 35%.[80]

Fewer than 15% of patients with thoracic injuries will require an operation; the vast majority can be managed successfully by simple procedures including tube thoracostomy, measures to relieve pain and maintain good pulmonary toilet, and occasional intubation and mechanical ventilation.[80] In a review of a large group of blunt thoracic injuries, it was found that more than 70% of injuries were to the chest wall, including a 13% incidence of flail chest. There was a 21% incidence of lung injury, and the heart, esophagus, and diaphragm were each affected in only 7% of cases. Pneumothorax and hemothorax were frequent sequelae of chest trauma, each occurring in approximately 20% of patients. Injuries to the thoracic aorta and great vessels occurred in only 4% of patients, though it must be kept in mind that these injuries may account for many of the deaths in nonsurvivors who never reach the hospital.[79]

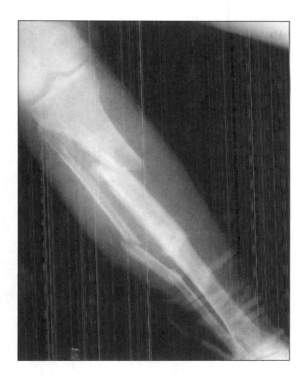

Figure 6–11 A 55-year-old pedestrian struck by a car sustained severe traumatic brain injury, blunt chest trauma, and this comminuted fracture of his right tibia and fibula.

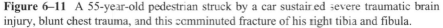

The initial management of thoracic trauma should be directed toward the early detection and correction of life-threatening injuries during the process of resuscitation. There are five mechanisms of early death after thoracic trauma: airway obstruction, loss of oxygenation and ventilation, exsanguination, cardiac failure, and cardiac tamponade.[79] Unless the primary injury resulting in these clinical states is appropriately treated, the patient can quickly succumb. Rapid detection of these injuries is especially critical for the patient with traumatic brain injury. Any delay in the acute management can further compromise neurologic outcome by subjecting the already injured brain to further hypotension and hypoxia.

The most common cause of upper-airway obstruction in the obtunded trauma patient is the tongue as it falls back into the hypopharynx. Blood or secretions in the airways, broken teeth or other foreign objects, or direct laryngeal or tracheobronchial injury can also lead to airway obstruction. The airway must be expediently secured, sometimes by simple maneuvers such as chin lift or jaw thrust, but more often in the multiply injured patient by intubation. Loss of proper oxygen-

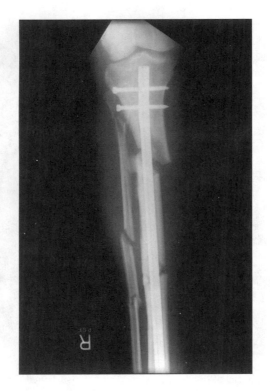

Figure 6–12 A completion radiograph following open reduction and internal fixation of the lower-extremity fracture demonstrates good alignment of the tibia and fibula. This repair was performed three days after the patient's initial injury, once his hemodynamic and pulmonary status had stabilized.

---

ation or ventilation can result from a tension pneumothorax, open pneumothorax, hemothorax, flail chest, or severe pulmonary contusion. Once a patent airway is ensured, these injuries frequently mandate the need for tube thoracostomy or mechanical ventilation (Figure 6–13). Exsanguination with a massive hemothorax resulting from great vessel, pulmonary, cardiac, or chest wall vascular disruption will necessitate prompt tube thoracostomy, possibly followed by emergent surgical intervention to stop the source of hemorrhage. Cardiac failure from severe cardiac contusion is rare but must be managed by aggressive supportive measures while other sources of shock are being excluded. Finally, patients with cardiac tamponade following cardiac perforation will require immediate surgical intervention in the emergency department if they are to survive. All of these injuries have the potential to lead to acute hemodynamic instability or cardiopulmonary arrest.[79-81] Without prompt intervention, survival is seriously jeopardized.

Specific Thoracic Injuries

Pleural Injuries

Pneumothorax and hemothorax following blunt trauma are usually the result of rib fractures that puncture the pleura and underlying lung or the direct result of pulmonary or bronchial laceration. In a tension pneumothorax, as air enters the pleural space, it cannot exit. As the intrathoracic pressure increases, hemodynamic instability can result from impaired venous return to the heart and mediastinal shift to the contralateral side. The patient will present with respiratory distress and diminished breath sounds on the affected side. In clinically suspected cases, even prior to chest radiograph, a needle thoracentesis through the second intercostal

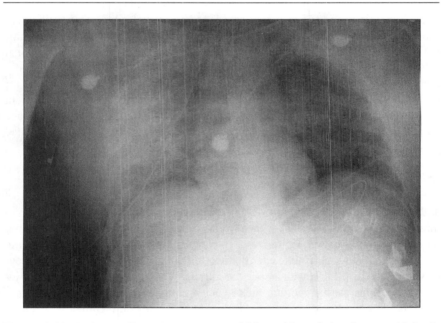

Figure 6–13 A chest radiograph of a motor vehicle accident victim shows multiple rib fractures associated with an underlying right pulmonary contusion. Bilateral chest tubes have been placed for pneumothorax. These chest injuries, along with other systemic injuries, have resulted in the need for intubation and mechanical ventilatory support.

space at the midclavicular line followed by immediate tube thoracostomy can be lifesaving.[80,81]

An open pneumothorax occurs with large wounds of the chest wall. Usually it is associated with penetrating high-velocity missiles, but on occasion it may result from major blunt trauma. If the size of the defect is greater than two thirds the size of the tracheal diameter, with each inspiratory effort, air will pass preferentially through the lower-resistance chest wall defect rather than through the normal airways. Treatment consists of a tube thoracostomy at a separate clean site as well as occlusion of the open wound with a dressing taped on three sides, effectively creating a one-way valve to allow air to egress from the pleural space without permitting more air to enter through the chest wound.[80,81]

Hemothorax is usually the result of bleeding from an intercostal or internal mammary vessel that has become disrupted from a fractured rib. On occasion, laceration of the thoracic viscera will lead to a significant hemothorax. Hemodynamic instability may result from both hypovolemia associated with the hemorrhage and impaired venous return with increasing intrathoracic pressure. Usually a hemothorax is successfully managed by simple tube thoracostomy and volume resuscitation.[80] As in all trauma situations, a large chest tube, 36 to 40 French, should be used. Occasionally massive or ongoing hemorrhage, as seen by an initial chest tube output of greater than 1,200 to 1,500 mL or continued bleeding of at least 100 to 200 mL per hour, will mandate an open thoracotomy to surgically ligate bleeding points.[80] Sometimes closed-tube thoracostomy will not allow for the evacuation of a large amount of intrathoracic clot. This may subject the patient to impaired pulmonary mechanics as well as contamination of the pleural space with empyema formation. To prevent these complications, thoracoscopic guided evacuation of the clot should be considered.[82]

Flail Chest

Flail chest represents a loss of stability of the chest wall resulting from direct high-energy impact. For there to be a flail segment, multiple ribs must be fractured, with at least two breaks in each rib. Sternal fractures or costochondral separations can combine with rib fractures to create a flail segment. It is important to recognize that the high kinetic energy imparted to the chest to create the flail segment can also result in severe associated intrathoracic as well as nonthoracic injuries. Indeed, the most important factor causing impaired ventilation in these patients is the underlying pulmonary parenchymal contusion (see below).[83] Other factors can also contribute to impaired pulmonary mechanics and respiratory compromise. One proposed theory is that during normal inspiration, the intact portion of the chest wall expands as intrapleural pressure becomes more negative. However, in the unstable flail segment, external atmospheric pressure exceeds the negative pleural pressure, causing the flail segment to move inward. During expiration, the reverse occurs; the intrathoracic pressure exceeds atmospheric pressure, and the flail segment is pushed outward while the rest of the chest contracts normally. Hence, the classic paradoxical chest wall motion of the flail segment.[80] Another possible explanation of impaired ventilation is that during inspiration, air from the higher-resistance injured lung may move to the expanding, more compliant contralateral lung. Then during expiration, air from the uninjured lung may move to the paradoxically expanding injured lung. The net result of this back-and-forth movement of air is an increase in dead space and mismatch, with overall impaired ventilation.[80]

The management of a flail chest is that of effective analgesia, aggressive pulmonary toilet, and selective intubation for those patients with multisystem trauma and worsening respiratory distress.[80] Mechanical stabilization of the flail segment is no longer a mainstay of treatment, as it was in the 1950s. Without proper analgesia, the patient will exhibit splinting and a poor inspiratory effort, which can lead to hypoventilation and atelectasis. Parenteral narcotics are useful in some patients but may cause respiratory depression. Intercostal nerve blocks and now, more recently, continuous epidural analgesia can very effectively control pain without the adverse consequences of respiratory depression. Aggressive pulmonary toilet/chest physical therapy includes frequent suctioning, incentive spirometry, postural drainage, occasional bronchoscopy, percussion and vibration, and cough stimulation techniques to reverse segmental lung collapse.[80,83]

Parenchymal Pulmonary Injuries

Parenchymal pulmonary injuries include pulmonary contusion, pulmonary hematoma, and pulmonary laceration.[80] The injuries result from high-energy impact to the chest and are frequently associated with multiple thoracic and other systemic trauma. Pulmonary contusion is the most common of the three and is seen histologically as interstitial hemorrhage with leakage of blood into the alveoli. The ensuing interstitial edema and increased airway secretions result in atelectasis and consolidation of the lung.[80] The patient frequently presents with evidence of respiratory distress: tachypnea, dyspnea, chest pain, splinting, and occasional hemoptysis. The chest radiograph can lag behind the patient's clinical condition, although variable findings from a patchy nonspecific infiltrate to consolidation will usually appear within several hours of injury.[84] As in flail chest injuries that are associated with pulmonary contusions, treatment is directed toward aggressive pulmonary toilet, pain control, and selective intubation for mechanical ventilation as necessary.[80,83] Prophylactic antibiotics and systemic steroids have no role in the treatment of these patients and may in fact lead to the development of nosocomial infections.[84] These patients must be closely monitored for evidence of respiratory deterioration with clinical observation, arterial blood gases, and continuous pulse oximetry.

Pulmonary hematomas usually appear as sharply defined 2- to 5-cm lesions on chest X-ray. They can cause pulmonary consolidation as they displace normal lung parenchyma. By themselves, they require no specific treatment unless the hematoma progresses into an abscess with an air/fluid level.[80]

With pulmonary lacerations, treatment is directed toward the resulting hemopneumothorax, using tube thoracostomy. Operative intervention is reserved for those patients with significant ongoing hemorrhage (1,200 to 1,500 mL initially, followed by 100 to 200 mL/h). This can be the case if the laceration extends into the hilar vessels of the lung, necessitating repair or ligation with a vascular stapler or, if exsanguinating hemorrhage exists, hilar cross clamping with possible pneumonectomy.[85,86]

Tracheobronchial Injuries

Fortunately, injuries to the trachea and bronchi are rare, making up less than 1% of injuries after blunt trauma.[84] The majority of these injuries, about 80%, occur within 2 to 3 cm of the carina. An explanation for this might be that a sudden increase in airway pressure occurs as the chest is compressed while the glottis is closed. According to Laplace's law, this places the greatest amount of tension in the larger-diameter airways, leading to rupture at these sites.[80] Rapid changes in the anteroposterior diameter of the chest can also lead to overstretching of the mainstem bronchi as they are pulled away from the relatively fixed midline trachea and carina.[80]

The clinical presentation will vary depending upon the location and extent of injury. If the disrupted bronchus communicates with the pleural cavity, a large tension pneumothorax, prominent pneumomediastinum, and subcutaneous emphysema, along with severe hemoptysis and respiratory distress, can result. Immediate intubation and tube thoracostomy followed by bronchoscopy to confirm the injury should be quickly done. Operative repair may then be necessary.[80] If, on the other hand, a small disruption of the distal trachea or proximal mainstem bronchi is confined to the mediastinum, symptoms can be much more subtle and in fact may be delayed by several days, at which time granulation tissue at the site of injury may lead to stricture formation and partial airway obstruction.[80] Radiographic findings such as pneumomediastinum or subcutaneous emphysema should prompt investigation with endoscopy of the aerodigestive tract in these situations. Some of the smaller injuries may be managed conservatively and heal spontaneously, though complications such as bronchial stenosis, bronchopleural fistula, and empyema can occur.[87]

Injuries to the larynx and cervical trachea likewise are very rare and result in severe respiratory distress in the face of partial or near-total upper-airway obstruction. Blind intubation must never be attempted, since it can lead to complete obstruction or disruption of the airway. Intubation by fiber-optic bronchoscopy should be attempted, and, if this is unsuccessful, the airway must be secured by tracheostomy. Cricothyroidotomy is unfortunately not a good option, since it may directly violate the injury site. Despite laryngeal reconstruction, many of these patients go on to develop stenosis at the site of injury.[87] Trauma to the trachea and bronchi carries a high mortality rate: about a third of these patients die, not only because of the life-threatening nature of the injury itself, but also because of the multiple injuries associated with it.[84]

Esophageal Injury

Trauma to the esophagus is more often the result of penetrating injuries; however, severe blunt trauma in rare circumstances can lead to a linear disruption, usually located in the lower esophagus.[80] The danger with esophageal injuries is that they frequently go unrecognized until signs of systemic sepsis have developed. Initial radiographic signs such as mediastinal air and a small pleural effusion should prompt evaluation with esophagoscopy and/or an esophagram. If an esophageal injury is confirmed within 24 hours of injury, direct repair of the laceration and wide drainage of the mediastinum and pleural space can be performed. Otherwise, if the injury is discovered late, local contamination and sepsis prohibit primary closure. In this case, antibiotics must be given, and diversion with cervical esophagostomy and gastrostomy, followed by eventual late reconstruction, must be done.[80] Late mortality with these injuries is primarily due to overwhelming sepsis and multiple organ failure.

Myocardial Contusion

Myocardial contusion usually results from a direct blow to the chest and is most commonly found among unrestrained occupants of motor vehicles. Deceleration forces may propel the heart forward against the sternum, or the heart may be crushed between the sternum and vertebral column. Wojcik and Morgan looked at sternal fractures as a specific risk factor for myocardial contusion. They found the incidence of myocardial contusion to be 18% (12/66) among patients with blunt sternal fracture. None of these seven patients went on to develop any ill sequelae in terms of life-threatening arrhythmias or hemodynamic instability.[88]

The right ventricle, since it makes up most of the anterior surface of the heart, is the region most at risk for injury.[84] Mitral and aortic valves, being located in the higher-pressure region of the left ventricle, are also more at risk compared to the tricuspid and pulmonic valves. Histologically, the lesion appears as myocardial cell rupture with hemorrhage into the interstitium.[84]

Myocardial contusion can result in widely variable clinical states, from the asymptomatic patient to the one in whom potentially fatal arrhythmias and hemodynamic instability arise.[89,90] Clinically significant myocardial contusions are fortunately very rare; most patients are admitted for a period of observation and monitoring and then sent home without any long-term sequelae. The problem has been how to identify which patients are at high risk for the development of arrhythmias and pump failure. Most trauma centers are now focusing on physical examination and electrocardiography (ECG) as the most important diagnostic criteria. Although no specific ECG abnormalities exist, persistent tachycardia, ectopy or arrhythmias, and nonspecific ST-T wave abnormalities will identify those patients who deserve cardiac monitoring.[91] Additional ECGs at 24 to 48 hours may help screen for infarction in older individuals or those with a history of coronary artery disease. Serum myocardial enzymes and radionuclide studies are not useful in that they are not predictive of cardiac complications. In those patients who go on to develop cardiac sequelae, echocardiography may assist in diagnosing specific cardiac abnormalities and guiding subsequent therapy.[91]

Aortic Dissection

Rupture of the thoracic aorta is the most common cause of death after blunt chest trauma from a motor vehicle accident. Eighty percent to 90% of these patients sustain full-thickness rupture of the aortic wall and die at the scene. Of the 10% to 20% who reach the hospital, another 50% will die within the first 24 to 48 hours if the injury goes unrecognized.[80] This occurs as a partial-thickness disruption through the intima and media progresses to include the outer thin adventitia of the aortic wall. The mechanism of injury is that of rapid deceleration; shearing forces occur between the relatively mobile ascending and descending aorta and the fixed aortic root and transverse aortic arch. Clinically, this results in the most common site of injury being at the level of the ligamentum arteriosum just distal to the left subclavian artery, and the second most common site being the ascending aorta just beyond the aortic root.[80,84]

The mechanism of injury remains the most important factor in alerting the physician as to the possibility of a major intrathoracic vascular injury. Clinical signs and symptoms such as obvious chest trauma, chest pain, midscapular back pain, dyspnea, and alteration in peripheral pulses may not be present and are unreliable in the multiply injured patient.[84,92] Further, other more obvious injuries might be distracting. Chest radiograph is the best initial screening tool: pertinent findings include widened mediastinum, an obscure aortic knob or aortopulmonary window, apical pleural capping, depression of the left mainstem bronchus, and deviation of the trachea and esophagus to the right.[80,84] If suspicions are heightened, one should proceed to aortic angiography as soon as other life-threatening problems have been stabilized. Aortography remains the definitive means of establishing the diagnosis.[92] Although transesophageal echocardiography has been developed as a more recent diagnostic technique, it does have certain limitations in terms of proper visualization of the distal ascending aorta and aortic arch, in addition to ready availability and technical expertise in its use.[93] Dynamic CT of the chest can also be used to look for mediastinal hematoma and can be followed by aortography if positive. Once the diagnosis of a major arterial injury is confirmed, it must be repaired without delay before full-thickness rupture of the vessel wall leads to exsanguination.

Diaphragmatic Injuries

Diaphragmatic rupture is also quite rare, having an incidence of 1% to 3% among blunt chest trauma victims. It occurs far more frequently on the left side and is often associated with injuries to the spleen and stomach.[84] The chest X-ray may demonstrate an obscured or elevated hemidiaphragm and sometimes hollow abdominal viscera within the left hemithorax. If the diagnosis is missed initially, the patient may go on to a latent phase in which he or she develops vague abdominal symptoms, followed by a late phase when herniated abdominal contents become obstructed or strangulated.[84]

In a review of 44 patients with blunt diaphragmatic injury, Morgan et al observed several important points.[94] First, diaphragmatic injury is a marker of a high-energy impact and, as a consequence, is associated with other serious injuries. Most commonly, these include intra-abdominal viscera (59%), orthopaedic (68%), and thoracic injuries (46%).[94] Although thoracic injuries are very common, it appears that disruption of the diaphragm results from a sudden impact to the abdomen. As the victim braces for the accident in a Valsalva position, the diaphragm offers the weakest point of release for the increased pressure created from the blow to the abdomen against the steering column or dash.[94]

Second, although 93% of the patients in this series had the diagnosis of diaphragmatic rupture established within six hours of admission, in only about half of these patients was the diagnosis made preoperatively by abnormal chest X-ray or by the visualization of intraperitoneal lavage fluid or omentum extruding from a thoracostomy tube. In 42% of patients, the diaphragmatic injury was an incidental finding during celiotomy, and in an additional 11%, the diagnosis was made during thoracotomy.[94]

A positive diagnostic peritoneal lavage is a common indication for proceeding with celiotomy in these patients; however, as a specific method to diagnose diaphragmatic injury, DPL is notoriously inaccurate. In this series, DPL carried a false-negative rate of 21%.[94] A disruption of the posterior diaphragm may cause bleeding confined to the lesser omental sac, resulting in a clear effluent on DPL if no other intra-abdominal viscera are injured. Whether the diagnosis is established preoperatively or incidentally, a transabdominal approach generally offers the simplest access to direct repair of the diaphragmatic injury as well as other intra-abdominal visceral injuries.[84,94]

ABDOMINAL INJURIES

Abdominal injuries can have a significant impact on the management and outcome of the patient with brain injury. The majority of these combined injuries are the result of motor vehicle accidents. It has been estimated that 20% of patients involved in vehicular accidents will have sustained an intra-abdominal injury.[95] Such injuries can be a major source of hemorrhage and shock, thereby putting the patient with brain injury at risk for secondary brain injury. The rapid restoration of adequate blood pressure and tissue perfusion is of paramount importance in minimizing this effect. Diagnostic maneuvers such as DPL, CT, and now ultrasonography are frequently used to detect abdominal injuries.[96,97] Emergent laparotomy may then be necessary in the unstable multiply injured patient to control sources of hemorrhage and repair the injuries. These diagnostic and surgical interventions can be potentially lifesaving, but they must be used with discretion and performed in such a way as to minimize delays in the evaluation and treatment of the primary brain injury.

Several anatomic features are important when considering blunt abdominal trauma. The abdomen can be divided into four main regions. The most cephalad portion of the abdomen is surrounded by the diaphragm superiorly and the thoracic cage circumferentially. This portion includes the liver, spleen, stomach, and transverse colon. Just caudal to this, the intra-abdominal cavity contains the majority of the small bowel, mesentery, and parts of the colon. The third region is the pelvis, which is surrounded by a bony ring and contains the rectum, bladder, iliac vessels, and female genitalia. Finally, the retroperitoneum contains the aorta and vena cava and their major tributaries, the pancreas, duodenum, kidneys, ureters, and portions of the colon.[96,97]

Once again, the mechanism of injury has significant implications in the multiply injured patient. Decelerating forces, as may occur in a motor vehicle accident or fall, can cause compression and torsion of intra-abdominal structures. Solid organs such as the liver, spleen, and kidney are subject to stretching and shearing forces. Tearing of solid organs may extend through major associated elastic vessels. Hollow viscus injuries can occur near points of relative fixation as the result of shearing forces and sudden increases in intraluminal pressure. Retroperitoneal structures, including the pancreas, duodenum, kidney, and major vascular conduits, are also at risk following crushing blows such as those that might occur during impact to the abdomen from a lap belt or steering column.[96,97]

Although a detailed discussion of all blunt abdominal injuries goes beyond the scope of this chapter, a brief discussion of liver and splenic trauma is worth conducting. Situated in the upper abdomen, the liver and spleen are relatively noncompressible solid organs surrounded by a thin capsule. Ligamentous attachments keep these organs relatively fixed in relation to the diaphragm, gastrointestinal tract, and large blood vessels. Although partially protected by the overlying ribs of the lower chest, these anatomic and structural features put the liver and spleen at risk for injury following crushing blows to the abdomen.[58] As the largest solid organ in the abdomen, the liver is particularly vulnerable and, not surprisingly, is the most commonly injured organ in both blunt and penetrating abdominal trauma.[98]

Much has been written on the nonoperative management of both liver and splenic injuries following blunt abdominal trauma.[97–103] Nonoperative treatment in physiologically stable patients is now widely accepted among trauma surgeons. But it is important to remember that hemodynamic stability is not the only criterion used in selecting observational management. Other factors include the grade of injury as determined by CT, the absence of associated intra-abdominal injuries, neurologic integrity, age, and the need for no more than two abdominal-related units of blood transfusion.[97–103]

The major criterion as related to the patient with brain injury is, of course, neurologic integrity. Nonoperative management of blunt hepatic and splenic injuries necessitates continuous monitoring of the patient's hemodynamic status as well as serial physical examinations for the first two to three days following the trauma. The development of a worsened abdominal examination or peritoneal signs is one of the criteria used as an indication for surgery.[97–103] Patients in whom reliable assessment of the abdomen is precluded because of associated trauma such as brain injury frequently cannot be safely managed nonoperatively. To a certain extent, clinical judgment will depend on the severity of brain injury: those patients with minor or moderate brain trauma resulting in only a slightly depressed mental status may be able to be safely observed. However, if there is any doubt as to the reliability of examination, surgical intervention for the abdominal injury is justified. The actual methods used to control hemorrhage and salvage parenchyma, as for example is done with splenorrhaphy, goes beyond our discussion. Suffice it to say that ensuring direct control of abdominal hemorrhage is the critical factor for the patient with brain injury.

Diagnosis of Intra-Abdominal Injuries

In an evaluation of the multiply injured blunt trauma victim, the patient's physiologic status is the most important determinant of the route of diagnosis and management. A hemodynamically unstable patient who presents with tachycardia and possibly hypotension will require immediate steps to find and stop sources of hemorrhage. Potential bleeding sites include the chest, abdomen, pelvis, and extremities. The leader of the trauma team, usually a general surgeon, must expeditiously ascertain whether the source of hemorrhage is within the abdominal cavity. In rare situations, physical signs such as a distended or expanding abdomen in the face of hemodynamic instability will convince the trauma surgeon to proceed immediately with emergent exploratory laparotomy. More often, however, physical signs are much less obvious or equivocal. Further, the patient with brain injury cannot be assessed reliably for subjective abdominal tenderness or objective peritoneal signs. The majority of patients will therefore require some form of diagnostic evaluation of their abdomens.

Diagnostic Peritoneal Lavage

DPL has become one of the standard methods of evaluating blunt abdominal trauma. It has gained widespread use since it was first introduced by Root et al in 1965.[97,104] It has its greatest application among hemodynamically unstable patients in whom physical examination is equivocal or cannot be relied upon because of obtundation or intoxication.[96–98] DPL can be performed in the emergency department quickly and safely by inserting a DPL catheter into the peritoneal cavity through a small infraumbilical incision.[96] A positive result consists of 10 mL of gross blood aspirated through the catheter or a microscopic cell count of greater than 100,000 red blood cells per cubic milliliter. Also the presence of bile, elevated amylase above that of serum, vegetable or fecal matter, or lavage fluid draining from a Foley catheter or chest tube will constitute a positive result.[96] Those patients with the finding of gross blood on aspiration are most at risk for exsanguinating hemorrhage within the peritoneal cavity and should be taken to the operating room for emergent exploration of their abdomens.[96] The test is quite accurate, with a false-positive rate of 0.2% and a false-negative rate of 1.2% as reported by Fischer et al in a series of 2,586 patients over a 14-year period.[105] Limitations include occasional false positives, as with pelvic retroperitoneal hematomas, and false negatives, as might occur with diaphragmatic ruptures.[96–98,106] Overall, DPL is an expedient and preferred method to evaluate the abdomen as a potential source of hemorrhage in the hemodynamically unstable blunt trauma victim.

Ultrasonography

More recently, abdominal ultrasonography is being evaluated as a potential diagnostic method for blunt abdominal trauma. It has already gained widespread use in Europe, and some trauma centers in the United States are now finding it useful as a noninvasive tool that might replace DPL.[96,97] Many studies have found ultrasonography to carry high sensitivity and specificity, comparing favorably with DPL.[96,97] In the setting of blunt trauma, sonography can detect evidence of a hemoperitoneum. It may be especially applicable for pregnant patients and those having had previous abdominal surgery. However, because of uncertainty in terms of operator dependence and the detection of hollow viscus injuries, ultrasonography has not yet gained widespread popularity in the United States.[98] But as interested clinicians become trained in its use, ultrasonography promises to become a valuable tool in detecting intraperitoneal and retroperitoneal hemorrhage in the hemodynamically unstable blunt trauma patient.

Computed Tomography

CT plays an important role in the evaluation of blunt abdominal trauma, but it must be restricted to those patients who are hemodynamically stable. Critical delays in definitive management can be incurred by sending an unstable patient to the CT scanner. Yet under physiologically acceptable conditions, CT scanning can often accurately delineate the nature and extent of both intra-abdominal and retroperitoneal injuries.[96,97,106] First popularized by Federle et al, CT scanning has since become a valuable method for the assessment and management of abdominal and retroperitoneal injuries.[107] Certain solid viscus injuries, including those of the liver, spleen, and kidney, are now frequently managed nonoperatively using CT scanning as an initial diagnostic tool and subsequent adjunct to physiologic monitoring of the patient (Figure 6–14).[97,99–101,108] CT scanning, however, does not reliably exclude hollow viscus injury, and for that reason must be used in conjunction with physiologic and physical findings.[96,97]

Priority in the Treatment of Abdominal and Brain Injury

Prioritizing the diagnosis and treatment of abdominal injury versus primary brain injury can pose a difficult challenge to the trauma surgeon. In the case of a hemodynamically stable patient with brain injury, one has the luxury of being able to perform CT scanning of the head after the initial primary and secondary surveys. From that point, a diagnostic plan to exclude abdominal injury can be formulated on the basis of the severity of brain injury. CT scanning of the abdomen and pelvis can follow the head CT if surgery is not considered necessary for the brain injury. In the event of a severe brain injury requiring immediate decompression of a hemorrhagic mass lesion, the abdomen can be evaluated by performing a DPL in the operating room as the craniotomy is getting under way.[96]

If a patient with major head trauma has a nonoperative injury, such as severe brain contusions, then strong consideration should be given for an ICP device to monitor the patient's neurologic status during subsequent surgical procedures and during the postinjury period. If, for example, an abdominal CT scan demonstrates an operative injury, an ICP monitor can be placed in the operating room as the laparotomy is proceeding. While the patient is under a general anesthetic for either abdominal or thoracic exploration or fixation of orthopaedic injuries, it is impossible to follow his or her clinical neurologic examination. Therefore, an ICP monitor can be a useful method to detect early rises in the ICP such as those that might be caused by an underlying expanding hematoma.[109] Care must be taken by both

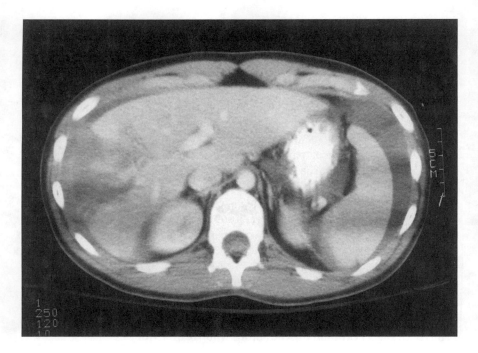

Figure 6–14 CT scan demonstrates blunt hepatic injury with intraparenchymal hemorrhage involving the right lobe of the liver associated with a hemoperitoneum; free intraperitoneal blood can be seen around the liver and spleen and in the pelvis on lower cuts (not shown).

the operative surgeon and the anesthesiologist to avoid and treat excessive blood loss and hypotension during these procedures in order to minimize secondary brain injury.

Special consideration must be given to the multiply injured obtunded patient who presents with hemodynamic instability. This situation creates a dilemma for the trauma surgeon, who must balance the possibility of an intracranial hemorrhagic mass lesion with that of ongoing hemorrhage and shock from an untreated abdominal or thoracic injury.[109] Frequently, hypotensive blunt trauma victims present with an altered or depressed mental status. The difficulty lies in knowing whether this is indicative of a central nervous system mass lesion that might necessitate emergent craniotomy.

Often, initial hypotension in the field or upon arrival in the emergency department can be successfully corrected with resuscitation. In this situation, it may be possible to perform head CT after initial survey and DPL without deleterious delays in treatment.[109] On the other hand, persistent hypotension, despite aggressive resuscitation, is usually an indication of ongoing hemorrhage, which must be controlled surgically if the patient is to survive. Because a head CT would waste valuable time, a rapid neurologic assessment in the emergency department can be a critical guide to detecting an intracranial mass lesion.[109] Lateralizing signs such as ipsilateral pupillary dilation can indicate that tentorial herniation is imminent, in which case diagnostic and therapeutic burr holes can be placed while definitive control of hemorrhage in other body sites is obtained.[109,110] Without clinical signs of impending herniation, head CT can usually safely be deferred until immediately following surgical treatment of the abdominal injuries.[109] Whether intraoperative ICP monitoring is used depends upon the degree of neurologic deficit. If a patient has a depressed mental status but is awake and following commands, the risk of significant intracranial pathology is low, and these patients do not generally require ICP monitoring during the operative procedure. Alternatively, if the patient presents in coma or with a Glasgow Coma Scale score of 8 or less, intraoperative ICP monitoring is prudent [109,110]

In a study designed to determine the frequency of emergency craniotomy and urgent laparotomy or thoracotomy, Thomason et al prospectively reviewed 734 blunt trauma patients presenting with initial hypotension. Emergency craniotomy for intracranial hemorrhage was performed on 2.5% of patients, while 21% required urgent laparotomy, thoracotomy, or both. The frequency of urgent laparotomy or thoracotomy was 8.5 times greater than emergent craniotomy.[109] These data should not, however, minimize the importance of detecting intracranial hemorrhagic mass lesions. It remains the ultimate responsibility of the trauma surgeon to prioritize diagnostic and treatment decisions in these critically injured patients. The control of hemorrhagic shock must be carefully balanced against the possible risk of delaying definitive surgical treatment of severe brain injury.

REFERENCES

1. Gutierrez PA, Young RR, Vulpe M. Spinal cord injury: an overview. *Urol Clin North Am.* 1993;20:373–382.

2. Sonntag VKH, Douglas RA. Management of spinal cord trauma. *Neurosurg Clin North Am.* 1990;1:729–750.

3. Dollfus P. Rehabilitation following injury to the spinal cord. *J Emerg Med.* 1993;11:57–61.

4. Selecki BR, Berry G, Kwob B, et al. Experience with spinal injuries in New South Wales. *Aust NZ J Surg.* 1986;56:567–576.

5. Reiss SJ, Raque GH Jr, Shields CB, et al. Cervical spine fractures with major associated trauma. *Neurosurgery.* 1986;18:327–330.

6. Hills MW, Deane SA. Head injury and facial injury: is there an increased risk of cervical spine injury? *J Trauma.* 1993;34:549–554.

7. Kirshenbaum KJ, Nadimpalli SR, Fantus R, et al. Unsuspected upper cervical spine fractures associated wtih significant head trauma. *J Emerg Med.* 1990;8:183–198.

8. O'Malley KF, Ross SE. The incidence of injury to the cervical spine in patients with craniocerebral injury. *J Trauma.* 1988;28:1476–1478.

9. Kennedy FR, Gonzalez P, Beitler A, et al. Incidence of cervical spine injury in patients with gunshot wounds to the head. *South Med J.* 1994;87:621–623.

10. Thal ER. Advanced Trauma Life Support Program. *Spine Spinal Cord Trauma.* 1988;19:161–171.

11. Bohlman HH. Acute fractures and dislocations of the cervical spine. *J Bone Joint Surg Am.* 1979;61:1119–1142.

12. Bunegin L, Hung T-K, Chang GL. Biomechanics of spinal cord injury. *Crit Care Clin.* 1987;3:453–470.

13. Kaye JJ, Nance EP. Thoracic and lumbar spine trauma. *Radiol Clin North Am.* 1990;28:361–377.

14. Denis F. The three column spine and its significance in the classification of acute thoracolumbar spinal injuries. *Spine.* 1983;8:817–831.

15. McAfee PC, Yuan HA, Lasda NA. The unstable burst fracture. *Spine.* 1982;7:365–373.

16. Sipski ML, Hendler S, DeLisa JA. Rehabilitation of patients with spinal cord disease. *Neurol Clin.* 1991;9:705–725.

17. Anderson DK, Hall ED. Pathophysiology of spinal cord trauma. *Ann Emerg Med.* 1993;22:987–992.

18. De La Torre JC. Spinal cord injury: review of basic and applied research. *Spine.* 1981;6:315–335.

19. Young W. The role of calcium in spinal cord injury. *Cent Nerv Syst Trauma.* 1985;2:109–114.

20. Hsu SY, Halushka PV, Hogan EL, et al. Increased thromboxane level in experimental spinal cord injury. *J Neurol Sci.* 1986;74:289–296.

21. Janssen L, Hansebout RR. Pathogenesis of spinal cord injury and new treatments: a review. *Spine.* 1989;14:23–32.

22. Hilton G, Frei J. High-dose methylprednisolone in the treatment of spinal cord injuries. *Heart Lung.* 1991;20:675–680.

23. Bracken D, Shepard M, Collins W, et al. A randomized, controlled trial of methylprednisolone or naloxone in the treatment of acute spinal cord injury. *N Engl J Med.* 1990;322:1405–1411.

24. Hall ED, Braughler JM. Glucocorticoid mechanisms in acute spinal cord injury: a review and therapeutic rationale. *Surg Neurol.* 1982;18:320–327.

25. Hall ED, Braughler JM, McCall JM. New pharmacologic treatment of acute spinal cord trauma. *J Neurotrauma.* 1988;5:81–89.

26. Faden AI, Jacobs TP, Smith MT, et al. Comparison of thyrotropin-releasing hormone (TRH), naloxone and dexamethasone treatments in experimental spinal injury. *Neurology.* 1983;33:673–678.

27. Faden AI, Jacobs TP, Smith MT. Evaluation of the calcium channel antagonist nimodipine in experimental spinal cord ischemia. *J Neurosurg.* 1984;60:796–799.

28. Villaneuva, PA. Management of vertebral column injuries in connection with brain injuries. Presented at Advances in Acute Neurotrauma Care Conference; June 1994; Hartford, Conn.

29. White AA III, Panjabi MM. The role of stabilization in the treatment of cervical spine injuries. *Spine.* 1984;9:512–522.

30. Marshall LF, Knowlton S, Girfin SR, et al. Deterioration following spinal cord injury: a multicenter study. *J Neurosurg.* 1987;66:400.

31. Heiden JS, Weiss MH, Rosenberg AW, Apuzzo ML. Management of cervical spinal cord trauma in southern California. *J Neurosurg.* 1975;43:732.

32. Levi L, Wolf A, Rigamonti D, et al. Anterior decompression in cervical spine trauma: does the timing of surgery affect the outcome? *Neurosurgery.* 1991;29:216–222.

33. Murphy KP, Opitz JL, Cabanela ME, et al. Cervical fractures and spinal cord injury: outcome of surgical and nonsurgical management. *Mayo Clin Proc.* 1990;65:949–959.

34. Krengel WF III, Anderson PA, Henley MB. Early stabilization and decompression for incomplete paraplegia due to a thoracic-level spinal cord injury. *Spine.* 1993;18:2080–2087.

35. Lemons VR, Wagner FC, Montesano PX. Management of thoracolumbar fractures with accompanying neurologic injury. *Neurosurgery.* 1992;30:667–671.

36. Guha A, Tator CH. Endrenyi L, et al. Decompression of the spinal cord improves recovery after acute experimental spinal cord compression injury. *Paraplegia.* 1987;25:324–339.

37. Frost FS. Role of rehabilitation after spinal cord injury. *Urol Clin North Am.* 1993;20:549–559.

38. Carlsson GS, Svardsudd AK. Carlsson S, et al. A study of injuries during life in three male populations. *J Trauma.* 1986;26:364–372.

39. Jerrard DA. Pelvic fractures. *Emerg Med Clin North Am.* 1993;11:147–163.

40. Mucha P, Farnell M. Analysis of pelvis fracture management. *J Trauma.* 1984;24:379–386.

41. Moreno C, Moore E, Rosenberger A. Hemorrhage associated with major pelvic fracture: a multispecialty challenge. *J Trauma.* 1986;26:987–994.

42. Trafton PG. Pelvic ring injuries. *Surg Clin North Am.* 1990;70:655–669.

43. Kricun ME. Fractures of the pelvis. *Orthop Clin North Am.* 1990;21:573–590.

44. Young JWR, Resnik CS. Fractures of the pelvis: current concepts of classification. *AJR.* 1990;155:1169–1175.

45. Bucholz R. The pathologic anatomy of Malgaigne fracture–dislocations of the pelvis. *J Bone Joint Surg Am.* 1987;63:400.

46. Pennal GF, Tile M, Waddell JP, et al. Pelvic disruption: assessment and classification. *Clin Orthop.* 1980;151:12–23.

47. Tile M. *Fractures of the Pelvis and Acetabulum.* Baltimore, Md: Williams & Wilkins; 1986.

48. Young JWR, Burgess AR. *Radiologic Management of Pelvic Ring Fractures.* Baltimore, Md: Urban and Schwartzenberg; 1987.

49. Dalal SA, Siegel JH. Burgess AR, et al. Pelvic fractures in multiple trauma: classification by mechanism is key pattern of organ injury, resuscitative requirements and outcome. *J Trauma.* 1989;29:981–1002.

50. Ben-Menachem Y, Coldwell DM, Young JWR, Burgess AR. Hemorrhage associated with pelvic fractures: causes, diagnosis and emergent management. *AJR.* 1991;157:1005–1014.

51. Agnew SG. Hemodynamically unstable pelvic fractures. *Orthop Clin North Am.* 1994;25:715–721.

52. Hubbard SG, Bivins BA, Sachatello CR, et al. Diagnostic errors with peritoneal lavage in patients with pelvic fractures. *Arch Surg.* 1979;114:844–846.

53. Burgess AR, Eastridge BJ, Young JWR, et al. Pelvic ring disruptions: effective classification system and treatment protocols. *J Trauma.* 1990;30:848–856.

54. Seibel R, LaDuca J, Hassett JM, et al. Blunt trauma (ISS36), femur traction, and the pulmonary failure–septic state. *Ann Surg.* 1985;202:283–295.

55. Wu CC, Shih CH. Femoral shaft fractures associated with unstable pelvic fractures. *J Trauma.* 1993;34:76–81.

56. Latenser BA, Gentilello LM, Tarver AA. Improved outcome with early fixation of skeletally unstable pelvic fractures. *J Trauma.* 1991;31:28–31.

57. Hirvensalo E, Lindahl J, Bostman O. A new approach to the internal fixation of unstable pelvic fractures. *Clin Orthop.* 1993;297:28–32.

58. Leenen LPH, Vander Werken, Schoots F, et al. Internal fixation of open unstable pelvic fractures. *J Trauma.* 1993;35:220–225.

59. Faringer PD, Mullins RJ, Feliciano PD, et al. Selective fecal diversion in complex open pelvic fractures from blunt trauma. *Arch Surg.* 1994;129:958–964.

60. Fallon WF. The present role of colostomy in the management of trauma. *Dis Colon Rectum.* 1992;35:1094–1102.

61. Rosenthal RE. Lower extremity fractures and dislocations. In: *Trauma.* 2nd ed. Norwalk, Conn: Appleton and Lange; 1991:623–638.

62. Bochner RM, Pellicci PM, Lyden JP. Bipolar hemiathroplasty for fracture of the femoral neck. *J Bone Joint Surg Am.* 1988;70:1001.

63. Swiontkowski MF, Winquist RA, Hansen ST Jr. Fractures of the femoral neck in patients between the ages of 12 and 49 years. *J Bone Joint Surg Am.* 1984;66:837.

64. Schwartz JT Jr, Brumback RJ, Lakatos R, Poka A. Acute compartment syndrome of the thigh: a spectrum of injury. *J Bone Joint Surg Am.* 1989;71:392–400.

65. Brumback RJ, Uwagie-Ero S, Lakatos RP, et al. Intramedullary nailing of femoral shaft fractures. *J Bone Joint Surg Am.* 1988;70:1453–1462.

66. Bynoe Rp, Miles WS, Bell RM, et al. Noninvasive diagnosis of vascular trauma by duplex ultrasonography. *J Vasc Surg.* 1991;14:346–352.

67. Caudle RJ, Stern PJ. Severe open fractures of the tibia. *J Bone Joint Surg Am.* 1987;69:801–807.

68. Belsole RJ, Hess AV. Concomitant skeletal and soft tissue injuries. *Orthop Clin North Am.* 1993;24:327–331.

69. Ecker J, Sherman R. Soft tissue coverage of the distal third of the leg and ankle. *Orthop Clin North Am.* 1993;24:481–488.

70. Gulli B, Templeman D. Compartment syndrome of the lower extremity. *Orthop Clin North Am.* 1994;25:677–684.

71. Mabee JR, Bostwick TL. Pathophysiology and mechanisms of compartment syndrome. *Orthop Rev.* 1993;22:175.

72. McGee DL, Dalsey WC. The mangled extremity: compartment syndrome and amputations. *Emerg Med Clin North Am.* 1992;10:783–800.

73. Alexander JJ, Piotrowski JJ, Graham D, et al. Outcome of complex vascular and orthopedic injuries of the lower extremity. *Am J Surg.* 1991;162:111–116.

74. Poole GV, Agnew SG, Griswold JA. The mangled low extremity: can salvage be predicted? *Am Surg.* 1994;60:50–55.

75. Levy D. The fat embolism syndrome: a review. *Clin Orthop.* 1990;261:281–286.

76. Ganong RB. Fat emboli syndrome in isolated fractures of the tibia and femur. *Clin Orthop.* 1993;291:208–214.

77. Svenningsen S, Nesse O, Finsen V, et al. Prevention of fat embolism syndrome in patients with femoral fractures: immediate or delayed operative fixation? *Ann Chir Gynaecol.* 1987;76:163.

78. Marion DW, Gruen GS, Clyde B. Intraoperative hypotension during repair of lower-extremity long bone fractures. Presented at Eastern Association for the Surgery of Trauma; January 14, 1995; Sanibel, Fla.

79. Feliciano DV. The diagnostic and therapeutic approach to chest trauma. *Semin Thorac Cardiovasc Surg.* 1992;4:156–162.

80. Cooper C, Militello P. The multi-injured patient: the Maryland Shock Trauma Protocol approach. *Semin Thorac Cardiovasc Surg.* 1992;4:163–167.

81. Westaby S, Brayley N. Thoracic trauma—I. *Br Med J.* 1990;300:1639–1643.

82. Calhoom JH, Grover FL, Trinkle JK. Chest trauma: approach and management. *Clin Chest Med.* 1992;13(1):55–67.

83. Ciraulo DL, Elliott D, Mitchell KA, et al. Flail chest as a marker for significant injuries. *J Am Coll Surg.* 1994;178:466–470.

84. Jackimczyk K. Blunt chest trauma. *Emerg Med Clin North Am.* 1993;11:81–96.

85. Sayers RD, Underwood PC, Porter KM. Surgical management of major thoracic injuries. *Injury.* 1994;25(2):75–79.

86. Tominaga GT, Waxman K, Scannell G, et al. Emergency thoracotomy with lung resection following trauma. *Am Surg.* 1993;59:834–837.

87. Campbell DB. Trauma to the chest wall, lung and major airways. *Semin Thorac Cardiovasc Surg.* 1992;4:234–240.

88. Wojcik JB, Morgan AS. Sternal fractures: the natural history. *Ann Emerg Med.* 1988;17:912–914.

89. Cachecho R, Grindlinger GA, Lee VW. The clinical significance of myocardial contusion. *J Trauma.* 1992;33:68–73.

90. McLean RF, Devitt JH, McLellan BA, et al. Significance of myocardial contusion following blunt chest trauma. *J Trauma.* 1992;33:240–243.

91. Christensen MA, Sutton KR. Myocardial contusion: new concepts in diagnosis and management. *Am J Crit Care.* 1993;2(1):28–34.

92. Fisher RG, Chasen MH, Lamki N. Diagnosis of injuries of the aorta and brachiocephalic arteries caused by blunt chest trauma: CT vs aortography. *AJR.* 1994;162:1047–1052.

93. Karalis DG, Victor MF, Davis GA, et al. The role of echocardiography in blunt chest trauma: a transthoracic and transesophageal echocardiographic study. *J Trauma.* 1994;36:53–58.

94. Morgan AS, Flancbaum L, Esposito T, Cox EF. Blunt injury to the diaphragm: an analysis of 44 patients. *J Trauma.* 1986;26:565–568.

95. Trunkey DD, Hill AC, Schecter WP. Abdominal trauma and indications for celiotomy. In: *Trauma.* 2nd ed. Norwalk, Conn: Appleton & Lange; 1991:409–426.

96. Thal ER, Meyer DM. The evaluation of blunt abdominal trauma: computed tomography scan, lavage or sonography? *Adv Surg.* 1991;24:201–228.

97. Morgan AS, Lane-Reticker A, eds. Blunt and penetrating abdominal trauma, part 1. *Top Emerg Med.* 1993;15(1):1–50.

98. Reed RL II, Merrell RC, Meyers WC. Continuing evolution in the approach to severe liver trauma. *Ann Surg.* 1992;216:524–538.

99. Pachter HL, Hofstetter SR. The current status of nonoperative management of adult blunt hepatic injuries. *Am J Surg.* 1995;169:442–454.

100. Goff CD, Gilbert CM. Nonoperative management of blunt hepatic trauma. *Am Surg.* 1995;61:66–68.

101. Cogbill TH, Moore EE, Jurkovich GJ. Nonoperative management of blunt splenic trauma: a multicenter experience. 1989;29:1312–1317.

102. Feliciano PD, Mullins RJ, Trunkey DD. A decision analysis of traumatic splenic injuries. *J Trauma.* 1992;33:340–348.

103. Smith JS, Wengrovitz MA. Prospective validation of criteria, including age, for safe, nonsurgical management of the ruptured spleen. *J Trauma.* 1992;33:363–369.

104. Root HD, Keizer PJ, Perry JF Jr. Peritoneal trauma: experimental and clinical studies. *Surgery.* 1967;62:679–685.

105. Fischer RP, Beverlin BC, Engrav LH. Diagnostic peritoneal lavage. *Am J Surg.* 1978;136:701–704.

106. Goins WA, Rodriguez A, Lewis W. Retroperitoneal hematoma after blunt trauma. *Surg Gynecol Obstet.* 1992;174:281–290.

107. Federle MP, Crass RA, Jeffrey RB. Computed tomography in blunt abdominal trauma. *Arch Surg.* 1982;117:645–650.

108. Herschorn S, Radomski SB, Shoskes DA. Evaluation and treatment of blunt renal trauma. *J Urol.* 1991;146:274–277.

109. Thomason M, Messick J, Rutledge R. Head CT scanning versus urgent exploration in the hypotensive blunt trauma patient. *J Trauma.* 1993;34:40–45.

110. Andrews B, Pitts L, Lovely M. Is computed tomographic scanning necessary in patients with tentorial herniation? *Neurosurgery.* 1986;19:408–411.

CHAPTER 7

Physical Therapy in the Intensive Care Unit

Severe brain injury may cause posturing, increased tone, weakness, and/or paralysis. These deficits, if left untreated, will cause deformities, contractures, and an inability to function. Immobility may result in complications such as pressure sores, pneumonia, and deep-vein thromboses (DVTs). Physical therapy addresses these motor problems and reduces secondary physical complications.

Historically, physical therapy is ordered for stable patients who require extended time in the intensive care unit (ICU) as a result of complications arising from severe brain injury or for other medical reasons. Increasingly, however, physicians in trauma centers are referring patients for therapy while the patient is still "unstable" (before stabilization of the brain injury), creating a need for physical therapists with a different knowledge level and a different approach to treatment. Edema of the brain, bleeding within the brain, fluctuations in the intracranial pressure (ICP), variances in the cerebral perfusion pressure (CPP), alterations in oxygenation of the brain, and fluctuations in vital signs significantly affect the brain during the first few days post injury. This is considered the unstable period for the patient with severe brain injury. Aggressive rehabilitation intervention with patients with severe brain injury (Glasgow Coma Scale[1] score below 8) should be initiated within one to three days of admission to the hospital. This approach decreases sensory deprivation, prevents contractures, stimulates the patient to a higher level of alertness, and results in a shorter hospital length of stay and an improved functional outcome.[2,3]

Physical therapists are trained to provide range of motion for immobilized patients to prevent or decrease contractures or to provide pulmonary toilet for patients who develop pneumonia. The therapist providing early intervention must know which therapeutic interventions will help prevent secondary insults to the already compromised brain. Vital signs and their relationship to the brain's functioning must be understood. Within this therapeutic environment, the therapist

271

must have a thorough understanding of the patient's medical status, equipment used, and medications. These areas can have significant effects on the provision of and benefits from physical therapy.

ASSESSMENT

Ideally, the physical therapist should be part of the interdisciplinary ICU team, attending rounds and discussing the patients and the therapeutic interventions needed, but for the new therapist treating this patient population, an understanding of the information that will affect the way the patient is evaluated or treated is necessary. A thorough chart review must be completed before initiation of the evaluation. The therapist must know the patient's status, the extent of the brain injury, and the neurologic, orthopaedic, or pulmonary injuries or surgical procedures that may affect therapy intervention or future mobilization of the patient.

Multidisciplinary Input

After a thorough chart review and before patient treatment, the physical therapist should contact the primary care nurse to obtain current information and clearance to evaluate or treat at that particular time. The latest information in the chart may be several hours old, whereas the nurse or critical care intensivist is aware of the most current information on the patient. Information that can be obtained includes

- overall neurologic stability
- changes in physical and behavioral responses secondary to nursing care activities
- variations and ranges in vital signs
- presence of eye opening
- display of agitated behavior
- following of commands
- attempts at communication
- use of medications
- identification of sleep/wake cycles
- use of precautions with patient

Patient observations during rest or treatment procedures should be reviewed. Noting the medication schedule and potential side effects will help determine when sessions should be deferred. Postponement of therapy sessions may also be needed due to frequent procedures, X-rays, and other patient care activity.[4–6]

The respiratory therapist or the nurse can provide information on the patient's respiratory status and response to suctioning. The physical therapist should obtain information regarding the type of ventilator support and the amount of secretions. The therapist trained in auscultation should evaluate the breath sounds. Therapists trained in suctioning but not familiar with severe brain injury should not suction this patient population until they are familiar with unstable severe brain injury, the precautions, and the techniques (protocols) for suctioning these patients. If the physical therapist is responsible for pulmonary toilet, this information will apprise the therapist of the need for treatment to be initiated.

The physical therapist may also obtain necessary information from other team members. The intensivist can provide overall information on the patient's orthopaedic, neurosurgical, and pulmonary needs and concerns. The orthopaedic surgeon can provide specific input regarding any contraindications to movement resulting from orthopaedic injuries. The neurosurgeon provides input regarding any contraindications resulting from secondary brain injury or, if present, a spinal cord injury with neurologic involvement. The occupational therapist and speech/language pathologist can also provide input from their respective assessments.

Universal precautions should be used during the evaluation of the patient. Gloves should be donned before handling patients who have sustained trauma, since blood or bodily fluids may be present. Abrasions or lacerations, surgical incisions, or pin sites from traction or external fixators may be bleeding or oozing. Movement of the patient may result in a need to replace the ventilator tube. Tears may be present when the eyes are opened, or secretions may be present when the therapist repositions the patient's head. Intubated patients will not project sputum when coughing, but extubated patients may have projectile coughing or vomiting. Circumstances may even arise when the therapist may need to apply pressure emergently to an artery if an A-line detaches.

Equipment

Upon entering the patient's room, the physical therapist should note the equipment being used. Is the patient on a ventilator, and what type of ventilatory support is being used? Is the patient not in phase with the ventilator? What is the number of respirations per minute? Is the patient orally or nasally intubated or tracheostomized? In the presence of coughing or increased secretions, the nurse or respiratory therapist should be asked to suction the patient if the therapist is not familiar with suctioning this patient population. The therapist should observe any patient response to suctioning. Care should be taken not to pull on the intubation tubes when moving the patient, since this may cause discomfort. Such discomfort may cause increased posturing, increased ICP, or fluctuations in the patient's vital signs or cerebral perfusion.

The therapist should also be aware of the vital signs displayed on the monitor. The heart rate should be checked and characterized as fast, normal, or slow and as regular or irregular. The presence of an irregular rhythym or premature atrial or ventricular contractions should be noted. The therapist should document if the blood pressure is high, within the normal range for the patient, or low and if the mean arterial pressure is sufficient to maintain adequate cerebral perfusion (normal range is 50 to 170 mm Hg, but in patients with brain injury the desired range is 60 to 150 mm Hg). Too low a mean arterial pressure (<60 mm Hg) or too high a mean arterial pressure (>150 mm Hg) will cause a disruption in the autoregulation of blood flow to the brain.

The oxygen saturation range allowed for the patient and the parameters allowed for the other vital signs (pulse, blood pressure, mean arterial pressure, and respirations per minute) have been programmed into the monitor. An alarm should sound if any levels drop below or rise above the parameters established. A probe recording the oxygen saturation level may be on a finger, earlobe, or toe and can frequently fall off during movement. The probe may need to be replaced or placed on an alternate site until therapy on that extremity is completed.

Rest may be needed if vital signs fluctuate. Calming the patient and removing the stimulus may be adequate to restore the vital signs to baseline. If vital signs do not return to baseline levels after a rest period, cessation of that treatment may be warranted. If vital signs improve during therapy, the therapist should document the benefits obtained.

The ICP monitoring device restricts the amount of head movement allowed. The therapist should refrain from turning the head until the device is removed. The presence of ICP monitoring also prevents raising or lowering the head of the bed beyond what is prescribed by the physician. The appropriate elevation of the bed should be documented in the chart.

The therapist should not provide range of motion of the neck when lines have been inserted there unless this is cleared by medical staff. The therapist should note the location of the A-line placement if it is present. Arterial lines in the wrist or groin restrict the movements that the therapist is allowed to perform, since movement may dislodge the line or "dampen" (alter) the signal. During movement of the extremity with an A-line in place, the signal on the monitor may flatten or vary. Repositioning the wrist or leg should return the signal to baseline.

The use of a cooling blanket alerts the therapist to the presence of a temperature probe. If the temperature is elevated, the therapist may be asked, or may decide, to defer treatment, since an increased temperature may affect brain metabolism.[7] Care should be taken during movement not to dislodge the probe or cause discomfort. Movement of the legs or body may cause discomfort if urinary catheters or fecal collection bags are being used. The therapist must ensure that these devices are not pulled at the insertion or attachment point. Cardiac monitor leads may detach during movement of the arms but are easily reattached. Chest tubes, if present, should be watched during movement of the arms to avoid crimping, which may cause improper drainage of the system.

Patient Observation

Following assessment of equipment, the physical therapist should observe the patient at rest. The following questions provide a framework for observation:

1. Is the patient moving or remaining still? Is the movement purposeful, random, or characteristic of posturing? What type of posturing is occurring: decerebrate or decorticate? Are both sides moving or posturing symmetrically?
2. Are restraints present, and if so, which extremities are restrained?
3. Are the eyes open or closed? If the eyes are open, is the patient fixating, tracking, or staring blankly?
4. Are the eyes conjugate or dysconjugate? If they are closed, is there eye movement present under the lids, or are the lids flickering?
5. Is there any facial movement?
6. In what position is the head: neutral, turned left or right, laterally flexed left or right, on a pillow, or resting on the bed?

Depending upon the patient's neurologic stability, the initial evaluation may be limited to observing the patient during nursing care rather than conducting a thorough hands-on evaluation. Observing the patient's reactions to routine nursing procedures such as washing, moving, rolling, or neurologic checks gives the therapist an opportunity to observe the entire patient. The patient should be observed for responses to potentially noxious stimuli such as placement of intravenous or arterial lines, suctioning, insertion of Dobhoff tubes, and dressing changes. Viewing the patient from different positions (including the head and foot of the bed) may reveal responses that are difficult to view from the typical side-of-the-bed position.

Direct Assessment

When full evaluation is allowed, the therapist should interact and talk to the patient, observing any changes.

1. Does the patient arouse to voice with head movement? Is there head movement toward the voice?
2. Is there any eye movement?

3. Does the patient follow any simple commands?
4. Do vital signs change when the patient hears speech?
5. Does the patient move purposefully or randomly or demonstrate posturing?
6. Does the patient startle or demonstrate agitated behaviors?

Before touching a comatose patient, the therapist should tell the patient what he or she is about to do so as to avoid startling the patient. Startling may increase posturing, agitation, or ICP or may change vital signs, sometimes requiring termination of the session. The therapist should encourage all team members to use this approach with patients.

Posturing

Head position and posturing are the two most important areas to be addressed early by the physical therapist. If the head is not maintained in a neutral position, jugular vein compression may occur, resulting in increased ICP.[5,6,8–15] Posturing may facilitate increased ICP (normal range 0 to 15 mm Hg)[10,13–16] and/or unstable vital signs, such as an increased heart rate, elevated blood pressure, changes in the mean arterial pressure, and an increased respiratory rate.

Decorticate posturing is the result of injury to the hemispheres, internal capsule, cerebral peduncle, basal ganglia, or thalamus.[17,18] Decorticate posturing is referred to as a *flexor pattern* because the upper extremities position in elbow flexion. Additionally, increased tone in adduction, internal rotation at the shoulder, and flexion of the wrist and fingers are noted. The thumb is classically tucked under the flexed fingers. The lower extremities are in extension at the hips and knees, with adduction of the legs and plantarflexion.

Decerebrate posturing is indicative of greater impairment, demonstrating injury to the mid- and upper brainstem.[18] Decerebrate posturing is referred to as an *extensor pattern* because of the extension of all four extremities. The upper extremities demonstrate increased tone in shoulder and elbow extension, adduction, internal rotation, pronation, and wrist and finger flexion (thumb tuck may also be present). The lower extremities demonstrate increased tone in extension of the hips and knees, with adduction and internal rotation of the legs and plantarflexion with inversion. The characteristic positions seen in decorticate and decerebrate posturing are shown in Figure 7–1.

Evaluation of posturing should include the type and consistency of posturing. Is it constant, on arousal of the patient, or only upon painful stimulation? Does the use of inhibitory techniques decrease the posturing and allow movement to occur, either passively or by the patient? The practitioner may decrease posturing, both decerebrate and decorticate, simply by talking to the patient, using inhibitory techniques during movement, or using positioning techniques. In patients with elevated ICP (consistently over 20 mm Hg) or unstable vital signs, positioning to

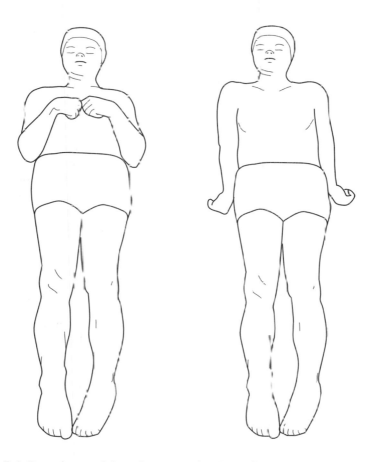

Figure 7–1 Decorticate and decerebrate posturing. Decorticate posturing (left) is termed *flexor pattern*, and decerebrate posturing (right) is termed *extensor pattern*, on account of the position of the arms.

---

decrease posturing may be the only intervention possible. The therapist should demonstrate and explain techniques that may decrease posturing with the nurse, emphasizing the importance of using these techniques 24 hours a day.

Range of Motion

Passive range of motion of the joints not limited by orthopaedic injuries or invasive lines should also be assessed. This assessment establishes a baseline of the range of motion and associated muscle tone. Any evidence of pain should be documented. Pain may be communicated through facial grimacing, thrashing, resistance to a specific movement, increased tone or posturing, or changes in vital signs. The physical therapist may identify orthopaedic injuries, soft tissue injuries, or peripheral injuries that may have escaped notice during the initial life-sustaining resuscitation. These injuries may include clavicle fractures; acromioclavicular separations; wrist, hand, ankle, or foot injuries; and knee instability.

Active Movement

An assessment of the patient's ability to perform active movements on request is essential. Regardless of eye opening or posturing, the patient may still be able to perform simple active movements, such as squeezing with the hand or wiggling the toes. Adequate time must be given because of the potential for delayed responses. The need for repeated requests and the ability to follow simple versus complex commands should be noted. Care must be taken to ensure that hand grasp or toe wiggling is not a reflex.

Eye Movement

To evaluate eye movements, the therapist may need to physically open the eyelids in patients who have no spontaneous or directed eye opening. Eye injuries or orbital fractures may impair eyelid opening. Severe edema secondary to facial injuries may also preclude eye opening. The therapist should assess and document the position of the eyes (conjugate or dysconjugate), movement of the eyes (roving, fixed; movement to left, right, up, and down of each eye), and any attempts to close the eyelids. Eye movement should be observed with the patient at rest and in reaction to voice and to touch. If no movement is seen, painful stimulation can be applied to an extremity on the same side as the eye being assessed.

Pain Stimulus

If vital signs remain stable following stimulation and/or movement, a painful stimulus can be given to assess responses. If the patient is highly agitated, a painful stimulus should not be used. To apply a painful stimulus, the therapist should apply pressure on the nailbed of a finger or toe of each extremity with a fingernail or the side of a pen (Figure 7–2). Central painful stimulus (sternal rub or orbital pressure) may elicit movement of all four extremities, whereas painful stimuli to each extremity may show differences in the ability to move or may demonstrate decreased sensation in the extremity. Briskness or slowness, the degree and type of each movement, and changes in tone and posturing should be noted. Documentation per extremity is necessary when variations are noted.

In patients with concomitant neurologically compromised spinal cord injury, the evaluation should indicate the level of sensory and/or motor dysfunction. Patients with orthopaedic injuries should be cleared by the orthopaedist before painful stimulus is given to the injured extremity. Documentable or questionable pe-

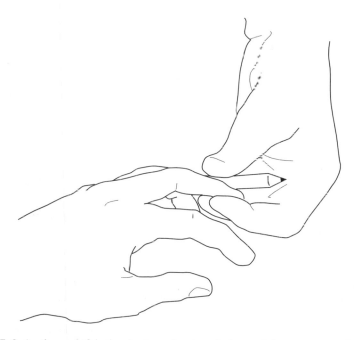

Figure 7–2 Apply a painful stimulus to each extremity by applying pressure to the nailbed of a finger or toe. The examiner may use his or her own fingernail or a pen or pencil to apply the pressure.

ripheral nerve injuries may be identified when there is no reaction to painful stimulation in one extremity or when part of an extremity does not demonstrate a motor response to painful stimulation.

Cognitive Level

The approach that a physical therapist uses in treatment is affected by the patient's cognitive level, as well as neurologic and physical stability. Assessment and consideration of all these areas promote a treatment approach that encompasses the total patient.

The Rancho Los Amigos Scale of Cognitive Functioning[19] (RLA) should be used to assess the behavioral and cognitive level, since it is one of the simpler scales commonly used by rehabilitation specialists in the trauma center, rehabilitation facilities, and state funding agencies. It is common for patients in the early postinjury period to experience fluctuations in medical and neurologic status, with resultant variations in level of alertness and ability to respond. An interdisciplinary approach in determining the RLA level will most accurately reflect the patient's status.

FOCUS OF PHYSICAL THERAPY SERVICES

The primary areas of focus for physical therapy in the ICU are

1. improvement in arousal, alertness and orientation
2. normalization of tone
3. full range of motion of joints not limited by injuries
4. motor control

Additional areas addressed by the physical therapist include prevention of pulmonary complications, skin breakdown, and DVTs.

Individual areas of focus are not treated in isolation. The prevention of skin breakdown and DVTs is accomplished through positioning and moving the patient. These techniques are also used to address arousal, alertness, tone, range of motion, and motor control. The therapist may be required to perform chest physical therapy if atelectasis or pneumonia develops during the first few days post injury, while the patient is still too unstable to mobilize. Moving the patient to the side or to the sitting or upright position helps with the pulmonary toilet in patients who can be mobilized. These movements may also assist with tone, motor control, and skin integrity.

The development of goals during the early stages of recovery often involves creative combinations of these areas of focus. Affective goals are generally based upon both cognitive/behavioral and physical issues. Examples based upon RLA level are outlined in Table 7–1.

TREATMENT

Benefits of Multidisciplinary Treatment Sessions

The physical therapist, occupational therapist, and speech/language pathologist frequently work together during treatment of patients in coma or in an agitated state. The speech/language pathologist may wish to see the patient in coma with either the physical or occupational therapist because his or her evaluation or treatment is enhanced when the patient is in his or her most aroused state. Subtle responses may be more easily observed during joint treatment sessions. The speech/language pathologist may obtain valuable input regarding development of a communication system by observing the physical or occupational therapist performing exercises. The therapists may be helpful in suggesting positions and inhibitory

Table 7–1 Example of Goals Based on a Patient's RLA Level

RLA Level	Goals
I	1. The patient will demonstrate vital sign changes to a painful stimulus. 2. The patient will demonstrate a generalized response to a painful stimulus.
II	1. The patient will open his or her eyes to a tactile or painful stimulus. 2. The patient will perform a controlled generalized movement on request. 3. The patient will follow a simple command three times.
III	1. The patient will open his or her eyes to voice. 2. The patient will follow simple commands five times.
IV–V	1. The patient will calm on request. 2. The patient will perform automatic functional activities on request. 3. The patient will attend to a 30-minute therapy session with redirection as needed.

techniques that the speech/language pathologist can use during therapy. The physical and occupational therapists may need to work together in positioning or moving the patient with multiple injuries. Agitated patients may benefit from two therapists working together because restraints may be removed, allowing the patient to move more freely and thereby reducing agitation and calming the patient.

Level of Alertness and Orientation

Patients with severe brain injury vary in their levels of alertness. Patients in coma may show no arousal (RLA I), generalized responses (RLA II), or localized responses (RLA III). Variations in alertness are affected by sleep/wake cycles, the amount of stimulation given by the therapist, and medications.

Patients in coma need periods of controlled stimulation throughout the day. All therapists create the potential for some level of arousal in most patients by providing auditory, visual, tactile, painful, kinesthetic, and proprioceptive stimulation. This sensory stimulation is applied by talking to the patient, moving the patient, opening the patient's eyes, and using visual stimuli. The physical therapist and occupational therapist must schedule treatment sessions that allow for adequate rest periods. If cotreatments are used, a morning and afternoon session should be scheduled to maximize the frequency of stimulation.

Orientation should be provided throughout treatment sessions. Family members, nurses, and other care providers should be instructed to provide orientation during their interactions. The therapist should first greet the patient, introduce himself or herself, and orient the patient to place, date, reason for hospitalization, and length of stay. Negative information should be avoided at this stage of recovery, especially with patients who are restless, agitated, or exhibiting posturing. If restraints or tubes are in place, a simple description of the device should be given. At times the therapist may note a decrease in elevated blood pressure, pulse rate, respiratory rate, posturing, thrashing, or agitation after orientation information is provided. However, even if there is no response, the therapist should continue to provide orientation regularly.

Visual stimulation should be included in treatment. If the patient cannot open his or her eyes, the therapist may open them, barring any contraindications. Requests to focus visually on the therapist from both the left and right sides should be attempted. Manual blinking of the eyelids will be periodically needed to moisturize the eyes and allow for rest. Patients with dysconjugate gaze should have one eye opened at a time, since double or blurred vision may increase restlessness or agitation.

During range of motion, the therapist should tell the patient what he or she is going to do before performing the movement. Informing the patient may result in increased or decreased resistance, tone, or posturing, depending on the individual patient's level of alertness and level of motor control.

The therapist should take a holistic approach by including the patient's active participation in therapy. Patients who are posturing may be able to relax the extremity on request or may be able to perform a gross motor activity, such as extending the knee after it has been flexed. If the patient extends the entire leg, this may demonstrate that the patient has some control of the extremity and some ability to comprehend. Once a response is elicited, the patient should be encouraged to repeat the response. Refinement of the movement is addressed later. Because responses may be delayed, the therapist must allow adequate time to elapse. The therapist must observe the total patient, since the patient may move an arm or the head instead of a leg and since the vital signs may change when the patient attempts to do what was asked.

A painful stimulus should be used to increase arousal only when other methods (ie, verbal, tactile, movement) have been unsuccessful. Again, the therapist should tell the patient what he or she is going to do before applying the stimulus. The therapist observes for a response before presenting the painful stimulus. After no observed response, the painful stimulus is applied. Again, the therapist observes for any response, including vital sign changes. In the stable patient, the painful stimulus may be repeated if needed. The therapist should monitor the vital signs of unstable patients before repeating the stimulus. When the therapist repeats the verbal statement, he or she should note if the patient moves or attempts to withdraw before the painful stimulus is applied.

The therapist should be aware of the type of brain injury and its potential effect on patient performance. It is not uncommon for patients with bithalamic injury to show no initial responses except for changes in vital signs or pupillary responses because of the nature of injury at the arousal center of the brain. Considerable stimulation may be needed to arouse the patient. It may be beneficial to use cotreatments with the speech/language pathologist with these patients. Increased arousal and alertness allow the speech/language pathologist to better assess comprehension and level of response.

As patients become more responsive, sleep/wake cycles become easier to identify. These cycles can vary, with patients alert for one therapy session and less arousable for another. Nursing may report that the patient was restless all night, thereby explaining why the therapists were unable to arouse the patient during daytime therapy sessions. If the patient's sleep/wake cycle is reversed, prolonging therapy sessions may arouse the patient and achieve the responses desired. Good communication among all team members helps everyone become aware of the patient's level of alertness during the entire 24-hour period.

The family may be the first to report eye opening, movement, or following a command. The therapist should identify if the patient response was reflexive or purposeful. If the action appears to be reflexive, the therapist should explain and demonstrate to the family how the reflex occurs. Patients in coma frequently respond to familiar people first; therefore, the therapist should encourage the family to continue to stimulate the patient.

As the patient progresses from RLA II to III and IV, a focus of treatment is to increase consistency of responses. When agitation is present, the objectives are to calm rather than stimulate the patient and to orient him or her to the environment. If possible, restraints should be removed during therapy, since these may increase agitation. Care must be taken that the patient does not pull on any vital tubes or lines. If agitation is significant, the therapist may be limited to removing only one restraint at a time. As previously stated, cotreatments may be helpful, allowing for better control and management of behavior and the removal of all restraints.

Increased distractibility and decreased attention may also be noted as the patient becomes more alert. Closing the door to the room, turning off music, speaking softly, dimming lights, pulling the shades on windows, or turning off the television may help calm the patient and increase attending. The family should also be taught methods of decreasing agitation. Limiting the number of visitors, allowing frequent rest periods, refraining from playing loud music, and not frequently testing the patient on orientation information are appropriate approaches for the family to use.

Normalization of Tone

A patient at RLA I shows no motor response to stimulation, including posturing, tone, and random or purposeful movements. Range of motion and painful stimulus should be provided by the physical therapist to elicit motor or physiologic responses. Heart rate, blood pressure, and respirations must be monitored for fluctuations during range of motion or when giving a painful stimulus. The physical therapist may be the only consistent rehabilitation team member working with a patient at RLA I. As the patient progresses to RLA II, the physical therapist should inform the occupational therapist and speech/language pathologist so that other interventions may be initiated.

At RLA II, a patient's generalized responses may be manifested as decerebrate or decorticate posturing, primitive reflexes, increased tone, or extraneous movement during attempts to perform purposeful movement. Posturing and tone increase when the patient feels pain, is startled, or feels that a part of the body is unsupported. Decerebrate or decorticate posturing and increased tone must be inhibited.

In response to a perceived lack of support in a supine position, the patient's shoulders will retract and the knees hyperextend. The retraction of the shoulders facilitates additional posturing or increases in tone in the upper extremities. The increased extension of the knees results in a similiar pattern in the lower extremities.[20] Proper supported positioning to decrease high tone or posturing is accomplished by placing towel rolls behind the shoulders (Figure 7–3). Latching the foot of the bed will support the legs in a slightly flexed position. The patient should not have a pillow behind his or her head; rather, a towel or blanket roll should be placed behind the neck to support its normal curve (Figure 7–3). A soft surface behind the head stimulates further extension of the neck as the back of the head pushes into the pillow, searching for firm support.[21] Slight flexion of the neck may help decrease posturing if the neutral position does not affect it. A roll may be placed perpendicular to this roll, if needed, to help keep the patient's head in a neutral position (Figure 7–4). These guidelines can be applied to positioning in bed and in a chair. In the ICU, the patient is often first seated in a recliner to allow the cardiovascular system to adjust to the sitting position. If the seated position results in orthostatic hypotension, the chair can be reclined to stabilize the vital signs.

Body alignment must be evaluated and maintained. With acute brain injury, proper alignment of the head helps control cerebral perfusion by preventing venous outflow problems that occur when the head is turned left or right.[7–15] If the

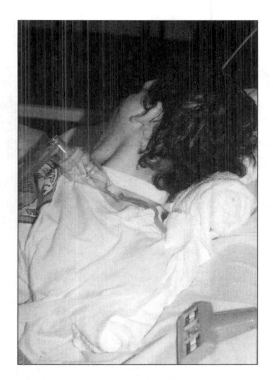

Figure 7–3 Rolls placed behind the neck and shoulders to support them.

head is not in a neutral position, it may influence tone or primitive reflexes or may increase posturing of the extremities.[12,22] Positioning the head in a neutral position also helps prevent later neck contractures (Figure 7–5). Rolling followed by proper positioning can help decrease high tone. Early mobilization, including sitting and standing, is also important. Proper body alignment and support in these positions can also reduce high tone or posturing. All effective techniques should be communicated to the nurse for carryover.

Inhibitory techniques should be used to decrease the tone or posturing before and during range of motion of the extremity. Key areas of control for the arms and legs may be found proximally or distally.[22] Relaxation techniques for the upper extremity are discussed in Chapter 8.

Proper hand placement is important when working with lower extremities when increased extensor tone or decorticate or decerebrate posturing is present. Placement of the hand on the medial side of the plantar surface of the foot will stimulate internal rotation of the leg, as well as inversion and plantarflexion of the foot. The

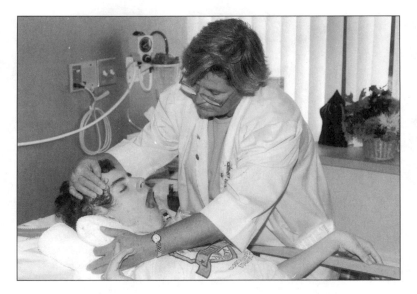

Figure 7–4 A roll may be placed next to the head to maintain it in a neutral position if it tends to turn.

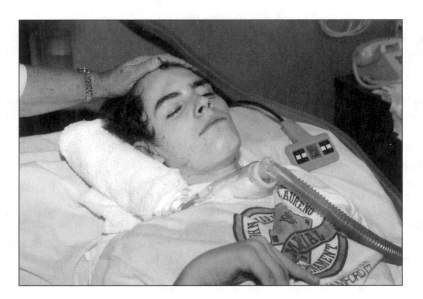

Figure 7–5 Following positioning of towels, the head is in proper alignment in a neutral position.

hand should be placed on the lateral plantar aspect of the foot to facilitate eversion, dorsiflexion, and external rotation of the leg.[22] If this does not result in flexion of the hip and knee, the therapist may try external rotation of the leg, with hands placed medially above and below the knee. Table 7–2 explains techniques to decrease tone and posturing for the upper and lower extremities.

Maintenance of Range of Motion

Maintaining range of motion during the early stages of recovery can significantly affect function and outcome for the individual with a severe brain injury. The therapist should never force an extremity through range of motion. The therapist should be cognizant that grimacing, thrashing, resisting, or exhibiting changes in vital signs during the range of motion may be indicative of a preexisting problem or previously undetected injury. The therapist should also be aware of the incidence of heterotopic ossificans (HO) in patients with severe brain injury[7,23–28] who posture or have high tone and patients who have spasticity following spinal cord injury. The actual reason that HO develops is unclear, but in both patient populations, prolonged or strong muscle contractions are present. The incidence of HO in severe brain injury is estimated to be between 11% and 76%.[23,24,26] Forcefully moving the extremity through the range of motion when there is high tone or posturing may well be a factor in causing HO to occur.

In the unstable patient, forceful movement will cause changes in vital signs, including ICP. Standard practice should include gentle range of motion, following relaxation techniques. To prevent contractures, full range of motion of all joints that are not limited by injury, edema, or equipment must be completed. If high tone or posturing develops during range of motion, the therapist should not try to resist it, but should rather allow the reaction to occur. Before proceeding, the therapist should encourage the patient to relax the arm or leg. The therapist should also assess the accuracy of the techniques used. Was hand placement incorrect, was the extremity moved too quickly, was the patient startled, or did pain occur? Going through range of motion may be a slow process, but it is necessary to prevent pain or injury.

Trauma may also occur if the physical therapist aggressively performs range of motion on edematous extremities. If edema is present, care should be taken to provide as full range of motion as possible without force, since this may cause soft tissue or joint injuries. The extremity should be elevated to decrease edema. Fluid retention secondary to fluid resuscitation, kidney failure, or positional edema may limit full range of motion, but the therapist should provide range of motion through the allowable range. Range of motion is prohibitive with edema caused by DVT, until the patient is treated and cleared for further activity by the physician. If anticoagulation therapy is used, exercise or range of motion of the extremity

Table 7–2 Techniques To Decrease Posturing and Primitive Reflexes

Area	Positioning	Handling
Head	1. Neutral position 2. Roll placed behind neck to support head and neck curvature 3. Roll parallel to head to prevent lateral flexion and rotation	1. Gentle range of motion when ICP and cerebral perfusion stable 2. Hands at base of skull or on sides of head
Trunk	1. Rolls behind shoulders 2. Roll behind hip if rotation is occurring 3. Normal alignment needs to be maintained	1. Hand on scapula, arm supported, rhythmical protraction/retraction, elevation/depression 2. Hand on posterior pelvis, leg supported, rhythmical elevation and depression (rotation) 3. When patient stable: rolling segmentally
Upper extremity	1. Roll behind shoulder 2. Cone in hand if fingers in flexion 3. Wedges between fingers if adducted 4. When stable: turn onto side for weight bearing into arm	1. Relaxation of scapula (1 above) 2. Hand placed in patient's hand from ulnar side to help decrease flexor tone of elbow, wrist, and hand 3. Range of motion of fifth finger or thumb to help break up flexor tone 4. Hand placed over biceps when increased extensor tone and over the triceps when increased flexor tone
Lower extremity	1. Hips and knees supported in a slightly flexed position 2. No pressure on ball of foot medially 3. Roll between legs if strong adduction or internal rotation	1. Hand on lateral side sole of foot for range of motion of foot, knee, and hip 2. Hands placed above and below knee, medially for external rotation, hip and knee flexion 3. Hand behind knee for flexion and external rotation of hip, flexion of knee

should not be completed until therapeutic blood levels have been reached. Many facilities use Greenfield filters for DVT management, because of increased risk for bleeding in the brain with anticoagulation therapy. These filters can be placed to prevent emboli from traveling to vital areas, thereby decreasing the threat to the patient's life. After the placement of a Greenfield filter, the physical therapist may continue range of motion and exercise.

Ankle range of motion can affect standing, transferring, and ambulation skills. If full range is not maintained, these skills may be lost, sacrificed because of plantarflexion contractures or foot deformities.[29] Gentle anterior and posterior mobilizations of the ankle joint can be completed with the foot resting on the therapist's hand. Gentle pressure should be maintained on the heel cord if dorsiflexion is limited. Abduction of the toes or extension of the great toe may help reduce plantar flexor tone, facilitating range of motion into dorsiflexion. The foot range of motion should include eversion, since this is necessary for standing and walking. Range of motion of the toes is often not addressed but is essential with this patient population. Patients with decerebrate or decorticate posturing or increased extensor tone also have increased flexor tone of the toes. When the toes lack extension, balance may be problematic, as well as pushing off during walking. Persons with severe brain injuries frequently have balance problems from vestibular and visual problems, further complicating their ability to walk safely. Full range of motion of the toes should be maintained. If tone is problematic, abduction wedges between the toes may be helpful in reducing tone before contractures develop.[22]

Chemical Paralysis

Patients may need to be chemically paralyzed to decrease the ICP, prevent being out of phase with the ventilator, or prevent further injury. Agitated patients with unstable spinal fractures may be chemically paralyzed until stabilization can be performed. Patients with severe posturing or agitation may be chemically paralyzed to help maintain cerebral perfusion, ICP, vital signs, or ventilator support. Patients with flail chest or those who develop sepsis or acute respiratory distress syndrome (ARDS) may require high-frequency ventilation.[30] Jet ventilation is the most commonly used form of high-frequency ventilation. Over 100 breaths per minute may be delivered under high pressure. A patient with motor control would fight this treatment, so the patient is chemically paralyzed.

When patients are chemically paralyzed, range of motion should still be provided two to three times a week to all joints not restricted by injury or equipment. Range of motion is necessary to prevent capsule tightness and to maintain joint integrity. Joint deformity may also occur if the surrounding muscles that normally support the joint lack tone. Splinting may also be recommended while the patient is maintained on the paralyzing agents. Care should be taken not to force any movement, since the patient cannot display pain but may feel it. Additionally, because of the flaccidity, injury may occur from forcing movement. The patient should not be overstimulated, since he or she may start fighting the ventilator or may become restless as the chemical paralysis wears off. Input from the nurse can be helpful to coordinate treatment with peak medication effects.

Splints/Casts

A role exists for the use of splints and casts with critically ill patients with brain injuries. Improper and unjustified use, however, can result in harm to the patient. Appropriate recommendations and application of these devices should be based on the sound clinical judgment of an experienced physical therapist.

Footboards, sneakers, and standard splints should not be used on patients with high tone or posturing, since these may stimulate increased tone/posturing.[29,31,32] A standard drop foot splint placed on a posturing patient or a patient with increased extensor tone can result in limitations in dorsiflexion in 24 to 48 hours. These limitations may require a week or more of physical therapy to resolve. These splints may also stimulate increases in inversion and plantarflexion tone resulting in pressure sores. These sores develop on the lateral surface of the foot, especially at the base of the fifth toe and over the Achilles tendon. A standard resting splint applied to the hand to maintain a neutral position may have a similiar effect, causing pressure sores and increased tone in the arm.

Certainly, regular, aggressive range of motion by rehabilitation and nursing staff is preferable over casting. Casting can cause sensory deprivation, as well as pressure sores and increased tone if not applied properly. However, casting is the treatment of choice if the physician has major concerns about "drop foot" or if the range of motion into dorsiflexion is decreasing even with therapy.[33-36] Casting should only be performed by therapists experienced in techniques and application. If the physical therapist is not experienced in casting (regularly applying and removing casts), an orthopaedic technician may be used. The therapist, however, must communicate the special needs of the patient, including suggestions as to where pressure should be applied to help inhibit high tone. During casting, padding amounts are reduced from those used with fractures. This reduction reduces the potential for movement due to padding compression, which may stimulate increased tone.[37]

Serial casts should be applied over one major joint rather than the entire leg. When a short leg cast is applied to maintain dorsiflexion, the cast should extend beyond the toes on the plantar surface to decrease stimulation of the toes, which can result in increased tone. The cast should be applied in the patient's *present* range of dorsiflexion. Forcing further dorsiflexion may result in discomfort for the patient. The use of sedation before casting may result in achievement of more dorsiflexion, but once the sedation wears off, increased discomfort and agitation may be present. Pressure should be applied to the base of the fifth-toe side of the plantar surface while the cast is hardening to maintain the foot in a neutral position and prevent inversion and plantarflexion. The cast should not be bivalved or removed for five to seven days unless a change in the patient's status necessitates removal.

Because patients in coma cannot functionally communicate pain, the therapist and nurse must be cognizant of other physiologic signs. Fluctuations in vital signs, an increase in ICP, or an increase in tone or posturing may be the only indication that discomfort or pain is present. An agitated patient may develop increased agitation. Such increases in agitation may necessitate sedation, which may be warranted to facilitate functional use of an extremity.

After five to seven days, the cast should be bivalved to allow for range of motion. The skin must be checked for pressure areas. If tone is still present, the cast can be reapplied as needed. A new cast should also be applied if satisfactory range of motion has not been obtained.[31]

It may be necessary to apply stockinette material and/or padding to the exterior of the cast to prevent skin breakdown of the other leg due to rubbing. Casts may be fabricated of plaster or fiberglass. Fiberglass is more expensive but hardens more quickly than plaster. Fiberglass is also stronger and more durable for use with agitated patients.

Many facilities use pneumatic stockings to help prevent DVTs. Since many physicians recommend that these stockings be used on both lower legs, casting may be problematic. The therapist, however, can recommend that pneumatic stockings be placed on an arm and a leg rather than on both lower extremities. Neither splints nor bivalved casts should be applied under or over pneumatic stockings since discomfort and pressure sores may develop.[32]

Air splints, used to maintain extension of the elbow or knee, allow the skin to be observed while the splint is in use.[31] Again, sensory deprivation occurs with this type of splinting; therefore, it should not be overused. Air splints should not cause abrasions to surrounding areas, as casting may. Increased perspiration from continuous skin contact can occur. The rehabilitation therapist should educate nursing staff on monitoring the area regularly for skin irritation.

Normal Motor Control

With many patient populations, the physical therapist's primary goal is to help the patient achieve independence in physical mobility, including bed mobility, transfers, and ambulation. Regaining motor control is a prerequisite for patients who have sustained a severe brain injury. Independent physical mobility, if achievable, must be considered a very long-term goal, more appropriately achieved in the inpatient rehabilitation or outpatient stage of recovery.

The patient should experience normal and functional movement patterns while in coma to help stimulate purposeful and normal movement. Moving the patient's leg to kick objects or touch the other leg is a functional activity that can be done with the legs. As with all activities, the patient should be told what is going to be done before the movement. If a patient is unable to participate actively in therapy, the therapist must use approaches that stimulate the muscles of the extremities, including weight bearing, bilateral movements, tapping, vibration, and quick stretch.

The patient should be mobilized as early as possible to help prevent complications, including rolling and sitting (Figure 7–6). Out-of-bed orders should be pursued as soon as the patient is stable. The upright position can be felt through standing or use of a tilt table if feasible. The therapist should identify and communicate the best transfer techniques, proper seating, and supports that are necessary to maintain proper anatomical alignment. Seating needs must be reevaluated as changes in posturing, tone, and motor control occur. Ongoing assessment and ongoing education are vital to patient recovery in the ICU and throughout the hospital course.

Many facilities use high-back wheelchairs with customized seating components to maintain proper alignment and support. When specialized equipment is not available, the physical therapist must be innovative in using available supplies to provide a similar support system. Wheelchairs are preferable over recliners in that they are narrower, have a more appropriate seat depth, provide better support to the legs, and have armrests that allow attachment of trays for upper-extremity support and positioning. A firm seat cushion and back support may be added to the chair. When indicated, the seat cushion can be jackknifed to increase hip flexion, which decreases extensor tone.[38] If the chair must be partially reclined, the anterior part of the seat cushion can be angled to maintain a degree of hip flexion. Again, blanket or towel rolls may be used for lateral trunk support, abduction of the legs, and head positioning. A seat belt applied when the buttocks are properly leveled and positioned should hold the patient in hip flexion and maintain contact with the back of the chair if this is not contraindicated by other injuries.[36]

Head control may be more difficult to maintain in a sitting position. Limited success is noted with a "headband" for control of neck flexion. A reversed baseball cap secured to the chair may be of benefit. Again, monitoring for increased flexor tone in the neck should be done, since the patient may develop increased flexor tone from this stimulus, negatively affecting positioning of the arms and legs. Lateral supports will prevent the head from laterally flexing. A firm cervical collar is preferable and maintains the head in proper alignment and the neck in a neutral postion. The therapist must monitor skin condition, however, since break-

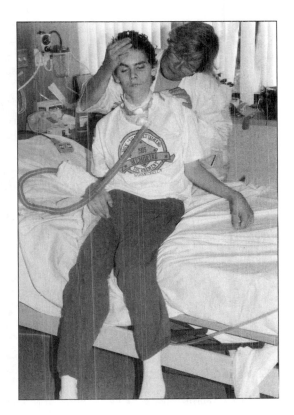

Figure 7–6 The patient should be mobilized as early as possible to help prevent complications.

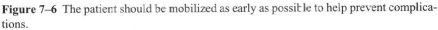

down may occur from the collar. Head control and sitting control should be addressed during therapy sessions. As soon as the patient can be mobilized, activities to increase head and trunk control can be initiated.

It is important for the patient in coma to feel weight shifting, weight bearing into the extremities, and trunk movements. Cotreatments are very helpful at this stage in that two people are often needed to move the patient safely, to provide adequate support, and to monitor lines and equipment (Figure 7–7). Coordination of physical and occupational therapies also facilitates carryover and viewing of the "whole" patient from a functional perspective.

Patients with focal brain injuries may exhibit a hemiplegia. Large subdural or subarachnoid hematomas, which may be focal in nature, press on the brain and may cause injury to brain cells. Hematomas or contusions that create a shift of the

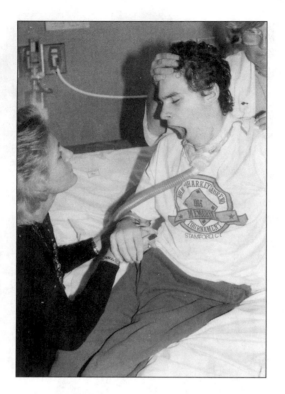

Figure 7–7 The use of two therapists, when working on sitting, allows for safer handling of the patient.

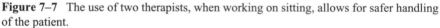

midline structures may cause injury to the brain on the same and/or opposite side. Patients who have sustained a severe brain injury, especially from a motor vehicle accident, usually have diffuse injuries rather than simple hemiplegia. Patients who have been in coma are likely to have sustained injuries to the midbrain and/or brainstem. The therapist should not assume the type and location of physical deficit purely on the basis of location of a focal injury. The therapist must assess the patient during each treatment session to identify any motor control problems. Hemiplegia may not be seen until the patient is moving purposefully on the cortical level. These deficits should be treated with the same techniques as those used on patients who have had cerebral vascular accidents.

With motor control problems, automatic movement may be easier to stimulate than specifically detailed movements. Automatic movements are considered movements that the person does not have to think through how to perform, whereas requested, on-command movements involve the person's having to follow the steps requested to do the movement. This phenomenon may be seen even with patients who are in lighter stages of coma. Automatic knee extension may be stimulated by supporting the leg behind the knee, with the hip and knee flexed, and asking the patient to kick the therapist's hand. Asking the patient to straighten his or her knee while the therapist taps on the quadriceps may show no results. To stimulate extension of the leg, the therapist may push on the sole of the foot while holding the patient's hip and knee flexed and tell the patient to push the therapist away (Figure 7–8). The therapist may need to use different verbal commands or cues to stimulate an automatic response from the patient. At times, the more the therapist clarifies each step, the less the patient is able to follow the directions. With cognitively impaired patients, the focus is on producing an automatic movement with the fewest verbal cues.

Patients who have had a significant hypoxic event may have athetoidlike movements. Primitive reflexes, such as tonic neck reflex, may be present, as well as spasticity, high tone, clonus, or low tone. Coordination problems may be present once the patient begins purposeful movement. Frequently movement is delayed. Reflex-inhibiting patterns may be used to reduce the effects of primitive reflexes and spasticity.[22] The therapist should remember the "key points of control,"[22] which are the optimal control points for the individual patient. The shoulder or

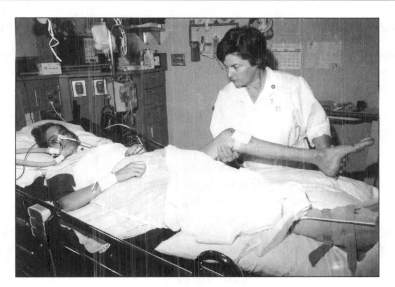

Figure 7–8 Automatic movements may be stimulated by asking the patient to push into the therapist's hand.

pelvis may be a key spot for some patients, whereas for others it may be the toes or fingers. The position of the head may also interfere with particular movements. The most successful therapist is not one specialized in a specific technique but rather one demonstrating basic knowledge and skill level with several different therapy techniques.

For the patient who is able to participate actively, short-arc movements may be used to help regain coordination.[22] The therapist's hands should be placed at either end of the arc for the range of motion desired. The patient should be encouraged to move slowly and to alternate touching the therapist's hands. Constant, calm, verbal cueing may be necessary. Visual feedback by observing the movements, in addition to tactile and verbal cues, is important for retention and increasing accuracy and attention to the activity. As the patient gains control, the range can be increased.

Proprioceptive neuromuscular facilitation (PNF) patterns may be used for range of motion, but straight movements should also be completed. The use of PNF techniques for active exercise is too complicated for the patient with a severe brain injury to comprehend or to tolerate because of the constant verbal commands. Use of these techniques may also result in increased frustration and agitation for the patient.

Motor control in severe brain injury progresses through many stages, from no movement or generalized responses to performance on command. Cognitive skills also progress through stages of agitation, decreased attending, and inability to learn new information.[39] This progression must be remembered when addressing motor control. The patient may regain function without the need for a developmental approach to therapy but may need therapy because of cognitive/behavioral deficits. The patient may be unable to carry through on his or her own, needing constant verbal cueing or demonstration. Decreased attention and agitation impede carryover with these patients.

Skin Integrity

It is appropriate for the physical therapist to assist the nurse in addressing skin integrity because of the therapist's knowledge of the impact of tone, posturing, and agitation on the skin. The patient with a severe brain injury is generally maintained in the supine position, with or without head elevation, until stabilization (standard recordings of ICP less than 20 mm Hg and adequate cerebral perfusion) occurs. The therapist should provide recommendations on positioning to decrease tone and posturing, thus reducing the risk of skin breakdown. Pressure on the heels may be relieved through placement of intravenous fluid bags under the Achilles tendons or through positioning of the heels off the bed with towels. Padding may be placed between the feet or knees to prevent rubbing and contact. Sacral pressure may be relieved by slightly rotating the entire body either left or right while maintaining body and neck alignment. To decrease pressure and edema, elbows and fingers may be elevated on pillows. Ischemia of the skin and soft tissues causes pain and increases tone and posturing and should therefore be prevented. Special beds may be used in the intensive care unit to help reduce skin breakdown. Information on the use of specialized beds is discussed in Chapter 5.

COMPLICATIONS

Orthopaedic and Spinal Injuries

Often the severity of the brain injury makes stabilization of orthopaedic injuries impossible until the patient has stabilized neurologically. The therapist must be careful to maintain alignment of any unfixated fractures during therapy.

External fixation devices may affect physical therapy. Pelvic external fixators may limit rolling or sitting upright if 90 degrees or more of hip flexion is desired. External fixators on a leg are potential sources of injury to the other leg if agitation or posturing is present. Recommendations for positioning and/or padding should be made. Towel rolls may be placed around the pins of a pelvic external fixator, or a pillow may be wrapped around a lower- or upper-extremity fixator and secured with tape or gauze to prevent injury. The therapist may also make suggestions regarding sedation or chemically paralyzing the patient to prevent further injuries. The agitated or confused patient may disassemble the fixator if left unattended. Patients in posttraumatic amnesia will not remember the purpose of the device but will be aware of the resulting discomfort. Close communication with the nurse must be maintained to emphasize the need for observation of the agitated or confused patient. Patients may attempt to climb out of bed, not remembering that a fracture is present and that bearing weight is not allowed.

Stabilized orthopaedic injuries may or may not affect physical therapy. Frequently, fractures are stabilized while the patient is still in coma or on bed rest. The orthopaedic physician may not document weight-bearing status at the time of surgery because of the patient's level of consciousness. The therapist must therefore consult with the orthopaedist regarding weight-bearing status and movement limitations before progressing with rehabilitation.

The therapist must be especially aware of spinal injuries and knowledgeable about equipment used to maintain alignment. Equipment should be checked before each session and monitored during the session to ensure that alignment is maintained. If traction is used, the therapist must safeguard alignment and ensure that the traction is continually applied throughout the therapy session. These techniques are used for skeletal traction as well. The therapist should consult with the physician to identify any limitations for range of motion. With unstable cervical spine injuries, no range of motion of the neck should be performed. Limitations will also be placed on range of motion of the shoulders. With lumbar injuries, limitations may be placed on hip movements. Skeletal traction for an acetabular or femur fracture may limit hip and possibly knee movements. If the patient is thrashing, or if posturing or increased tone prevents alignment and traction from being maintained, the therapist may recommend sedation until stabilization is possible.

Edema

Edema in the lower leg may cause compartment syndrome, especially if tibia and/or fibula fractures are present. Changes in foot sensation are generally the initial sign of compartment syndrome. Numbness at the web space, between the first and second toe, is an early sign of compartment syndrome in the lower leg. Identification of compartment syndrome may be difficult in this early stage because of impaired cognition and behavior. The therapist, however, may first note that longer painful stimulus is required to elicit a reaction. If a compartment syndrome is not released during this phase, coolness of the foot will occur, with an inability of the great toe to move into extension. Paralysis will then develop, with an inability to dorsiflex the foot.

Pulmonary Complications

In some facilities, the physical therapist rather than the respiratory therapist may be responsible for performing pulmonary toilet. Conflicting studies exist regarding the use of postural drainage with positioning in the unstable patient with severe brain injury. Studies have shown minimal risk in lowering the head for proper positioning during postural drainage as long as the head is not turned or the neck flexed.[9,31] Other studies have demonstrated an increase in ICP if the head is level with the body and have recommended elevating the head to 30 degrees.[12]

Studies have demonstrated increases in ICP due to suctioning when oxygen supplementation was not provided.[8,10] Reports also state that if suctioning is provided for less than 10 seconds, no maintained increase in ICP is seen.[7,8,10] The ICP and CPP must be monitored during suctioning. It is of utmost importance for these to return to safe ranges before suctioning and between suctionings. Pulmonary complications, such as pneumonia and its resultant temperature increases, can also have a detrimental effect on the injured brain. The patient with pneumonia often experiences delays in extubation. These prolonged periods on a ventilator can delay or interfere with receiving intensive rehabilitation.

Physical therapists performing postural drainage on patients with unstable severe brain injury must follow defined protocols, including close monitoring of vital signs during treatment. Monitoring the ICP and mean arterial pressure during positioning is especially important. The head must remain in neutral alignment. Therapy should be ceased if the ICP increases and remains elevated or if an alarm sounds, indicating that safe established parameters have been exceeded. The therapist must identify the presence of any rib, sternum, or scapular fractures, since percussion and vibration may be painful for the patient.

Pulmonary or chest injuries may limit the patient's ability to participate in active therapy. The patient may be unable to compensate for the increased oxygen demands during activity because of pulmonary contusions, hemothorax or pneumothorax, diaphragmatic repairs, atelectasis, ARDS, prolonged time on the ventilator, or injury to the brain affecting respiratory control. The physical therapist may work on breathing exercises and energy conservation techniques with the patient if the patient is able to follow directions.

Fractures of the ribs may limit the patient's ability to take deep breaths during exertion. Rolling or sitting may not be possible because of the pain from the rib fractures. Sternal fractures and scapular fractures may also affect breathing. The physical therapist may suggest a trial of transcutaneous electrical nerve stimulation for pain control for the patient who is cognitively and communicatively able to participate. An analgesic may be necessary for the patient to tolerate manual techniques with rib and sternal injuries. Decreasing pain will help improve pulmonary function and increase the patient's ability to move.

Narcotics are one method used for pain control. Because this method suppresses coughing, it may result in pulmonary complications, including pneumonia. Drowsiness or lethargy from narcotics also affects the patient's ability to participate in therapy. Administration of medication through a line in the epidural space of the spinal canal is another method of pain control. Regardless of the method, the therapist should be aware of medications used in pain control. Some medications block all sensory feedback, an effect that may prevent moving the patient safely.

Other Complications

The physical therapist must be aware of any changes occurring during therapy sessions. A patient who initially was able to quickly dorsiflex a foot but who now exhibits sluggish movements or no movement should have the position of his or her leg analyzed. Peripheral nerve injuries may develop from pressure on the nerve exerted by positioning or from objects on, or near, the patient. The therapist must evaluate the leg at rest and assess whether the peroneal nerve is subjected to pressure from the position. Pneumatic stockings, splints, or rolls may also put pressure on the nerve, causing "drop foot" or paralysis.[32]

Patients who develop infections, a common complication in this population, may show deterioration in their level of alertness and their ability to participate in therapy. The metabolic requirements necessary to overcome an infection reduce the energy available for arousal, attending, and moving. The physical therapist should reduce the demands placed on the patient who has developed an infection, although treatment should not be stopped completely. The patient with severe brain injury will physically and cognitively deteriorate if stimuli and treatment are stopped. The amount of stimuli and treatment must be adjusted according to the patient's condition, regardless of cause.

Surgery may also affect therapy. Surgeries may limit activity (as in the case of skin grafts), decrease movement (as in the case of fixation of a fracture with extensive casting applied), or reduce responses for a period of time (as in the case of anesthesia or pain medication given postoperatively). Surgery may cause increased pain, which will increase tone, posturing, and agitation. The patient may also be placed on bed rest following surgery. Placement of feeding tubes (whether a simple procedure such as percutaneous endoscopic gastrostomy or more complex procedures such as jejunostomy) may cause discomfort. Most forms of abdominal discomfort can increase tone or posturing in the extremities and may also increase agitation.

INTERACTIONS WITH THE FAMILY

The physical therapist, like other members of the rehabilitation team, must educate the patient's family and loved ones. It should be standard procedure, once the evaluation has been completed, to allow family members to observe treatment. The family is often intimidated by equipment and the condition of the patient and may be quite apprehensive about touching the patient. Observation of therapy educates the family that the patient may be moved without causing harm or jeopardizing his or her life. Family members can be instructed in specific therapy techniques that can be performed with the patient. Families should not, however, be forced to treat the patient. Each person has different ways of handling a crisis, and the therapist must be sensitive to each individual's needs. The therapist may also suggest reading cards or notes to the patient or playing tapes. The physical therapist, like all members of the team, must develop a rapport with the family to facilitate the family's acceptance and assimilation of education regarding brain injury and the rehabilitation needs of the patient.

SUMMARY

The physical therapist is an integral member of the team caring for the patient with severe brain injury. The physical therapist must be familiar with the equipment in the ICU and must have theoretical and clinical knowledge of brain injury. The therapist must also be keenly aware of the other injuries seen in this population and how these injuries affect the brain injury and its treatment. Evaluation and treatment of persons with brain injury who are still unstable medically are vital to normalize tone, decrease posturing, and maintain or gain full range of motion; otherwise, contractures and deformities will develop. These complications will interfere with, or delay, ongoing rehabilitation as well as future mobility and ambulation skills. Early physical therapy helps ensure that sensory deprivation will not occur and helps prevent secondary complications, such as skin breakdown, pulmonary complications, and DVTs. Additionally, the patient may be better able to participate in rehabilitation because of improvement in arousal or alertness.

For the safety and progress of the patient, the therapist must respect and be respected by other team members. The physical therapist should not be the only rehabilitation team member treating these patients in the ICU. He or she must facilitate involvement of occupational therapy and speech/language pathology in the treatment process to maximize a patient's functional recovery.

REFERENCES

1. Teasdale G, Jennet B Assessment of coma and impaired consciousness: a practical scale. *Lancet.* 1974:2:81–84.

2. Morgan AS, Chapman P, Tokarski L. Improved care of the traumatically brain injured. Presented at First Annual Conference of the Eastern Association for Surgery of Trauma; January 1988; Longboat Key, Fla.

3. Mackay LE, Bernstein BA, Chapman PE, Morgan AS, et al. Early intervention in severe head injury: long-term benefits of a formalized program. *Arch Phys Med Rehabil.* 1992;73:635–641.

4. Parsons LC, Wilson MM. Cerebrovascular status of severe closed head injured patients following passive position changes. *Nurs Res.* 1984;33:68–75.

5. Mitchell PH, Ozuna J, Lipe HP. Moving the patient in bed: effects on intracranial pressure. *Nurs Res.* 1981;30:212–218.

6. Mitchell PH. Intracranial hypertension: implications of research for nursing care. *J Neurosurg Nurs.* 1980;12:145–154.

7. Mitchell PH. Central nervous system I: closed head injuries. In: Cardona VD, Hurn PD, Mason PJ, Scanlon A, et al, eds. *Trauma Nursing from Resuscitation through Rehabilitation.* 2nd ed. Philadelphia, Pa: WB Saunders Co; 1994:383–434.

8. Jess LW. Assessing your patient for increased I.C.P. *Nursing.* 1987;17:34–42.

9. Lee ST. Intracranial pressure changes during positioning of patients with severe head injury. *Heart Lung.* 1989;18:411–414.

10. Boortz-Marx R. Factors affecting intracranial pressure: a descriptive study. *J Neurosurg Nurs.* 1985;17:89–94.

11. Snyder M. Relation of nursing activites to increases in intracranial pressure. *J Adv Nurs.* 1983;8:273–279.

12. Palmer M, Wyness MA. Positioning and handling: important considerations in the care of the severely head-injured patient. *J Neurosci Nurs.* 1988;20:42–49.

13. Mitchell PH. Intracranial hypertension: influence of nursing care activities. *Nurs Clin North Am.* 1986;21:563–576.

14. Sherman DW. Managing an acute head injury. *Nursing.* April 1990:47–51.

15. Lipe HP, Mitchell PH. Positioning the patient with intracranial hypertension: how turning and head rotation affect the internal jugular vein. *Heart Lung.* 1980;9:1031–1037.

16. Feldman Z, Reichenthal E. Intracranial pressure monitoring. *J Neurosurg.* 1994;81:329–330. Letter to the editor.

17. Griffith ER, Mayer NH. Hypertonicity and movement disorders. In: Rosenthal M, Griffith ER, Bond MR, Miller JD, eds. *Rehabilitation of the Adult and Child with Traumatic Brain Injury.* 2nd ed. Philadelphia, Pa: FA Davis Co; 1990:127–147.

18. Caronna JJ. The neurologic evaluation. In: Rosenthal M, Griffith ER, Bond MR, Miller JD, eds. *Rehabilitation of the Head Injured Adult.* Philadelphia, Pa. FA Davis Co; 1983:59–73.

19. Hagen C. Language disorders secondary to closed head injury: diagnosis and treatment. *Top Lang Disord.* September 1981:73–87.

20. Bobath B. *Abnormal Postural Reflex Activity Caused by Brain Lesions.* London, England: William Heinemann Medical Books Ltd; 1974.

21. Manzi DB, Weaver PA. *Head Injury: The Acute Phase.* Thorofare, NJ: Charles B Slack Inc; 1987.

22. Bobath B. *Adult Hemiplegia: Evaluation and Treatment.* London, England: William Heinemann Medical Books Ltd; 1981.

23. Kalisky Z, Morrison DP, Meyers CA, Von Laufen A. Medical problems encountered during rehabilitation of patients with head injury. *Arch Phys Med Rehabil.* 1985;66:25–29.

24. Garland DE, Blum CE, Waters RL. Periarticular heterotopic ossification in head-injured adults: incidence and location. *J Bone Joint Surg Am.* 1980;62:1143–1146.

25. Lehmkuhl LD, Thoi LL, Baize C, Kelley CJ, et al. Multimodality treatment of joint contractures in patients with severe brain injury: cost, effectiveness, and integration of therapies in the application of serial/inhibitive casts. *J Head Trauma Rehabil.* 1990;5:23–42.

26. Rogers RC. Heterotopic calcification in severe head injury: a preventive programme. *Brain Inj.* 1988;2:169–173.

27. Cherry DB. Review of physical therapy alternatives for reducing muscle contracture. *Phys Ther.* 1980;60:877–881.

28. Powell JN, Chapman P. The impact of early orthopedic management on patients with traumatic brain injury. *J Head Trauma Rehabil.* 1994;9:57–66.

29. Leahy P. Equinus deformity in adults with severe traumatic brain injury: a pilot study examining incidence over time. *Neurol Rep.* 1990;14:16–19.

30. Hurn PD, Hartsock RL. Thoracic injuries. In: Cardona VD, Hurn PD, Mason PJ, Scanlon A, et al, eds. *Trauma Nursing from Resuscitation through Rehabilitation.* 2nd ed. Philadelphia, Pa: WB Saunders Co; 1994:466–511.

31. Boughton A, Ciesla N. Physical therapy management of the head-injured patient in the intensive care unit. *Top Acute Care Trauma Rehabil.* 1986:1–18.

32. Gill-Body KM, Giorgetti MM. Acute care and prognostic outcome. In: Montgomery J, ed. *Clinics in Physical Therapy: Physical Therapy for Traumatic Brain Injury.* New York, NY: Churchill Livingstone Inc; 1995:1–31.

33. Anderson D. Management of decreased ROM from overactive musculature or heterotopic ossification. In: Montgomery J, ed. *Clinics in Physical Therapy: Physical Therapy for Traumatic Brain Injury.* New York, NY: Churchill Livingstone Inc; 1995:81–86.

34. Sullivan T, Connie TA, Goodman M, Mackie T. Serial casting to prevent equinus in acute traumatic head injury. *Physiother Can.* 1988;40:346–350.

35. Booth BJ, Doyle M, Montgomery J. Serial casting for the management of spasticity in the head-injured adult. *Phys Ther.* 1983;63:1960–1966.

36. Roush JS, Emory N. Positioning the coma-emergent patient through the use of orthotics and wheelchair seating systems. *Neurol Rep.* 1990;14:20–23.

37. Davies PM. *Starting Again.* Berlin, Germany: Springer-Verlag; 1994.

38. Chiu ML. Wheelchair seating and positioning. In: Montgomery J, ed. *Clinics in Physical Therapy: Physical Therapy for Traumatic Brain Injury.* New York, NY: Churchill Livingstone Inc: 1995:117–136.

39. Jennett B, Teasdale G. *Management of Head Injuries.* Philadelphia, Pa: FA Davis Co; 1982.

CHAPTER 8

Occupational Therapy for Severe Brain Injury

The occupational therapist is an integral member of the brain injury team treating patients with severe brain injury. Areas of expertise and intervention include oculomotor function, vision, movement, integration of sensory stimuli, perception, and cognition. In some intensive care units (ICUs), however, the occupational therapist may not receive referrals for evaluation and treatment of the patient with severe brain injury unless the patient is stable and weakness of an upper extremity is present or unless splinting is required to prevent or correct contractures.

The occupational therapist addresses sensory, cognitive, perceptual, and motor problems. Integration of sensory stimuli is necessary for perception. Perception and the ability to move are necessary for motor control. Cognition is not possible without perceptual awareness. Sensory integration, perception, cognition, and motor control are necessary for function. Severe brain injury may cause visual, perceptual, motor, and cognitive problems. A lack of stimulation during coma may cause sensory deprivation. Lack of early rehabilitation intervention may cause complications, including compensatory techniques for visual problems that will affect later posture, balance, and function. Contractures may develop that will prolong the rehabilitation process and interfere with function. Patients who have sustained severe brain injury, scoring below 9 on the Glasgow Coma Scale,[1] must receive early rehabilitation intervention, including occupational therapy. Initiation of rehabilitation, within one to three days of admission, is imperative to decrease length of stay and to maximize the potential for functional recovery.[2,3]

The occupational therapist must have the knowledge and clinical skills necessary to treat this medically and neurologically unstable patient population. Knowledge of equipment, physiologic monitoring, the meaning of monitored information, safe parameters, and equipment limitations placed on evaluation and treatment is necessary before interaction with the patient is possible. The occupational therapist must understand the medical information in the chart and its relationship to the brain injury and to the treatment of the patient. The therapist must have knowledge of the medications used and their effects on the patient. Because this patient population is usually unstable, the therapist must know when to stop a treatment, when to work with the patient, and when not to treat the patient.

ASSESSMENT

Evaluation is not initiated until a thorough chart review has been completed. In addition to information regarding the brain injury, the occupational therapist should note any orbital or eye injuries, cranial nerve injuries affecting the eyes, cervical or upper thoracic injuries, and shoulder or upper-extremity injuries. These specific areas directly affect the occupational therapist's assessment and treatment of the patient.

Multidisciplinary Input

Following the chart review, the occupational therapist should discuss the patient's case with his or her nurse or the intensivist before therapy is initiated. The therapist must know the most current information on the patient's medical stability, neurologic status, vital signs, and the allowable ranges for vital signs. Patient responses during various nursing care activities, such as presence or absence of eye opening, fixating, or tracking of movement, following of commands, and attempts at communication, should be discussed with the nurse. Additionally, information should be sought regarding medication use and schedule, identification of sleep/wake cycles, and patient precautions.

The primary care nurse may also have information on responses to procedures that have been scheduled or recently completed and information regarding the patient's family or loved ones that may be beneficial in treatment. The nurse also has knowledge of vital sign fluctuations and potential triggers for these fluctuations. The therapist must know what will quickly normalize and what will not. The nurse may request that the therapist return later because the patient is showing increased fatigue or instability from too many procedures recently being done with him or her.[4,5]

The occupational therapist may also obtain information regarding the patient from other team members. The intensivist, orthopaedic surgeon, neurosurgeon, or oromaxillofacial (OMF) surgeon may be contacted for information on the patient's condition, precautions, and concerns. Specific input regarding contraindications to movement because of orthopaedic injuries or concomitant spinal cord injury is essential, as is information regarding facial or orbital injuries. The physical therapist and speech/language pathologist also provide input regarding their respective assessments.

Equipment

The therapist must be familiar with the equipment used in the ICU (refer to Chapters 5 and 7). The mean arterial pressure should be between 60 mm Hg and 150 mm Hg for adequate cerebral perfusion.[6] The therapist should note physiologic data during rest and should monitor throughout the therapy session to ensure that they remain stable. The parameters for the allowed variations in the vital signs are set, and an alarm will sound if any fluctuation beyond those parameters occurs. Treatment must be stopped if the vital signs fluctuate too much. If vital signs do not return to normal after stimulation is removed and attempts are made to calm the patient, the session must be terminated.

Cardiac monitor leads should be checked to be sure there is enough slack for arm range of motion. Leads are easily replaced if they become unattached, however. Lines in the neck or an intracranial pressure (ICP) monitor will limit the ability to move the head and neck. A pulse oximeter may be attached to a finger. The therapist should move this probe to another site while performing range of motion on that extremity or be sure that there is enough line to perform range of motion without its detaching. A radial arterial line (A-line) may restrict range of motion of that wrist. Sufficient slack must be present in an A-line so that range of motion of the extremity may be completed without pulling it out. The signal may dampen during movement of the extremity but should return when the arm is brought back to the resting position. If the signal does not return, repositioning of the arm is necessary until the signal successfully returns. Intravenous lines must also be checked to be sure their placement will not restrict movement. The tubing for the ventilator should be observed to ensure that there is enough room to move the shoulder and head and neck through the range of motion. Pulling on the tubing (oral or nasal) at the insertion to the patient will cause discomfort and may alter the patient's vital signs. Additionally, the tubing must be examined for any accumulation of water. If water is present, it should be removed before movement of the patient begins to prevent the chance of water entering the patient's airway with movement.

Chest tubes may cause discomfort during shoulder range of motion. The therapist must also determine the location of the chest tube drainage system so that he or she does not kick it during therapy. Drainage systems are usually placed on the floor next to the bed.

The presence of a cooling blanket should alert the therapist to the possibility of an elevated temperature. If the temperature is elevated, the therapist should consult the nurse before treating the patient. Alternately, the therapist may consider seeing the patient when the temperature is in the normal range. An elevated temperature in an unstable patient with a severe brain injury may cause secondary insult to the brain[7] and should be considered more serious than one occurring in a stable patient.

Observation

The patient should be observed, and what is seen should be documented before stimulation is provided (see Chapter 7). Documentation should include whether both sides are moving or posturing symmetrically. Generalized random movement or any purposeful movement, such as turning the head, following movement, holding onto objects, or scratching, should be documented. The use of restraints on any extremities should also be mentioned.

The therapist should document whether the eyelids are open or closed, whether the patient is staring blankly, whether there are random or roving eye movements, or whether the patient is fixating or tracking. Conjugate or dysconjugate eye movement should also be noted. If the eyelids are closed, the therapist should note whether there is eye movement present under the lids or whether the eyelids are fluttering.

Documentation of facial movement, head position, and movement is necessary. Oral movement, spontaneous swallowing, or grimacing should be noted if present. Head position should be characterized as neutral, rotated left or right, laterally flexed left or right, on a pillow, or resting on the bed.

The therapist should observe for and document any edema, ecchymosis, or deformity present around the eyes or in the face, neck, trunk, or upper extremities. Any known fractures, dressings, splints, casts, external fixator devices, or sutures should also be documented.

Direct Assessment

Direct assessment should begin with evaluation of the patient's response to auditory, light tactile, firm tactile, visual, proprioceptive, and kinesthetic stimulation (through movement of the patient). If these stimuli do not arouse the patient, a painful stimulus may be employed. Patients with severe brain injury may respond to their environment (arousal) with increased posturing, restlessness, random movement, or eyelid opening.

When assessment involves physical contact with the patient, the therapist should wear gloves and practice universal precautions. Trauma patients may have lacerations or abrasions that are still bleeding. Body fluids may be present. With so many lines present, the chance for contact with body fluids, especially blood, is high.

Response to Auditory Stimulation

The occupational therapist should interact with and talk to the patient, observing for any responses to the auditory stimulation. Patient responses to voice may include head or eye movement toward or away from the sound, posturing, moving randomly or purposefully, agitated behaviors, following of simple commands, and vital sign changes.

Response to Tactile Stimulation

Tactile stimulation should be provided after observation and auditory stimulation. Telling the patient what the therapist is going to do before doing it should be a standard with this patient population to prevent startle responses. Startling may cause fluctuations in the vital signs, especially the ICP. The patient's response to touch should be documented on the evaluation.

Firm tactile stimulation may be applied by tapping on the extremity or face, applying firm pressure, such as squeezing the hand, or firmly rubbing the patient's hand. Again, the therapist should note the patient's response to this type of stimulation. Arousal (posturing, changes in the vital signs, eye opening, or movement) may occur in response to one or more types of stimulation.

Response to Visual Stimulation

The eyelids should be opened by the occupational therapist if they are not already open and if there are no contraindications. The therapist should observe any responses to eyelid opening. An object, such as a familiar photograph, should be placed in the patient's visual field, or the therapist may place himself or herself in the patient's visual field. Any responses to the stimulus should be noted.

Response to Proprioceptive and Kinesthetic Stimulation

Proprioceptive and kinesthetic stimulation is provided through range of motion and weight bearing into the joints of the upper extremity. Range of motion of the neck, if not limited by injury or lines, should be performed carefully within a limited range so as not to affect the ICP. Gentle flexion, extension, lateral flexion, and rotations should be done. Observation of the patient's response to these movements is difficult, but the therapist may see eyelid or eye movement, movement of the arms, or restlessness occur. Following range of motion of the neck, the therapist should perform range of motion of the upper extremities, again documenting any changes that occur. The therapist may push down on the shoulder, elbow, or wrist joints to stimulate weight bearing into the joints.

Response to Painful Stimuli

Painful stimuli should be used only after all previous stimuli have failed to arouse the patient. Agitated patients and those with injuries that prohibit movement should not have painful stimulation applied. Again, the patient should be told, before the stimulus is applied, that painful stimulus is going to be applied and where. The therapist should note any changes. The therapist should give the painful stimulus to each extremity by applying pressure to the nailbed of a finger or toe of each extremity with his or her fingernail or the side of a pen and then document the reaction (Figure 7–2). The appropriateness of the response must be evaluated. An arm in extension that goes into flexion because of painful stimulation should also have painful stimulation provided when in flexion. Further flexion is considered an inappropriate response, whereas extension may be considered an appropriate withdrawal from the painful stimulus. Extension of the arm would be considered an appropriate but generalized response for that extremity. This would be a higher level of response than the entire body's responding to the stimulus. Localized responses include withdrawal of the fingers from the stimulus. Generalized painful stimulation, such as sternal rub, may result in generalized movement of all four extremities, whereas a painful stimulus given to each extremity better clarifies function. One extremity may respond sluggishly, whereas another may respond briskly. Posturing or delayed responses may be elicited in only one extremity.

In patients with a concomitant spinal cord injury, the therapist must consider the dermatomal levels involved when providing tactile and painful stimulation. Documentation of the level of sensory and/or motor impairment is necessary, allowing the therapist to assess recovery, lack of recovery, or deterioration of function from the spinal injury. Peripheral nerve injuries may be directly related to the initial trauma the patient sustained or may develop over time from positioning or edema. Secondary injuries such as positional ulnar nerve injury may be detected sooner following a thorough initial evaluation of upper-extremity movement and sensation.

Assessment of Motor Control

Motor control should be assessed initially through observation followed by stimulation. Patients progress from no movement, to movement on stimulation, to random/generalized movement, to purposeful movement, and finally to following of commands.

The patient may not move his or her head, may thrash with constant head movement, may turn the head to the location of the stimulus, or may follow commands for head movement. Head movement to the left and/or to the right should be documented. The therapist must evaluate the cause for lack of turning to one side. Lack of head turning may be the result of neglect, decreased sensation, muscle imbalance, or soft tissue injury. Additionally, a hearing impairment may cause lack of head turning. Verbal requests to turn the head, therefore, should be given from both sides of the bed in case hearing is impaired in one ear. Tactile stimulation to the arm on the side the patient is being asked to turn to may not produce the desired effect if there is decreased sensation in that arm. Tactile stimulation to other areas (ie, the face and neck) may result in the requested movement. Visual cues may also be helpful. Head position is one of the most important areas to be addressed early in the rehabilitation process. The head must be positioned in neutral, at rest, to avoid jugular vein compression, which results in increased ICP.[4,5,8–15]

The therapist should evaluate whether there is random, generalized, or purposeful movement of the extremities and whether the patient is able to follow simple commands. The following of commands progresses from a gross motor activity, such as squeezing the therapist's hand, to releasing it, and then to straightening the fingers, pointing one finger, and tapping one, two, or three fingers. Both upper extremities must be compared for the degree of tone, including passive range of motion, and active movement. Variances in spontaneous movement between the arms should alert the therapist to the potential for a hemiparesis.

Tone/Posturing

Tone is evaluated bilaterally during range of motion. Patients with a space-occupying lesion may have decreased tone on one side. Decreased tone may occur on the same side of the lesion or on the opposite side because of brain shift. Increased tone, or spasticity, may also be present. If tone variations are secondary to primitive reflexes, the therapist must determine the positioning necessary to decrease the frequency of occurrence.

Posturing is evaluated by observation, stimulation, and movement of the patient. Figure 7–1 in the previous chapter shows decorticate and decerebrate posturing. Decorticate posturing, referred to as a *flexor pattern*, is exhibited by flexion of the elbows, wrists, and fingers. Additionally, increased tone in adduction and internal rotation at the shoulder and pronation of the forearm are noted. Decerebrate posturing denotes a lower level of brain injury and therefore greater impairment and is referred to as an *extensor pattern*. The upper extremities demonstrate increased tone in shoulder extension, internal rotation and adduction, elbow extension, pronation, and wrist and finger flexion, frequently with thumbs tucked under the fingers. The lower extremities are in extension in both forms of posturing. Evaluation should include the type of posturing, if present, and the consistency. A thorough assessment should identify whether any inhibitory techniques decrease the posturing yet allow movement to occur. Posturing may occur constantly or intermittently, in response to being startled or in pain. The patient may have random or purposeful movement with intermittent posturing. The therapist can decrease posturing by talking to the patient or by using inhibitory techniques or positioning, although some patients may be unresponsive to all attempts at control. In patients with an elevated ICP (constantly over 20 mm Hg) or whose vital signs are unstable, positioning to decrease posturing may be the only intervention allowed. Posturing may result in increased ICP.[10,13-16] The therapist must discuss effective positioning techniques with the nurse for adequate carryover. The orthopaedist should be consulted if any orthopaedic injuries are present, since these may directly affect early positioning as well as later mobilization of the patient.

Posturing may facilitate instability of the vital signs. Increased heart rate, elevated blood pressure, and alterations in the mean arterial pressure may occur. An increase in the respiratory rate may also occur from posturing. All of these factors must be addressed in the unstable patient who is posturing.

Range of Motion

Range of motion of the head and neck and upper extremities is assessed, after first informing the patient. All joints not limited by injury or invasive lines must be evaluated. Differences in tone, limitations in range of motion, and differences between the two extremities should be documented.

The therapist must monitor the patient to ensure that no signs of discomfort occur. Discomfort may be manifested by grimacing, eye opening, generalized increases in posturing or tone, increases in restlessness, changes in the vital signs, or resistance to movement. Due to the severity of the brain injury and other potentially life-threatening injuries, lesser injuries may be first discovered by the rehabilitation team or nurse. Injuries such as wrist and hand fractures, acromioclavicular separations, clavicle fractures, elbow fractures, peripheral nerve injuries, or soft tissue injuries such as whiplash may be present and first noted by the occupational therapist. The occupational therapist must communicate with the physicians any question of injuries found during the evaluation so that appropriate evaluation and treatment may occur.

The baseline evaluation of range of motion and of the patient's responses during these activities assists the occupational therapist in evaluating any changes that may occur. A patient who shows no signs of discomfort during early range of motion but later develops pain and swelling in the arm as he or she starts moving it may have a deep-vein thrombosis (DVT) diagnosed and treated expeditiously.

Purposeful, On-Command Movement

The patient's ability to move on request must be evaluated. The patient may squeeze a hand on request or move his or her head when there is no eye opening or when posturing is present. Hand squeezing may be a reflex that occurs when the palm of the hand is stimulated; therefore, the therapist must make certain that the movement occurred on command. Placing the therapist's hand in the patient's hand and pausing, with no further stimulus to the hand, before asking the patient to squeeze should prevent reflexive grasp. Repetition of the action can also be requested. Delays in response time and difficulty in following or inability to follow complex requests are frequently seen in this patient population. Simple one-step commands should be used, and adequate response time should be allowed. Gross movements occur before specific movements. The therapist must ascertain if a gross movement observed was the result of the patient's attempt to follow commands or spontaneous movement. Gross or spontaneous movements may include posturing.

Visual-Motor Assessment

The occupational therapist addresses ocular motor function, which relates to vision. It is essential to determine that no eye or facial injuries are present that would contraindicate opening of the eyelids. Patients initially at level I or II of the Rancho Los Amigo Scale of Cognitive Functioning[17] (RLA) do not demonstrate eyelid opening. When the eyelids are opened by the therapist, the eyes may be in a fixed conjugate or dysconjugate position or may be roving. Patients at RLA III may or may not open their eyes, but eye movement may be present. If no movement of the eyes is seen, firm tactile or painful stimulation can be applied to the same side of the body as the eye being assessed to stimulate eye movement. Other team members benefit from the occupational therapist's input regarding ocular motor function and visual skills. The therapist must assess and document movement of each eye (fixed, roving, or random movement to the right, the left, upward, and downward) and whether the movement is conjugate or dysconjugate. The occupational therapist must assess each eye individually when the eyes are dysconjugate because of possible diplopia. The occupational therapist assesses whether the patient fixates on objects presented in the visual field, tracks the movement of objects in the visual field, or scans the environment. Impaired convergence may result in diplopia and depth perception problems later. Double vision may cause increased agitation in patients at RLA level IV or V. Impaired convergence may affect the patient's interpretation of where he or she is in relation to the environment during later stages of rehabilitation, resulting in holding the head to one side, balance problems, leaning to one side in order to see the horizon as level, or seeing the floor as uneven.

The occupational therapist must have an understanding of the cranial nerves that affect vision and eye movement. Table 8-1 lists the cranial nerves affecting vision, eye movements that the nerve controls, and the potential impairment. Assessment of eye movement may indicate that a cranial nerve injury, a disruption in central neural control,[18] or a muscle entrapment resulting from an orbital fracture exists. With a disruption in central neural control, the patient may present with no ocular movement or may exhibit ocular movement without conjugate function. The dysconjugate gaze shown in Figure 8–1 may result from central neural control problems, muscle entrapment, or cranial nerve injury. Determination of the cause of the problem is necessary to determine the approach to treatment.

Visual information is transmitted by the optic nerve from the eyes to various areas of the brain for interpretation. If the optic nerve is injured, visual field defi-

Table 8–1 Cranial Nerves Affecting the Eyes and the Potential Impairments If Injury Occurs

Cranial Nerve	Eye Muscles, Function	Impairment
Optic (II)	Carries information from eye to brain for interpretation	Visual field deficits, cortical blindness Bilateral pupillary dilation when light stimulus to eye with optic nerve injury
Oculomotor (III)	Medial, superior, inferior rectus; inferior oblique. Eyelid opening, pupil constriction. Eye movement toward nose downward, upward, and up away from nose.	Eye will be laterally and inferiorly positioned. Eyelid ptosis. Dilated pupil
Trochlear (IV)	Superior oblique moves downward and lateral—away from nose.	Diplopia
Abducens (VI)	Lateral rectus moves eye lateral–away from nose	Eye will be medially positioned
Facial (VII)	Orbicularis oculi closes eyelid.	Unable to close eye, causing irritation and drying of eye if no intervention taken

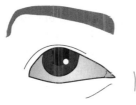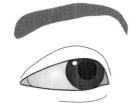

Figure 8–1 Dysconjugate gaze.

cits or blindness may result. Bilateral optic nerve, chiasmal, or optic tract injuries may result in cortical blindness. The eyes and the processing areas of the brain are not injured, but the visual information is not being received for interpretation; therefore, the patient may state, if asked, that he or she can see. Only with continued questioning and testing regarding what the patient sees will it be apparent that a problem is present. The occupational therapist may suggest that visual evoked potentials be performed if there is suspicion of cortical blindness. Optic nerve injury will also cause unilateral pupillary dilation. Pupillary response to light testing will show bilateral constriction to a light stimulus on the side with an intact optic nerve. Bilateral pupillary dilation occurs when a light stimulus is given to the eye with optic nerve injury.[19]

Cranial nerve III (oculomotor nerve) injuries, from direct injury or from herniation secondary to edema or brain shifting, result in ptosis of the eyelid, a dilated pupil that is unreactive to light, and inability to move the eye inferior and medially toward the nose.[19,20] Injury to this nerve results in an outward and downward eye and diplopia. The occupational therapist may suggest that objects be placed in the visual field of that eye, laterally and caudally, so that the patient may focus on the object.

Cranial nerve IV (trochlear nerve) injury results in impaired downward gaze and vertical diplopia. Cranial nerve VI (abducens nerve) injury results in an eye positioned medially with diplopia.[20] These are the more common cranial nerves affected by brain injury, edema, and brain shifting. The therapist should suggest appropriate locations for placing objects in the patient's visual field. Cranial nerves affecting the corneal reflex are the trigeminal and facial nerves (V and VII). Additionally, facial nerve injury may cause paralysis to the orbicularis oculi, which is necessary for closure of the eyelid. Decreased blinking results from injuries to these nerves, which may cause irritations or injury to the eye resulting from lack of sensation and lack of moisture. The occupational therapist may suggest ophthalmologic or optometric consultation for prevention of further eye injury or evaluation of visual function.

Orbital injuries causing muscle entrapment must not be confused with cranial nerve injury. A retracted globe, enophthalmos, results from a "blowout" fracture or fracture of the maxillary sinus secondary to a blow to the orbit. Symptoms include subconjunctival hemorrhage and vertical diplopia.[20] Consultation with the OMF surgeon may be of benefit in developing a treatment program to best meet the patient's needs. Papilledema, or swelling of the optic disc, may occur secondary to increased ICP and may result in diplopia from cranial nerve VI (abducens nerve) paralysis.

Eye alignment can be tested whether the patient is able to participate or not. The therapist observes where light reflects on the eyes. If the eyes are aligned, the light will reflect on the same spot of each cornea.[21] Eyes that are not aligned will result in diplopia or head tilt, to align the horizon.

Pupil size and reaction to light should be noted and monitored throughout the hospital stay. Anisocoria, or unequal pupil size, exists in 17% of the normal population.[20] A patient with a dilated pupil that is nonreactive to light may have visual problems resulting from decreased accommodation and may be photophobic (sensitive to light). Pupil size and reaction to light may be the result of medication; therefore, the therapist should discuss unusual findings with the nurse or intensivist to be sure that medication is not the cause. Nystagmus may also be caused by medications such as Dilantin or certain barbiturates.

The results of the visual assessment should be communicated with other team members. Suggestions for interaction and strategies for any visual problems should be shared. The therapist may suggest patching an eye, shielding one lens of the patient's glasses, or taping to shield specific areas of the lens of glasses, if double vision is present, to decrease agitation. Suggestions as to where to position stimuli, such as pictures, may be made, depending on findings of muscle entrapment or cranial nerve involvement.

Cognitive Level

The occupational therapist, in consultation with the physical therapist and speech/language pathologist, assists in determining the RLA level. Patients fluctuate in their level of responsiveness early post injury; therefore, each discipline may evaluate the patient at a different level of arousal or alertness. Additionally, medications may affect the patient's ability to respond to commands as well as to stimulation. The RLA scale should be used by rehabilitation team members throughout the hospital course to facilitate consistency in patient interaction.

OCCUPATIONAL THERAPY GOALS

The primary areas of focus for occupational therapy in the ICU are

1. improvement in arousal, alertness, orientation, attention
2. improvement in oculomotor function
3. improvement in neuromuscular skills (normalization of tone, full range of motion of joints not limited by injury, motor control)
4. improvement in sensorimotor integration (neuromuscular skills and sensory integration, including visual spatial, body integration, awareness of midline, movement of the body in space, and ability to cross midline)

In some facilities, the occupational therapist may be involved in the evaluation and treatment of dysphagia, including prefeeding therapy and feeding programs (see Chapter 11).

The patient with severe brain injury has complex cognitive/behavioral and physical issues. Fluctuations in cognition, as demonstrated by fluctuating RLA levels, are frequently seen. Therapy goals must therefore be broadly written and varied daily according to the patient. Specific goals should be based on the RLA levels and must be measurable. Table 8–2 illustrates various ways of measuring goals. These percentages and durations are not standard measurements; rather, they are used to show different means of measuring goals.

Therapy may address multiple goals at once. Movement stimulates arousal, alertness, oculomotor skills, improvement in neuromuscular skills, and improvement in sensorimotor integration. Asking the patient to track a photograph addresses oculomotor skills as well as arousal, alertness, neuromuscular skills, and sensorimotor integration.

Remedial or adaptive techniques can be used in therapy. Visual problems secondary to a nerve injury or muscle entrapment require an adaptive approach to therapy. Special glasses, eye patching, or teaching the patient to focus within the limited range of motion of the involved eye are adaptive approaches. Adaptive approaches are necessary until the nerve injury repairs or the entrapment is released. Imbalance of the muscles due to the brain injury is treated with a remedial approach. Exercises to strengthen and coordinate movement are done until eye movements and convergence improve and accommodation occurs.

TREATMENT

Benefits of Multidisciplinary Treatment Sessions

The occupational therapist frequently works with the physical therapist or the speech/language pathologist in treatment of the patient in coma or in an agitated state. Arousal of the comatose patient may occur during occupational or physical therapy; therefore, the speech/language pathologist may wish to be present during those treatments. Occupational and physical therapists may jointly treat the agitated patient, since two people may be required to remove restraints safely. Mobilization of the comatose, posturing, high- or low-tone patient may also require two people. If the speech/language pathologist is working on swallowing and feeding, the occupational therapist may assist the patient in bringing the food to the mouth or with positioning. Subtle responses may be more easily observed with two rehabilitation specialists. The speech/language pathologist may be able to develop a communication system as a result of observing patient responses during occupational or physical therapy. Inhibitory techniques or positioning may be suggested for carryover during speech therapy sessions.

Table 8–2 Various Methods Used for Goal Measurement

Goal	Measurement
Arousal	
1. Patient will arouse. To voice For 5 seconds	To painful stimulus
Eyes	
1. Patient will open his or her eyelids.	To stimulus Once during therapy session For 2–3 seconds 50% of therapy session
2. Patient will look at objects.	When placed in visual field Spontaneously Inconsistently vs consistently With cueing For 10 seconds 75% of the time
Attending	
1. Patient will attend to a task.	For 5 seconds 20% of the time With redirection as needed Inconsistently vs consistently
Movement	
1. Patient will respond to stimulus.	With generalized response of the entire body With generalized response of the extremity being stimulated With a localized response
Following of Commands	
1. Patient will open fingers.	To stimulus Once vs 5 repetitions Inconsistently vs consistently 80% of time

Improvement in Arousal, Alertness, and Orientation

Stimulation is necessary for arousal and alertness of comatose patients. The stimulation must be controlled so as not to alter significantly the vital signs. The amount of required stimulation varies according to the patient's RLA level. Chapter 7 discusses the approach used in physical therapy for patients at RLA I and II.

Auditory stimulation may be provided by talking to the patient throughout the treatment session, using different sounds, playing music, or turning on the television. Orientation should be provided regularly. An explanation of the equipment may be provided while touching it with the patient's hand. Additionally, family members or friends should be encouraged to talk to the patient to stimulate arousal and alertness.

The patient's eyelids should be opened unless there are contraindications. The therapist should present objects familiar to the patient in the visual field. Photographs of the patient, family, or special events are beneficial since they have personal meaning to the patient. If fixation occurs, the therapist should move the object slowly to see if tracking occurs, while telling the patient to look at the object. The therapist should ask the patient from each side of the bed to look at him or her. Tapping on the arm, on the side on which movement is desired, may assist in getting the patient to look in that direction. The therapist should periodically close the patient's eyes for lubrication and rest. Patients with dysconjugate eyes may benefit from having only one eyelid opened at a time.

The therapist should explain to the patient, before and during range of motion, what is going to be done. The patient may respond to the verbal statement with resistance, increased tone or posturing, or initiation of movement, depending on his or her level of alertness. The therapist should orient the patient to areas of his or her body, facilitating tactile cueing. An example would be, "Your right hand is touching your left arm. . . . Feel your left arm. . . . Rub your left arm," while moving the hand up and down the arm. The patient may automatically start moving the hand up or down the arm, resist the movement, or pull away.

Responses may occur even during posturing. The patient may be able to squeeze a hand or point a finger, even though posturing is present. This demonstrates some control of movement and some comprehension. Responses may be delayed; therefore, adequate time must be allowed. Additionally, the therapist must observe the entire patient when requesting movement since a leg may move or the vital signs may change when the patient is asked to perform a movement.

Variances in temperature and texture should be used for stimulation. Quick strokes with ice may add awareness to a movement desired, whereas prolonged contact with ice will be noxious, possibly causing arousal or movement away from the stimulus. Stroking with soft materials versus coarse materials may have the same effect. Painful or noxious stimulus may be used to increase arousal.

Factors That Affect Arousal

Arousal may be affected by the area of brain injury, sleep/wake cycles, and medications. The therapist must understand brain injuries and their impact on arousal. The brainstem controls sleep/wakefulness. The reticular activating system controls consciousness.[7] Prolonged periods of stimulation may be necessary to arouse patients with bithalamic injury. Once aroused, the patient may be able to participate in therapy. The occupational therapist may want to cotreat with the physical therapist or speech/language pathologist. Together, they may provide sufficient stimulation to arouse the patient.

Sleep/wake cycles affect arousal. Rehabilitation specialists need to communicate patient responses to therapy with each other. One therapist may observe no arousal during treatment, whereas another may observe arousal and following of simple commands. Sleep/wake cycles become easier to identify as the patient becomes more responsive. The team must communicate so that all are aware of the sleep/wake cycles and the patient's level of alertness and performance when "awake."

The family must be included in stimulation of the patient. They should be asked to bring in familiar or favorite objects and photographs They may be instructed in orienting and stimulating the patient with these objects. Education must be provided on what can and cannot be done with the patient. Demonstration of range-of-motion and stimulation techniques should be provided. Family members should be allowed to watch and participate in treatment sessions. Patients with severe brain injury frequently respond to the familiar first, so family members may be the first to observe movements on command or eyelid opening.

The patient's progression from RLA II to III or IV alters the approach/focus of treatment. Consistency of responses is the focus at RLA III. Calming rather than stimulating is the focus with patients at RLA IV. Orienting the patient to his or her environment may help reduce agitation. Reducing noise and visual stimulation may also help reduce agitation and distractibility. Turning off the radio or television, dimming the lights, closing the door, and allowing only one person to talk may help increase attending during this period. Cotreatments may be necessary with the agitated patient so that restraints may be removed without jeopardizing patient safety.

Improvement in Oculomotor Function

A patient at RLA I has no eyelid opening. The occupational therapist should open the patient's eyelids if this is not contraindicated. The sequence for eye opening is first to painful stimulus, then to touch, to voice, and finally spontaneously. Objects should be placed in the visual field, and an explanation as to what an object is should be given. Bright colors should be used. Familiar photographs of a single subject may also be used. Photographs of groups or a scene are often too difficult to focus on at this phase. Initially, attempts are made to elicit a response, whether changes in vital signs or generalized movement. The response sequence begins with fixating on the stimulus with one eye, then with both eyes, and then progresses to tracking the object.

The occupational therapist addresses visual skills, including focusing, tracking, saccadic movements, and eye-hand coordination, as the patient progresses through RLA levels II, III, and IV. Treatment must be different for patients with cranial nerve injuries affecting the muscles of the eyes. The therapist must know what eye movements will cause diplopia. The therapist may address each eye separately for fixating, tracking, shifting gaze, and eye-hand activities. The therapist should also address vision within the area that the eyes are able to work together. The occupational therapist should inform other team members where to position objects so that the patient is able to focus clearly. Agitation may be reduced with elimination of double vision. Patching or shielded glasses may be beneficial in reducing agitation but should not be used excessively since the eyes need exercise together to develop the ability to focus again.

Improvement in Neuromuscular Skills

The occupational therapist addresses tone, posturing, primitive reflexes, range of motion, and motor control. Patients at RLA I show no motor activity; therefore, physical and occupational therapists may treat these patients together, or they may alternate treating the patient so that each may monitor any changes resulting from his or her intervention. Range of motion to the neck and both upper extremities and painful stimuli are used to elicit movement, tone, or physiologic responses.

Patients at RLA II (generalized response) may show primitive reflexes, decerebrate or decorticate posturing, or increased tone. The occupational therapist, as well as the physical therapist, must provide positioning techniques that will inhibit primitive reflexes, increased tone, and posturing.

Proper head alignment is mandatory to prevent jugular vein compression, thereby helping maintain adequate cerebral perfusion.[4,5,8–15] Proper head positioning and support also help decrease primitive reflexes and decerebrate or decorticate posturing,[23] a cause of increased ICP.[10,13–16] A pillow should not be placed behind the head since a soft surface stimulates further extension of the neck as the head seeks firm support.[24] Proper positioning to maintain head alignment is described in Chapter 7. (Also refer to Figures 7–3, 7–4, and 7–5.) This positioning is necessary to prevent development of neck contractures.

The patient's shoulders must be supported to prevent retraction, which may stimulate further posturing or increased tone. A roll should be placed behind each shoulder to support a neutral or slightly protracted position.[25] Cones (Figure 8–2) or splints with finger separators (Figure 8–3) may help reduce decerebrate or decorticate posturing or increased flexor tone in the arm, as well as the hand.[26] Once the necessary cone size is established, moleskin may be used to cover the cone, and a strap may be added to keep it in place. When the patient can be moved to a chair, these techniques should be continued if increased tone or posturing is present. In the ICU, the patient initially is placed in a recliner to allow cardiovascular adjustment to the upright position. If vital signs fluctuate, the nurse can recline the patient to help stabilize the vital signs. Early mobilization of the patient, including rolling, sitting, and standing, is important but is usually not done until the vital signs are stable. Proper body alignment and support in each position can also reduce high tone or posturing. All effective techniques should be shared with other team members.

Inhibitory techniques should be used before and during range of motion. Key areas of control for the arms may be found proximally or distally.[23] Relaxation of the shoulder girdle is necessary before range of motion of the shoulder. Rhythmical elevation and depression, then protraction and retraction of the scapula, may reduce tone in the entire arm. Likewise, range of motion of the fingers, starting with the fifth finger, may help decrease decerebrate posturing. Thumb abduction may help reduce finger flexor tone.[23,26]

Proper hand placement is another inhibitory technique used to decrease tone and posturing. In patients with decorticate posturing, the therapist's hand should be placed in the patient's hand from the ulnar side, with greater pressure applied at

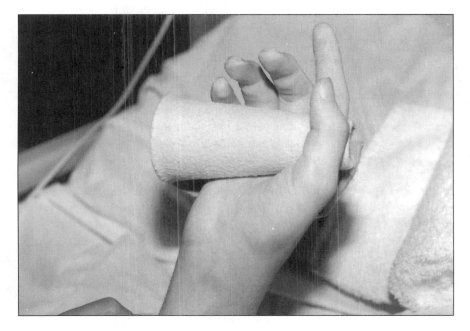

Figure 8–2 Cones may be used to help decrease flexor tone in the hand.

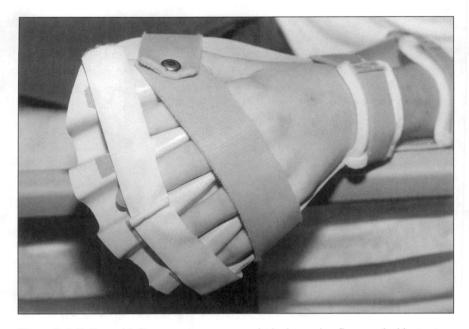

Figure 8–3 Splints with finger separators may assist in decreasing flexor and adductor tone in the hands.

the base of the fifth finger, to help decrease flexor tone at the elbow, wrist, and fingers. The therapist's other hand is placed over the triceps to stimulate extension of the elbow (Figure 8–4). Avoiding stimulation of the biceps is imperative, since this will cause increased flexor tone. In the patient with decerebrate posturing, the therapist's other hand is placed over the biceps to stimulate flexion.

Following inhibition of tone/posturing, full range of motion of all joints not limited by injury or equipment should be done. Maintenance of range of motion affects future rehabilitation and outcome. Forceful range of motion should never be done in the early stage since it may produce changes in the vital signs secondary to pain, necessitating termination of the treatment session. Forced range of motion when high tone or posturing is present may be a factor in heterotopic ossificans (HO) development. The incidence of HO is high in patients with severe brain injury who posture, have high tone, or have spinal cord injury with spasticity.[27–33] In brain injury, the incidence is estimated to be between 11% and 76%.[30] Standard practice should be gentle range of motion. The therapist should not resist tone or posturing if it develops during range of motion. Rather, the therapist should allow the extremity to move within the posture. Once relaxation occurs, the

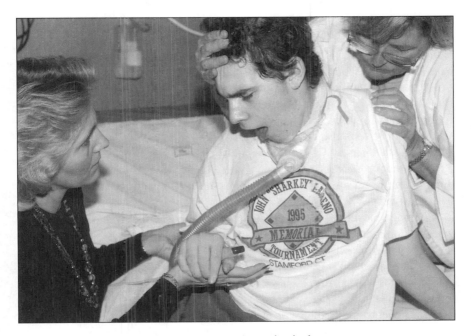

Figure 8–4 Hand placement to decrease tone/posturing in the arm

extremity can be ranged again. The therapist may need to assess hand placement, speed of movement, and discomfort if unable to perform range of motion.

Edema in the extremity will affect the degree of range of motion that the therapist can perform. Forcing range of motion when edema is present may cause soft tissue or joint injury. The occupational therapist must determine the cause of the edema. Edema secondary to fluid overload, dependent positioning of the extremity, or kidney failure does not limit range of motion within the allowable range. Edema secondary to a DVT prohibits range of motion until the DVT is treated. The therapist should be in communication with the physician so that range of motion may be reimplemented as soon as this is safe.

Range of motion should be completed several times per week for patients who are chemically paralyzed to prevent capsule tightness and to maintain joint integrity. Joint deformity may occur if joints are not maintained in proper alignment or if the muscles around them have no tone. Therefore, functional position resting splints for the wrists and fingers should be provided if the patient is to remain paralyzed for extended periods. These functional position resting splints should not be used in nonparalyzed patients if increased tone or posturing is present, since pressure sores and increased tone and posturing will develop.

The occupational therapist should allow the patient to experience normal movement by having the patient touch objects or perform activities, even passively. The patient's hand can be moved to wash the face with a washcloth or to smooth the hair. The patient should experience touching other parts of the body. Motor control progresses through different stages, from no movement to generalized responses, followed by automatic and purposeful responses and progressing to performance on command. Cognitive behaviors also progress through different stages, from no response, to agitation, to low level of attending, and better level of attending but inability to learn new information.[34] These progressions must be remembered when treating this patient population. Normal motor control may return without being addressed with a developmental approach but may be affected by cognitive/behavioral problems.

Automatic movement may be easier to stimulate than movement on command when motor control problems exist. Automatic activities such as handing the patient a ball may produce the activity desired, whereas asking the patient to do the specific movement may produce no result. At times, the more the therapist tries to clarify what is wanted, the less the patient is able to perform. The cognitive/behavioral impairment may cause agitation instead of the requested movement.

Some patients may exhibit a hemiplegia from a space-occupying lesion (subdural or subarachnoid hemorrhage). The majority of patients with severe brain injury have injury to multiple areas of the brain. Comatose patients usually have injury to the midbrain or brainstem. The therapist should not assume that the only deficit is a hemiplegia when a space-occupying lesion is present. Assessment is done at each treatment session so that identification of any motor control problems can be quickly made and addressed. Hemiplegia may not be apparent until the patient starts moving purposefully on the cortical level. If hemiplegia is present, techniques and approaches used with patients who had cerebral vascular accidents should be used. Following of commands may be difficult for the patient because of other injuries to the brain. Weight bearing, bilateral movements, tapping, icing, vibration, and quick stretch are some of the techniques that may assist in treatment.

Primitive reflexes, delay in movement, spasticity, high or low tone, clonus, or coordination problems may be present. Reflex-inhibiting patterns[23] may be used to reduce the effects of primitive reflexes and spasticity. The therapist should remember the "key points of control."[23] The occupational therapist must find the optimal control points for each patient as well as for each treatment session, since the patient may vary from day to day. The therapist who has basic knowledge and skill level with multiple therapy techniques will be successful in treating this patient population.

The patient should be mobilized as early as possible. Rolling and sitting help prevent complications. Feeling weight shifting, trunk movement, and weight bear-

ing into the extremities is important for the patient in coma. Early out-of-bed orders should be pursued. Head and trunk control cannot be addressed until mobilization is allowed. Proper alignment should be maintained and discussed with the
patient's nurse for follow-through. A high-back reclining wheelchair should be
provided for sitting as soon as possible. A wheelchair provides better support for
the entire body than does a recliner. Head and trunk alignment and support and
positioning of the upper extremities should be established when the patient is
seated properly in the wheelchair. Blanket rolls to support the trunk laterally also
provide positioning and support for the upper extremities in abduction and/or
some shoulder flexion. Support for the head may include a soft or firm cervical
collar if the patient has increased flexor tone in the neck. Head and trunk control
activities must be part of the treatment program (Figure 8–5). Visual and functional activities may assist in regaining head control. When eyelid opening is not
present, the therapist should manually hold the eyelids open while performing
head and trunk movements.

Patients who are able to participate actively in therapy may benefit from the use
of short-arc movements to regain coordination.[23] The therapist places his or her
hands on each end of the arc of movement desired and asks the patient to touch
one hand and then the other. The patient should see the movement, as well as
receive verbal cues, to assist attention and increase accuracy. The range is increased as the patient develops coordination.

Complications

Cervical Spinal Cord Injuries

In the presence of cervical spine instability, proper alignment is essential until
stabilization can be performed. Traction, if in use, must be continually applied.
The therapist should be sure that weights are free from contact with the bed or
floor and that the alignment of the traction is maintained during each treatment
session. Shoulder flexion and abduction should not extend beyond 90 degrees, and
resistive exercises to the shoulders should not be performed. No range of motion
to the neck or scapula is allowed. If the patient is restless or posturing, the occupational therapist may recommend sedation until stabilization is possible. Following
cervical stabilization, mobilization of the scapula and full shoulder range of motion should be performed once approved by the physician.

Infections

The presence of an infection in patients with severe brain injury is common.
The level of alertness and the ability to participate in therapy may decrease. The
demands placed on the patient must be decreased, since the metabolic require-

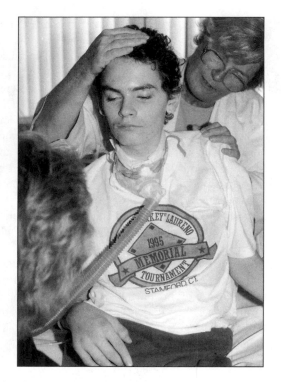

Figure 8–5 Head and trunk activities, sitting to increase control.

ments to overcome the infection reduce the energy available for therapy participation. Treatment should continue, but with fewer demands placed on the patient.

Improvement in Sensorimotor Integration

The occupational therapist addresses sensorimotor integration throughout treatment for oculomotor, visual, and motor problems. Visual-spatial integration and body integration are addressed during range of motion, active movements, and visual activities and exercises. Integration of movement of the eyes and the extremities helps with awareness of midline, movement of the body across midline, and movement in space (Figure 8–6). Movement requires interaction with the environment.[35] The exercise of reaching for an object or touching an object addresses motor activity, eye-hand control, and figure-ground and position-in-space awareness.[22]

Sensory integration is divided into three integrative levels[36]:

1. organization of vestibular and proprioceptive input, resulting in postural and ocular control
2. body perception and motor planning using both sides of the body
3. eye-hand coordination visual perception, and purposeful activity[37]

Sensory integration includes coordination of sensory input, motor output, and sensory feedback. Sensory awareness, visual-spatial awareness, and body integration are included in sensory integration.[38] Sensorimotor integration involves neuromuscular and sensory integrative skills, including perceptual motor skills.[38]

INTERACTIONS WITH THE FAMILY

The occupational therapist must interact with the patient's family and significant others to provide ongoing education. Following evaluation, all team members should allow family members to observe treatment. This involvement helps the family become more comfortable with the equipment and the ICU setting. As

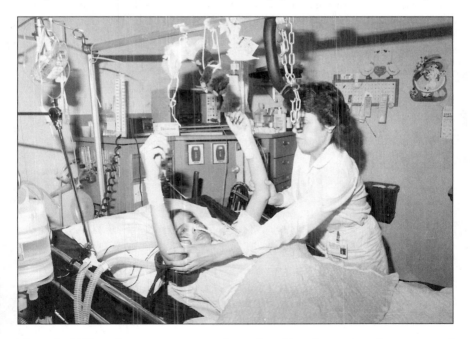

Figure 8–6 Bilateral arm movements may be used to address integration of movement and movement in space. This may also address eye-hand control.

family members begin to understand the surroundings, they will feel less intimidated and begin interacting with the patient. Instruction in what can and cannot be done with the patient is essential. The therapist must be sensitive to each person's needs and must not force involvement on individuals not comfortable with that role. It is important to develop rapport with the family to educate it effectively on brain injury and the present and future needs of the patient. Family members must be considered important members of the patient care team.

SUMMARY

The occupational therapist is an integral member of the team caring for the patient with severe brain injury in the ICU. The therapist must have knowledge of brain injury, the equipment used in the ICU, the safe parameters for vital signs, complications and their effects on brain injury, and how to treat patients with brain injury. Clinical skills must be adapted to this unstable patient population. The occupational therapist must be aware of all injuries that the patient sustained and must know the impact that other injuries have on the brain injury and treatment. Occupational therapy is necessary to increase alertness, prevent sensory deprivation, maintain or improve range of motion, prevent contractures, decrease posturing and normalize tone for improved neuromuscular control, and improve visual motor skills and sensory integration. Occupational therapy helps improve sensorimotor function so that the patient is better able to participate in his or her rehabilitation at discharge.

REFERENCES

1. Teasdale G, Jennett B. Assessment of coma and impaired consciousness: a practical scale. *Lancet.* 1974;2:81–84.
2. Morgan AS, Chapman P, Tokarski L. Improved care of the traumatically brain injured. Presented at First Annual Conference of the Eastern Association for Surgery of Trauma; January 1988; Longboat Key, Fla.
3. Mackay LE, Bernstein BA, Chapman PE, Morgan AS, et al. Early intervention in severe head injury: long-term benefits of a formalized program. *Arch Phys Med Rehabil.* 1992;73:635–641.
4. Mitchell PH, Ozuna J, Lipe HP. Moving the patient in bed: effects on intracranial pressure. *Nurs Res.* 1981;30:212–218.
5. Jess LW. Assessing your patient for increased I.C.P. *Nursing.* 1987;17:34–42.
6. Butterworth JF, Prough DS. Head trauma. In: Rippe JM, Irwin RS, Alpert JS, Fink MP, eds. *Intensive Care Medicine.* 2nd ed. Boston, Mass.: Little, Brown and Co; 1991:1459–1478.
7. Mitchell PH. Central nervous system I: closed head injuries. In: Cardona VD, Hurn PD, Mason PJ, Scanlon A, et al, eds. *Trauma Nursing from Resuscitation through Rehabilitation.* 2nd ed. Philadelphia, Pa: WB Saunders Co; 1994:383–434.

8. Mitchell PH. Intracranial hypertension: implications of research for nursing care. *J Neurosurg Nurs.* 1980;12:145–154.

9. Lee ST. Intracranial pressure changes during positioning of patients with severe head injury. *Heart Lung.* 1989;18:411–414.

10. Boortz-Marx R. Factors affecting intracranial pressure: a descriptive study. *J Neurosurg Nurs.* 1985;17:89–94.

11. Snyder M. Relation of nursing activities to increases in intracranial pressure. *J Adv Nurs.* 1983;8:273–279.

12. Mitchell PH. Intracranial hypertension: influence of nursing care activities. *Nurs Clin North Am.* 1986;21:563–576.

13. Lipe HP, Mitchell PH. Positioning the patient with intracranial hypertension: how turning and head rotation affect the internal jugular vein. *Heart Lung.* 1980;9:1031–1037.

14. Sherman DW. Managing acute head injury. *Nursing.* 1990;20:46–51.

15. Palter MD, Dobkin E, Morgan AS, Previost S. Intensive care management of severe head injury. *J Head Trauma Rehabil.* 1994;9:20–31.

16. Feldman Z, Reichenthal E. Intracranial pressure monitoring. *J Neurosurg.* 1994;81:329–330. Letter to the editor.

17. Hagen C, Malkmus D, Burditt C. Intervention strategies for language disorders secondary to head trauma. Presented at American Speech-Language-Hearing Association Convention Short Course, November 1979; Atlanta, Ga.

18. Warren M. A hierarchical model for evaluation and treatment of visual perceptual dysfunction in adult acquired brain injury, part 1. *Am J Occup Ther.* 1993;47:42–54.

19. Karesh J, Keyes BJ. Ocular injuries. In: Cardona VD, Hurn PD, Mason PJ, Scanlon A, et al, eds. *Trauma Nursing from Resuscitation through Rehabilitation.* 2nd ed. Philadelphia, Pa: WB Saunders Co; 1994:616–638.

20. Leitman MW. *Manuel for Eye Examination and Diagnosis.* 3rd ed. Oradell, NJ: Medical Economics Books; 1988.

21. Warren M. A hierarchical model for evaluation and treatment of visual perceptual dysfunction in adult acquired brain injury, Part 2. *Am J Occup Ther.* 1993;47:55–66.

22. Dow PW. Traumatic brain injuries. In: Trombly CA, ed. *Occupational Therapy for Physical Dysfunction.* 3rd ed. Baltimore, Md: Williams & Wilkins; 1989:484–509.

23. Bobath B. *Adult Hemiplegia: Evaluation and Treatment.* 2nd ed. London, England: William Heinemann Medical Books Ltd; 1981.

24. Manzi DB, Weaver PA. *Head Injury: The Acute Phase.* Thorofare, NJ: Charles B Slack Inc; 1987.

25. Bobath B. *Abnormal Postural Reflex Activity Caused by Brain Lesions.* 2nd ed. London, England: William Heinemann Medical Books Ltd; 1974.

26. Palmer M, Wyness MA. Positioning and handling: important considerations in the care of the severely head-injured patient. *J Neurosci Nurs.* 1988;20:42–49.

27. Kalisky Z, Morrison DP, Meyers CA, Von Laufen A. Medical problems encountered during rehabilitation of patients with head injury. *Arch Phys Med Rehabil.* 1985;66:25–29.

28. Garland DE, Blum CE, Waters RL. Periarticular heterotopic ossification in head-injured adults: incidence and location *J Bone Joint Surg Am.* 1980;62:1143–1146.

29. Lehmkuhl LD, Thoi LL, Baize C, Kelley CJ, et al. Multimodality treatment of joint contractures in patients with severe brain injury: cost, effectiveness, and integration of therapies in the application of serial/inhibitive casts. *J Head Trauma Rehabil.* 1990;5:23–42.

30. Rogers RC. Heterotopic calcification in severe head injury: a preventive programme. *Brain Inj.* 1988;2:169–173.

31. Cherry DB. Review of physical therapy alternatives for reducing muscle contracture. *Phys Ther.* 1980;60:877–881.

32. Powell JN, Chapman P. The impact of early orthopedic management on patients with traumatic brain injury. *J Head Trauma Rehabil.* 1994;9:57–66.

33. Citta-Pietolungo, TJ, Alexander MA, Steg NL. Early detection of heterotopic ossification in young patients with traumatic brain injury. *Arch Phys Med Rehabil.* 1992;73:258–262.

34. Jennett B, Teasdale G. *Management of Head Injuries.* Philadelphia, PA: FA Davis Co; 1982.

35. Trombly CA. Motor control therapy. In: Trombly CA, ed. *Occupational Therapy for Physical Dysfunction.* 3rd ed. Baltimore, Md: Williams & Wilkins; 1989:72–95.

36. Hus AJ. Sensorimotor and neurodevelopmental frames of reference. In: Hopkins HL, Smith HD, eds. *Willard and Spackman's Occupational Therapy.* 7th ed. Philadelphia, Pa: JB Lippincott Co; 1988:114–127.

37. Silberzahn M. Integration in sensorimotor therapy. In: Hopkins HL, Smith HD, eds. *Willard and Spackman's Occupational Therapy.* 7th ed. Philadelphia, Pa: JB Lippincott Co; 1988:127–142.

38. American Occupational Therapy Association, Inc, Practice Division. *AOTA Head Injury Information Packet.* 1985:73–75.

CHAPTER 9

Respiratory Management of the Brain-Injured Patient

PULMONARY FUNCTION AND RESPIRATORY SUPPORT

Assessment of pulmonary status of the patient with brain injury must begin from the first response on scene and continue throughout the treatment and recovery process in the intensive care unit (ICU). Adequate ventilation, oxygenation, and circulation are fundamental to the process of gas exchange and are essential to resuscitation. Abnormalities in other bodily systems will also be reflected in ventilatory dysfunction and acid-base imbalance. Life-threatening abnormalities are usually apparent on gross physical examination and can be dealt with immediately. Beyond the initial injuries, respiratory management of initial and subsequent complications is one of the primary determining factors of outcome for the injured patient. This is particularly true with brain injury.

The respiratory system provides gas exchange in order to regulate and maintain the respiratory component of acid-base homeostasis. Respiration is a rapid buffering mechanism that achieves this delicate balance. The coordinated functions of the neuromuscular, cardiovascular, and respiratory systems create pressure gradients within the thorax, drawing air into and out of the lungs. This process allows for the movement of oxygen into and the removal of carbon dioxide from the blood in order to maintain the narrow range of pH in the blood needed to maintain homeostasis. The renal system, which provides the metabolic component to acid-base balance, removes the fixed acid that was not converted to carbon dioxide by the bicarbonate buffering system. This process is much slower than the respiratory process.

Normal Respiratory Control and Mechanics of Breathing

The integration of respiratory control and respiratory mechanics is achieved through the action of six functional divisions within the respiratory system:

(1) central nervous system, (2) peripheral nervous system, (3) chest wall, (4) muscles, (5) upper airway, and (6) lung. Many of the components of respiration are complicated and not completely understood. Both afferent and efferent signals are sent through the central nervous system in response to chemical, reflex, or mechanical stimuli. The medulla is responsible for the rhythmic cycle of inspiration and expiration. Dorsal neurons appear to be the source of inspiratory effort, probably through efferent stimulation of the phrenic nerve and afferent stimulation of the vagal and glossopharyngeal nerves. A ventral group of neurons receives no afferent signals but sends efferent stimuli that result in active exhalation.[1-3] The pons can influence the medullary function of respiration by stimulating or inhibiting inspiration through the pneumotaxic and apneustic centers. The cerebral cortex can consciously control breathing pattern in a limited fashion but generally cannot override the medullary centers of control.[1-3] Central chemoreceptors located in the medulla will respond to arterial Pco_2 and the cerebrospinal fluid pH.

Peripheral chemoreceptors located in the carotid bodies respond to decreases in Pao_2 and pH and to increases in Pco_2 and are the sole response to arterial hypoxemia.[1-3] Proprioceptors respond to reflex stimuli. The gamma-efferent feedback system controls the timing and coordination of contractions of the muscles of respiration. The integration of the autonomic and somatic controls occurs in the motor neurons of the spinal cord

The purpose of the chest wall is to protect the internal vital organs. The chest wall expands as the muscles used for respiration contract, creating the pressure differences necessary to allow gas to flow into and out of the lung. Muscular contractions will vary the amount of volume stimulated in response to respiratory control innervation. The diaphragm and the intercostal muscles are the primary muscles of respiration. Accessory muscles are used when an increased ventilatory demand is present.

The upper airway functions to warm, filter, and humidify the inspired gas. The lower airways act as the conducting tubes for the gas to enter and exit the lungs. The lungs provide the surface area for gas exchange to occur and have a dual circulatory system that maintains them and provides the capillary network for gas exchange. The lungs also act as the blood reservoir for the left ventricle of the heart. The pleurae act as the link between the chest wall and the lung. The process of ventilation occurs because of the pressure gradients that are created to overcome the elastic (compliance) and frictional (resistance) forces opposing lung and thoracic expansion.

Hemoglobin and cardiac output provide the supply and transport of oxygen to the cells for internal respiration and the transport of carbon dioxide to the lungs for external respiration. Normally, this process functions very efficiently and effectively. Efficient ventilation is achieved with minimal work of breathing, requiring little oxygen and producing the minimum amount of carbon dioxide. Effective ventilation occurs when this process meets the body's needs for oxygen uptake and carbon dioxide removal. Efficiency is determined or measured by tidal volume (V_T), the amount of gas inspired or expired with each breath; respiratory rate, the number of breaths taken in a minute; and the product of these two factors, *minute ventilation* ($\dot{V}_e$). Effectiveness can be determined only by blood gas analysis. Any alteration in either efficiency or effectiveness will cause respiratory compromise.

In normal rhythmic breathing, in which breaths are usually almost equal in depth and duration, the tidal volume is approximately 5 to 7 mL/kg of body weight (approximately 500 mL), the frequency is about 12 to 20 breaths per minute, and minute ventilation is 5 to 10 L/min. Alveolar ventilation ($\dot{V}_A$), the amount of gas that reaches the alveoli in the lungs and experiences gas exchange, is approximately 4.2 L.

Dead space ventilation ($\dot{V}_{DS}$) is unused gas that either remains in the airways or goes to nonperfused areas of the lungs (approximately 1.8 L). The dead space–to–tidal volume ratio, normally 2% to 4%, is used to indicate the efficiency of ventilation. Shunting is the portion of cardiac output that does not exchange with alveolar air. Shunting and dead space are the factors that create ventilation-perfusion ($\dot{V}/\dot{Q}$) mismatching. The functional residual capacity is the content of gas remaining in the lungs at the end of normal exhalation, approximately 2.4 L of the 6-L total lung capacity. Oxygenation is very dependent upon functional residual capacity. The balance of alveolar ventilation and carbon dioxide production is seen in the P_{CO_2} in the arterial blood gas analysis and reflects the effectiveness of ventilation relating to gas exchange. Gas exchange occurs through diffusion due to the pressure gradients present at the alveolar-capillary membrane. The lung has regional differences that allow different areas to be preferentially ventilated (upper) and perfused (lower). Anatomic shunts exist in the pulmonary circulation that never come into contact with gas exchange areas. Normally, these variations balance out, but pathologic factors will detrimentally affect these variations.

Blood Gas Physiology

Blood gas analysis is used to determine acid-base status and the influence of ventilation, oxygenation, dead space, shunting, and metabolism upon that status. Ventilation must occur to achieve oxygenation. Oxygenation is accomplished by having adequate $\dot{V}/\dot{Q}$ matching in the lung, diffusion across the alveolar-capillary membrane, and transfer of oxygen from the capillaries to the tissues. The transfer requires adequate hemoglobin and cardiac output to circulate oxygen to the body for aerobic cellular use in metabolism.

A normal ambient-air arterial blood gas would be as follows:

- hydrogen ion concentration (pH): 7.35 to 7.45, indicative of acid-base status
- partial pressure of arterial carbon dioxide ($Paco_2$): 35 to 45 mm Hg, indicative of effective ventilation
- partial pressure of arterial oxygen (Pao_2): 80 to 100 mm Hg, indicative of blood oxygen level
- bicarbonate (HCO_3^-): 22 to 26 mEq/L, indicative of metabolic buffering
- base excess or deficits: ± 2 mEq/L, indicative of the magnitude of metabolic contribution to acid-base status
- oxygen saturation: 95% to 100%, indicative of oxygen in the hemoglobin and the relationship of Pao_2 and oxygen content

A decrease or increase in pH is indicative of an acidotic or alkalotic state, the cause of which can be respiratory or metabolic. Acidemia tends to decrease oxygen content and decrease the oxygen affinity of the hemoglobin, allowing for transfer to the tissues. Although this allows for better oxygen uptake at the tissues, the lower oxygen content results in hypoxemia. Alkalosis tends to increase oxygen content and increase the oxygen affinity, being less effective in transferring the oxygen to the tissues. The oxyhemoglobin dissociation curve (Figure 9–1) demonstrates what happens with oxygen transport when a shift to the right or left occurs.

Assessment of Respiratory Insufficiency

Injury can cause abnormalities or dysfunction of any or all of the integrated systems that provide for adequate oxygenation and ventilation. Pulmonary dysfunction, which can present at various times and in a variety of forms from mild to life threatening, is a common complication of brain injury. The primary injury to the brain may cause abnormal autoregulation. A secondary injury may result in hypotension, hypoxia, or intracranial hypertension. Initial resuscitation and prevention and management of secondary injury are paramount. The initial evaluation of patients with suspected brain injury is essential in determining the extent of damage to the brain and other vital organs. The assessment will also dictate the method of treatment and provide input regarding prognosis.[4] Evaluation must concurrently focus on obtaining vital signs, protecting the airway, observing the pattern of ventilation, controlling any hemorrhage, and determining the level of consciousness. These initial findings categorize the severity of brain injury and direct treatment response; they also serve as a reference of comparison for future evaluations. Following brain injury, many cells are left dysfunctional but not permanently disrupted, so the course of treatment is to provide the best possible environment for recovery.

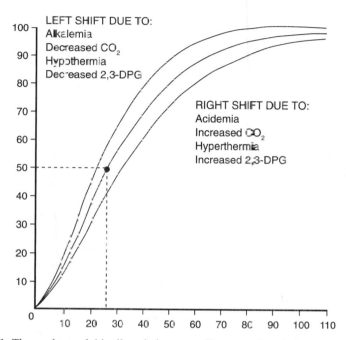

Figure 9–1 The oxyhemoglobin dissociation curve illustrates the relationship of the percent saturation (% SAT) of the hemoglobin to the amount of oxygen (Po$_2$) dissolved in plasma. The P50 is the level of oxygen (Po$_2$) at 50% oxygen saturation. A shift to right raises the P50 and lowers the hemoglobin affinity for oxygen. A shift to the left lowers the P50 and raises the affinity for oxygen.

Abnormal breathing patterns are frequently seen immediately following brain injury or may develop later.[5] Plum and Posner[6] have described six respiratory patterns resulting from lesions in the central nervous system: eupneic or normal respiration, Cheyne-Stokes respiration, central neurogenic hyperventilation, apneustic respiration, ataxic respiration, and apnea. Eupneic or normal respiration may be seen even in the presence of small lesions. Cheyne-Stokes respiration is characterized by waxing and waning tidal volume with a period of apnea prior to the next cyclic start in a rhythmic pattern and is associated with bilateral hemispheric disease. Central neurogenic hyperventilation is characterized by a consistent increase in rate and depth of breathing that may be indicative of injury at the pontine level. Apneustic respiration involves a long gasping inspiration with insufficient expiration, also reflecting damage to the pons. Ataxic respiration occurs when both rhythm and rate are irregular. An apneic period may exist as well.

Biot's pattern, a form of ataxic respiration caused by medullary dysfunction, is characterized by deep breaths with apneic periods in no rhythmic consistency. Apnea is the complete absence of breathing, caused by overwhelming damage to the medulla.

In mild or moderate brain injury (ie, Glasgow Coma Scale[7] [GCS] score between 9 and 15), normal breathing patterns or hyperventilation can occur, with hypoxemia potentially evident on blood gas analysis.[5,8] The intracranial pressure and ventilatory response mechanisms will remain intact and reactive if the initial injury has caused minimal disruption to the autoregulation controls of breathing in the brain. In this scenario, only oxygenation support may be necessary for hypoxia. In the presence of severe brain injury (GCS $\leq$8), hypoventilation or apnea can be present, reflected in the increased $Paco_2$ and severe hypoxemia of respiratory failure. This situation requires immediate intubation, oxygenation, and ventilatory support. Initial hypoxemia appears to correspond to the location and magnitude of the brain injury[5] and can be caused by neurologically induced increases in $\dot{V}/\dot{Q}$ mismatching that accompany the varying durations of loss of consciousness, associated apnea, aspiration, and decreased diffusion from pulmonary edema.[9] Most severe brain injuries are the result of acceleration or deceleration of the head, resulting in shearing injuries that can result in loss of consciousness and apnea. The greater the movement, the longer the apneic period that is responsible for the hypoxemia. Frost et al[10] have shown that early $\dot{V}/\dot{Q}$ mismatch correlates with the GCS and can be used as a prognostic indicator in brain injury. A hypermetabolic state that increases oxygen consumption or direct lung injury can also produce significant hypoxemia in the presence of $\dot{V}/\dot{Q}$ mismatch.[8,11] The venous blood mixing with the arterial blood is more desaturated. Supplemental oxygen, aggressive respiratory therapy, and ventilatory support, if necessary, should be initiated in an attempt to prevent secondary complications (ie, intracranial hypertension, pneumonia, impending respiratory failure, and acute respiratory distress syndrome).

Preferred Method of Airway Management

Management of the upper airway is a crucial part of therapy in persons with severe brain injury. Most patients arrive in the ICU with an endotracheal tube inserted. Intubation is performed at the scene of the injury, in the trauma bay, in the operating room, or in the ICU. Often this procedure is performed emergently. Occasionally, patients may require a cricothyroidotomy. A cricothryoidotomy is used when an obstructed airway or severe maxillofacial trauma is present or when there is difficulty establishing a conventional airway via endotracheal intubation.

As a rule, oral endotracheal intubation is the technique of choice when immediate control of the airway is required. Laryngoscopy, followed by oral intubation, is usually faster than the nasal technique or even cricothyroidotomy and requires the least disruption of resuscitative efforts. However, the patient with an associated cervical spine injury should be approached cautiously when the oral route is used. A two-person technique is required, with one person stabilizing neck position and the other inserting the oral tube.

In an adult comatose patient, the oral route is ideal. An 8-mm tube in the adult is the preferred size (Figure 9–2), particularly when fiber-optic bronchoscopy is used. Because the oral tube in inserted under direct vision, it can be inserted fairly precisely below the vocal cords about 2 cm above the carina, ensuring adequate ventilation of both lungs. However, if the oral tube is inadvertently advanced beyond the carina, it will usually lodge in the right mainstem bronchus, resulting in an atelectatic left lung. A substantial shunt is produced as perfusion to the affected lung persists, while gas exchange is severely impaired. In an awakening patient, the oral route can precipitate problems of stress, leading to agitation. Agitation can cause an elevation of mean arterial pressure, an increase in heart rate, and a potential increase in intracranial pressure (ICP). The agitated person with brain injury invariably requires sedation, which effects a blunting of mentation. At times, paralysis is required, which compromises the assessment of neurologic status. Addi-

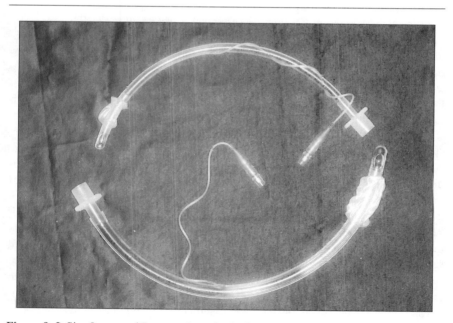

Figure 9–2 Size 8-mm and 7-mm endotracheal tubes. Size 8 is for oral intubation, and size 7 is for nasotracheal intubation.

tional problems with the oral route are gagging and the inability to implement adequate mouth care. In the less sedated or seizing patient, the oral route can be obstructed by the patient's biting down on the tube. Insertion of a bite block will prevent the patient from biting down.

Nasotracheal intubation is not the technique of choice in the comatose patient. The technique can be time consuming, and the potential hypoventilation is not well tolerated by patients with severe brain injury, who are extremely sensitive to hypoxia. Nasotracheal intubation is an adequate safe technique for the patient who does not require brief periods of anesthesia or muscle relaxation. In an awake patient with cervical spine injury, the nasal route does not require manipulation of the head and neck and is thus a safer technique. The patient who is a candidate for the nasal route is usually awake, and the surrounding clinical situation is relatively stable. The nasal route can be performed blindly and is more secure than the oral route. The oral route does not have the advantage of bony structure of the nasal passageways, which stabilize the position of the tube.

The nasal route is, however, limited by size. A tube less than 8 mm in diameter is generally required (Figure 9–2). Nasal intubation is not performed under direct vision and is dependent on the clinical situation. This procedure is not recommended for patients with severe maxillofacial trauma or basilar skull fractures. There is risk of tissue necrosis and epistaxis.

Both techniques present a number of common problems in the ICU. Obstruction caused by mucous plug or blood clots is a major complication of endotracheal tubes. A cuff leak is also a common problem. Often the cause of the leak is migration of the endotracheal tube superiorly, elevating the cuff into the glottis, where it is difficult to achieve a seal. The tube may malfunction to account for the leak. If the cuff is compromised, lung volume cannot be maintained and positive end-expiratory pressure (PEEP) may be lacking.[12]

Early problems with endotracheal intubation include self-extubation, difficulty suctioning, aspiration, malpositioning of the tube, pain, laryngospasm, sinusitis, supraglottic/glottic edema, vocal cord paresis, tracheal stenosis, serous otitis media, and reports of pneumothorax.[14,15] Complications seen with prolonged use of endotracheal intubation include many of the above, and may lead to vocal cord granulation, vocal cord paralysis (usually unilateral), dysphonia, and dysphagia.[16] The person with brain injury who is subjected to prolonged endotracheal intubation is at increased risk of incurring an airway complication. The risk is increased when the patient is subjected to tracheostomy. Chronic laryngeal and tracheal stenosis are common in patients undergoing tracheostomy following prolonged endotracheal intubation.[15] Laryngotracheal stenosis can be seen as early as four days in the endotracheal intubated patient and is more commonly seen after periods of intubation in excess of seven days.[17] These airway injuries are prevalent in those patients who have significant degrees of gross motor movement and suffer restlessness while intubated. The incidence of major laryngopathology is not uncommon in the person with brain injury who has rigid posturing, coughing, and head movement.[18]

Tracheostomy

Timing of Tracheostomy

The patient with a brain injury who is posturing is at the greatest risk of airway complication with an endotracheal tube. Statistically, persons with severe brain injury (ie, GCS ≤8) are highly likely to require a tracheostomy.[19] Early tracheostomy is prudent for patients requiring greater than three to five days of ventilatory support.[20] A 5% complication rate exists with tracheostomy.[20] The complication rate is less with early tracheostomy than with tracheostomy at greater than five to seven days post injury.[17] Additional advantages include (1) early weaning from the ventilator, (2) reduced incidence of nosocomial pneumonia, (3) decreased length of stay in the ICU, (4) decreased overall hospital days, and (5) no mortality associated with early tracheostomy. Early tracheostomy benefits the patient with severe brain injury, providing a safe technique with low morbidity and no significant mortality.[20-23]

Percutaneous Dilational Tracheostomy

Percutaneous dilational tracheostomy (PDT), performed at the bedside of a critically ill or injured patient, is a relatively new technique of tracheal cannulation. PDT is derived from the classical method of open tracheostomy, described in 1909 by Chevalier Jackson.[24] However, tracheostomy as a procedure reportedly dates back to Egyptian times, approximately 3,500 years ago, and was described in the *Rig Veda,* a book of the Hindu scriptures, some 1,000 years or more BC. Percutaneous tracheostomy itself was described in 1955,[25] and alternative techniques were studied in 1969.[26] These early techniques were not at all accepted by the surgical community. Since 1985, PDT, as described by Ciaglia et al, has become increasingly popular in the surgical/critical care community.[27] The current highly popular technique combines PDT with the use of bronchoscopic guidance.[28-29]

With PDT, the patient's positioning is similar to that for conventional tracheostomy, with the neck in neutral position with slight extension. Under direct bronchoscopic guidance, the endotracheal tube is partially withdrawn at the level of the larynx. The endotracheal tube should not impede the use of the needle, guidewire, dilators, or eventual tracheostomy tube. The cricoid is identified after the skin is cleansed and anesthetized, and a 2-cm midline incision is made 2 cm below the cricoid. By use of blunt dissection, the pretracheal tissue is identified. A prefilled 16-gauge saline cannulated syringe is inserted into the trachea posteriorly and caudally (Figure 9–3).

The needle and syringe are removed once there is assurance that the trachea has been safely entered, again under direct vision of the bronchoscope. With the cannula in place, a guidewire is inserted, followed by a Teflon guiding catheter. There are two markings on the Teflon catheter at the insertion level to protect the posterior trachea from injury (Figure 9–4). Sequential dilators, from no. 12 to no. 36 French dilators, are passed into the guidewire, guiding catheter assembly until the tip reaches the double-line mark (Figure 9–5). The entire assembly is then advanced into the trachea two to three times until the black mark and the tapered dilator reach the skin level. At the completion of the dilation, a size 8-mm tracheostomy tube is loaded over a no. 24 French dilator and advanced into the trachea, under the direct vision via the bronchoscope (Figure 9–6). Following insertion of the tracheostomy tube, the dilator, guidewire, and guiding catheter are all removed, followed by the endotracheal tube and bronchoscope. The trachea is aspirated, the cuff inflated, and the tracheostomy tube attached to the ventilator. At completion of the procedure, the stoma should be dressed and a chest X-ray completed.

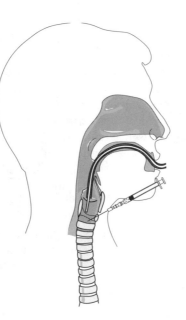

Figure 9–3 A saline cannulation syringe is inserted caudally and posteriorly.

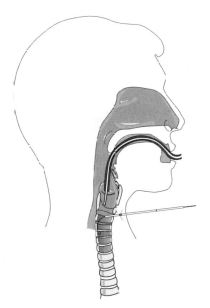

Figure 9–4 Via a guidewire, a Teflon guiding catheter is passed.

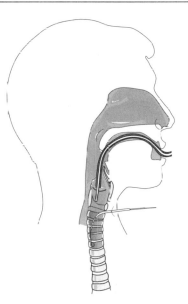

Figure 9–5 With nos. 12 to 16 French graduated dilators, the guidewire, guiding catheter assembly, is inserted.

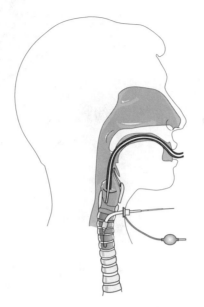

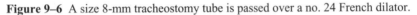

Figure 9–6 A size 8-mm tracheostomy tube is passed over a no. 24 French dilator.

The primary advantage of PDT is the avoidance of transporting the patient, who may or may not have associated complicating injuries, to the operating suite. PDT completed at the bedside is a fast procedure, requiring fewer staff.[27,28] The complication rate for PDT varies from 15% to 1%, comparing favorably with open tracheostomy.[30–37] Insignificant complications have been found, and the cosmetic result with PDT is far superior to that of the open tracheostomy.[34] Additionally, the overall cost of PDT is significantly less than that of open tracheostomy due to the avoidance of the operating suite, the lower need for personnel and equipment, and the lower morbidity associated with the procedure.

The only disadvantage of PDT is that long-term complications, if they exist, have yet to be adequately identified and quantified. Concerns about tracheal stenosis have been reported,[38] but in some studies this was not identified.[35]

Ventilatory Support

Artificial ventilation is initiated to support the patient until the underlying problem is resolved and the patient can independently maintain adequate ventilation. The goals of artificial ventilatory support are (1) to support or manipulate gas exchange by improving alveolar ventilation and arterial oxygenation, (2) to increase lung volume by increasing end inspiratory lung inflation and functional residual volume, and (3) to reduce or manipulate the work of breathing.[39]

Complications of mechanical ventilation include (1) adverse physiologic effects, such as decreased cardiac output, increased intracranial pressure, gastric distension and stress ulcers, and impaired renal function; (2) ventilator malfunction; (3) pneumothorax or bronchopleural fistula; and (4) nosocomial pneumonia.[40]

All modes of ventilatory support inflate the lung by increasing the transpulmonary pressure gradient. Positive-pressure ventilation (PPV) reverses the pressure gradients seen in spontaneous breathing. PPV increases the transpulmonary pressure, which in turn causes decreased cardiac output, especially with the use of PEEP.[41] In the presence of brain injury, PPV may impair cerebral blood flow and pose a potential threat to secondary injury.[42] A balancing act exists between the need for ventilatory support and risks involved in providing it.

The extent of support, full or partial, should be the first consideration when initiating artificial ventilation. In the case of severe brain injury, respiratory failure and the resulting need for sedation and paralytics to facilitate intubation and control ventilation require full ventilatory support.

There are four possible control or phase variables on a ventilator: volume, pressure, flow, and time. Inspiration is triggered, limited, or cycled by one or a combination of these factors. There are two possible breath types: *mandatory*, which can be either machine or patient triggered, and *spontaneous*, which is patient triggered. An understanding of these concepts is necessary to determine ventilatory mode settings and any subsequent changes necessary to adjust oxygenation and ventilation support.[41]

The primary conventional ventilatory controls of oxygenation are fractional inspired oxygen (FIO_2) and PEEP. PEEP is used to increase FRC, thereby improving oxygenation. The primary controls of ventilation are tidal volume and rate, or minute ventilation. Continuous mandatory ventilation (CMV) or assist/control (A/C) and normal-rate synchronized intermittent mandatory ventilation (SIMV) provide full support and a guaranteed $\dot{V}e$. FIO_2 and PEEP are set at levels to maintain an oxygen saturation of at least 90%. In the presence of probable brain injury, a normal tide volume (7–15 mL/kg) and a higher-than-normal (>8–12 beats per minute) rate are instituted to achieve a Pco_2 at approximately 30 mm Hg. Flow rate (normal, 40–100 L/min) is set to meet patient demand and determines normal inspiratory time. Flow rate and frequency determine inspiratory to expiratory (I/E) ratio (normal, 1:2). Humidification must be provided to help prevent drying of airway secretions, destruction of airway epithelium, and atelectasis. Airway and alveolar pressure, a product of ventilator settings and lung compliance and resistance, must be monitored closely. The American College of Chest Physicians (ACCP) recommends keeping plateau pressures below 35 cm H_2O to avoid ventilator-induced barotrauma.[39]

Variations of these initial settings are based upon the specific pathologic problems that are encountered. Blood gas analysis is absolutely essential for making the proper adjustments.

FIO_2 should be lowered gradually, always with an attempt to maintain a saturation greater than 90% in order to maintain adequate ventilation and oxygenation. Optimal PEEP levels are achieved by monitoring cardiovascular function, barotrauma, and lung compliance. A PEEP level of 10 cm H_2O is considered a safe level for patients with brain injury because of the potential impairment to cerebral blood flow.[42] Airway pressures must be monitored, since they may indicate alterations of patient status. Increases in pressure may indicate a reduction of lung compliance or an increase in resistance due to the need for suctioning or the patient's biting down on the tube. Decreases may indicate an improvement in the patient's condition or possibly a leak.

Agitated patients may exhibit asynchrony with the ventilator and therefore require more sedation. Agitation may be indicative of an emergency situation, such as pneumothorax or pulmonary emboli. Both the patient and the ventilator must be monitored to track gradual or sudden changes in order to make necessary adjustments. At times, conventional volume ventilation and the adjustments of its parameters cannot maintain adequate ventilation and oxygenation. When the patient requires high FIO_2 and PEEP levels, exhibits high airway pressures, and is still unable to maintain adequate gas exchange, pressure control ventilation (PCV) is an alternative.[41] With PCV, the controls of ventilation become pressure and time, and tidal volume is variable. PCV can be accomplished with normal I/E ratios or when inspiratory time is increased to create an inverse I/E ratio, creating some auto-PEEP in the hopes of improving gas exchange. PCV is frequently used in the presence of acute respiratory distress syndrome (ARDS). Later in this chapter, ARDS will be discussed at length as a pulmonary complication.

High-frequency jet ventilation (HFJV) is also used for patients in ARDS or those who fail conventional ventilation.[41] The pressure gradients created with standard ventilation may perpetuate $\dot{V}/\dot{Q}$ mismatching. Jet ventilation delivers a rapid succession of pulses of small quantities of gas that create a constant intraalveolar pressure and enhance gas exchange by maintaining stability of the alveolar membrane. Jet ventilation also uses pressure and time for ventilation. Increasing I/E ratio and drive pressure increases the FRC and V_T. Increasing frequency decreases V_T and increases $Paco_2$ in stiff lungs. Patients with significant brain injury are usually unstable from a respiratory standpoint and frequently require these alternative means of ventilation.

Independent lung ventilation is another alternative to standard ventilation and may be indicated for use in the presence of unilateral lung injury or bronchopleural fistula, seen in multiple trauma. Each lung is ventilated separately and differentially through a double-lumen tube, using two ventilators.[43] The noncompliant lung will be ventilated less than the more normal, compliant lung in the hopes of allowing healing and closure. Jet ventilation is often initiated under the same circumstances but does not require two ventilators. With these complications, no one alternative mode of ventilation improves a patient's condition more than another, and morbidity and mortality do not appear to be affected.[43]

Monitoring is the key to successful patient management in the acute setting. Monitoring helps detect a catastrophic event before the clinical signs present and potentially before the event can alter the patient's outcome. The accuracy of monitoring devices has been studied and has proven reliable. The challenge becomes the interpretation and clinical decision making based upon clinical observation and the information that monitoring provides. Responses to manipulation of physiologic variables can be predicted, but the amount of response is variable and patient specific. A variety of invasive and noninvasive interfaces are used. Hemodynamic monitoring is achieved by means of a pulmonary artery or Swan-Ganz catheter. This monitoring helps to distinguish problems in fluid volume, right and left heart function, and pulmonary function. Differential problem solving is facilitated when hemodynamic monitoring is combined with monitoring for arterial blood gases (ABG) via arterial line, cardiac output (CO), pulmonary artery pressure (PAP), and pulmonary capillary wedge pressure (PCWP). The effects of mechanical ventilation on these variables must also be taken into account. Wedge pressure will help distinguish between cardiogenic shock and neurogenic pulmonary edema and can determine the effects of PEEP. Mixed venous blood sampling provides information on lung function and oxygen consumption. Cardiac output, hemoglobin values, and blood gas sampling results allow for calculation and evaluation of oxygenation. The ventilator and ABG provide the data for assessing ventilatory function. Many ventilators have the ability to display pressure, volume, and time waveforms, which provide data concerning lung mechanics, the presence of auto-PEEP, and work of breathing. The Bicore CP-100 Pulmonary Monitor is used to assess the patient's respiratory condition and allows for intervention before the onset of fatigue or failure. It directly measures airway pressure, esophageal pressure, tidal volume, and flow through two transducers. It provides information on the patient's work of breathing, as well as strength and endurance. ICP monitoring and its benefits have already been discussed. Pulse oximetry uses light transmission and reception, through a noninvasive finger or ear probe, to measure arterial oxygen saturation, providing real-time oxygenation response. End-tidal carbon dioxide monitoring provides information on the relationship between ventilation and ICP. The Hewlett Packard Component Monitor[44] has the capacity to formulate, with inputs, all of this information. The management team can also manually calculate it (Table 9–1). Rapid determination and response to various data are important. Metabolic monitoring, though somewhat limited in the ventilated patient, can provide valuable data concerning oxygen consumption,

Table 9–1 Manual Calculations for Physiologic Variables

Physiologic Variables	Calculation Method	Normal Ranges
Arterial oxygen content (Cao_2)	$(1.34 \times \text{hemoglobin} \times Sao_2/100) + (.0031 \times Pao_2)$	17–20 mL/dL
Venous oxygen content (Cvo_2)	$(1.34 \times \text{hemoglobin} \times Svo_2/100) + (.0031 \times Pvo_2)$	12–15 mL/dL
Arteriovenous oxygen difference ($avDo_2$)	$Cao_2 - Cvo_2$	4.2–5.0 mL/dL
Oxygen availability (O_2AV)	$Cao_2 \times \text{cardiac output (CO)} \times 10$	950–1,150 mL/min
Oxygen consumption ($\dot{V}o_2$)	$avDo_2 \times \text{cardiac output} \times 10$	
Shunt (Qs/Qt)	$100 \times (1.34 \times \text{hemoglobin} + .0031 \times Pao_2 - Cao_2)/(1.34 \times \text{hemoglobin} + .0031 \times Pao_2 - Cvo_2)$	3%–5%
Volume of dead space (Vds)	$(Paco_2 - PEco_2) \times Vt/Paco_2$	145–155 mL
Dead space to tidal volume ratio	Vds/Vt	.25–.40
Alveolar ventilation ($\dot{V}a$)	$(\dot{V}t\dot{V}ds) \times \text{respirations}$	

carbon dioxide production, energy expenditure, and nutritional support needs. Vital signs, electrocardiogram (ECG) monitoring, daily chest X-ray, and daily patient weight are essential standards of monitoring. Information from any of these monitoring methods will identify trends of deterioration or improvement long before the patient may exhibit clinical symptoms and are useful tools for identifying problems and determining corrective treatment, particularly in the patient with brain injury.

Providing aggressive respiratory care to improve lung function is essential in the ventilated patient with severe brain injury. These compromised patients are at high risk for aspiration, infection, and pneumonia. Pulmonary infection is the most common serious form of infection seen in these patients. Pneumonia is discussed later in this chapter. The risk of aspiration leading to infection must be kept at a minimum. A flat lying position should be avoided, and gastric decompression should be provided. Proper cuff inflation of the tube, 20 cm H_2O or less, should be monitored to ensure adequate defense of the airway, yet not cause necrosis of the tissue. Suctioning of oral secretions pooled above the cuff should be completed to reduce colonization.

Endotracheal suctioning can be detrimental in that it can cause increased ICP and hypoxemia. However, clearing secretions is a necessary task. Suctioning can transiently stimulate high levels of ICP, and rebounding can be slow. The effects, with some patients, can be cumulative with each pass.[45,46] Recommendations for suctioning a patient with brain injury are as follows:

1. Negative suction pressure should not exceed 120 mm Hg.
2. The suction catheter should not occlude the airway, and a 14F catheter should be adequate.
3. Hyperoxygenation should precede suctioning.
4. Suction duration should not exceed 10 seconds.
5. Catheter insertion should be limited to just below the tube.
6. The number of catheter insertions should not exceed two in any one suction procedure.[26,27]

A closed catheter system eliminates the need to disconnect the patient from the ventilator and the lost effect of PEEP on the FRC but may create enough negative pressure and decrease FRC also.[45] Suctioning is a necessary part of respiratory management for this patient population and can be done in a manner that has a limited negative impact.

Bronchodilator therapy and chest physiotherapy are also used as aids in airway and secretion management. Normal bronchomotor tone is maintained through the equal opposing forces of the sympathetic and parasympathetic systems. In altered respiratory states, the balance of tone is weakened, allowing one system to override the other. Beta-adrenergic and anticholinergic drug intervention attempts to return bronchial tone to balance by stimulating the beta-adrenergic receptors or by inhibiting the cholinergic receptors. Albuterol is the most widely used beta-2 adrenergic bronchodilator, with quick onset and a duration of up to six hours. Atrovent is a commonly used anticholinergic bronchodilator. Occasionally, anti-inflammatory glucocorticosteroid in the aerosolized form is needed for clinical situations, such as aspiration pneumonitis. This medication inhibits the formation and release of inflammatory mediators. All of these medications are administered to optimize mucociliary clearance. Chest physiotherapy uses some combination of postural drainage, chest wall percussion and vibration, coughing or suctioning, and breathing exercises in an attempt to facilitate clearance of secretions. Suctioning is completed by either respiratory therapists or physical therapists. Postural drainage, the use of body position and gravity to improve secretion removal, can be difficult, at best, in a ventilated patient. In the person with severe brain injury, performing postural drainage may be hazardous if ICP becomes elevated and systemic blood pressure increases. Benefit versus risk must be weighed carefully. Percussion is the rhythmic striking of the chest wall with the hands in a cupped position to mechanically jar and dislodge retained secretions. Waves of mechanical energy are transmitted to the lung from the chest wall. Vibration with chest compression, done on exhalation, moves the mucus toward a larger airway for clearance. A modification to flat or semi-Fowler position can be used in combination with percussion and vibration, and appropriate sedation, to improve the clearance of secretions. These techniques can be beneficial for patients with brain injury because they are at risk for aspiration, which leads to pneumonia even in later stages of recovery.

Weaning from the Ventilator

Once the patient exhibits consistent signs of improvement for a period of several days, such as stable hemodynamics, improved lung function, and neurologic stability, the process of weaning from the ventilator can begin. Patients with brain injury are some of the most complex patients to wean. The amount of intact neurologic function and the need for sedation determine success. Sedation should be discontinued or kept at a minimum as the patient's neurologic function improves.

The ventilator, now supplying only partial support, should be set in the SIMV mode at a normal rate. A gradual reduction of machine breaths will allow patients to increase their own spontaneous breathing. Pressure support ventilation (PSV) is used in weaning to decrease the work of spontaneous breathing. The ventilator assists the spontaneous inspiratory effort of the patient to a preset level of inspiratory pressure. Inspiration is terminated when peak inspiratory flow rate reaches a minimum level or percentage of initial inspiratory flow.[39] Tidal volume is supplemented to help maintain adequate minute ventilation and still use and strengthen the muscles of respiration. With gradual reduction of rate, the PSV will allow for exercise and improvement in the mechanics of breathing. FIO_2 should be at or less than 50%, and PEEP should be no more than 5, while maintaining at least 90% saturation. This process can be protracted for the patient with brain injury, particularly when agitation is present and when spontaneous hyperventilation necessitates sedation, making weaning difficult.

Clinical signs of diaphoresis and hyperventilation are not always related to muscle fatigue but can be indicative of continued neurologic dysfunction. Weaning, at that time, should be discontinued. Eventually, a continuous positive airway pressure (CPAP) trial of all spontaneous breathing is attempted. At a constant level of positive pressure, the patient does all spontaneous breathing, and respiratory mechanics and gas exchange are assessed. The respiratory rate should be 30 or less. Tidal volume should be at least 5 mL/kg or 350 mL. The minute ventilation should be less than 10 L. A negative inspiratory force (NIF), the pressure created with inspiration, should be at least 20 cm H_2O within 20 seconds. A static compliance, the change in volume over the change in pressure at a point of no air movement in the lung, should be 30 to 33 mL/cm H_2O. Meeting these parameters is considered necessary to achieve successful weaning and discontinue artificial ventilation.[43] Trials of continuous flow or blow-by with supplemental oxygen to the endotracheal tube or trach mask allows for spontaneous breathing without positive pressure. This method, alternated with supported ventilation and gradually increasing the time off the ventilator, provides another possible weaning process. The discontinuation of mechanical ventilatory support greatly reduces the risk of secondary pulmonary complications and must be achieved as soon as the patient's condition allows.

PULMONARY COMPLICATIONS

Pneumonia

Following electrolyte imbalance, pneumonia is the second most frequent complication in the person with a brain injury.[11,42] Pneumonia has a significant influence as an extracranial complication in the overall outcome of persons with brain injury.

The mortality figures for mechanically ventilated patients who develop pneumonia range from 30% to 60%.[45–47] In the surgical ICU, there is an 18% incidence of pneumonia in the trauma population. However, in the general surgical, nontrauma population, the incidence of pneumonia is significantly lower, 3%.[48] Within the trauma population, the person with a brain injury is at the greatest risk of developing pneumonia.[47,49–51] The majority of these pneumonias are defined as nosocomial. The nosocomial pneumonias present themselves at 48 hours or more after admission.[52]

Trauma patients in general are at an increased risk for incurring serious infections such as pneumonia. May patients who have sustained major trauma suffer immunologic disturbances. T-cell count suppression, which occurs as early as 24 hours after injury, can last up to 10 days.[53,54] T cells are responsible for cell-mediated interactions between macrophages (monocytes) and B cells. B cells are lymphocytes that are primarily responsible for the production of immunoglobulins or antibodies.[55] Along with T-cell suppression, there can be suppression of lymphocyte function, but few changes have been noted in the function of B cells.

Pulmonary Defense

The lung possesses a complex defense system against infection. The prevention of pneumonia depends on the defense status and the immediate environment of the patient. The nature of the infecting organism also plays a significant part in the development and successful eradication of the offending organism.

The pulmonary defense system begins with the removal of potentially infective debris by nasopharyngeal filtration. The normal host harbors numerous, mainly nonvirulent, bacteria in the oropharynx. These nonvirulent resident flora normally prevent pathogenic organisms from colonizing the area. This preventative function is called *bacterial interference.* Additional upper-airway defenses are mucosal integrity/adherence and saliva. From an immunologic standpoint, immunoglobulin A (IgA) predominates in the upper airway. The secretion of IgA into mucosal surfaces facilitates clearance of invading organisms by mucosal macrophages and neutrophils (white blood cells that protect the body against pyogenic infections). When IgA levels are low, the incidence of secretory infection rises.[56]

The protection of the lower airway begins with a normal cough reflex. In the normal host, the cough reflex is extremely effective in preventing aspiration. The normal lung clears bacteria from the tracheobronchial tree by a highly efficient mucociliary clearance system. Other lower-airway host defenses are humoral (antibodies) and cellular (T cell–dependent) factors. Immunoglobulin G is dominant in the lower respiratory tract. Cellular defenses in the lower respiratory tract include alveolar macrophages, neutrophils, and bronchial-associated lymphoid tissue.

The most common complication of a dysfunctional immune system is infection. Immunoglobulins G, M, and A are most vital to normal opsinization (the process by which bacteria are made more susceptible to ingestion). IgG activates the complement system. Complement activation is accomplished through the classic and alternate pathways. The complement system is capable of producing a broad series of inflammatory actions, including cell lysis, chemotaxis (drawing white cells into an area of bacterial infection), opsinization, anaphylactoid reactions, and anti-inflammatory effects.[57]

Susceptibility

The person with severe brain injury who requires prolonged ventilatory support (>48 hours) lacks the normal response to combat pulmonary infection.. The ability to remove potentially infective material from nasal and nasopharyngeal surfaces can be impaired by nasotracheal intubation, suction catheters, and nasogastric tubes.[58] Lower-airway infections can result from small repetitive aspirations of upper-airway secretions. The upper airway becomes susceptible to colonization (presence and proliferation of organisms on a surface with no tissue invasion and/ or inflammatory response) of bacteria due to microaspiration of oral secretions.[59]

Aspiration pneumonia can result from gastroesophageal reflux associated with the presence of a feeding tube. The feeding tube relaxes the lower esophageal sphincter, further creating a nidus for reflux. The incidence of pneumonias in patients who are receiving nasoenteral feeding and whose tracheas are intubated is 20%.[60] The person with a severe brain injury is at significant risk of aspiration due to a depressed level of consciousness. This depressed level of consciousness can result in a diminished or absent gag or cough reflex and swallowing disorders. Swallowing disorders frequently lead to chronic aspiration, with an incidence of 41% in patients with severe brain injury.[61] The person with brain injury is usually receiving some form of acid prophylaxis. Antacids and H2 blockers can cause overgrowth of bacteria in the stomach.[62,63] Decreased gastric acidity increases gastric and tracheal colonization, particularly when a nasogastric tube is in place.[60-64] If patients are given some other form of ulcer prophylaxis (eg, sucralfate), the incidence of pneumonia goes down precipitously.[53,65,66]

Mechanical ventilation has its own inherent risks for the development of pneumonia. Several studies have concluded that intubation increases the risk of pneumonia 7- to 21-fold.[46,67,68] Many mechanical ventilators have air that is heated and moistened by a cascade humidifier. Some organisms, like *Pseudomonas*, prove to be ubiquitous and thrive in moist environments.[69] Studies show that ventilator circuit changes done every 24 hours, rather than every 48 hours, increase the incidence of pneumonia.[53,70] The risk of pneumonia with 24-hour ventilator circuit changes is probably the result of increased manipulation of the patient, the endotracheal tube, or the ventilator tubing, which could result in inadvertently pushing colonized bacteria into the tracheal-bronchial region.[71]

The misuse or overuse of antibiotics can precipitate deleterious effects on the host immune response to infection.[72,73] Antibiotics can create a shift in the flora, thereby altering colonization and selecting out organisms. The greatest risk is producing resistant strains, or casing a superinfection.

Early-Onset Pneumonia

Many studies have shown that airway colonization with bacteria usually takes place within 2 to 3 days after endotracheal intubation, with subsequent clinical infection occurring 3 to 7 days later.[57,74] The person with brain injury who is unconscious at the scene of the injury can experience an initial aspiration of oropharyngeal contents. Many of these patients have consumed a meal prior to their injuries, placing them at enormous risk of aspiration, and later in the course may develop lower-airway colonization following intubation.[74] All of these factors play a principal role in the development of early-onset pneumonia.

Pneumonia in the person with severe brain injury occurs earlier than in other trauma patient groups.[50,51,75] Early pneumonia has been described as occurring from 3 to 7 days after injury.[47,51,75–77] The incidence of early-onset pneumonia at post–injury day 3 can be 40%; at day 4, 60%; and at day 7, 80%.[75] The more common bacterial types for all pneumonias seen in trauma patients are *Staphylococcus aureus*, *Haemophilus influenzae*, and *Pseudomonas aeruginosa*.[48,75,78–81] With early-onset pneumonia, the dominant organisms are *Staphylococcus aureus* and *Haemophilus influenzae* (40.6% and 19%, respectively).[75] *Pseudomonas aeruginosa* is usually the dominant organism in later-onset pneumonias.[75] The consequences of developing early-onset pneumonia in the severely brain injured who are on mechanical ventilation are (1) increased days on the ventilator, (2) longer stay in the ICU, (3) prolonged hospitalization, and (4) increased morbidity and mortality.[75–79] The risk factors for the development of early-onset pneumonia are intubation at the scene of the injury, GCS scores lower than or equal to 5, associated swallowing disorders (documented following extubation), and aspiration.[75]

Signs and Symptoms

The typical symptoms of impending pneumonia are tachypnea (more than 20 breaths per minute) and fever. On auscultation, rales may be heard. Purulent sputum or frothy sputum can be an indication of some form of pneumonitis. Tachycardia is a common symptom for many infections, like pneumonia. Occasionally, a bradycardia may be noted in those patients who have an atypical pneumonia such as *Legionella* or *Mycoplasma*. Pleural effusions are particularly common in pneumonias caused by *Haemophilus influenzae*, pneumococcal, and streptococcal species.

Diagnosis

The finding of a leukocytosis greater than 20,000 cells per cubic centimeter, with the presence of immature forms (left shift), suggests infections. The use of a chest X-ray in the diagnosis of pneumonia in the critically ill is of extreme importance. Focal infiltrates seen on chest X-ray are typical for the critically ill person with pneumonia (Figure 9–7). Acute focal infiltrates are due to *Staphylococcus aureus*, pneumonococcus, and gram-negative bacilli.

Gram's stain evaluation of sputum has been the traditional first step in the assessment of the patient suspected of having pneumonia. Ideally, the secretions to be Gram stained should come from the deep lower airways. The specimen should have more than 25 leukocytes and fewer than 10 squamous cells per low-power field. Unfortunately, the sensitivity of Gram stain is between 40% and 60%, and 75% of samples obtained are usually inadequate.[82,83] In short, Gram's stain has the

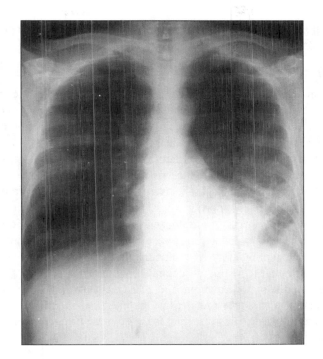

Figure 9–7 Pulmonary infiltrate found in the left lower lobe

luxury of being easy to perform, rapidly available, and inexpensive, but it possesses high rates of both false positives and false negatives.

Conclusive evidence of pneumonia can be obtained only through a good expectorated sputum and/or a positive blood culture that are consistent with the clinical picture. Sputum culture is simple to obtain, but it also comes with a significant rate of false positives and false negatives. More invasive techniques can improve the odds of confirming a diagnosis of pneumonia. Transtracheal aspiration involves a cricothyroid membrane puncture with a polyurethane catheter. Transtracheal needle aspiration is performed with an 18- or 25-gauge needle. The technique has fewer false negatives but has high false positives due to colonization of bacteria[84] and can cause bleeding, violent coughing, and cervical and mediastinal emphysema. Bronchoscopy aspirates with a protected catheter brush have proven useful in ventilated patients in that they carry a low morbidity and mortality and a high specificity. However, this method is not useful if the patient is on antibiotics or is bacteremic. A high risk of pneumothorax is present, especially in the ventilated patient. Therefore, obtaining aspirates during bronchoscopy is not practical in the person with severe brain injury[85] who is potentially bacteremic and on ventilatory support.

Treatment

Treatment of pneumonia must always begin with attempts at prevention. First and foremost is environmental control. Hand washing is crucial because many infections are caused by lack of adequate hygiene. Attention should be paid to respiratory equipment, with proper disinfection after each use. The use of heat moisture exchange along with ventilator circuit changes every 48 hours, as opposed to every 24 hours, can reduce risk of bacterial colonization.[73–75] Avoid, when possible, the use of nasogastric tubes to limit the risk of aspiration. Providing adequate nutritional support is crucial in maintaining host defense fortification. Avoid using histamine type 2 blockers and antacids, which neutralize gastric pH and add to the risk of developing pneumonia.[66,69] Prophylactic antibiotics may play a role in preventing early-onset pneumonia.[75] Topical antibiotics have been used successfully in preventing nosocomial pneumonia. However, this technique may be unsafe due to the emergence of resistant bacteria.[86] Selective digestive decontamination is an attempt to sterilize the intestine and oral cavity, on the assumption that the gastrointestinal tract is the source of the organisms that cause pneumonia.[87–89]

Nutritional support in the form of total parenteral nutrition (TPN) or preferably in the form of enteral feedings is of paramount importance,[90,91] particularly in preventing host defense impairments due to malnutrition. The use of a small-bore tube placed in the jejunum is felt by many to be the ideal feeding method for the severely brain injured.[92,93] It has been demonstrated in the moderate and severely brain injured that within the first two weeks post injury, there is prolonged gastric emptying,[94] implying that patients who are prone to aspiration would be at some risk if they were subjected to gastric feedings. An additional factor that places the person with brain injury at great risk of aspiration is the integrity of the lower esophageal sphincter (LES). Some investigators have shown that in moderate and severe brain injury, the LES is relaxed, thereby increasing the risk of aspiration in those persons receiving gastric feedings.[95]

Chest physiotherapy, an additional supportive measure, can enhance the evacuation of tenacious viscid secretions from the bronchial tree. The person with a severe brain injury who has an ineffective cough may benefit from percussion, vibration, and postural drainage, especially when the secretions are purulent. Patients who have viscid sputum can also benefit from aerosols and humidifiers, which reduce sputum viscosity and promote mucociliary clearance.[96]

Antibiotic therapy has both empiric and curative components. From the empiric point of view, the person with severe brain injury who may or may not have associated injuries is a potentially compromised host for developing pneumonia. A patient with a fever, leukocytosis, and a positive infiltrate by chest X-ray is probably a prime candidate for empiric therapy. The empiric antimicrobial regimen should be tailored to treat the most likely offending organisms: *Staphylococcus aureus*, *Haemophilus influenzae*, and *Pseudomonas aeruginosa*.[75,80,81] Cephalosporin, aminoglycosides, antipseudomonal penicillin, or erythromycin in appropriate combinations can adequately treat most gram-positive and gram-negative organisms. More recent antibiotics, such as ampicillin-sulbactam and ticarcillin-clavulanic acid, can be useful empiric therapies in covering a broad spectrum of organisms.

When a specific pathogen or pathogens have been identified, the antibiotic therapy with a narrow and focused regimen should be implemented. Many pneumonias can be polymicrobial, particularly in the person with severe brain injury who is being mechanically ventilated. Single agents or combinations of antibiotics may be acceptable depending on the clinical situation (eg, positive sputum and blood cultures). In these situations , or when circumstances do not allow a definitive diagnosis, the administration of broad-spectrum antibiotics should be entertained.

In the opinion of many investigators, if pneumonia could be eliminated from persons with severe brain injury, then 3% of this population could shift from a poor outcome to a much improved outcome.[44] If pneumonia could be abated or kept in check, many associated complications, such as septic shock, acute respiratory distress syndrome, systemic inflammatory response syndrome, and hypoxia, could be prevented, thereby increasing the percentage of improved outcomes. The role of antibiotic prophylaxis and routine culture surveillance, along with increasing awareness of risk factors, can probably result in fewer complications and improved survival.[44,75]

Pulmonary Empyema

The word *empyema*, derived from Greek and Latin, means "suppuration." Hippocrates is credited with being the first to describe in detail the symptomatology and management of empyema.[97]

Thoracic empyema develops usually as a consequence of another process, such as pneumonia, trauma, or some thoracic surgical procedure. Thoracic empyemas are common, resulting in a significant morbidity and mortality.[98] The overall incidence of empyema due to pneumonia is about 5%.[99] Interestingly, posttraumatic empyema of the thorax has increased in the last 20 years, from a reported low of 5% to a high of 15%.[100-103] Mortality figures associated with empyema vary from 7.3% to 21.7%.[100,104-114] The two factors associated with excess mortality are the presence of gram-negative rods or anaerobes in the empyema and the presence of associated diseases. Mortality figures are doubled with the presence of gram-negative rods or anaerobes (33%, 42%),[100,115] whereas the mortality figure associated with gram-positive cocci (*Staphylococcus aureus*) is less than half (15%).[115] These mortality figures are difficult to decipher, since the vast majority of these patients have comorbid medical conditions such as chronic pulmonary disease, cardiac disease, and associated pulmonary infections.[104,11,112,116–119]

Clinical Picture

Thoracic empyema is not unusual in patients with brain injury who have associated injuries. Many of these patients have drug problems, which place them at risk. The nature of their associated injuries, such as chest trauma and the need for surgical intervention, places them at additional risk. Aspiration pneumonia is also a principal risk factor in the development of an empyema or lung abscess.

The most common signs and symptoms of empyema, albeit nonspecific, are fever, chest pain, cough, dyspnea, pleural effusion, and leukocytosis.[100,116] These signs and symptoms tend to be more common in the younger patient than in the older patient who may have a comorbid disease. The most common bacteria isolated are anaerobes and aerobes. The more common organisms isolated from the pleural fluid are streptococcal, gram-negative bacilli; *Staphylococcus aureus*; and *Bacteroides fragilis*.[100,104] Pleural fluid pH is generally less than 7.2 with positive cultures. Mean white blood cell counts range from 79,000 to 117,000.[100] Glucose levels within the pleural fluid are low, less than 100 mg/dL. Additionally, laboratory assessments of the pleural fluid will commonly show protein levels greater than 3 g/dL, corroborating the exudative component of the fluid. Lactate dehydrogenase values are most times significantly elevated, with means of 3,979 U/mL (normal, 225 U/mL).[100] Chest X-rays are really the major marker for identifying a pleural effusion (Figure 9–8), and thoracentesis documents that the effusion is an empyema after laboratory analysis. The chest computed tomograpy (CT) scan provides further information as to whether the empyema is loculated or multiloculated (Figure 9–9).[116]

Treatment

The usual therapies for thoracic empyema are empiric antibiotic coverage and a drainage procedure. The antibiotics chosen should have a broad spectrum, either singularly or in combination. The usual drainage procedure is a closed thoracostomy (chest tube thoracostomy). For the uncomplicated acute empyema, closed thoracostomy has been advocated.[98,109,117–119]

Image-directed catheters using a small-bore "pigtail" catheter can be placed by either ultrasound or CT guidance. The success rate varies from 60% to 90%.[120,121] However, the drawbacks are cost, inadequate drainage, and poor lung reexpan-

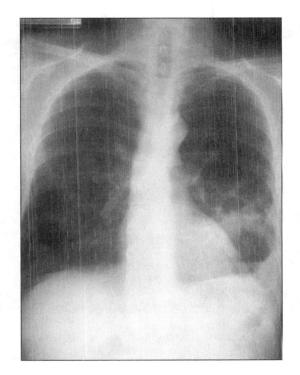

Figure 9–8 Identified as empyema post thoracentesis.

sion.[115] Renewed interest in the use of intrapleural thrombolytics exists currently. Several decades ago, their use was attempted, with mixed results and unacceptable adverse effects.[122]

There are reports of successful use of streptokinase and a single chest tube placement under ultrasonic guidance with few complications,[123–125] usually with multiloculated uncomplicated thoracic empyema. When closed drainage of any form fails, open thoracostomy and debridement should be entertained.[108,118,126]

Closed- or open-method drainage results in failure 20% to 30% of the time.[109,111,118,126] With failure of both closed and open techniques, the patient should undergo early, rather than later, surgical decortication.[105] There are reports of thoracoscopic debridement and drainage, but success rates are only 60%,[127–129] due to the inability to perform decortication adequately. The more thorough and acceptable procedure is open thoracostomy with decortication.[116]

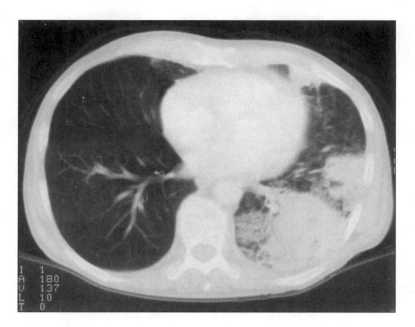

Figure 9–9 CT confirmation of a multiloculated empyema.

Lung Abscess

A primary lung abscess is a necrosis of pulmonary tissue caused by aspiration-induced microbial infection. The area of necrosis is about 2 cm or greater in diameter. Two thirds of these abscesses are found in the right lung,[130] probably due to the anatomic take off of the right mainstem bronchus. The bacteriology of lung abscess is commonly anaerobic bacteria, gram-negative rods, and, occasionally, gram-positive cocci.[131–133]

Most patients with lung abscess are chronically very ill. They are anemic and febrile, sometimes suffer from hemoptysis, and have purulent sputum and an elevated white blood cell count. A lung abscess takes approximately two weeks to develop after aspiration. The diagnosis of lung abscess is based on the presence of virulent pathogens in the sputum. Occasionally, there is associated pleural effusion (Figure 9–10). This fluid should undergo a laboratory analysis. The most crucial support for the diagnosis is radiographic evidence of a solitary cavitary lesion in a gravity-dependent section of the lung (Figure 9–11).

Many clinicians consider drainage to be the most crucial component of treatment for lung abscesses. Historically, drainage has been accomplished through the use of bronchoscopy, postural drainage, or surgical intervention. The need for

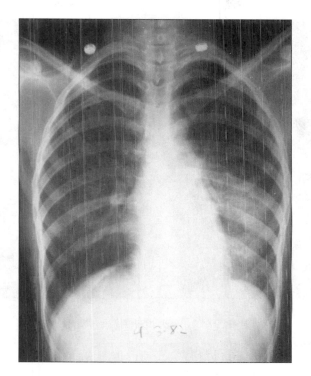

Figure 9–10 Following laboratory analysis, pleural effusion noted to be a lung abscess.

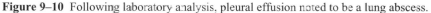

surgical intervention occurs only about 10% of the time.[34] Early in the course of developing a lung abscess, there may actually be spontaneous drainage into the bronchus. Antimicrobial therapy is an important facet of treatment.[135–137] Some form of drainage of the lung abscess is necessary with patients who are resistant to standard therapy of antibiotics and postural drainage. Recent evidence strongly favors the use of CT-guided catheter drainage as an effective method of treating most lung abscesses.[138,139]

Persons with brain injury do not commonly incur lung abscesses, even though their risk of aspiration is high. These patients tend not to be chronically ill and debilitated. In the critically ill or injured, the sequence of treatment should be a course of antimicrobials that are able to cover anaerobic, gram-negative, and gram-positive cocci species. Adjunctive therapy should include postural drainage and bronchoscopy if anatomically feasible. Depending on the condition of the patient, CT-guided catheter drainage should be implemented sooner rather than later. If CT-guided catheter drainage fails, then surgical intervention must be performed.

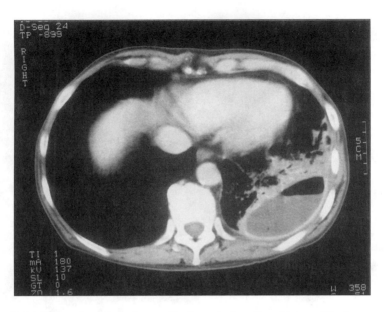

Figure 9–11 CT confirmation of a gravity-dependent cavitory lesion of the lung.

Neurogenic Pulmonary Edema

Impaired pulmonary function can be seen in a variety of central nervous system (CNS) insults: (1) injury to the brain,[140,141] (2) subarachnoid hemorrhage,[142,143] (3) intracerebral bleeds,[144] and (4) grand mal seizures.[145] The pathophysiology of neurogenic pulmonary edema (NPE) is not well elucidated. NPE was first described in 1874 in animals and in 1918 in humans.[146,147] Earlier in the 1900s, pulmonary edema was documented in humans following epilepsy and injury to the brain.[148–150]

Current Thinking

It is accepted that the common denominator for NPE is some form of CNS insult. Classically, NPE is categorized as noncardiogenic, that is, normal capillary wedge pressure with an abnormally elevated protein content within the edema, particularly evident in the intermediate or late phase of NPE.[151]

The edema that occurs is due to a shift of pulmonary fluid. The shift is related to changes in the net filtration of fluid as described by Starling.[152] The Starling equation explains movement of fluid out of any vascular bed:

$$Q = k[(Pmv - Pi) - \delta(\pi mv - \pi i)]$$

where Q = net filtration, k = fluid filtration coefficient, Pmv = microvascular hydrostatic pressure, Pi = interstitial hydrostatic pressure, δ = protein reflection coefficient, πmv = microvascular osmotic pressure, and πi = interstitial osmotic pressure. Under normal conditions, a state of near-equilibrium exists between osmotic pressure and opposing hydrostatic pressures. Fluid filtered out through the arterial capillaries is equivalent to the amount of fluid reabsorbed at the venous end of the capillaries. The fluid that is not fully reabsorbed is drained into the vascular system by the lymphatics. The probable associations between CNS insults and pulmonary edema are (1) increase in pulmonary microvascular hydrostatic pressure (Pmv), (2) the endothelial permeability to protein is increased (the protein reflection coefficient [δ][53]), and (3) recruitment of microvasculature, causing an increase in protein-rich lymph.[154,155] Animal studies have supported all three mechanisms as causes of pulmonary edema.[155–158]

Animal studies suggest that the "edemogenic" center exists in the CNS. When the preoptic nucleus of the hypothalamus is experimentally injured, one of the results is pulmonary edema.[159] In other animal studies, injury to the caudal brain bilaterally also produced pulmonary edema.[160] The CNS injury induces a massive sympathetic discharge (blast injury theory), or a "catecholamine storm." The "blast injury theory"[161,162] proposes that cerebral injury causes a massive sympathetic release that leads to both venous and arterial vasoconstrictions. The vasoconstriction increases venous return and shunts blood to the lungs. Arterial constriction results in elevated systemic blood pressure.

The proposed alpha-cholinergic–mediated response causes not only systemic hypertension but also peripheral vasoconstriction, increased pulmonary artery pressure, pulmonary microvascular vasoconstriction, and a failure of left ventricular relaxation.[163] These factors result in an increase in capillary pressure. The "blast effect" causes hydrostatic pulmonary edema during the period of high pressure and directly damages the pulmonary capillary endothelium. The endothelial damage creates a defect, resulting in a continuation of the pulmonary edema, even though the pulmonary capillary pressure returns to normal[164] (Figure 9–12).

Some investigators have looked at the role of beta-adrenergic–mediated mechanisms.[165,166] These mechanisms result in an increase in epinephrine release and pulmonary lymphatic constriction, which results in an increase in filtration and a decrease in removal. There is increase in platelets and fibrinogen, precipitating pulmonary intravascular clotting, which results in pulmonary capillary endothelial damage. The release of bradykinin or histamine is another possible cause of endothelial damage.

Significant elevation of mean arterial pressure is noted, suggesting a cardiogenic component, the end result being pulmonary edema. The question remains as to whether NPE results from high pressures in the pulmonary vascular bed with eventual hydrostatic and mechanical injury or from neuromediated-induced in-

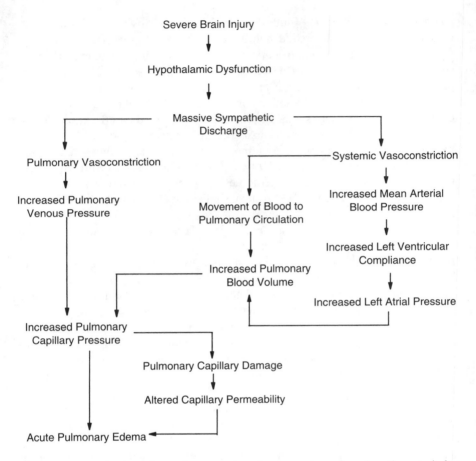

Figure 9–12 Pathophysiology of neurogenic pulmonary edema, based on the catecholamine storm theory.

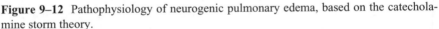

creased permeability alone. The laboratory and clinical scientific evidence suggests that NPE is probably caused by some combination of both mechanisms.

Incidence

The frequency of NPE continues to be questionable. The reported incidence has varied from 10% to 70%.[150,167,168] This disparity is due to lack of large autopsy series in NPE and in part to failure in recognizing the clinical relevance of NPE in nonfatal brain injuries. Nonfatal NPE has been thought to be a rare occurrence. In one fairly significant series of 686 deaths due to brain injury or spontaneous CNS hemorrhage, the incidence of pulmonary edema was 65% in the brain-injured sample and 75% in the nontraumatic intracranial hemorrhage sample.[158] This report also looked at the rapidity of NPE after CNS injury. Seventy-three patients died within one hour of injury from spontaneous hemorrhage. Of that number, 60% had evidence of pulmonary edema at autopsy.

In a recent study looking at traumatic brain injuries alone, both fatal and nonfatal, the reported incidence of NPE was 32% for victims who died within 96 hours.[169] Their criterion for considering NPE is those patients who died at the scene or who died within 96 hours was weight of the lungs. They found a significant increase in weight of the lungs, but not of other organs. Therefore, lung weight, in conjunction with edema, congestion, and hemorrhage, was felt to be consistent with NPE.

Signs and Symptoms

There appear to be two distinct forms of the NPE syndrome. In one form, NPE develops within minutes to several hours; in the other, it develops after several days.[170]

The signs and symptoms in the early form of NPE include tachypnea, cough, hemoptysis, rales, copious amounts of frothy sputum, and tachycardia. Low-grade fever is common. Hypoxemia, mild leukocytosis, and bilateral infiltrates may be present, with normal heart size on chest X-ray. The chest X-ray may show pulmonary infiltrates in a "butterfly" pattern or confined to the upper lobes. In many instances, transient changes in mean arterial pressure and pulmonary artery pressure can occur.[163,171–174]

Current evidence suggests that in traumatic brain injury, a marked decrease in the partial pressure of oxygen (Pao_2) to fractional inspired oxygen (Fio_2) ratio occurs, particularly when elevated ICP and low cerebral perfusion pressure (CPP) are present. All of these factors strongly suggest that intracranial hypertension may be an important component in the development of NPE.[169]

The delayed form of NPE occurs more insidiously, progressing over 12 hours to several days following the CNS insult.[175–177] Characteristic features of delayed NPE are not dissimilar to the early forms of NPE. In delayed NPE, there is slow development of hypoxemia, abnormal chest X-rays, and dyspnea over several days. It is important to note that many of these patients require ventilatory support.

Treatment

An essential principle in the clinical management of NPE is early suspicion of the syndrome, with the knowledge that NPE may present in the early or delayed form. An early possible marker is a Pao_2/Fio_2 ratio of less than 300 mm Hg, particularly in the absence of thoracic injury or aspiration.[169] The basis of management for suspected NPE is mechanical ventilation and the reduction of intracranial hypertension.[164,169,178,179]

Treatment for patients with severe NPE is based on recommendations for patients with ARDS. Ventilatory PEEP is usually used for both situations. PEEP is effective in the management of hypoxia secondary to alveolar leak and $\dot{V}/\dot{Q}$ mismatch. Improved arterial oxygenation and increased functional residual capacity and intrathoracic pressure are accomplished with PEEP. The use of PEEP in patients with intracranial hypertension has come into question because of concerns among some investigators that PEEP can decrease cerebral venous outflow, thereby worsening ICP.[180-182]

Rises in ICP secondary to PEEP have been found to correlate with worsening of neurologic function and a decrease in cerebral perfusion pressure.[179-183] Used with caution, PEEP can be a successful adjunct to treating NPE, provided that there is ICP monitoring and close attention paid to mean arterial pressure, arterial oxygenation, and cerebral perfusion pressure.[183-185]

High-frequency ventilation or high-frequency jet ventilation involves acceleration of gas through an injected cannula during inhalation at 100 to 150 breaths per minute. HFJV is of questionable use in NPE. Jet ventilation lowers airway pressures more than conventional ventilators, but it can have adverse effects on cerebral perfusion pressure.[185] Therefore, the role of HFJV remains uncertain.[186]

Evidence supports the theory of massive sympathetic discharge as a factor in the development of NPE. Therefore, alpha-adrenoceptor blockade becomes a logical choice in combating NPE. Alpha-receptor blocking agents such as nitroprusside, chlorpromazine, phenoxybenzamine, and phentolamine have been shown to be effective when used early.[169,187-189] Droperidol, an alpha-receptor blocking agent, has been shown not only to block the "catecholamine storm" but also to reduce cerebral metabolism.[173] There is some evidence in the subarachnoid hemorrhage model that dobutamine causes regression of severe NPE and that the reduction in total peripheral vascular resistance and the increase in cardiac contractility account for the observed beneficial effects.[190]

Acute Respiratory Distress Syndrome

ARDS is a disease state manifested by severe pulmonary dysfunction, often accompanied by systemic complications such as sepsis and nonpulmonary organ failure.[191-193] ARDS is a frequent cause of acute respiratory failure among critically ill patients and affects approximately 200,000 patients per year in the United States.[192] Severely injured trauma patients make up a substantial subset of patients afflicted with ARDS. These patients face up to a 50% mortality rate, and, in fact, ARDS is the most common cause of death following multiple trauma not related directly to the initial injury.[192,193]

Ashbaugh and Petty are credited with first describing the entity and coining the term *adult respiratory distress syndrome* in 1967.[191,194] However, the disease was recognized, if not by name, by clinical observation, much earlier in the 20th century. In his *Textbook of Medicine* published in 1927, Osler wrote that "uncontrolled septicemia leads to frothy pulmonary edema that resembles serum, not the sanguineous transudative edema fluid seen in dropsy or congestive heart failure."[191] For these patients in Osler's time and for many decades to follow, what we now know as an early manifestation of ARDS was seen as a terminal event.

The pulmonary dysfunction seen in ARDS is characterized by initial tachypnea and hypoxemia.[192–193] The oxygenation deficit can be quantified by the ratio of the measured arterial oxygen tension to the fraction of inspired oxygen (Pao_2/Fio_2). A Pao_2/Fio_2 lower than or equal to 150 or lower than or equal to 200 or a PEEP of at least 5 cm H_2O is indicative of significant hypoxemia.[151,193] The increased minute ventilation associated with the tachypnea may initially result in hypocapnia and a respiratory alkalosis; however, mixed acid-base disorders are common, especially in the clinical setting of sepsis or shock. As the disease progresses, carbon dioxide elimination also becomes impaired. The chest X-ray reveals diffuse infiltrates involving all lung fields.[191,192] There should be no clinical evidence of congestive heart failure, and if a pulmonary artery catheter is present, the pulmonary capillary wedge pressure should be less than 18 mm Hg. A more detailed discussion of the pathophysiology and clinical manifestations of ARDS will follow later in this section.

Patients at Risk for ARDS

As previously mentioned, trauma patients represent a specific group at risk for the development of ARDS. Yet the disease may afflict a variety of critically ill patients. Systemic inflammation is thought to be the common pathway by which diverse patient populations develop the lung injury process of ARDS.[195–198] The cascade of systemic inflammatory response can trigger the onset of multiple organ failure often seen as the final phase before death in ARDS patients.[199]

It is important first to identify disease states associated with overwhelming systemic inflammation and thus a high incidence of ARDS. Hudson et al have defined the following clinical conditions that have been associated with ARDS:[200]

- *Sepsis syndrome:* defined as a clinical picture of serious infection or inflammation with a concurrent, deleterious systemic response. Specific objective criteria such as body temperature, white blood cell count, positive blood cultures, known or suspected sources of infection, metabolic acidosis, hypotension, and reduced systemic vascular resistance contribute to the definition of sepsis. Of note, sepsis syndrome does not necessarily require the presence of an infection. For the patient lacking positive bacterial cultures, the term *sys-*

temic inflammatory response syndrome (SIRS) is more appropriately applied.

- *Aspiration:* occurs with the inhalation of gastric contents, documented either by direct observation by medical personnel or by suctioning of gastric contents from the trachea.
- *Drug overdose:* defined as the ingestion or parenteral injection of narcotics, aspirin, tricyclic antidepressants, or sedative hypnotic drugs that results in a depressed mental status and need for ICU monitoring.
- *Near-drowning:* involves a serious immersion resulting in loss of consciousness and either significant acidosis (pH <7.25) or hypothermia (core temperature <32°C).
- *Pulmonary contusion:* results from blunt trauma to the chest and can be seen as a localized infiltrate on chest X-ray within 6 hours of injury. There is clinical evidence of overlying chest wall trauma such as rib fractures, flail chest, or soft tissue ecchymosis.
- *Multiple transfusion:* Although the number of blood products transfused may vary, Hudson et al define multiple transfusion as at least 15 units of blood within 24 hours for the purpose of emergency resuscitation.
- *Multiple fractures:* defined as the fracture of two or more major long bones; an unstable pelvic fracture; or one major long bone and a major pelvic fracture.

Severe traumatic brain injury has previously been thought of as a separate risk factor for ARDS. In Hudson et al's study, 165 patients had severe brain injury as their sole clinical risk. Traumatic brain injury was defined as injury resulting in a loss of consciousness for more than 2 hours, intracranial hemorrhage, depressed skull fracture, lateralizing signs on neurologic examination, or evidence of elevated ICP by CT scan. Of these 165 patients, only 6 (3.6%) went on to develop ARDS.[200] Therefore, as an isolated finding, traumatic brain injury cannot be considered a major risk factor for ARDS. However, traumatic brain injury may indirectly lead to ARDS because of associated multiple trauma, pulmonary contusions, long bone fractures, the need for multiple transfusions, or aspiration secondary to loss of protective airway reflexes.[200,201] In addition, the patient with brain injury and neurogenic pulmonary edema may be at higher risk for pulmonary complications, including the developments of pneumonia and ARDS.

Over a three-year period, Hudson et al prospectively found 695 patients with at least one of the aforementioned seven risk factors. ARDS developed in 25.7% of the total,[200] occurring most frequently among patients with sepsis syndrome (42.6%; 75 of 176 cases) and multiple transfusions (40%; 46 of 115 cases). Two or more risk factors occurring in combination carried a much higher incidence of ARDS than did an isolated risk alone. There was a 25.5% (69 of 271 cases) incidence of ARDS among those patients with one or more trauma-related risk factors: pulmonary contusion, multiple fractures, and multiple transfusions. Once again, multiple transfusions occurring in combination with one of the other trauma risks led to a significantly higher rate of ARDS (47.3%; 18 of 38 cases). The development of sepsis increased the risk of ARDS nearly threefold among trauma patients. Mortality was significantly higher when ARDS was present (62%) as compared to that for patients with clinical risks who did not develop ARDS (19%). This marked difference in mortality rate held true among trauma patients who developed ARDS (58%) and trauma patients who did not (12.9%).[200]

Physiologic Alterations Leading to ARDS

Although our understanding of the systemic response and immunologic alterations that follow these clinical disease states is still evolving, it appears that excessive uncontrolled activation of inflammatory cells and their mediators, known as *cytokines*, leads ultimately to the development of organ injury and dysfunction. This systemic inflammatory response is the basis of ARDS and multiple organ dysfunction syndrome.[195,201–207] Infusion of endotoxin, the virulent component of gram-negative bacteria, results in the early appearance of several cytokines, initially tumor necrosis factor (TNF) and interleukin-1 (IL-1), followed later by IL-6 and IL-8, among others.[195,202,203] It has been proposed that translocation of gram-negative bacteria and endotoxin from the intestine occurs after trauma and hemorrhagic shock as a result of intestinal hypoperfusion and gut mucosal ischemia. This theory remains controversial, however, since endotoxin and TNF are not detected in the systemic or portal blood after severe trauma.[195,202] Small amounts of endotoxin may possibly be bound to lipopolysaccharide-binding proteins, which are then engulfed by phagocytic macrophages in the liver, spleen, and other organs. Once there, beyond detection, endotoxin may stimulate a cascade of inflammatory events.[195]

Other inflammatory mediators such as the complement fragment C5a and platelet-activating factor are increased immediately after trauma and can induce the generation of IL-6 and IL-8, apparently without the need of endotoxin.[195,202,203,205] Indeed, marked increases in these later two cytokines can be detected within a few hours of severe trauma. IL-6 induces hepatic production of acute-phase proteins such as C-reactive protein, complement components, fibrinogen, and α_1-antitrypsin.[195,202,203] Although these factors may not necessarily promote organ dysfunction, they appear to contribute to the overall systemic inflammatory state. IL-8 probably also plays an important role in the development of ARDS and systemic inflammation, inducing migration of neutrophils into the lungs and, along with other inflammatory mediators, enhancing neutrophil activation and respiratory burst.[195,202,203,205] Multiple factors, many beyond our understanding, are responsible for an overwhelming and uncontrolled systemic inflammatory response.

The net result, however complex, is that of cellular injury in both the lungs and other organs.

Pulmonary Pathology in ARDS

The pulmonary injury in ARDS is one of severe damage to the alveolar-capillary interface. Histologically, the disease can be divided into three evolving and interrelated phases: (1) the *exudative phase* of edema and hemorrhage; (2) the *proliferative phase* of organization and repair; and (3) the *fibrotic phase* of end-stage fibrosis.[206]

The exudative phase is pronounced by pulmonary bed capillary congestion, with leakage of plasma proteins and neutrophils from the injured endothelium. Initially, there is marked interstitial and alveolar edema as well as intra-alveolar hemorrhage. It is during this phase, which occupies approximately the first week after the onset of respiratory failure, that dense eosinophilic hyaline membranes, composed of plasma proteins, become prominent along the alveolar surface.[206] Even more pronounced than capillary endothelial damage is the extensive necrosis of type 1 cells of the alveolar epithelium. Although type 1 cells make up only 8% of parenchymal lung tissue, they make up the majority of the large surface area of the lung. As these cells slough from the alveolar surface, denuded basement membrane is left, to which hyaline membranes, fibrin, and cellular debris adhere.[206] With the loss of the alveolar epithelial barrier, interstitial fluid floods the alveolar space. Type 2 surfactant-producing alveolar cells are also susceptible to injury.[206,207] The net effect of these changes occurring in the exudative phase of ARDS is that of alveolar collapse and consolidation.

The proliferative phase begins as alveolar epithelial cells start to regenerate in an attempt to cover the previously denuded basement membrane. Type 2 cells proliferate along the alveolar surface. It is likely that these surfactant-producing cells are capable of differentiating into type 1 alveolar epithelial cells.[206] Within the regenerating alveolar wall, fibroblasts and myofibroblasts proliferate and then migrate through breaks in the alveolar basement membrane. Combining with the intra-alveolar exudate, fibroblasts then create granulation tissue and deposit collagen, generating a sparsely cellular dense fibrous tissue.[206] This pattern of lung remodeling leads to the fibrotic phase, which is seen in patients who have survived beyond three to four weeks from the onset of ARDS. By this time, the affected lung parenchyma is almost entirely remodeled into sparsely cellular collagenous tissue.[206]

The pulmonary vasculature in ARDS parallels this pattern of parenchymal reorganization. In the early phases of ARDS, pulmonary vasoconstriction, thromboembolism, and interstitial edema are prominent but reversible. Blood clots within the pulmonary vasculature may arise from both systemic venous emboli and intrapulmonary thrombi forming directly on injured endothelial cells.[206] As the disease progresses beyond several weeks, more permanent changes, including fibrous obliteration of the microcirculation and increased endothelial smooth muscle proliferation, may lead to pulmonary hypertension.[206]

Although lung injury in ARDS is commonly referred to as a diffuse process, there is actually marked heterogeneity of both structure and function within different areas of the lung.[208] The more gravity-dependent areas—for instance, the posterior lung fields in a supine patient—become more severely edematous and consolidated, participating minimally in chest expansion and gas exchange. Conversely, the anteriorly located lung fields exhibit near-normal elastance and ventilation. The stiff, noncompliant, dependent areas receive disproportionately greater blood flow, while forced positive-pressure airflow naturally follows the path of least resistance, leading to overexpansion of the more anteriorly located, compliant alveoli.[208] The net effect is a heightened $\dot{V}/\dot{Q}$ mismatch. This asymmetry may not be readily apparent on a supine portable plain chest radiograph, by which the lungs are often described as having "diffuse patchy infiltrates" (Figure 9–13). The regional differences are better illustrated with CT: transverse cuts of the chest CT demonstrate a pattern of dense consolidation in the gravity-dependent posterior areas of the lung, whereas anteriorly the lung parenchyma appears well aerated.[208]

Pulmonary Mechanics

What, then, do these histologic and macroscopic changes of ARDS translate into, in terms of functional pulmonary mechanics? The overall compliance of the lung and thorax, that is, the change in volume per unit change of pressure ($\Delta V/\Delta P$), is markedly reduced.[208] This stiffness of the entire thoracic cavity is the result of the edematous boggy changes along with collapsed alveoli within the gravity-dependent areas of the lung parenchyma. Initially, one is effectively dealing with reduced lung volume: that is, significant areas of regional alveolar collapse lead to a diminished FRC.[208] In this early stage of ARDS, the application of PEEP may recruit many collapsed alveolar units, with an overall improvement in FRC, compliance, and gas exchange. However, as the lung injury progresses and fibrosis sets in, it becomes increasingly difficult to maintain adequate oxygenation and carbon dioxide elimination despite high levels of supplemental oxygen, minute ventilation, and applied PEEP.[208] At this stage, one may face extremely high airway pressures as a result of deteriorating compliance. Often it becomes necessary to sedate and paralyze patients to reduce any degree of chest wall stiffness from the musculoskeletal thoracic cage.

Attempts at improving ventilation are often complicated by regional overdistension of the more compliant alveolar units. In the face of high peak and mean airway pressure, this hyperexpansion may lead to the potentially disastrous consequence of barotrauma.[208] Any clinical signs of acute deterioration in terms of he-

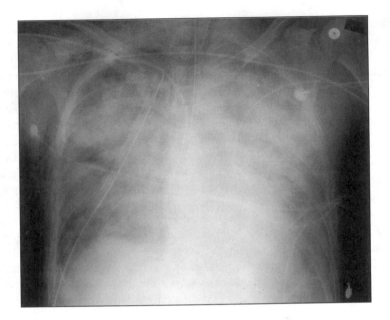

Figure 9–13 Typical radiographic pattern of "diffuse patchy infiltrates" consistent with ARDS.

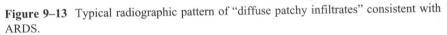

modynamics or pulmonary mechanics should therefore arouse the suspicion of a tension pneumothorax in the patient with ARDS, prompting an immediate clinical evaluation and chest X-ray, with possible need for emergent chest tube insertion.

Mechanical Ventilation

In view of the above discussion, patients with ARDS inevitably require intubation and mechanical ventilation. Although this measure will not alter the course of the disease, it does allow time for the lungs to recover following the acute injury of ARDS. The goal of mechanical ventilatory support is to maintain gas exchange while avoiding the complications associated with it, namely, barotrauma, oxygen toxicity, and structural damage to the upper tracheobronchial tree.[209] Different modes of ventilation have been tried and advocated, but it appears that none carries an advantage over the rest in terms of rate of recovery, complications, or overall prognosis.[209]

The most frequently used mode is that of conventional volume-controlled ventilation. Because of diminished lung compliance, it is often necessary to reduce the delivered tidal volume while increasing the frequency (respiratory rate) in order to limit excessive airway pressures and maintain an adequate minute ventilation.[209] The benefits of PEEP have already been discussed, but to review, PEEP reestablishes alveolar patency with improvement in FRC while promoting acceptable arterial oxygen saturation at a minimal inspired oxygen concentration (FIO_2)[208,209] The lowest PEEP necessary to maintain an FIO_2 below 0.5 should be used in order to avoid barotrauma and hemodynamic embarrassment as a result of reduced venous return to the right side of the heart.[209]

Several unconventional ventilatory modes have gained acceptance and may be tried in patients who fail initial conventional ventilatory management. PCV is a method by which the inspiratory pressure is preset in order to limit excessively high peak airway pressures. Tidal volumes (which are not preset) and hence minute ventilation therefore follow as a function of the patient's dynamic pulmonary compliance.[209–211] Inverse-ratio ventilation may be used to supplement this mode, whereby the inspiratory (I) time is prolonged and expiratory (E) time shortened, resulting in an I:E ratio of greater than 1, in contrast to conventional ventilation, as well as normal spontaneous ventilation, in which expiratory time is longer and the I:E ratio is on the order of 1:2 or 1:3. The goal is to maximally recruit collapsed alveoli while minimizing the adverse effects of high airway pressures.[209–211] When using this mode, however, one must be cautious of air trapping and overdistension at the alveolar level from an inadequate expiratory time. This auto-PEEP phenomenon may lead to barotrauma, hemodynamic deterioration, and even worsened gas exchange.[209–211]

HFJV is another method by which ventilation and oxygenation are achieved without large volume or pressure excursions.[209,212] The basic premise is to deliver gas at high pressures through a narrow tube (1–4 mm) placed within the endotracheal tube. Gas flow is very rapidly and repetitively interrupted by a timer-regulated valve (frequency). The tidal volume delivered by the jet flow is proportional to the driving pressure and is at, or near, dead space [209,211] Despite much initial enthusiasm for being able to maintain gas exchange, HFJV has not been found to be superior to conventional ventilation. As with all the different types of mechanical support, successful ventilation is dependent of the specific pulmonary mechanics of the individual patient as well as the clinician's experience.

Pharmacologic Treatment of ARDS

Several pharmacologic therapies have been studied in the treatment of sepsis syndrome and ARDS, including corticosteroids, nonsteroidal anti-inflammatory agents, and prostaglandin E_1 (PGE_1). Despite initial encouraging antidotal reports, none of these agents has been conclusively proven to prevent the development of ARDS, hasten its reversal, improve pulmonary function, or decrease mortality rate.[213] Surfactant has been successfully used in infants with hyaline membrane disease, but its role in adults with ARDS is yet unknown [213] The use of monoclonal antibodies toward endotoxin and inflammatory cytokines, such as TNF, is being evaluated to halt the uncontrolled systemic inflammatory response that precedes the onset of sepsis and ARDS.[213] Results of some animal and human trials have been encouraging, but more work is needed before definitive conclusions can be drawn. Any benefit of these expensive immunologic modulators will be based on careful patient selection and proper timing of administration.

More recently, inhaled nitric oxide has shown potential therapeutic value in the management of ARDS.[214] Nitric oxide is endogenously produced by endothelial cells and acts as a potent vasodilator by stimulating guanylic cyclase in vascular smooth muscle cells to produce increased levels of cyclic guanosine monophosphate (cGMP).[214] Frequently used intravenous drugs such as nitroglycerin and nitroprusside exert their vasodilatory effects through the release of nitric oxide. The mode of delivery of nitric oxide, that is, inhalation at very minute concentrations, is the key to its success in improving oxygenation in patients with ARDS.[214] Preferential delivery to well-ventilated areas of the lung appears to be the mechanism by which nitrous oxide works. The resulting vasodilation enhances regional blood flow to these areas, thereby improving $\dot{V}/\dot{Q}$ matching and hence oxygenation.[214] Intravenous vasodilators, on the other hand, offer very little benefit in the treatment of ARDS because they will primarily dilate areas of greatest hypoxic pulmonary vasoconstriction. As a consequence, blood flow to poorly ventilated areas of the lung is increased, and gas exchange is worsened.[214] Many logistic aspects of the use of inhaled nitric oxide are yet to worked out; the optimal method of delivery and standards of measurement among these. Moreover, whether nitric oxide will prove to be of benefit in terms of recovery and survival in these critically ill patients remains to be seen. Nonetheless, inhaled nitric oxide seems to hold promise as a future tool in the treatment of ARDS.

Conclusion

ARDS remains a serious complication in a subset of trauma patients, including patients with brain injury. Care is largely supportive during the acute phases of lung injury, and during this time early rehabilitative efforts are limited. Patients are often kept heavily sedated or paralyzed while on full mechanical ventilatory support. Even simple turning of the patient may promote further V/Q mismatching and arterial oxygen desaturation. Health care workers must work in concert to support these critically ill patients toward eventual pulmonary recovery and survival.

Deep-Venous Thrombosis

Acute deep-venous thrombosis (DVT), with or without pulmonary embolism (PE), is the most common vascular complication following major surgical procedures. DVT is a dangerous and frustrating entity because it may develop insidiously and, once in tiated, may have an unpredictable and occasionally fatal outcome. The true prevalence is uncertain due to inaccurate diagnosis and erratic reporting. Approximately 5 to 6 million cases of DVT are diagnosed yearly in the United States, leading to 650,000 to 700,000 cases of acute PE.[215-217]

It is generally accepted that the risk of DVT and PE is increased in the trauma patients. The reported incidence has varied widely: 10% to 90% for DVT and 5% to 50% for PE.[218-220] The risk is increased in multiple trauma, spinal cord injury with paraplegia, pelvic and lower-extremity fractures, advanced age, immobilization, and brain injury.[221] The estimated frequency of postoperative venous thrombosis in the calves of neurosurgical patients, ranges from 29% to 43%.[222] The incidence of clinically evident DVT is considerably lower, creating one of the difficulties in the management of this disease.

On the basis of anatomic, experimental, and clinical investigations that remain valid today, Virchow proposed that the essential features of DVT are (1) activation of platelets and the coagulation mechanism (thrombogenesis), (2) injury of the vein's endothelial lining, and (3) decreased velocity of blood flow (stasis).[218] Although the relative balance of these three factors will vary in each patient, origination and propagation of venous thrombi will not occur unless all three are present to some degree. Thrombogenesis involves a complicated but integrated series of reactions between circulating platelets and coagulation factors on an abnormal flow surface. The adherence of platelets to the surface of veins where the endothelium has been structurally or functionally injured will promote a series of chemical reactions that will enhance platelet aggregation and the formation of a thrombus.[217,223] The enlargement and stabilization of a thrombus depends on the formation of thrombin. Thrombin is generated by an intrinsic coagulation pathway via contact activation with subendothelial collagen or by activation of the extrinsic coagulation pathway with tissue factor, or by both pathways.[217] The explanation of these reactions is beyond the scope of this chapter. However, when thrombin is formed, the synthesis of thromboxane A_2 and the release of adenosine diphosphate are stimulated from platelets, thus promoting platelet aggregation.[224] There are several inherent control mechanisms limiting thrombogenesis: activated protein C, antithrombin III, and plasmin. The reactions involving these factors will ordinarily be sufficient to limit growth of the thrombus and even dissolve the clot, if the initial procoagulant stimulus is removed. However, in patients with DVT, the balance shifts in favor of progressive thrombogenesis unless anticoagulant or thrombolytic therapy is initiated.

The endothelial cells that line the vessel walls play an important role in regulating the coagulation process. Thrombus formation may result either when there is an unfavorable alteration in endothelial cell function or when morphologic injury exposes subendothelial surfaces. The endothelial cells have the potential for controlling local thrombus generation by the expression of both anticoagulant and procoagulant factors on their luminal surfaces.

Stasis, or markedly reduced venous flow, has long been implicated in the genesis of DVT. Although it may be a contributing factor, stasis has never been shown to initiate thrombus formation independently.[225] Conditions that decrease venous flow are associated with an increased risk of venous thrombosis.[217] If endothelial injury and coagulation system activation are present, then decreased flow will facilitate thrombosis by not physically removing procoagulant factors from local areas and by increasing time for blood-vessel interaction.

Thrombi preferentially form at selected foci. The specific site is principally determined by the venous anatomy, endothelial cellular function, and local flow conditions. Clinical studies suggest that the deep calf veins are the most common sites for thrombi to originate in patients who have not had surgical trauma to their hips or retroperitoneum.[226,227] A higher incidence of iliofemoral thrombosis, with and without distal thrombi, is found in patients who have undergone surgery involving trauma to the veins in those areas.[217] The essential step for thrombogenesis to occur is the local generation of thrombin, which will then stimulate platelet aggregation and transform fibrinogen into fibrin. Approximately 20% of patients have progression of the thrombi from the calf to the popliteal vein.[217]

Prophylactic Therapy

Patients with brain injuries are at a higher risk to develop DVT. The best strategy against this disorder and its complications, especially PE, is to prevent the onset of venous thrombogenesis. Some have suggested that while the per-patient dollar cost of prophylaxis is greater than that of treating thromboembolic events, the additional expense is justified by the lives saved.[222,228] The routine use of prophylaxis therapy in all patients who might be at risk for DVT has been advocated by a Consensus Development Conference of the National Institutes of Health.[229]

In 1950, de Takats noted that less heparin was required to prevent clotting than to treat a formed clot and suggested minidose heparin (5,000 U subcutaneously twice daily) as a prophylactic measure.[222] Heparin in this dosage inhibits factor X activation, thereby interrupting both intrinsic and extrinsic clotting mechanisms,[217,222,230] but causes only minor changes in the conventional measurements of clotting capacity. Since then, low-dose heparin administered subcutaneously every 8 or 12 hours has been shown by many to be effective in preventing DVT in different groups of surgical patients. In the broad scope of general surgery, this therapy has reduced the rate of DVT by 60%, for a net decrease in incidence from 25% to 10%.[229] The risk of bleeding in the majority of studies has been related to the surgical wound. Warfarin is another anticoagulation therapy used in the prophylaxis of DVT. Warfarin inhibits the synthesis of vitamin K–dependent coagulation factors (II, VII, IX, and X).[217] In certain groups of patients undergoing orthopaedic surgery (hip, knee), warfarin reduces the incidence of DVT by a factor of two when compared to low-dose heparin.[225] To achieve therapeutic levels, warfarin agents must be administered for several days.

Patients with brain injury admitted to the ICU are usually at risk of developing intracranial bleeding as a progression of the original injury or after craniotomy. More than 60% of these patients have other systems involved, where bleeding is the primary cause of morbidity in the first few days after admission. There are a few reports indicating the safeness and effectiveness of low-dose heparin reducing the incidence of DVT in neurosurgical patients undergoing craniotomy.[230-232] Despite these few reports, the majority consider that patients with severe brain injury are not suitable candidates for prophylaxis with anticoagulants, especially in the first few days after injury and when associated injuries are present. The point in time at which a patient with severe brain injury becomes a candidate for anticoagulation is not clear in the literature and is a matter of clinical judgment.

External or sequential pneumatic compression devices (SCDs) are another means of preventing DVT. The mechanism of this prophylactic measure is more complex than the mechanical induction of pulsatile flow. Intermittent pneumatic compression of the arms of surgical patients decreases the incidence of DVT in the legs and is found to prevent the usual decrease in fibrinolytic activity seen postoperatively.[233] This finding supports the concept that release of fibrinolytic activators may play a role in its prophylactic action,[234] but this theory has not been confirmed by many. Two large prospective randomized studies confirmed the reduction of DVT in patients receiving SCD treatment compared with no therapy.[222] Recently, the efficacy of SCDs to prevent DVT has been questioned in a small nonrandomized study.[235] Despite these controversies, SCDs are the recommended prophylaxis for DVT in patients with severe brain injury in the ICU, with or without associated injuries. SCD treatment should be initiated as soon as possible, using the lower extremities if possible. If the patient will be bedridden for a prolonged period, low-dose subcutaneous heparin is recommended. Timing of administration of low-dose heparin will depend on clinical judgment and is not recommended within the first five days post injury.

Diagnosis of DVT

Despite the use of SCDs or low-dose heparin in patients with severe brain injury, the risk of developing DVT is as high as 10% in this population.[217,222,229] A high index of suspicion is necessary to make the correct diagnosis of DVT in this population.

Clinical diagnosis of DVT is unreliable and should not be the basis for a full therapeutic course of anticoagulation. Homan's sign, long regarded as the classic indicator of DVT, has been refuted by studies that found no evidence of venous thrombosis in more than 50% of patients with a positive sign.[217,236] Pain and tenderness are the most common complaints but are not diagnostic, especially in patients with severe brain injury and associated injuries. Forty percent to 60% of patients with a history and physical examination compatible with venous thrombosis have actual thrombi confirmed by venography.[217] A clinical diagnosis of DVT is the least accurate and least cost effective of any modality. Therefore, a more objective evaluation must be pursued.

Doppler Ultrasonography. The Doppler ultrasound flow-velocity probe detects the presence and phasic qualities of venous blood flow. A diagnosis of venous obstruction is based on the presence or absence of phasic spontaneous flow, absence or respiratory variation in flow distal to the area of suspicion, and lack of augmented flow proximal to the occlusion.[237] The advantages of this technology are that the method is totally noninvasive, painless, and safe; it can be performed rapidly in most patients at the bedside and can be repeated as frequently as needed. In experienced hands, Doppler flow velocity is a sensitive technique for detecting proximal DVT, but below the knee it is less accurate, giving excessive false-positive results.[217,237,238]

Impedance Plethysmography. Plethysmography is a noninvasive method to detect blood volume changes in the calf. Plethysmographic methods depend on recognition of two physiologic parameters that occur when thrombi occlude major veins of the leg: decreased venous compliance and increased venous outflow resistance.[217] Blood volume changes in the calf, produced by inflation and deflation of a pneumatic thigh cuff, are measured by the change in electrical resistance (impedance). This technique is sensitive and specific for total occlusions of the popliteal, superficial femoral, common femoral, and iliac veins but is relatively insensitive to partial occlusion at any level and to thrombi formed below the knee.[239] Therefore, a normal impedance plethysmogram essentially excludes a diagnosis of proximal DVT but does not exclude a diagnosis of calf vein thrombosis, a partially occlusive thrombus, or a thrombus in a paired or well-collateralized venous system.[217] Plethysmography is portable, inexpensive, and noninvasive and can be repeated as frequently as needed. The major disadvantages of this method are its insensitivity to calf vein thrombi and the many potential sources of error for patients in a critical care environment (ie, elevation of central venous pressure, peripheral arterial insufficiency, vasoconstriction, hypothermia, or low–cardiac output states). Therefore, plethysmography has limited use in the patient with a severe brain injury and multiple trauma. Nevertheless, a positive examination can be used to make therapeutic decisions in the absence of clinical conditions that are known to produce false-positive results.[240]

Duplex Ultrasonography. Duplex ultrasonography overcomes many of the limitations of Doppler ultrasonography and plethysmography. This hybrid noninvasive technology allows simultaneous B-mode imaging and Doppler insonation of the structure and blood flow in both superficial and deep veins, primary veins and their tributaries (ie, internal iliac, deep femoral), and single and duplicated venous systems (tibial, popliteal) from the ankle through the inferior vena cava.[217] Three signs of DVT are accepted by most investigators. The first sign of thrombosis is the inability to compress the vein completely. The second sign is that Doppler insonation demonstrates no flow through the noncompressible portion of the vein. The third sign is based on the B-mode ultrasound image of the thrombus.[241,242] The reported sensitivity and specificity of this technique is over 90%.[213] The technique is noninvasive and repeatable, but the instrumentation is expensive and technician dependent.

[125]I-Fibrinogen Leg Scan. This technique requires active incorporation of labeled fibrinogen as fibrin into the thrombus. It can detect calf vein thrombosis in more than 90% of patients but is insensitive to thrombi in the upper thigh and the pelvis.[243] It is rarely used to detect DVT due to the expense, radiation exposure, and insensitivity to proximal thrombus.

Radiographic Methods. Contrast venography is still the standard for providing an objective diagnosis of DVT. Ascending venography with good technique should outline the entire deep-venous system of the lower extremity, including the external and common iliac veins. Deep femoral and internal iliac veins are rarely visualized with this examination.[218] The patient must be transported to a radiologic suite, creating a problem in the patient with severe brain injury. Although considered the standard for diagnosis of DVT, venography should be reserved for use when noninvasive studies are equivocal, are technically inadequate, or cannot be performed.

CT and magnetic resonance imaging (MRI) are increasingly being applied to the diagnosis of DVT.[217] Both techniques provide a noninvasive assessment of the anatomy of the vena cava, the presence and extent of thrombus, and any associated extravascular pathology. MRI is advantageous in that it is noninvasive, does not require contrast injection, and can be repeated as needed. Both techniques are expensive and require the mobilization of a critical care patient to specialized areas, with associated risk.

For a patient in the ICU with severe brain injury, where the index of suspicion is high for DVT, and when associated injuries are present (ie, long bone fractures, spinal cord injuries, major abdominal procedures), duplex ultrasonography is recommended. There is no accepted guideline in determining the frequency of this examination in this population except sound clinical judgment. If this technique is not available, Doppler ultrasonography is an accepted alternative screening technique. The advantages of these methods include noninvasiveness and portability of the examination. CT or MRI may be reserved when suspicion of DVT is high in the iliofemoral area (ie, pelvic fracture, retroperitoneal hematoma) because the use of contrast venography is limited in these types of patients.

Management of DVT

The main goal of DVT therapy is to prevent PE. Thrombi at any level can cause PE, but most investigators agree that thrombi in the thigh are the most threatening.[218,244,245] When thrombi remain confined to the tibial veins, conservative management, including bed rest, leg elevation, and heat application, can be employed in the patient with severe brain injury. Regular screening surveillance by one of the methods discussed previously should accompany initial efforts to detect proximal extension into the popliteal and iliofemoral segments.

Standard management of proximal DVT includes anticoagulation with heparin initially and warfarin for up to three to six months. The safety of full anticoagulation treatment in the patient with severe brain injury, especially in the early days after trauma, has not been established. Furthermore, hemorrhage during heparin therapy can appear unpredictably in spite of close laboratory monitoring.[223] Judicial use of anticoagulation in the patient suffering severe brain injury is recommended. Some investigators suggest that anticoagulation use should be prohibited within five days of the craniotomy or the brain trauma.[222,231] The severity and nature of the intracranial damage, the presence of intracranial blood, and the extent of the associated injuries are important factors to consider before initiating anticoagulation therapy. If anticoagulation is contraindicated or is judged too risky in the patient with severe brain injury, methods to prevent PE by interruption of the inferior vena cava (IVC) should be employed in those patients with proven DVT. Several methods for IVC interruption have been developed. The most frequently used and tested are the Kim-Ray Greenfield filter[246] and, lately, the bird's nest filter.[247] These filters can be inserted through the jugular, axillary, or femoral vein and, when in proper position, are highly efficient in trapping emboli. Small emboli (diameter less than 3 mm) pass through the filter, but these are significant in less than 2% of patients. The mortality rate for the vena cava filter is less than 2% and is usually attributed to the underlying disease rather than the filter itself. Complications of filter insertion, such as wound or retroperitoneal hematoma, air embolism, vocal cord paralysis, infection, and filter malposition or migration, have been reported in less than 2% of patients.[217] The long-term results in filter durability and migration, prevention of emboli, and patency are unknown, however. Despite these uncertainties, IVC filters are recommended in those patients with DVT in the early period after severe brain injury because anticoagulation is considered risky in this population.

Pulmonary Embolism

Pulmonary embolism is the most devastating sequela of DVT, occurring in approximately 10% to 15% of patients with documented DVT.[217] However, usually a part of the thrombus embolizes, so the majority of patients with proved PE have residual thrombus on venography. PE develops when a loosely adherent or free-floating segment of a thrombus lying in the deep-venous system, the right side of the heart, or the main pulmonary artery is carried into the mainstream of the pulmonary circulation, thereby causing partial or complete occlusion of a major pulmonary artery or extensive obstruction of multiple small pulmonary arteries. PE can be caused by thrombi at any level but is more likely to be clinically significant in patients with thrombi in the deep veins of the leg.[217,222] Fewer than 10% of emboli arise from thrombi located in the axillary or the subclavian vein. The most common causes of axillary-vein thrombosis are repeated trauma and malignant disease.

A PE will either lyse, fragment, and shower distally or become organized, with chronic obstruction of the pulmonary artery. The ideal prevention of PE is an effective prophylaxis of DVT. The treatment of PE is designed to prevent recurrent emboli and to support cardiopulmonary function.

The mortality rate from a single PE has been reported to be as high as 20% after a single episode[222] and increases with any subsequent episode. Most patients survive if they are treated promptly and aggressively before a definitive diagnosis. PE is a frequent cause of death in hospitalized patients and has been reported in up to 10% of autopsies of patients who died postoperatively. The incidence of deaths among neurosurgical patients has been reported to be as high as 3%.[222,229] The incidence of fatal PE is unknown in patients with severe associated trauma. Death occurs almost exclusively in patients with initially compromised cardiac or pulmonary function, with massive or recurrent PE, or, most frequently, in patients who are not suspected of having PE and who therefore are neither diagnosed nor treated. The effects of PE depend on the size, the location, and, most important, the cardiorespiratory status of the patient. A large alveoloarterial difference occurs as areas are well ventilated but not perfused. Significant hypoxemia that is refractory to high doses of oxygen occurs. The acute obstruction in the pulmonary circulation and blood return to the left side of the heart may cause a severe pump failure, usually fatal if the underlying cardiovascular status of the patient is compromised. Small emboli in patients with normal cardiopulmonary function rarely result in death. However, similar emboli in patients with compromised cardiorespiratory function are associated with a 10% to 20% mortality.[217] Not only does preexisting cardiovascular disease determine the outcome of patients with PE, it also influences the course of the disease by slowing the rate of recovery of pulmonary artery blood flow.

Diagnosis of Pulmonary Embolism

The clinical presentation of PE depends on the size of the embolus, the status of the cardiopulmonary system, and the neurohumoral response to the embolism.

The clinical diagnosis of PE is even less accurate than that of DVT.[222] The principal symptom is intense chest pain that occurs at the time of embolization and frequently dissipates in a few hours. However, chest pain may be absent in up to 40% of patients with documented PE.[248] Dyspnea and tachypnea occur frequently; patients are usually tachycardic with or without supraventricular arrhythmias and may exhibit right ventricular gallop, rales, pleural friction rub, diaphoresis, or cyanosis.[217] Hypotension is observed in approximately 10% to 15% of patients with major emboli. Arterial hypoxemia is always more pronounced than would be expected for the patient's general condition. The chest X-ray and ECG may show nonspecific changes. The classic radiographic wedge-shaped or truncated cone density is very uncommon but, when seen, is specific for PE.[249] An ECG demonstrating an S in lead I and a Q in lead III along with tachycardia suggests PE. Although confirmation of DVT increases the risk of PE, failure to document DVT in the extremities does not rule out the possibility that an embolus has caused the acute symptoms.[217] Because the clinical diagnosis of PE is in error 50% to 60% of the time, a high index of suspicion is the only factor necessary to start a diagnostic workup for PE or even treatment of these patients. Confirmatory results by radiologic methods can follow later.

Lung Ventilation-Perfusion Scan. The perfusion lung scan is the most widely used technique for diagnosing PE (Figure 9–14). The scan uses intravenous injection of technetium-labeled macroaggregated human albumin microspheres. The perfusion lung scan images the blood flow in the pulmonary arterioles. To enhance the sensitivity and specificity of the scan, patients inhale a radioactive aerosol (generally an isotope of krypton, such as xenon-133) during the procedure to trace the distribution of ventilation. The hallmark of PE as seen on ventilation-perfusion lung scans is a segmental or larger perfusion defect (Figure 9–15) associated with a relatively normal chest X-ray and relatively intact ventilation. This finding is associated with a positive angiogram in 85% to 90% of patients.[217,250] The results of these studies are grouped into high, intermediate, or low probabilities. A high-probability scan accurately detected PE in more than 90% of cases, although sensitivity was low. An intermediate-probability scan was associated with a 30% rate of PE; even normal and low-probability scans were associated with an 11% rate of PE.[251]

Pulmonary Angiogram. Pulmonary angiogram remains the best tool to diagnose PE. This invasive technique has acceptably low mortality and morbidity rates, even in the presence of pulmonary hypertension.[217] The diagnosis is based on detecting intravascular filling defects or an abrupt arterial cutoff (Figure 9–16). The test is both sensitive and specific, and the false-negative rate is low.

The clinical condition of the patient is of utmost importance in deciding which diagnostic test to use in the patient with severe brain injury. Most of these patients

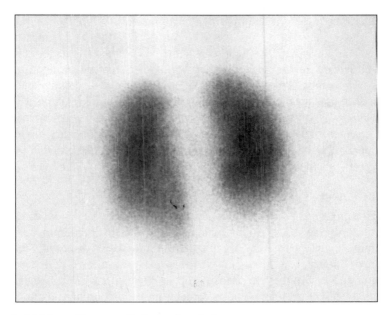

Figure 9–14 Normal lung ventilation and perfusion scan.

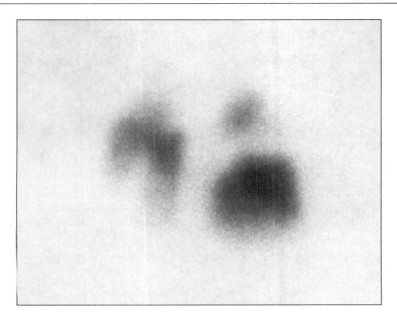

Figure 9–15 Large perfusion defect.

are intubated, and the ventilation part of the nuclear scan is less than optimal. If the patient is stable and the clinical suspicion for PE is not high, it is recommended that the ventilation-perfusion lung scan be the first method for diagnosis of PE. If the result is low probability, no further workup is necessary. A high-probability scan is sufficient basis to start therapy for PE if there are no contraindications. An intermediate scan should be followed by a pulmonary angiogram unless DVT has been diagnosed by one of the tests previously discussed. If the patient is hemodynamically unstable or if the chest X-ray is abnormal, pulmonary angiogram is recommended as the first diagnostic tool for diagnosing PE due to the low rate of false results.

Management of Pulmonary Embolism

Initial management of PE includes administration of oxygen, with endotracheal intubation in some cases, to treat hypoxia. Requirements for respiratory support will diminish rapidly as pulmonary blood flow returns toward normal. Fluid resuscitation to replace volume deficits is important to minimize peripheral hypoperfusion and to avoid hyperviscosity of the blood. Right heart catheterization with the Swan-Ganz thermodilution catheter provides a proper monitoring tool, especially for those patients with limited cardiorespiratory reserve or evidence of significant PE.

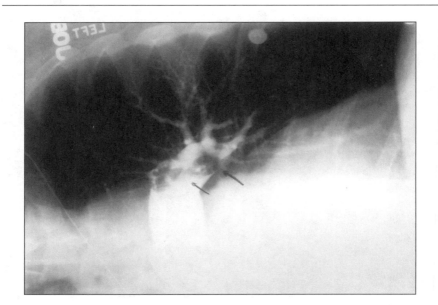

Figure 9–16 Significant intravascular filling defect in the left pulmonary artery.

Anticoagulation with intravenous heparin given initially as a bolus (5,000 to 10,000 U) and subsequently as a continuous infusion is the definitive therapy in those patients in whom the risk of intracranial bleeding is minimal. Heparin is usually continued for 7 to 10 days, maintaining the partial thromboplastin time at up to twice normal levels. Oral anticoagulation with warfarin is started soon after heparin and is continued for three to six months. The risk of further or recurrent intracranial bleeding in the patient with severe brain injury makes sound clinical judgment extremely important in the treatment of PE.

Thrombolytic therapy has been used successfully to augment endogenous fibrinolysis in a number of thrombotic conditions. Streptokinase, urokinase, and recombinant tissue–type plasminogen activator have proven very useful in these conditions. The use of this therapy in cases of severe brain injury is contraindicated in patients with injuries of less than two months' duration.[251]

Patients who suffer massive PE rarely become candidates for operative therapy. Most patients who die will succumb within one hour of the event.[217] In only a few patients is there sufficient time to consider pulmonary embolectomy and prepare the patient for surgery. Resuscitation in the ICU will obviate the need for operative intervention in most patients. However, persistence of a peripheral low flow state secondary to right heart failure constitutes an indication for heroic measures such as embolectomy. A pulmonary angiogram is mandatory in the patients for whom pulmonary embolectomy is considered. Surgical embolectomy with extracorporeal circulation is the best procedure, but the need of anticoagulation could be contraindicated in the patient with severe brain injury. Embolectomy, without thoracotomy using a suction catheter device, is possible but has not been widely accepted.

After sublethal PE has occurred, vena caval interruption can be used as a prophylactic measure to prevent further PE. This technique has been described above. Because of the potential for catastrophic hemorrhagic complications attendant to other therapies, vena caval interruption is frequently the only form of therapy used in the patients with PE and severe brain injury.

CONCLUSION

The vast majority of persons with severe brain injury will require some form of ventilatory support. A basic knowledge of airway management and respiratory physiology is crucial. An understanding of ventilatory mechanics and an awareness of different ventilatory options can have a direct influence on patient outcome.

Patients who are subject to a prolonged course of ventilator dependence will invariably incur some respiratory complications, the most common of which is pneumonia. Identifying risk factors for pulmonary complications can facilitate prevention or early treatment, which may affect mortality and morbidity.

REFERENCES

1. West JB. *Respiratory Physiology: The Essentials.* 3rd ed. Baltimore, Md: Williams & Wilkins; 1990.

2. Scanlon CL, Spearman CG, Sheldon RL. *Eagan's Fundamentals of Respiratory Care.* 6th ed. St Louis, Mo: Mosby-Year Book; 1995.

3. Dailey RH, Simon B, Young GP, Stewart RD. *The Airway: Emergency Management.* St Louis,Mo: Mosby-Year Book; 1992.

4. Pitt LH, Wagner FC. *Craniospinal Trauma.* New York, NY: Thieme Medical Publishers; 1990.

5. Fink ME. Emergency management of head-injured patient. *Emerg Med Clin North Am.* 1987;5:783–795.

6. Plum F, Posner JB. *The Diagnosis of Stupor and Coma.* 2nd ed. Philadelphia, Pa: FA Davis; 1972.

7. Teasdale G, Jennet B. Assessment of coma and impaired consciousness: a practical scale. *Lancet.* 1974;2:81–84.

8. Demling R, Riessen R. Pulmonary dysfunction after cerebral injury. *Crit Care Med.* 1990;18:768–774.

9. Moss IR, Wald A, Ransohoff J. Respiratory functions and chemical regulation of ventilation in head injury. *Am Rev Respir Dis.* 1974;109:205–214.

10. Frost EA, Arancibia CU, Shulman K. Pulmonary shunt as prognostic indicator in head injury. *J Neurosurg.* 1979;50:768–772.

11. Bloomfield EL. Extracerebral complications of head injury. *Crit Care Clin.* 1989;5:881–892.

12. Kennedy SK. *Airway Management and Respiratory Support: Neurological and Neurosurgical Intensive Care.* 3rd ed. New York, NY: Raven Press; 1993:69–95.

13. Redan JA, Livingston DH, Tortella BJ, Rush BF Jr. The value of intubating and paralyzing patients with suspected head injury in the emergency room. *J Trauma.* 1991;31:371–375.

14. Stauffer JL, Olson DE, Petty TL. Complications and consequences of endotracheal intubation and tracheotomy. *Am J Med.* 1981;70:65–76.

15. Lanza DC, Parnes SM, Koltai PJ, Fortune JB. Early complications of airway management in head-injured patients. *Laryngoscope.* 1990;100:958–961.

16. Mason MF, Meehan K, Hollinger CD. Tracheostomy and tracheostomy tubes. In: Mason MF, ed. *Speech Pathology for Tracheostomized and Ventilator Dependent Patients.* Newport Beach, Calif: Voicing Inc; 1993:154–157.

17. Whited RE. A prospective study of laryngotracheal sequelae in long-term intubation. *Laryngoscope.* 1984;94:367–377.

18. Dunham CM, LaMonica C. Prolonged tracheal intubation in the trauma patient. *J Trauma.* 1984;24:120–124.

19. Lanza DC, Koltai PJ, Parnes SM, Decker JW, et al. Predictive value of the Glasgow Coma Scale for tracheotomy in head injured patients. *Ann Otol Rhinol Laryngol.* 1990;99:38–41.

20. Lesnik I, Rappaport W, Fulginiti J, Witzke D. The role of early tracheostomy in blunt, multiple organ trauma. *Am Surg.* 1992;58:346–349.

21. Boyd SW, Benzel EC. The role of early tracheotomy in the management of the neurosurgical patient. *Laryngoscope.* 1992;102:559–562.

22. Rodriguez JL, Steinberg SM, Luchetti FA, Gibbons KJ, et al. Early tracheostomy for primary airway management in the surgical critical care setting. *Surgery.* 1990;108:655–659.

23. Klingbeil GE. Airway problems in patients with traumatic brain injury. *Arch Phys Med Rehabil.* 1988;69:493–495.

24. Jackson C. Tracheostomy. *Laryngoscope.* 1909;19:285–290.

25. Shelde CH, Pudenz RH, Freshwater DB, Crue BL. A new method of tracheostomy. *J Neurosurg.* 1955;12:428–431.

26. Toye FJ, Weinstein JD. A percutaneous tracheostomy device. *Surgery.* 1969;65:384–389.

27. Ciaglia P, Firshing R, Synie C. Elective percutaneous dilational tracheostomy: a new simple bedside procedure. Preliminary report. *Chest.* 1985;87:715–719.

28. Fernandez L, Norwood S, Roettger R, Eass D, et al. Bedside percutaneous tracheostomy with bronchoscopic guidance in critically ill patients. *Arch Surg.* 1996;131:129–132.

29. Barba CA, Angood PB, Kauder DR, Latenser B, et al. Bronchoscopic guidance makes percutaneous tracheostomy a safe, cost-effective, and easy-to-teach procedure. *Surgery.* 1995;118: 879–883.

30. Toursarkissian B, Zweng TN, Kearney PA, Pofahl WE, et al. Percutaneous dilational tracheostomy: report of 141 cases. *Ann Thorac Surg.* 1994;57:862–867

31. Manara AR. Experience with percutaneous tracheostomy in intensive care: the technique of choice? *Br J Oral Maxillofac Surg.* 1994;32:155–160.

32. Friedman Y, Franklin C. The technique of percutaneous tracheostomy. *J Crit Ill.* 1993;8: 289–297.

33. Friedman Y, Mayer AD. Bedside percutaneous tracheostomy in critically ill patients. *Chest.* 1993;104:532–535.

34. Leinhardt DJ, Mughal J, Bowles B, Glew R, et al. Appraisal of percutaneous tracheostomy. *Br J Surg.* 1992;79:255–258.

35. Ciaglia P, Granieri KD. Percutaneous dilational tracheostomy: results and long-term follow-up. *Chest.* 1992;107:464–467.

36. Hazard P, Jones C, Bonitone J. Comparative clinical trial of standard operative tracheostomy with percutaneous tracheostomy. *Crit Care Med.* 1991;19:1018–1024.

37. Fischler MP, Kuhn M, Cantieni R, Frutiger A. Late outcome of percutaneous dilational tracheostomy in intensive care patients. *Intensive Care Med.* 1995;21:475–481.

38. McFarlane C, Denholm SW, Sudlow CL, Moralee SJ, et al. Laryngotracheal stenosis: a serious complication of percutaneous tracheostomy. *Anaesthesia.* 1994;49:38–40.

39. Slusky AS. American College of Chest Physicians' Consensus Conference: mechanical ventilation. *Chest.* 1993;104:1833–1859.

40. Pierson DJ. Complications associated with mechanical ventilation. *Crit Care Clin.* 1990;6:711–724.

41. Branson RD, Chatburn RL. Technical description and classification of modes of ventilator operation. *Respir Care.* 1992;37:1026–1044.

42. Cooper KR, Boswell PA, Choi SC. Safe use of PEEP in patients with severe head injury. *J Neurosurg.* 1985;63 552–555.

43. Kirby RB, Banner MJ, Downs JB. *Clinical Application of Ventilatory Support.* New York, NY: Churchill Livingstore; 1990.

44. Hewlett Packard, Inc. *Hewlett Packard Component Monitoring System User Guide.* 4th ed. 1990.

45. Kerr ME, Rudy EB, Brucia J, Stone KS. Head-injured adults: recommendations for endotracheal suctioning. *J Neurosci Nurs.* 1993;25:86–91.

46. Rudy EB, Turner BS, Baun M, Stone KS, et al. Endotracheal suctioning in adults with head injury. *Heart Lung.* 1991;20:667–674.

47. Piek J, Chesnut RM, Marshall LF, van Berkum-Clark M, et al. Extracranial complications of severe head injury. *J Neurosurg.* 1992;77:901–907.

48. Bryan CS, Reynolds KL. Bacteremic nosocomial pneumonia: analysis of 172 episodes from a single metropolitan area. *Am Rev Respir Dis.* 1984;129:668–671.

49. Cross AS, Roup B. Role of respiratory assistance devices in endemic nosocomial pneumonia. *Am J Med.* 1981;70:681–685.

50. Craven DE, Kunches LM, Kilinsky V, Lichtenberg DA, et al. Risk factors for pneumonia and fatality in patient receiving continuous mechanical ventilation. *Am Rev Respir Dis.* 1986; 133:792–796.

51. Sherry T, Morgan AS, Hirvela E. Traumatic versus non-traumatic pneumonias in the intensive care unit. *Crit Care Med.* 1990;18(suppl):S189.

52. Torres A, Aznar R, Gatell JM, Jimenez P, et al. Incidence, risk, and prognosis factors of nosocomial pneumonia in mechanically ventilated patients. *Am Rev Respir Dis.* 1990;142:523–528.

53. Chevret S, Hemmer M, Carlet J, Langer M. Incidence and risk factors of pneumonia acquired in intensive care units: results from a multicenter prospective study of 996 patients. European Cooperative Group on Nosocomial Pneumonia. *Intensive Care Med.* 1993;19:256–264.

54. Helling TS, Evan LL, Fowler DL, Hays LV, et al. Infectious complications in patients with severe head injury. *J Trauma.* 1988;28:1575–1577.

55. Caplan ES, Hoyt N. Infection surveillance and control in the severely traumatized patient. *Am J Med.* 1981;70:638–640.

56. Morgan AS. Risk factors for infection in the trauma patient. *J Natl Med Assoc.* 1992;84:1019–1023.

57. O'Mahony JB, Palder SB, Wood JJ, McIrvine A, et al. Depression of cellular immunity after multiple trauma in the absence of sepsis. *J Trauma.* 1984;24:869–875.

58. Renk CM, Long CL, Blakemore WS. Comparison between in vitro lymphocyte activity and metabolic changes in trauma patients. *J Trauma.* 1982;22:134–140.

59. Hershman MJ, Cheadle WG, George CD, Cost KM, et al. The response of immunoglobulins to infection after thermal and nonthermal injury. *Am Surg.* 1988;54:408–411.

60. Unanue ER, Allen PM. The basis for immunoregulatory role of macrophages and other accessory cells. *Science.* 1987;236:551–557.

61. Sackner MA, Landa JF, Greeneltch N, Robinson MJ. Pathogenesis and prevention of tracheobronchial damage with suction procedures. *Chest.* 1973;64:284–290.

62. Johanson WG Jr, Pierce AK, Sanford JP, Thomas GD. Nosocomial respiratory infections with gram-negative bacilli: the significance of colonization of the respiratory tract. *Ann Intern Med.* 1972;77:701–706.

63. Barish CF, Wu WC, Castell DO. Respiratory complications of gastroesophageal reflux. *Arch Intern Med.* 1985;145:1882–1888.

64. Mackay LE, Morgan AS. Early swallowing disorders with severe head injury: relationships between RLA and the progression of oral intake. *Dysphagia.* 1993;8:161.

65. duMoulin GC, Paterson DG, Hedley-Whyte J, Lisbon A. Aspiration of gastric bacteria in antacid-treated patients: a frequent cause of postoperative colonization of the airway. *Lancet.* 1982;1:242–245.

66. Atherton ST, White DJ. Stomach as source of bacteria colonising respiratory tract during artificial ventilation. *Lancet.* 1978;2:968–969.

67. Hastings PR, Skillman JJ, Bushness LS, Silen W. Antacid titration in the prevention of acute gastrointestinal bleeding: a controlled, randomized trial of 100 critically ill patients. *N Engl J Med.* 1978;298:1041–1045.

68. Driks MR, Craven DE, Celli BR, Manning M, et al. Nosocomial pneumonia in intubated patients given sucralfate as compared with antacids or histamine type 2 blockers: the role of gastric colonization. *N Engl J Med.* 1987;317:1376–1382.

69. Tryba M. Risk of acute stress bleeding and nosocomial pneumonia in ventilated intensive care unit patients: sucralfate versus antacids. *Am J Med.* 1987;83:117–124.

70. Celis R, Torres A, Gatell JM, Almela M, et al. Nosocomial pneumonia: a multivariate analysis of risk and prognosis. *Chest.* 1988;93 318–324.

71. Haley RW, Hooton TM, Culver DH, Stanley RC, et al. Nosocomial infections in US hospitals, 1975–1976: estimated frequency by selected characteristics of patients. *Am J Med.* 1981;70: 947–959.

72. Reinarz JA, Pierce AK, Mays BB, Sanford JP. Potential role of inhalation therapy equipment in nosocomial pulmonary infection. *J Clin Invest.* 1965;44:831–839.

73. Craven DE, Goularte TA, Make BJ. Contaminated condensate in mechanical ventilator circuits: a risk factor for nosocomial pneumonia? *Am Rev Respir Dis.* 1984;129:625–628.

74. Craven DE, Connolly MG Jr, Lichtenberg DA, Primeau PJ, et al. Contamination of mechanical ventilators with tubing changes every 24 or 48 hours. *N Engl J Med.* 1982;306:1505–1509.

75. Hauser WE Jr, Remington JS. Effect of antibiotics on the immune response. *Am J Med.* 1982;72:711–716.

76. Espersen F, Gabrielsen J. Pneumonia due to *Staphylococcus aureus* during mechanical ventilation. *J Infect Dis.* 1981;144:19–23.

77. Hsieh AH, Bishop MJ, Kubilis PS, Newell DW, et al. Pneumonia following closed head injury. *Am Rev Respir Dis.* 1992;146:290–294.

78. Woratyla SP, Morgan AS, Mackay L, Bernstein B, et al. Factors associated with early onset pneumonia in the severely brain-injured patient. *Conn Med.* 1995;59:643–647.

79. Stoutenbeek CP, van Saene HK, Miranda DR, Zandstra DF, et al. The effect of oropharyngeal decontamination using topical nonabsorbable antibiotics on the incidence of nosocomial respiratory tract infections in multiple trauma patients. *J Trauma.* 1987;27:357–364.

80. Langer M, Cigada M, Mandelli M. Mosconi P, et al. Early onset pneumonia: a multicenter study in intensive care units. *Intensive Care Med.* 1987;13:342–346.

81. Rello J, Ausina V, Castella J, Net A, et al. Nosocomial respiratory tract infections in multiple trauma patients: influence of level of consciousness with implications for therapy. *Chest.* 1992;102:525–529.

82. Rodriguez JL, Gibbons KJ, Bitzer LG, Dechert RE, et al. Pneumonia: incidence, risk factors, and outcome in injured patients. *J Trauma.* 1991;31:907–912.

83. Rello J, Quintana E, Ausina V, Puzo C, et al. Risk factors for *Staphylococcus aureus* nosocomial pneumonia in critically ill patients. *Am Rev Respir Dis.* 1990;142:1320–1324.

84. Miller EH Jr, Caplan ES. Nosocomial *Hemophilus* pneumonia in patients with severe trauma. *Surg Gynecol Obstet.* 1984;159:153–156.

85. Teasdale G, Jennett B. Assessment of coma and impaired consciousness: a practical scale. *Lancet.* 1974;2:81–84.

86. Rein MF, Gwaltney JM Jr, O'Brien WM, Jennings RH, et al. Accuracy of Gram's stain in identifying pneumococci in sputum. *JAMA.* 1978;239:2671–2673.

87. Leach RP, Coonrod JD. Detection of pneumococcal antigens in the sputum of pneumococcal pneumonia. *Am Rev Respir Dis.* 1977;116:847–851.

88. Winterbauer RH, Dreis DF. New diagnostic approaches to the hospitalized patient with pneumonia. *Semin Respir Infect.* 1987;2:57–66.

89. Tobin MJ. Diagnosis of pneumonia: techniques and problems. *Clin Chest Med.* 1987;8:513–527.

90. Feeley TW, DuMoulin GC, Hedley-Whyte J, Bushness LS, et al. Aerosol polymyxin and pneumonia in seriously ill patients. *N Engl J Med.* 1975;293:471–475.

91. Stoutenbeek CP, van Saene HK, Miranda DR, Zandstra DF. The effect of selective decontamination of the digestive tract on colonisation and infection rate in multiple trauma patients. *Intensive Care Med.* 1984;10:185–192.

92. Unertl K, Ruckdeschel G, Selbmann HK, Jensen U, et al. Prevention of colonization and respiratory infections in long-term ventilated patients by local antimicrobial prophylaxis. *Intensive Care Med.* 1987;13:106–113.

93. Ledingham IM, Alcock SR, Eastaway AT, McDonald JC, et al. Triple regimen of selective decontamination of the digestive tract, systemic cefotaxime, and microbiological surveillance for prevention of acquired infection in intensive care. *Lancet.* 1988;1:785–790.

94. Moore FA, Moore EE, Jones TN, McCrosky, et al. TEN versus TPN following major abdominal trauma: reduced septic morbidity. *J Trauma.* 1989;29:916–922.

95. Hadley MN, Grahm TW, Harrington T, Schiller WR, et al. Nutritional support and neurotrauma: a critical review of early nutrition in forty-five acute head injury patients. *Neurosurgery.* 1986;19:367–373.

96. Grahm TW, Zadrozny DB, Harrington T. The benefits of early jejunal hyperalimentation in the head-injured patient. *Neurosurgery.* 1989;25:729–735.

97. Kirby DF, Clifton GL, Turner H, Marion DW, et al. Early enteral nutrition after brain injury by percutaneous endoscopic gastrojejunostomy. *JPEN.* 1991;15:298–302.

98. Ott L, Young B, Phillips R, McClain C, et al. Altered gastric emptying in the head-injured patient: relationships to feeding intolerance. *J Neurosurg.* 1991;74:738–742.

99. Saxe JM, Ledgerwood AM, Lucas CE, Lucas WF. Lower esophageal sphincter dysfunction precludes safe gastric feeding after head injury. *J Trauma.* 1994;37:581–584.

100. Wanner A, Rao A. Clinical indications for and effects of bland, mucolytic, and antimicrobial aerosols. *Am Rev Respir Dis.* 1980;122:79–87.

101. Major RH. Hippocrates. In: *Classic Descriptions of Disease,* ed. Major RH. Springfield, Ill: Charles C Thomas; 1968.

102. Bartlett JG. Bacterial infections of the pleural space. *Semin Respir Infect.* 1988;3:308–321.

103. Light RW, Girard WM, Jenkinson SG, George RB. Parapneumonic effusions. *Am J Med.* 1980;69:507–512.

104. Kelly JW, Morris MJ. Empyema thoracis: medical aspects of evaluation and treatment. *South Med J.* 1994;87:1103–1110.

105. Eddy AC, Luna GK, Copass M. Empyema thoracis in patients undergoing emergent closed tube thoracostomy for thoracic trauma. *Am J Surg.* 1989;157:494–497.

106. Caplan ES, Hoyt NJ, Rodriguez A, Cowley RA. Empyema occurring in the multiply traumatized patient. *J Trauma.* 1984;24:785–789.

107. Arom KV, Grover FL, Richardson JD, Trinkle JK. Posttraumatic empyema. *Ann Thoracic Surg.* 1977;23:254–258.

108. Alfageme I, Munoz F, Pena N, Umbria S. Empyema of the thorax in adults: etiology, microbiologic findings, and management. *Chest.* 1993;103:839–843.

109. Ashbaugh DG. Empyema thoracis: factors influencing morbidity and mortality. *Chest.* 1991;99:1162–1165.

110. Berger HA, Morganroth ML. Immediate drainage is not required for all patients with complicated parapneumonic effusions. *Chest.* 1990;97:731–735.

111. Barragry TP, Humphrey EW. Management of adult postpneumonic thoracic empyema. *Infect Surg.* July 1990:5–8.

112. Muskett A, Burton NA, Karwande SV, Collins MP. Management of refractory empyema with early decortication. *Am J Surg.* 1988;156:529–532.

113. Van Way C III, Narrod J, Hopeman A. The role of early limited thoracotomy in the treatment of empyema. *J Thorac Cardiovasc Surg.* 1988;96:436–439.

114. Wehr CJ, Adams RB Jr. Empyema thoracis: a ten-year experience. *South Med J.* 1986;79:171–176.

115. Grant DR, Finley RJ. Empyema: analysis of treatment techniques. *Can J Surg.* 1985;28:449–451.

116. Lemmer JH, Botham MJ, Orringer MB. Modern management of adult thoracic empyema. *J Thorac Cardiovasc Surg.* 1985;90:849–855.

117. Frimodt-Moller PC, Vejlsted H. Early surgical intervention in non-specific pleural empyema. *Thorac Cardiovasc Surg.* 1985;33:41–43.

118. LeBlanc KA, Tucker WY. Empyema of the thorax. *Surg Gynecol Obstet.* 1984;158:66–70.

119. Weese WC, Shindler ER, Smith IM, Rabinovich S. Empyema of the thorax then and now: a study of 122 cases over four decades. *Arch Intern Med.* 1973;131:516–520.

120. LeMense GP, Strange C, Sahn S. Empyema thoracis: therapeutic management and outcome. *Chest.* 1995;107:1532–1537.

121. Sadigh M, Wassef W. Parapneumonic effusions and empyema. *Curr Opin Infect Dis.* 1990;3:189–194.

122. Moran JF. Surgical management of pleural space infections. *Semin Respir Infect.* 1988;3:383–394.

123. Mavroudis C, Symmonds JB, Minagi H, Thomas AN. Improved survival in management of empyema thoracis. *J Thorac Cardiovasc Surg.* 1981;82:49–57.

124. Lee KS, Im JG, Kim YH, Hwang SH, et al. Treatment of thoracic multiloculated empyema with intracavitary urokinase: a prospective study. *Radiology.* 1991;179:771–775.

125. Crouch JD, Keagy BA, Delaney DJ. "Pigtail" catheter drainage in thoracic surgery. *Am Rev Respir Dis.* 1987;136:174–175.

126. Tillet WS, Sherry S, Read CT. The use of streptokinase-streptodornase in the treatment of chronic empyema. *J Thorac Surg.* 1951;21:325–341.

127. Taylor RF, Rubens MB, Pearson MC, Barnes NC. Intrapleural streptokinase in the management of empyema. *Thorax.* 1994;49:856–859.

128. Henke CA, Leatherman JW. Intrapleurally administered streptokinase in the treatment of acute loculated nonpurulent parapneumonic effusions. *Am Rev Respir Dis.* 1992;145:680–684.

129. Aye RW, Froese DP, Hill LD. Use of purified streptokinase in empyema and hemothorax. *Am J Surg.* 1991;161:560–562.

130. Orringer MB. Thoracic empyema: back to basics. *Chest.* 1988;93:901–902.

131. Sendt W, Forster E, Hau T. Early thoracoscopic debridement and drainage as definite treatment for pleural empyema. *Eur J Surg.* 1995;161:73–76.

132. O'Brien J, Cohen M, Solit R, Lindenbaum G, et al. Thoracoscopic drainage and decorticiation as definitive treatment for empyema thoracis following penetrating chest injury. *J Trauma.* 1994;36:536–539.

133. Ridley PD, Braimbridge MV. Thoracoscopic debridement and pleural irrigation in the management of empyema thoracis. *Ann Thorac Surg.* 1991;51:461–464.

134. Pennza PT. Aspiration pneumonia, necrotizing pneumonia, and lung abscess. *Emerg Med Clin North Am.* 1989;7:279–307.

135. Finegold SM, George WL, Mulligan ME. Anaerobic infections: part I. *Dis Mon.* 1985;31:1–77.

136. Johanson WG Jr, Harris GD. Aspiration pneumonia, anaerobic infections and lung abscess. *Med Clin North Am.* 1980;64:385–394.

137. Clinical conferences at the Johns Hopkins Hospital: lung abscess. *Johns Hopkins Med J.* 1982;150:141–147.

138. Bartlett JG. Anaerobic bacterial infections of the lung. *Chest.* 1987;91:901–909.

139. Smith DT. Medical treatment of acute and chronic pulmonary abscess. *J Thorac Surg.* 1948;17:52–72.

140. Brook I, Finegold SM. Bacteriology of aspiration pneumonia in children. *Pediatrics.* 1980;65:1115–1120.

141. Estrera AS, Platt MR, Mills LJ, Shaw RR. Primary lung abscess. *J Thorac Cardiovasc Surg.* 1980;79:275–282.

142. Lambiase RE, Deyoe L, Cronan JJ, Dorfman GS. Percutaneous drainage of 335 consecutive abscesses: results of primary drainage with 1 year follow-up. *Radiology.* 1992;184:167–179.

143. van Sonnenberg E, D'Agostino HB, Casola G, Wittich GR, et al. Lung abscess: CT guided drainage. *Radiology.* 1991;178:347–351.

144. Wauchob TD, Brooks RJ, Harrison KM. Neurogenic pulmonary oedema. *Anaesthesia.* 1984;39:529–534.

145. Casey WF. Neurogenic pulmonary oedema. *Anaesthesia.* 1983;38:985–988.

146. Yabumoto M, Kuriyama T, Iwamoto M, Kinoshita T. Neourugenic pulmonary edema associated with ruptured intracranial aneurysm: case report. *Neurosurgery.* 1986;19:300–304.

147. Schell AR, Shenoy MM, Friedman SA, Patel AR. Pulmonary edema associated with subarachnoid hemorrhage. *Arch Intern Med.* 1987;147:591–592.

148. Carlson RW, Schaeffer RC Jr, Michaels SG, Weil MH. Pulmonary edema following intracranial hemorrhage. *Chest.* 1979;75:731–734.

149. Fredberg U, Botker HE, Romer FK. Acute neurogenic pulmonary oedema following generalized tonic clonic seizures: a case report and a review of the literature. *Eur Heart J.* 1988;9:933–936.

150. Benassi G. Traumatismes cranio-encephaliques et oedeme pulmonaire. *Paris Med.* 1937;103:525.

151. Moutier F. Hypertension et mort par œdema aigu chez les blessés cranio-encephaliques (relation de ces faits aux recherches recentes sur les fonctions des capsules surrenales). *Presse Med.* 1918;16:108–109.

152. Olmacher AP. Acute pulmonary edema as a terminal event in some forms of epilepsy. *Am J Med Sci.* 1910;139:417–422.

153. Shanakan WI. Acute pulmonary edema as a complication of epileptic seizures. *NY State J Med.* 1908;87:54–56.

154. Weisman BS. Edema and congestion of the lung resulting from intracranial hemorrhage. *Surgery.* 1939;6:722–729.

155. Harari A, Rabin M, Regnier B, et al. Normal pulmonary-capillary pressures in the late phase of neurogenic pulmonary oedema. *Lancet.* 1976;1:494.

156. Starling EH. On the absorption of fluids from the connective tissue spaces. *J Physiol.* 1896; 19:312–326.

157. Theodore J, Robin ED. Pathogenesis of neurogenic pulmonary oedema. *Lancet.* 1975;2:749–751.

158. Chen HI, Sun SC, Chai CY. Pulmonary edema and hemorrhage resulting from cerebral compression. *Am J Physiol.* 1973;224:223–229.

159. Newman MM, Kligerman M, Willcox M. Pulmonary hypertension, pulmonary edema, and decreased pulmonary compliance produced by increased ICP in cats. *J Neurosurg.* 1984;60:1207–1213.

160. Simon RP, Bayne LL, Tranbaugh RF, Lewis FR. Elevated pulmonary lymph flow and protein content during status epilepticus in sheep. *J Appl Physiol.* 1982;52:91–95.

161. Bean JW, Beckman DL. Centrogenic pulmonary pathology in mechanical head injury. *J Appl Physiol.* 1969;27:807–812.

162. Ducker TB, Simmons RL. Increased intracranial pressure and pulmonary edema. 2. The hemodynamic response of dogs and monkeys to increased intracranial pressure. *J Neurosurg.* 1968; 28:118–123.

163. Maire FW, Patton HD. Neural structures involved in the genesis of preoptic pulmonary edema, gastric erosions, and behavior changes. *Am J Physiol.* 1956;184:345–350.

164. Doba N, Reis DJ. Acute fulminating neurogenic hypertension produced by brainstem lesions in the rat. *Circ Res.* 1973;32:584–593.

165. Simmons RL, Martin AM Jr, Heisterkamp CA III, Ducker TB. Respiratory insufficiency in combat casualties. II. Pulmonary edema following head injury. *Ann Surg.* 1969;170:39–44.

166. Sarnoff SJ, Sarnoff LC. Neurohemodynamics of pulmonary edema. Part II. The role of sympathetic pathways in the elevation of pulmonary and systemic vascular pressures following the intracisternal injection of fibrin. *Circulation.* 1952;6:51–62.

167. Colice GL. Neurogenic pulmonary edema. *Clin Chest Med.* 1985 5:473–489.

168. Luisada AA. Mechanisms of neurogenic pulmonary edema. *Am J Cardiol.* 1967;20:66–68.

169. Malik AB. Pulmonary vascular response to increase in intracranial pressure: role of sympathetic mechanisms. *J Appl Physiol.* 1977;42:335–343.

170. Kellner M, Maklari E, Kovach AG, et al. The role of central nervous system in the pathomechanism of epinephrine-induced pulmonary oedema. *Acta Med Acad Sci Hung.* 1966; 22:335–340.

171. Ducker TB. Increased intracranial pressure and pulmonary edema. 1. Clinical study of 11 patients. *J Neurosurg.* 1968;28:112–117.

172. Weir BK. Pulmonary edema following fatal aneursym rupture. *J Neurosurg.* 1978;49:502–507.

173. Rogers FB, Shackford SR, Trevisani GT, Davis JW, et al. Neurogenic pulmonary edema in fatal and nonfatal head injuries. *J Trauma.* 1995;39:860–866.

174. Baigelman W, O'Brien JC. Pulmonary effects of head trauma. *Neurosurgery.* 1981;9:729–740.

175. Braude N, Ludgrove T. Neurogenic pulmonary oedema precipitated by induction of anaesthesia. *Br J Anaesth.* 1989;62:101–103.

176. Terrence CF, Rao GR, Perper JA. Neurogenic pulmonary edema in unexpected, unexplained death of epileptic patients. *Ann Neurol.* 1981;9:458–464.

177. Loughnan PM, Brown TC, Edis B, Klug GL. Neurogenic pulmonary oedema in man: aetiology and management with vasodilators based on haemodynamic studies. *Anaesth Intensive Care.* 1980;8:65–71.

178. Wrap NP, Nicotra MB. Pathogenesis of neurogenic pulmonary edema. *Am Rev Respir Dis.* 1978;118:783–786.

179. Mackersie RC, Christensen JM, Pitts LH, Lewis FR. Pulmonary extravascular fluid accumulation following intracranial injury. *J Trauma.* 1983;23:968–975.

180. Fein IA, Rackow EC. Neurogenic pulmonary edema. *Chest.* 1982;81:318–320.

181. Fisher A, Aboul-Nasr HT. Delayed nonfatal pulmonary edema following subarachnoid hemorrhage. *J Neurosurg.* 1979;51:856–859.

182. Wohns RN, Kerstein MD. The role of Dilantin in the prevention of pulmonary edema associated with cerebral hypoxia. *Crit Care Med.* 1982;10:436–443.

183. James HE, Tsueda K, Wright B, Young AB. The effect of positive end-expiratory pressure (PEEP) ventilation in neurogenic pulmonary oedema: report of a case. *Acta Neurochir.* 1978;43:275–280.

184. Luce JM, Huseby JS, Kirk W, Butler J. A Starling resistor regulates cerebral venous outflow in dogs. *J Appl Physiol.* 1982;53:1496–1503.

185. Luce JM, Huseby JS, Kirk W, Butler J. Mechanism by which positive end-expiratory pressure increases cerebrospinal fluid pressure in dogs. *J Appl Physiol.* 1982;52:231–235.

186. Appuzo JL, Wiess MH, Petersons V, Small RB, et al. Effect of positive end expiratory pressure ventilation on intracranial pressure in man. *J Neurosurg.* 1977;46:227–232.

187. Shapiro HM, Marshall LF. Intracranial pressure responses to PEEP in head-injury patients. *J Trauma.* 1978;18:254–256.

188. Colice GL, Matthay MA, Bass E, Matthay RA. Neurogenic pulmonary edema. *Am Rev Respir Dis.* 1984;130:941–948.

189. Kosnik EJ, Paul SE, Rossel CW, Sayers MP. Central neurogenic pulmonary edema: with a review of its pathogenesis and treatment. *Child's Brain.* 1977;3:37–47.

190. Grasberger RC, Spatz EL, Mortara RW, Ordia JI, et al. Effects of high-frequency ventilation versus conventional mechanical ventilation on IP in head-injured dog. *J Neurosurg.* 1984;60:1214–1218.

191. Wauchob TD, Brooks RJ, Harrison KM. Neurogenic pulmonary oedema. *Anaesthesia.* 1984;39:529–534.

192. Nathan MA, Ries DJ. Fulminating arterial hypertension with pulmonary edema from release of adrenomedullary catecholamines after lesions of the anterior hypothalamus in the rat. *Circ Res.* 1975;37:226–235.

193. Wohns RN, Tamas L, Pierce KR, Howe JF. Chlorpromazine treatment for neurogenic pulmonary edema. *Crit Care Med.* 1985;13:210–211.

194. Knudsen F, Jensen HP, Petersen PL. Neurogenic pulmonary edema: treatment with dobutamine. *Neurosurgery.* 1991;29:269–270.

195. Matthay MA. The adult respiratory distress syndrome: definition and prognosis. *Clin Chest Med.* 1990; 11:575–580.

196. Case SC, Sabo CE. Adult respiratory distress syndrome: a deadly complication of trauma. *Focus Crit Care.* 1992;19:116–121.

197. Walker ML. Trauma: adult respiratory distress syndrome. *J N M Assoc.* 1991;83:501–504.

198. Ashbaugh DG, Bigelow DB, Petty TL, Levine BE. Acute respiratory distress in adults. *Lancet.* 1967;2:319–323.

199. Rinaldo JE, Christian JW. Mechanisms and mediators of the adult respiratory distress syndrome. *Clin Chest Med.* 1990;11:621–632.

200. Hudson LD, Milberg JA, Anardi D, Maunder RJ. Clinical risks for the development of the acute respiratory distress syndrome. *Am J Respir Crit Care Med.* 1995;151:293–301.

201. Hoyt DB, Simons RK, Winchell RJ, Cushman J, et al. A risk analysis of pulmonary complications following major trauma. *J Trauma.* 1993;35:524–531.

202. Hoch RC, Rodriguez R, Manning T, Bishop M. Effects of accidental trauma on cytokine and endotoxin production. *Crit Care Med.* 1993;21:839–845.

203. Roumen RM, Hendriks T, van der Ven-Jongekrijg J, Nieuwenhuijzen GA, et al. Cytokine patterns in patients after major vascular surgery, hemorrhagic shock and severe blunt trauma: relation with subsequent adult respiratory distress syndrome and multiple organ failure. *Ann Surg.* 1993:218:769–776.

204. Dunham CM, Frankenfield D, Belzberg H, Wiles CE II, et al. Inflammatory markers: superior predictors of adverse outcome in blunt trauma patients? *Crit Care Med.* 1994;22:667–672.

205. Rivkind AI, Siegel JH, Guadalupi P, Littleton M. Sequential patterns of eicosanoid, platelet, and neutrophil interactions in the evolution of the fulminant post-traumatic adult respiratory distress syndrome. *Ann Surg.* 1989;210:355–372.

206. Tomashefski JF Jr. Pulmonary pathology of the adult respiratory distress syndrome. *Clin Chest Med.* 1990;11:593–619.

207. Pison U, Seeger W, Buchhorn R, Joka T, et al. Surfactant abnormalities in patients with respiratory failure after multiple trauma. *Am Rev Respir Dis.* 1989;140:1033–1039.

208. Marini JJ. Lung mechanics in the adult respiratory distress syndrome: recent conceptual advances and implications for management. *Clin Chest Med.* 1990;11:673–690.

209. Stoller JK, Kacmarek RM. Ventilatory strategies in the management of the adult respiratory distress syndrome. *Clin Chest Med.* 1990;11:755–772.

210. Tharratt RS, Allen RP, Albertson TE. Pressure controlled inverse ratio ventilation in severe adult respiratory failure. *Chest* 1988;94:755–762.

211. Lain DC, DiBenedetto R, Morris SL, Van Nguyen A, et al. Pressure control inverse ratio ventilation as a method to reduce peak inspiratory pressure and provide adequate ventilation and oxygenation. *Chest.* 1989;95:1081–1088.

212. Jonson B, Lachmann B. Setting and monitoring of high-frequency jet ventilation in severe respiratory distress syndrome. *Crit Care Med.* 1989;17:1020–1024.

213. Goldstein G, Luce JM. Pharmacologic treatment of the adult respiratory distress syndrome. *Clin Chest Med.* 1990;11:773–787.

214. Fink M, Pearl R. Nitric oxide: its role in sepsis and ARDS. *Point/Counterpoint Intensivist.* 1995;4:1–6.

215. Bauer, PT, Machovich R, Aranyi, P, Buki KG, et al. Mechanisms of thrombin binding to endothelial cells. *Blood.* 1983; 61:368–372.

216. Crandon AJ, Peel, KR, Anderson JA, Thompson V, et al. Prophylaxis of postoperative deep vein thrombosis: selective use of low-dose heparin in high risk patients. *Br Med J.* 1980;281:345–347.

217. Bush HL. Venous thromboembolic disease. In: Barie PS, Shires GT, eds. *Surgical Intensive Care.* Boston, Mass: Little, Brown and Co; 1993:477–518.

218. Knudson MM, Collins JA, Goodman SB, McCrory DW. Thromboembolism following multiple trauma. *J Trauma.* 1992;32:2–11.

219. Shackford SR, Moser KM. Deep venous thrombosis and pulmonary embolism in trauma patients. *J Intensive Care Med.* 1988;3:87–98.

220. Huisman MV, Buller HR, ten Cate JW, van Royen EA, et al. Unexpected high prevalence of silent pulmonary embolism in patients with deep venous thrombosis. *Chest.* 1989;95:498–502.

221. Monreal M, Ruiz J, Olazabal A, Arias A, et al. Deep venous thrombosis and the risk of pulmonary embolism. *Chest.* 1992;102:677–681.

222. Swann KW, Black PM. Deep vein thrombosis and pulmonary emboli in neurosurgical patients: a review. *J Neurosurg.* 1984;61:1055–1062.

223. Coller BS. Platelets and thrombolytic therapy. *N Engl J Med.* 1990;322:33–42.

224. Niewiarowski S, Regoeczi E, Stewart CJ, Senyl AF, et al. Platelet interaction with polymerizing fibrin. *J Clin Invest.* 1972;51:685–699.

225. Breddin HK. Thrombosis and Virchow's triad: what is established? *Semin Thromb Hemost.* 1989;15:237–239.

226. Thomas ML, O'Dwyer JA. Site of origin of deep vein thrombosis in the calf. *Acta Radiol Diagn (Stockholm).* 1977;18:418–424.

227. Stamatakis JD, Kakkar VV, Lawrence D, Bentley PG. The origin of thrombi in the deep veins of the lower limb: a venographic study. *Br J Surg.* 1978;65:449–451.

228. Salzman EW, Davies GC. Prophylaxis of venous thromboembolism: analysis of cost effectiveness. *Ann Surg.* 1980;191:207–218.

229. Prevention of venous thrombosis and pulmonary embolism: NIH consensus development. *JAMA.* 1986;256:744–749.

230. Kakkar VV, Bentley PG, Scully MF, MacGregor IR, et al. Antithrombin III and heparin. *Lancet.* 1980;1:103–104.

231. Barnett HG, Clifford JR, Llewellyn RC. Safety of mini-dose heparin administration for neurosurgical patients. *J Neurosurg.* 1977;47:27–30.

232. Cerrato D, Ariano C, Fiacchino F. Deep vein thrombosis and low-dose heparin prophylaxis in neurosurgical patients. *J Neurosurg.* 1978;49:378–381.

233. Knight MT, Dawson R. Effect of intermittent compression of the arms on deep venous thrombosis in the legs. *Lancet.* 1976;2:1265–1268.

234. Allenby F, Boardman L, Pflug JJ, Calnan JS. Effects of external pneumatic intermittent compression on fibrinolysis in man. *Lancet.* 1973;2:1412–1414.

235. Gersin K, Grindlinger GA, Lee V, Dennis RC, et al. The efficacy of sequential compression devices in multiple trauma patients with severe head injury. *J Trauma.* 1994;37:205–208.

236. Cranley JJ, Canos AJ, Sull WJ. The diagnosis of deep venous thrombosis. Fallibility of clinical symptoms and signs. *Arch Surg.* 1976;111:34–6.

237. Raghavendra BN, Rosen RJ, Lam S, Riles T, et al. Deep venous thrombosis: detection by high-resolution real-time ultrasonography. *Radiology.* 1984;152:789–793.

238. Comerota AJ, White JV, Katz ML. Diagnostic methods for deep vein thrombosis: venous Doppler examination. phleborheography, iodine-125 fibrinogen uptake, and phlebography. *Am J Surg.* 1985;150:14–24.

239. Comerota AJ, Katz ML, Grossi RJ, White JV, et al. The comparative value of noninvasive testing for diagnosis and surveillance of deep venous thrombosis. *J Vasc Surg.* 1988;7:40–49.

240. Huisman MV, Buller HR, ten Cate JW, Vreeken J. Serial impedance plethysmography for suspected deep venous thrombosis in outpatients: the Amsterdam General Practitioner Study. *N Engl J Med.* 1986;314:823–828.

241. Sullivan ED, Peter DJ, Cranley JJ. Real-time B-mode venous ultrasound. *J Vasc Surg.* 1984;1:465–471.

242. Comerota AJ, Katz ML, Greenwald LL, Leefmans E, et al. Venous duplex imaging: should it replace hemodynamic tests for deep venous thrombosis. *J Vasc Surg.* 1990;11:53–59.

243. Hirsh J, Gallus AS. 125-I-labeled fibrogen scanning: use in the diagnosis of venous thrombosis. *JAMA.* 1975;233:970–973.

244. Le Quesne LP. Current concepts: relation between deep vein thrombosis and pulmonary embolism in surgical patients. *N Engl J Med.* 1974;291:1292–1294.

245. Moreno-Cabral R, Kistner RL, Nordyke RA. Importance of calf vein thrombophlebitis. *Surgery.* 1976;80:735–742.

246. Greenfield LJ, Peyton R, Crute S, Barnes R. Greenfield vena caval experience: late results in 156 patients. *Arch Surg.* 1981;116:1451–1456.

247. Roehm JO Jr, Johnsrude IS, Barth MH, Gianturco C. The bird's nest inferior vena cava filter: progress report. *Radiology.* 1988;168:745–749.

248. Goodall RJR, Greenfield LJ. Clinical correlations in the diagnosis of pulmonary embolism. *Ann Surg.* 1980;191:219–223.

249. Sabiston DC Jr, Wolfe WG. Experimental and clinical observations on the natural history of pulmonary embolism. *Ann Surg.* 1968;168:1–15.

250. Value of the ventilation/perfusion scan in acute pulmonary embolism: results of the prospective investigation of pulmonary embolism (PIOPED). The PIOPED investigators. *JAMA.* 1990;263:2753–2759.

251. Thrombolytic therapy in thrombosis. *Stroke.* 1981;12:17–21.

CHAPTER 10

The Metabolic Response to Acute Traumatic Brain Injury and Associated Complications

Hypermetabolism, hypercatabolism, the acute-phase response, altered immune function, hyperglycemia, increase in counterregulatory and cytokine levels, and gastric atony are all manifestations of the metabolic response to traumatic brain injury that play a role in the development of several complications that commonly occur in these patients. Malnutrition resulting from excessive protein breakdown and frequent inability to provide adequate calories is commonly encountered. Nutritional intervention in this patient population has been shown to ameliorate the negative nitrogen balance caused by excessive protein catabolism.[1] Other complications that occur as a result of the metabolic response to traumatic brain injury include disturbances in electrolyte and acid-base balance, cardiovascular abnormalities, and extracranial and cranial infections. Although early intervention with rehabilitation improves ultimate outcome, its specific impact on the metabolic state is not known. It is therefore important for members of the critical care team and the rehabilitation team to be acutely aware of the metabolic status of the patient before and during acute rehabilitative intervention. The key to optimal management and maximum functional recovery of the critically ill patient with traumatic brain injury is a thorough understanding of these types of complications, which may affect the implementation and the goals of early rehabilitation.

METABOLIC RESPONSE TO ACUTE TRAUMATIC BRAIN INJURY

Hypermetabolism

Because traumatic brain injury results in early, profound, unchecked catabolism, the metabolic balance that normally exists between catabolism and anabolism is disrupted. The end result is a hypermetabolic state that causes protein breakdown and muscle atrophy. The existence of hypermetabolism following traumatic brain injury has been well documented in the literature since the 1980s,[2-4] and further supporting data continue to accumulate.[5-7]

The intense hypermetabolic response to traumatic brain injury was first recognized during the 1980s. During this time, indirect calorimetric devices in the form of portable bedside metabolic carts became available that could measure oxygen consumption and carbon dioxide production and calculate resting energy or metabolic expenditure through a series of assumptions and equations. On the basis of a series of indirect calorimetric measurements obtained in patients with acute traumatic brain injury, Clifton et al[8] developed a bedside nomogram that could be used to estimate metabolic expenditure in this patient population (Figure 10–1). Resting metabolic expenditures (RMEs) were found to be 200% or more of expected values in patients who exhibited posturing, sweating, increased muscle tone, and fever. Energy expenditures that were lower than expected were found primarily in patients who were given sedative or paralytic agents and in patients who were brain dead. The percentage of normal RME may also be predicted from a formula using Glasgow Coma Scale (GCS) score, heart rate (HR), and days since injury (DSI) (Exhibit 10–1). An inverse relationship exists between GCS score and measured energy expenditure.[8] This relationship can be used clinically to predict energy or caloric requirements. However, there may be tremendous variability in any individual patient's metabolic response to traumatic brain injury. Studies in critically ill patients that compare measured energy expenditure to predicted energy expenditure determined by standard predictive formulas such as the Harris-Benedict formula (Exhibit 10–2) have found a wide variation in the actual metabolic state of the patients.[9] The Harris-Benedict formula correctly predicted energy expenditure only in approximately 50% of cases. A similar study in patients with acute brain injury supports the notion that energy expenditure can be better estimated using indirect calorimetry from metabolic carts than from standard predictive formulas such as the Harris-Benedict formula.[5] Weekes and Elia demonstrated that measured energy expenditure in a small group of stable patients with severe brain injury (GCS ≤8) was up to 35% higher than predicted.[10] Another benefit of the indirect calorimeter is the derivation of the respiratory quotient (RQ). The RQ is the ratio of carbon dioxide produced to oxygen consumed (V_{CO_2}/V_{O_2}), which provides information concerning the percent substrate utilization by the body and can be used to adjust the percentage of fat and carbohydrate calories accordingly. However, indirect calorimetry also has its limitations. A variety of factors, such as hyperventilation, hypoventilation, pain, leaks in the respiratory circuit, and pressure surges from the ventilator; may cause artifactual changes in measured energy expenditure. Furthermore, indirect calorimetry should not be used if (1) the inspired concentration of oxygen exceeds 60%; (2) there is excessive air leak, as in the case of bronchopleural fistula; (3) the patient exhibits rapid, shallow breathing; (4) the patient is anesthetized with anesthetic gases; or (5) the

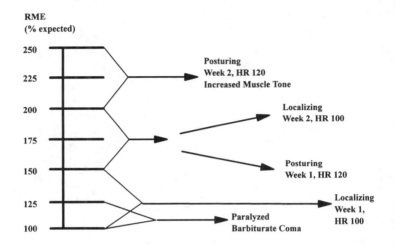

Figure 10–1 Nomogram used to estimate resting metabolic expenditure (RME) in comatose patients during the first two weeks after injury. *Source:* Reprinted with permission from G.L. Clifton, C.S. Robertson, and S.C. Choi, *Journal of Neurosurgery,* Vol. 64, p. 899, © 1986, American Association of Neurological Surgeons.

patient is undergoing concurrent hemodialysis. These situations alter the measurements of inspired oxygen and exhaled carbon dioxide, thereby adversely affecting the accuracy of the indirect calorimeter and thus precluding its use.

Several factors have been implicated in the hypermetabolic response to traumatic brain injury. Although the use of steroid therapy for acute traumatic brain

Exhibit 10–1 Formula Predicting Percentage of Resting Metabolic Expenditure (RME) for Patients with Acute Traumatic Brain Injury and GCS Scores of 7 or Less and 8 or Greater.

% RME = 152 – 14(GCS) + 0.4(HR) + 7(DSI)

GCS = Glasgow Coma Scale score
HR = heart rate
DSI = days since injury

Source: Reprinted with permission from G.L. Clifton, C.S. Robertson, and S.C. Choi, *Journal of Neurosurgery,* Vol. 64, pp. 898–899, © 1986, American Association of Neurological Surgeons.

Exhibit 10–2 Harris-Benedict Formula, Which Can Be Used To Estimate Basal Energy Expenditure in Hospitalized Patients

---

Harris-Benedict Equation: BEE

Males: $66 + (13.7 \times W) + (5 \times H) - (6.8 \times A)$

Females: $665 + (9.6 \times W) + (1.7 \times H) - (4.7 \times A)$

W = weight in kilograms

H = height in centimeters

A = age in years

BEE = basal energy expenditure

---

injury has largely been abandoned, corticosteroids are well known to increase protein catabolism.[11,12] Their effect on energy metabolism is less clear. Measured energy expenditure has been shown to be increased independent of steroid treatment in patients with brain injury.[12,13] Because of the thermogenic effect of food, enteral diets can increase metabolic rate, especially if they are administered in bolus form. The effect can be minimized by use of continuous enteral feedings. However, this does not appear to contribute in any significant fashion to the hypermetabolic state in either fed or nonfed patients with brain injuries.[13] Although sedatives and paralytic agents are known to decrease metabolic rate, certain patients show an increased measured energy expenditure despite pharmacologic sedation and/or paralysis.[2] This also suggests that the stimulation, activity, and posturing frequently seen in this patient population do not entirely explain the hypermetabolic state. Likewise, craniotomy and infection are not clearly associated with hypermetabolism.[13] Cytokines, a class of small proteins, have been implicated as a factor in hypermetabolism. Brain injury causes a significant localized inflammatory response at the site of damage, resulting in an accumulation of lymphocytes and macrophages, which release cytokines.[14] Cytokines affect systemic immunity, metabolism, hemodynamics, the central nervous system, and the endocrine system. They exert their effect by binding specific cell receptors in target organs and can also stimulate production of other cytokines locally and at distant sites. They function in a paracrine, autocrine, and endocrine fashion. The cytokines are broadly classified as tumor necrosis factors, interleukins, interferons, and colony-stimulating factors. These agents have been shown to mediate natural immunity, regulate lymphocyte function, activate inflammatory cells, and stimulate hematopoiesis. Interleukin-1, interleukin-6, and tumor necrosis factor may play an etiologic role in the hypermetabolism and hypercatabolism that accompany traumatic brain injury.[4,6,13,14] Another major contributor to the hypermetabolic state is the massive production of counterregulatory hormones such as epinephrine, norepinephrine, glucagon, and cortisol.[15] Levels of norepinephrine can be extremely high following traumatic brain injury.[16] Because the brain normally regulates metabolism through its effect on the sympathetic nervous system, the normal regulatory mechanisms of the brain are disrupted and a disordered hypermetabolic state ensues following brain injury. Blockade of the adrenergic system with agents such as the alpha-adrenergic antagonist prazosin and the beta-adrenergic antagonist propanolol has been shown to decrease the hypermetabolic state locally in the brain, as well as systemically.[17,18] The duration of the hypermetabolic phase following acute brain injury is controversial but has been reported to last from one week up to one year after injury.[19–21]

Hypercatabolism

Hypercatabolism following traumatic brain injury is characterized by increased protein turnover. Urinary nitrogen excretion rates in excess of 25 to 30 g/d are commonplace in patients with isolated severe brain injury[22] and are comparable to those seen in patients with multisystem traumatic injuries and burns (Figure 10–2). Stress such as that seen with traumatic brain injury induces a significant increase in glucose utilization by glucose-dependent organs such as the brain, blood cells, and bone marrow. Glycogen stores are rapidly depleted within 24 hours, and gluconeogenesis becomes the primary method of glucose production. A major source of the carbon skeletons required for gluconeogenesis is amino acids, which are derived from protein breakdown, primarily from skeletal muscle. During nonstressed states of starvation, fat stores are broken down to fatty acids and subsequently to ketone bodies, which can be used for energy by many organ systems. In this adapted state, protein is relatively conserved. The nonstressed starved person loses approximately 200 to 300 g of muscle tissue per day, but the stressed, acutely ill patient can lose up to 1,000 g/d because the glucose requirements are much higher and because adaptation to the use of ketone bodies for energy may not occur.[23] Without intervention, this profound, unchecked hypercatabolic response may lead to severe protein-calorie malnutrition and may ultimately contribute to poor immune function and increased risk of infection, resulting in increased morbidity and mortality. Despite exogenous administration of protein in the form of parenteral and/or enteral nutrition, positive nitrogen balance is very difficult to achieve. This is particularly true during the first two weeks following traumatic brain injury. Achieving the lowest level of negative nitrogen balance should be the goal during this early catabolic period.

The etiology of excessive protein catabolism secondary to brain injury is also multifactorial. These patients can lose a significant amount of weight and muscle mass for up to three months after the injury. Protein catabolism is required after injury for synthesis of acute-phase proteins. There is also a significant depression

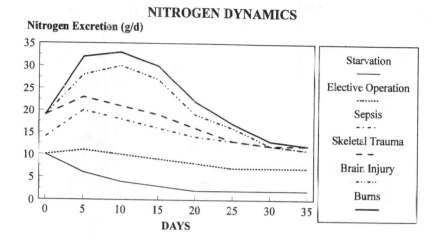

NITROGEN DYNAMICS

Figure 10–2 Nitrogen excretion curves showing association of degree of nitrogen excretion and type of injury, operation, or starvation. *Source:* Reprinted with permission from J. Rombeau and M.D. Caldwell, in *Clinical Nutrition: Enteral and Tube Feeding,* 2nd edition, B.A. Bivins and J.J. Fath, eds., © 1990, W.B. Saunders Company.

of the synthesis of visceral proteins such as albumin and transferrin. Prolonged immobilization has been well characterized as a factor in excessive protein turnover. However, negative nitrogen balance occurs only after five to six days of immobilization, whereas the excessive urinary nitrogen levels are seen almost immediately after brain injury.[13] Furthermore, many patients with brain injury display frequent movement and posturing and are not entirely immobile. This suggests the presence of an endogenous stimulation to protein catabolism. Although not commonly used, steroids potentiate the excessive nitrogen loss associated with brain injury in both children and adults,[11] but they are not the sole cause (Figure 10–3).

Acute-Phase Response

The acute-phase response is another metabolic manifestation of traumatic brain injury that may influence nutritional intervention. The acute-phase response to stress results in increased synthesis of the acute-phase proteins such as fibrinogen, alpha-1-acid glycoprotein, c-reactive protein, and ceruloplasmin, as well as decreased synthesis of proteins such as albumin, retinol-binding protein, and prealbumin. A significant decrease in serum zinc and iron levels, increased serum copper levels, and fever with leukocytosis are also characteristic of the acute-

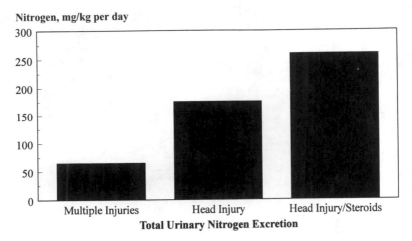

Figure 10–3 Comparison of total nitrogen excretion in patients with multiple injuries. head injuries, and head injuries treated with steroids. *Source:* Adapted with permission from E.G. Ford, L.M. Jennings, R.J. Andrassy, Steroid Treatment of Head Injuries in Children: The Nutritional Consequences. *Current Surgery,* Vol. 44, p. 312, © 1987, Williams & Wilkins.

phase response. The response may serve as a protective mechanism to prevent loss of primary host functions and seems to be mediated by the cytokines interleukin-1 and interleukin-6.[6] Patients with acute traumatic brain injury have diminished serum zinc levels and increased urinary losses of zinc.[24] There is a redistribution and redirection of zinc to the liver, spleen, and wound site due to an increased need for synthesis of the acute-phase proteins. Zinc is important for protein synthesis and wound healing, and deficiency of this trace element leads to a disorder of the skin and gastrointestinal tract called *acrodermatitis enteropathica*, as well as immune dysfunction. Because it is a cofactor for superoxide dismutase, an enzyme required for control of oxygen free radical formation, zinc may help prevent ischemia and reperfusion injury to tissues. Replacement of zinc has been shown to improve visceral protein stores and GCS scores in patients with acute traumatic brain injury.[24,25] Current recommendations to help counteract the effect of the acute-phase response on zinc metabolism include supplementation with 12 mg of zinc per day.

Immunosuppression

Infections following traumatic brain injury are unfortunately very common and a major cause of late deaths.[26] This has been directly attributable to dysfunction of the immune system, which is part of the metabolic response to traumatic brain injury. Cell-mediated immurity is significantly impaired and results in almost universal anergy following brain injury. [27,28] T-cell function, interleukin-2 production, and interferon-gamma production, all of which are necessary for cell-mediated immunity, are significantly depressed.[29] The specific cause of the immune depression has not clearly been established, but it is believed to be related to a deficit of some nutrient or mineral. It has not yet been established whether specific nutrient or mineral supplementation can improve immune status or decrease the incidence of infectious complications.[30] However, there is some evidence to suggest that supplementation of aggressive nutritional support with infusion of insulinlike growth factor prevents the derangement of the ratio of T-helper cells to T-suppressor cells associated with acute traumatic brain injury[31] and that this may translate into an improved infection rate.

NUTRITIONAL SUPPORT FOR ACUTE TRAUMATIC BRAIN INJURY

The deleterious effect of neurologic injury on nutritional status has been recognized for decades, but reports of early nutritional support in this patient population are not found in the literature until the 1980s. Until that time, initiation of nutrition was routinely delayed until the return of adequate gastrointestinal function permitted gastric feeding. Total parenteral nutrition (TPN) was at one time perceived to be detrimental to patients with traumatic brain injury because of excessive fluid volumes and the risk of precipitation or potentiation of cerebral edema. In addition, hyperglycemia and hyperosmolarity, which are known to be injurious to the already traumatized brain, were thought to be prohibitive risks of TPN. Hyperglycemia is common following experimental and clinical brain injury and has been shown to be directly correlated with worse outcome.[32] Interestingly, studies that have addressed the effect of elevated serum glucose levels on cerebral ischemia have conflicting results.[33] The hyperglycemia associated with brain injury is more related to excessive glucose production and relative resistance to endogenous insulin resulting from the stress response to injury and is not as much due to the delivered exogenous glucose delivered in the TPN. Gastric dysfunction following acute brain injury has long been recognized and was once felt to contribute significantly to the risk of aspiration pneumonia and gastric feeding intolerance. As much as a twofold reduction in the rate of gastric emptying and reflux has been documented in patients with traumatic brain injury when compared to normal controls.[10] Increased intracranial pressure (ICP), cytokines, opioids, corticotropin-releasing factor, and a direct effect of brain injury on the vagus nerve have all been implicated as causes of the gastric dysfunction. For these reasons, clinicians were reluctant in the past to initiate either enteral or parenteral nutritional support. Several studies have now shown that TPN does not cause significant hyperosmolarity, cerebral edema, or ICP.[34,35] Furthermore, enteral access distal to the stomach now can be more easily and reliably obtained, so early nutritional intervention is currently the rule rather than the exception.

Nutritional Requirements

Caloric Requirement

The previously described metabolic alterations have a profound effect on the nutritional requirements of critically ill patients with acute traumatic brain injury. Because metabolic expenditure varies greatly among these patients, the amount of daily calories required will vary from 25 to 50 kcal/kg per day. Standard formulas, such as the Harris-Benedict formula, have not been helpful when applied to patients with acute traumatic brain injury. To avoid severely underestimating or overestimating caloric requirements in individual patients, indirect calorimetry with a portable, bedside metabolic cart is recommended to determine total daily caloric requirements. Total daily calories are usually administered in an amount equal to the measured energy expenditure, although as much as 5% to 20% of the measured energy expenditure may be added to the total daily caloric need in order to account for the additional energy expended as a result of patient movement and nursing procedures.[30] Ideally, indirect calorimetry should be performed twice each week until the energy expenditure reaches a plateau or normalizes. As neurologic function improves, energy expenditure appears to normalize. A baseline measurement of energy expenditure is also useful during the recovery phase to prevent overestimation of caloric needs and subsequent detrimental overfeeding. Patients with frequent posturing and excessive diaphoresis will require the most caloric and protein input, as well as free water in order to avoid dehydration and hypernatremia.

As previously stated, the respiratory quotient can also be determined with this technique, which allows an estimation of the composition of fuels actually being utilized. Lipogenesis occurs at RQ values greater than 1.00, implying an excess of total calories or an excess of dextrose calories. Pure fat utilization occurs at RQ values of 0.70 or less, implying a deficiency of total calories. The RQ can therefore be used to adjust the ratio of fat to carbohydrate calories being administered to meet the total daily caloric requirement. Delivery of total daily calories with a high percentage of fat calories (>40% to 50%) has been implicated in immunosuppression due primarily to omega-6 fatty acids.[36] It is therefore recommended that fat calories be limited to 25% to 33% of total calories. Recently, administration of an enteral diet rich in omega-3 fatty acids has been associated with improved immunologic function and decreased incidence of infectious complications in critically ill patients and cancer patients.[37,38] However, more studies are needed before widespread recommendation of such expensive immunomodulating formulas can occur. Approximately 66% to 75% of total daily calories should be administered in the form of glucose or dextrose. The rate of glucose or dextrose infusion should be limited to 4 to 5 mg/kg per minute or a maximum of 7 g/kg per day to avoid hyperglycemia and excessive glucose load on the liver. Close monitoring of serum glucose levels is imperative and is achieved by fingerstick capillary glucose levels every 4 to 6 hours or more frequently if hyperglycemia is persistent. Insulin should be used if glucose levels approach 200 mg/dL, since hyperglycemia induces anaerobic cerebral metabolism and has been associated with an elevation in cerebral lactate levels. Lactic acid has been shown to produce neuronal injury.[39] Because hypoglycemia is also injurious to the brain,[33] continued frequent glucose determinations are necessary once insulin therapy has begun.

Protein Requirements

The standard adult recommended daily allowance (RDA) for protein is 0.8 g/kg per day. However, because of the excessive protein catabolism that occurs, the protein requirements for patients with severe traumatic brain injury during the acute phase may approach 2.0 g/kg per day or more. Although positive nitrogen balance is usually not attainable until postinjury day 10 or later,[22] nitrogen retention is improved in patients who receive a high percentage of protein.[40] It is reasonable to start protein supplementation in the range of 1.5 to 1.8 g/kg per day . Because optimal protein utilization greatly depends on adequacy of calories consumed, protein needs to be given in the proper ratio with calories. For patients with acute traumatic brain injury, a calorie-to-nitrogen ratio of 100:1 to 125:1 or more is most appropriate. Careful daily monitoring of serum urea nitrogen levels should be employed to signal excess protein administration. Weekly monitoring of prealbumin, a serum protein with a half-life of only 2 to 3 days, should aid in determining whether the amount of protein being administered is adequate. Changes in prealbumin can be expected to reflect protein supplementation within one week of beginning nutritional intervention. Weekly 24-hour urinary urea nitrogen levels and calculation of nitrogen balance can help guide protein supplementation as well. Nitrogen balance is defined as the difference between nitrogen intake and nitrogen excretion in urine, stool, and sweat. For each gram of nitrogen measured in the urine, 6.25 g of protein have been catabolized (Exhibit 10–3).

Parenteral Nutrition

Nutrition can be supplied either parenterally, via a central vein or peripheral vein, or enterally via a variety of access devices. Administration of parenteral nutrition by a peripheral vein avoids all of the complications associated with a central venous catheter. Peripheral parenteral nutrition (PPN) is the least appropriate in patients with acute traumatic brain injury because excessive volume is required

Exhibit 10–3 Formula for Calculating Nitrogen Balance. There are 6.25 g of protein per g of nitrogen. The addition of 4 g of nitrogen to UUN accounts for nitrogen lost in the stool and sweat.

Nitrogen Balance = (Nitrogen in) – (UUN + 4)
UUN = Urinary urea nitrogen in grams

---

to deliver adequate calories and protein due to the limit of the osmolality of a solution that can be given through a peripheral vein (800 mosm). There is no limit to the osmolality of a parenteral nutrition solution given centrally. Peripherally inserted central catheters (PICCs) now exist that can overcome the osmolality limitation. However, there are other risks and complications associated with TPN. TPN can induce volume overload, electrolyte imbalance, and catheter-related complications. Pneumothorax, arterial injury with or without hemothorax, chylothorax, and hydrothorax have all been described following placement of central venous access catheters. Right atrial rupture with infusion of TPN solution into the pericardium and cardiac tamponade have also occurred. Nerve injury, lymphatic injury, embolic events, and thrombosis are also possible. Fortunately, these major complications are rare.[41] Catheter-related sepsis is a potential complication of TPN that can add significant cost to the total care of the patient.[42] Other infectious complications have been associated with TPN. Findings from the Veterans Affairs Total Parental Nutrition Cooperation Study Group[43] showed that TPN, when given preoperatively for patients undergoing general and thoracic surgical procedures, actually increases the rate of infectious postoperative procedures. Enteral nutrition obviates the concern generated from potential catheter-related complications, is less costly than parenteral nutrition, and has less risk of hyperglycemia. Enteral nutrition also seems to be associated with fewer septic complications when compared to TPN in general surgical and multiple-trauma patients.[44,45] Whether these data should be extrapolated to patients with acute traumatic brain injury is not known at this time. It is known, however, that no nutrition or inadequate nutrition predisposes this patient population to infectious complications.[1] Neither parenteral nor enteral nutrition seems to offer an advantage with respect to infectious complications. Most clinicians agree that enteral nutrition should be employed whenever possible (ie, "If the gut works, use it!").

Enteral Nutrition

Enteral Access Devices

Enteral access can be obtained in a nasoenteric, percutaneous, or surgical fashion (Figures 10–4 through 10–6). The nasal route is the least invasive method.

Nasoenteric
Access

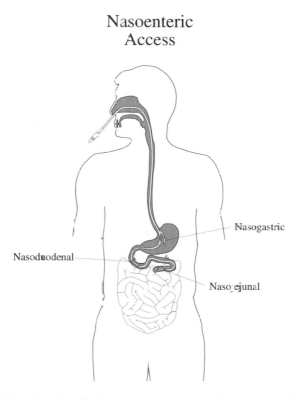

Nasogastric

Nasoduodenal

Nasojejunal

Figure 10–4 Methods of establishing nasoenteric access for enteral nutrition.

Nasoenteric tubes made of soft polyurethane are usually size 8 French to 12 French and can be placed in the stomach, postpylorically in the duodenum, and distal to the ligament of Treitz in the jejunum. Passage of the feeding tube beyond the pylorus usually requires techniques such as positioning the patient with the right side down. The addition of promotilant agents such as metoclopramide and erythromycin[46,47] has also been tried, with varying degrees of success. Cisapride has been shown to improve gastric emptying time in critically ill patients receiving gastric feedings, resulting in lower gastric residuals,[48] but its impact on postpyloric nasoenteric tube passage is not known. Fluoroscopic guidance can be employed, but this usually requires transport of a critically ill patient to the radiology suite, which is cumbersome and may be dangerous. Endoscopic techniques are available to assist the placement of the nasoenteric tube beyond the pylorus. Unfortunately, no technique can guarantee that the postpyloric position of the tube will be maintained. Frequent dislodgement of the tube is frustrating and may cause aspiration of feedings if the tube is withdrawn into the esophagus or pharynx.

Percutaneous
Enteral Access

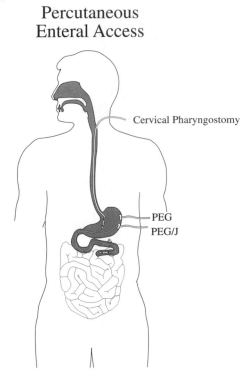

Cervical Pharyngostomy

PEG
PEG/J

Figure 10–5 Methods of establishing percutaneous access for enteral nutrition.

Because of the relatively small diameter of the tube, clogging may be a problem and may require replacement of the tube. Other complications include arrhythmias, sinusitis, otitis media, inadvertent tracheal-bronchial feeding, pneumothorax, epistaxis, pyriform sinus perforation, and knotted tubes. The presence of a tube passing through the pharynx has been linked to relaxation of the lower esophageal sphincter,[49] and lower esophageal sphincter dysfunction has been documented in patients with acute brain injury.[50,51] The risk of aspiration due to these factors alone may preclude the use of gastric feedings following traumatic brain injury. Since transpyloric placement of a feeding tube also renders the pylorus incompetent, reflux of the enteral feeding formula into the stomach may occur, even if the formula is instilled into the small bowel distal to the ligament of Treitz. Nasoenteric tubes should be limited to short-term access, defined as a period of less than three weeks.

The first report of percutaneous placement of a gastric feeding tube was published in 1980 by Gauderer et al.[52] Using endoscopic guidance, the practitioner

Surgical
Enteral Access

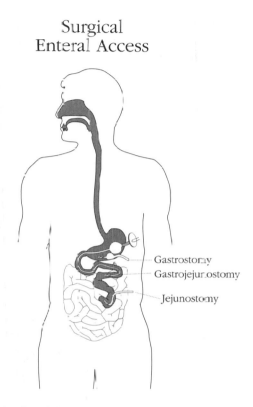

Gastrostomy

Gastrojejunostomy

Jejunostomy

Figure 10–6 Methods of establishing surgical access for enteral nutrition.

punctures the anterior abdominal and gastric walls with a needle, passes a guidewire through the needle into the stomach, withdraws the guidewire out the mouth with the endoscope, and then uses it to guide the passage of gastrostomy tube through the mouth, into the stomach, and out through the anterior abdominal wall (percutaneous endoscopic gastrotomy [PEG]). A modification of this technique can be used to place a tube into the jejunum (percutaneous endoscopic gastrojejunostomy [PEG/J]). These procedures require additional skill and are more invasive than the nasoenteric placement of feeding tubes. Bleeding, wound infection, abdominal wall necrosis, gastric wall necrosis, gastric leak, peritonitis, colon perforation, and gastrocolic fistula are some of the complications that have been reported following PEG or PEG/J. Fortunately, these are rare complications when appropriate patients are selected and the endoscopist is experienced. Because of transpyloric passage of the jejunal tube in PEG/J, aspiration is still a risk, as it is with PEG as well. A tube can be placed under direct endoscopic visualization into the jejunum (percutaneous endoscopic jejunostomy [PEJ]) and would be comparable to a surgically placed jejunal tube. However, this requires a longer endoscope and much more expertise and skill to identify an appropriate site in the proximal jejunum. Percutaneous access to the pyriform sinus of the pharynx can be obtained rather easily at the bedside under local anesthesia and can be used to pass a feeding tube into the stomach or beyond the pylorus.[53] Endoscopy is not required to place a cervical pharyngostomy. Since this technique removes the tube from the nasal passage, sinusitis is not a problem, and inadvertent dislodgement of the tube by the patient is less common, since it is affixed in the posterior neck. Complications of this type of enteral feeding access include clogged tubes, tube migration into the pharynx, aspiration, and local wound infection. Percutaneous cervical pharyngostomies can remain in place for longer than three months and can be replaced in a similar fashion to surgically placed gastrostomies once a tract has formed.[53]

Surgical access to the gastrointestinal tract can be obtained by either laparotomy or laparoscopy. A gastrostomy, jejunostomy, or a combined gastrojejunostomy can be created. A variety of tubes are used, including Foley catheters, T-tubes, red rubber catheters, Malecot catheters, and peritoneal dialysis catheters. A needle catheter (size 7 French) can be used to establish access to the jejunum rapidly and has been used extensively in trauma patients undergoing laparotomy for their injuries. These techniques usually require general anesthesia in the operating room and are subject to the same risks of any laparotomy or laparoscopy. Proper placement of surgical gastrostomy or jejunostomy is not perfectly guaranteed. Feeding tubes have inadvertently been placed in the colon and the distal small bowel.

Complications of Enteral Nutrition

Unfortunately, enteral feeding may also be fraught with complications. Many patients with brain injuries do not tolerate the early initiation of enteral feedings, and the time to achievement of full nutritional goals is prolonged if TPN is not initiated simultaneously. Indications of intolerance include high gastric residual volumes, abdominal distension, diarrhea, vomiting, and aspiration. Intolerance seems to be related to increased ICP and low GCS score on admission and may result from ablation of higher central nervous system (CNS) centers that affect neurointestinal reflexes.[54] Gastric atony, prolonged ileus, and stress gastritis are common gastrointestinal responses to brain injury and contribute to the inability to attain nutritional goals. Hypoalbuminemia, which is commonly seen following traumatic brain injury, may also play a role in enteral feeding intolerance. Aspiration, seen in 22% to 45% of patients with brain injuries who are enterally fed, is the most feared complication. Postpyloric placement of feeding tubes does not prevent aspiration in patients with acute brain injury.[55,56] The studies published to date concerning route of enteral feeding and subsequent aspiration rates are limited because of deficiencies in definition of aspiration, documentation of its occurrence, and methodologies and do not definitively prove benefit of jejunal feedings over gastric feedings.[57] Even though the risk of aspiration from a surgically placed jejunostomy is less than that for other access routes, and even though most people would recommend jejunostomy placement for long-term use in patients prone to aspiration, there are reported rates of aspiration for this procedure.[58] Unfortunately, comparisons of aspiration rates between different studies are difficult because of limitations and flaws. Despite this, enteral feeding beyond the ligament of Treitz is the "gold standard," and intuition, rather than exact science, guides the preference of jejunal over gastric feedings, particularly in patients with acute traumatic brain injury. Because access to the jejunum is difficult at best, practicality dictates the use of gastric or duodenal feeding, particularly early during the patient's course. Precautionary maneuvers should always be initiated in patients with traumatic brain injury when enteral feedings are begun proximal to the jejunum. Routine checking of gastric residuals, abdominal distension, and tracheal secretions for the presence of enteral feeds is paramount for the prevention of aspiration pneumonia. Also, all enterally fed patients should have the head of the bed elevated to a minimum of 30 degrees at all times. Figure 10-7 outlines a reasonable nutritional supplementation protocol for patients with acute traumatic brain injury within the first two to three weeks. After that, more permanent access should be obtained.

Nutritional Therapy and Outcome

Rapp et al[1] performed a study that was designed to compare enteral with parenteral nutrition in patients with traumatic brain injury. The enterally fed group received fewer calories and less protein than the TPN group because of significant difficulties encountered with gastrointestinal intolerance and, in effect, became a starvation control group. All patients remained in negative nitrogen balance throughout the study, but the degree of negative nitrogen balance was much less in the TPN group and was associated with improved survival. The study shows a benefit of nutritional supplementation over starvation. Additionally, it suggests that immunity is impaired in brain injury patients who receive inadequate nutrition, since the majority of deaths in the enterally fed group were due to sepsis and infectious complications. The study was later repeated by the same group of investigators, and benefit of early parenteral nutrition in terms of neurologic recovery was found up to three months following injury.[34] Although the enterally fed group met a greater percentage of nutrient goals than the same group in the earlier study, they still received less calories and protein than the TPN group. No conclusion can be reached about the benefit of TPN over enteral nutrition. No difference in mortality or neurologic recovery was seen after randomization of 45 patients to either

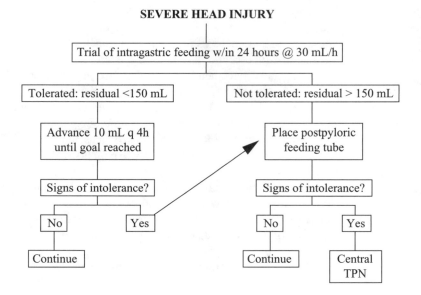

Figure 10–7 Algorithm for initiation of nutritional supplementation in patients with severe acute traumatic brain injury (GCS score of 8 or less). Requires vigilant monitoring for and prevention of aspiration.

TPN or enteral nutrition.[59] As in previous studies, the enterally fed patients received significantly less protein, a finding that underscores the difficulties encountered with enteral nutrition in patients with traumatic brain injury. Retrospective studies have also suggested that neurologic outcome is improved with less caloric deficit.[60,61] Infectious complications were found to be similar in TPN- versus enterally fed patients when both groups received isocaloric and isonitrogenous supplementation.[62]

To prove a beneficial effect of nutrition on morbidity, mortality, and neurologic outcome, a prospective, randomized, controlled trial would need to compare a fed group to a nonfed group of patients with brain injury. Ethically, this could not be undertaken. From the studies previously performed, it can be concluded that nutritional support early following acute brain injury versus inadequate or no nutritional support may have a favorable effect on neurologic recovery. Whether enteral nutrition is more beneficial than parenteral nutrition in this patient population has not yet been determined. Because of lower costs and complications, enteral nutrition should be attempted. Recognition of the propensity toward enteral feeding intolerance should alert clinicians to the likelihood that TPN may be required in addition to low rates of enteral feeding in order to allow attainment of metabolic requirements.

ELECTROLYTE ABNORMALITIES ASSOCIATED WITH TRAUMATIC BRAIN INJURY

Disturbances in serum electrolyte concentrations occur frequently following traumatic brain injury. Fifty-nine percent of all patients registered in the national Trauma Coma Data Bank (TCDB) have an electrolyte abnormality at least once during their hospital stay, but these disturbances do not seem to have prognostic significance.[63] Normally, plasma osmolality and serum sodium concentration are maintained within a very narrow range by fine adjustments in total body water. Total water balance is achieved by arginine vasopressin or antidiuretic hormone (ADH), a small protein manufactured in the anterior hypothalamus. It travels to the posterior pituitary gland and is secreted when increased osmolality and decreased intravascular volume are detected by osmoreceptors located in the anterior hypothalamus and volume receptors located in the heart. ADH functions at the distal convoluted tubules and collecting ducts of the kidneys, where it causes free water absorption. Up to 30 L of water each day is conserved by the action of ADH.[64] The thirst center, which is also located in the anterior hypothalamus, also plays a role in water balance. Since the majority of regulators of water balance are located in the brain, it is not surprising that abnormalities of serum sodium concentration are commonplace in patients with traumatic brain injury. Furthermore, nutritional supplementation via TPN or enteral formulas may upset water and electrolyte balance. Hyponatremia, defined as a serum sodium concentration less than 135 mEq/L, is a very common electrolyte abnormality encountered following traumatic brain injury. The stress response to trauma includes a significant release of ADH, which promotes water reabsorption by the distal tubules and collecting system of the kidneys and results in relative intravascular water excess. The serum sodium concentration decreases, as it does following any acute stress, including elective surgery. Beyond this, however, other factors such as the syndrome of inappropriate release of antidiuretic hormone (SIADH) and cerebral salt wasting may contribute to hyponatremia after traumatic brain injury. Pseudohyponatremia due to hyperlipidemia or hyperproteinemia should be ruled out before a search for the cause of true hyponatremia is undertaken. Hypernatremia, defined by a serum sodium concentration of greater than 145 mEq/L, may result from therapeutic use of mannitol, densely caloric enteral feedings, and excessive insensible water loss due to diaphoresis, tracheostomy, and posttraumatic diabetes insipidus (DI). Phenytoin, a potent inhibitor of ADH, may also cause hypernatremia in this patient population. Hypokalemia is seen usually in association with alkalosis induced by therapeutic or intrinsic hyperventilation. Excessive loss of potassium may occur as a result of the use of diuretics or steroids. Diagnosis and treatment of serum potassium abnormalities are relatively straightforward. However, the management of serum sodium abnormalities is a little more complex.

Hyponatremia

SIADH is the most frequent cause of hyponatremia after brain injury and is usually associated with a deterioration in neurologic status. ADH continues to be secreted despite low serum sodium and osmolality and hypervolemia. Criteria for the diagnosis of SIADH include a serum osmolarity of less than 135 mEq/L, a serum osmolality of less than 280 mEq/L, a urinary sodium greater than 25 mEq/L, and a high urinary osmolality, all in the absence of renal and adrenal dysfunction and diuretics. Hyponatremia will develop only if both increased levels of ADH and water intake occur. If extremely elevated levels of ADH are present, hyponatremia may occur even if normal amounts of maintenance fluid are given. The treatment of hyponatremia due to SIADH is fluid restriction. Intake should be limited to 1,000 mL of fluid per day. This is usually very difficult to accomplish in the intensive care unit (ICU) setting due to concerns regarding nutrition, antibiotic administration, and organ perfusion. The injured brain is exquisitely sensitive to ischemia, and therefore even transient periods of hypoperfusion are unacceptable. Demeclocycline, given enterally in a dose of 300 mg every six hours, will inhibit the action of ADH at the collecting duct and will correct the hyponatremia. Lithium may also be given at a dose of 900 mg/d. Both of these drugs have a delayed onset of action and are not appropriate for the rapid correction of severe hyponatremia. Hyponatremia can also occur from cerebral salt wasting syndrome. This is characterized by a profound natriuresis, which is stimulated by elevated circulating levels of atrial natriuretic factor[65] and results in hyponatremia and hypovolemia. In contrast to SIADH, cerebral salt wasting requires repletion of sodium and volume. Fluid restriction would exacerbate the hyponatremia. Table 10–1 outlines the differential diagnosis and treatment of variously caused hyponatremia and illustrates the utility of urinary sodium levels.

A more rapid approach to the correction of hyponatremia is necessary when severe hyponatremia (serum sodium less than 120 mEq/L) or symptoms such as seizures or cerebral edema develop. The mortality of symptomatic severe hyponatremia, when corrected slowly, approaches 50% but is reduced to 8% when corrected rapidly.[66] Hypertonic (3%) saline solutions can be given slowly at a rate of 500 mL over four to six hours. Since hypertonic saline may precipitate acute hypervolemia, concomitant administration of 1 mg/kg of furosemide intravenously may be necessary. Urine electrolytes should be monitored frequently and hypokalemia corrected. Concern has been generated over the rapid correction of

Table 10–1 Diagnosis and Treatment of Various Causes of Hyponatremia in Patients Following Acute Traumatic Brain Injury

Cause	ECV	Urinary Na⁺	Treatment
Extrarenal losses	Decreased	<10 mEq/L	Isotonic saline
Renal losses (cerebral salt wasting)	Decreased	>20 mEq/L	Isotonic saline
CHF, cirrhosis, nephrotic syndrome	Increased	<10 mEc/L	Water restriction
SIADH	Normal or increased	>20 mEq/L	Water restriction

hyponatremia because of its role in central pontine myelinolysis (CPM). CPM is characterized by rapidly progressive quadriparesis with dysarthria and dysphagia and variable level of consciousness. It was initially thought to be related to chronic alcoholism and malnutrition but has been reported in association with the use of hypertonic saline for correction of hyponatremia. The longer the severe hyponatremia has been present, the higher the risk that rapid correction will lead to CPM. It is recommended that rapid (greater than 0.6 mmol/L per hour) correction of severe hyponatremia probably outweighs the risk of CPM if the hyponatremia has been present for less than 48 hours.[66]

Hypernatremia

Hypernatremia is defined as a serum sodium greater than 145 mEq/L. Minimal elevation of 3 to 4 mmol/L will result in intense thirst. If there is no thirst response, or if the patient is not mentally alert enough to satisfy the thirst voluntarily, then hypernatremia results. Both of these situations are common in the patient with traumatic brain injury. The earliest symptom related to hypernatremia is lethargy, which may progress to coma and seizures. Muscular tremor, rigidity, and hyperreflexia are also seen. Slowly developing hypernatremia is much better tolerated than rapidly progressive hypernatremia. Sudden, severe hypernatremia overcomes cerebral volume autoregulation and causes such a profound osmotic shift of water from cerebral tissue that abrupt dehydration and shrinkage of the brain occur. Symptoms of hypernatremia are therefore the result of decreased cerebral intracellular volume. The total-body sodium content may be increased, normal, or decreased, depending on the cause. Total-body sodium remains normal when free water is lost in the absence of sodium intake, as in the case of untreated diabetes insipidus. When both salt and water are lost but water loss is greater, as with osmotic diuresis, osmotic diarrhea, sweating, or vomiting, hypernatremia with decreased total-body sodium content results. Most commonly, hypernatremia occurs in association with increased total-body sodium content because of chronic volume depletion, which stimulates aldosterone secretion and results in renal retention of sodium. Infusion of hypertonic saline will also result in hypernatremia with increased total-body sodium content. Treatment of hyperglycemia may result in hypernatremia as a result of extracellular free water in the intravascular space shifting into cells to maintain the osmotic equilibrium of the cell. Finally, hypernatremia may occur with treatment of hypokalemia, since a cellular exchange of sodium for potassium may occur if there is total-body depletion of potassium. The patient with acute traumatic brain injury may become hypernatremic because of mannitol therapy, diarrhea secondary to hyperosmolar tube feeding formulas with inadequate additional free water, excessive diaphoresis, hypovolemia, DI, or any combination of these. It is important to recognize the onset of DI because this may need therapy other than just free water replacement.

Neurogenic Diabetes Insipidus

Central or neurogenic DI is a cause of hypernatremia that results from excessive renal loss of free water due to a deficiency in ADH. It usually occurs as a result of disruption of the hypothalamic-hypophyseal axis and may be associated with basilar skull fractures in the region of the sella turcica,[67,68] minor brain injury, or severe brain injury and intracranial hypertension.[63] DI is frequently of grave prognostic significance, since its onset often heralds brain death. Hypernatremia due to DI is associated with profuse output of a very dilute urine. The diagnosis can be made if urine osmolality is considerably less than serum osmolality and serum sodium concentration continues to climb. Typically, the critically ill patient with DI following severe brain injury will make greater than 200 to 300 mL of urine hourly with a specific gravity of less than 1.005. Severe dehydration and hypernatremia will shortly follow unless treatment occurs. Even in the case of brain death, initiation of therapy is warranted if organ donation is being considered. Mild to moderate forms of DI should be treated by free water replacement, using urine output as a guide. However, because administration of large volumes of free water to patients with traumatic brain injury may worsen intracranial hypertension and convert central DI to nephrogenic DI, use of aqueous desmopressin acetate (dDAVP) is indicated. dDAVP is a synthetic analogue of vasopressin that is devoid of clinically significant pressor activity and acts to cause free water absorption by the distal tubules and collecting system of the kidneys. It should be given in a dose of 2 to 4 μg intravenously every 8 to 12 hours on a limited basis. If longer-term treatment is required, dDAVP can be given intranasally. In severe cases of DI when there is large urinary volume, uncontrollable intracranial hypertension, and hypotension, a continuous infusion of 1 to 2 U/h of synthetic arginine vasopressin

(Pitressin) is necessary. This will control the DI within 10 to 20 minutes and increase blood pressure without causing ischemia to potentially transplantable organs.

CARDIOVASCULAR COMPLICATIONS OF ACUTE TRAUMATIC BRAIN INJURY

It has long been recognized that the CNS under normal circumstances generates stimulatory and inhibitory influences on such cardiovascular parameters as blood pressure, cardiac output, vasomotor tone, heart rate, and metabolism. Injury to the CNS, then, could naturally be expected to lead directly to perturbations of the cardiovascular system. The cardiovascular system also exhibits an adaptive response to the hypermetabolic state caused by the injured brain. This is characterized by hypertension, tachycardia, and increased cardiac output, all of which are necessary to meet the increased metabolic demands caused by injury to the brain.[8] Failure of the cardiovascular system to supply adequate oxygen for metabolic needs may be fatal. Cardiovascular response occurs early following acute brain injury but does not seem to independently affect outcome.[59] The cardiovascular disturbances occur as a result of increased sympathetic nervous system activity secondary to the release of catecholamines such as epinephrine, norepinephrine, and dopamine. Levels of these hormones have been found to be elevated proportionally to the severity of brain injury and seem to predict outcome.[70,71] The types of complications seen as a result of the sympathetic hyperactivity include hypertension, myocardial ischemia, and cardiac arrhythmias. Severe brain injury may also cause increased vagal tone; therefore, profound bradycardia may occur. This is usually indicative of Cushing's triad of bradycardia, bradypnea, and hypertension and is not related to the excessive catecholamine release associated with other cardiovascular disturbances. It may be a grave prognostic sign and may portend severe intracranial hypertension. Of course, hypotension also occurs in multiply injured patients with concomitant traumatic brain injury, but the brain injury itself is usually not the cause unless brain death has occurred. Hypotension in a patient with acute traumatic brain injury dictates a rapid, diligent search to rule out hemorrhage or spinal cord injury as a cause.

Hypertension

Hypertension associated with traumatic brain injury is estimated to occur in 15% to 25% of affected individuals.[69,72,73] Clifton et al found it to be the most common disturbance of the cardiovascular system.[74] In this study, the average mean arterial blood pressure (MAP) was greater than 100 mm Hg, and both sustained and labile patterns were noted. Cardiovascular lability tended to improve with improving neurologic status. Although hypertension tends to occur early, it may be persistent in some patients and may still be a problem at the time of transfer to a rehabilitation facility.[73,75] It has also been associated with the new onset of normal pressure hydrocephalus after recovery from acute traumatic brain injury.[76] The etiology of hypertension has been related to a direct effect due to lesions or injuries to various sites in the medulla oblongata and hypothalamus,[77,78] since these regions, especially the hypothalamus, are the primary regulators of autonomic activity. Injuries to the orbitofrontal cortex[73] and increased ICP[72] also seem to play a role. It has been postulated that some degree of mechanical distortion, compression, and torsion on the medulla oblongata or mesencephalon results in a change in the normal CNS-vascular relationship that stimulates catecholamine release and subsequent hypertensive response. It may be a direct effect of increased ICP or a result of relative ischemia to these areas of the brain secondary to the intracranial hypertension.[72] However, hypertension may occur in traumatic brain injury in the absence of increased levels of catecholamines.[73]

Sustained systemic hypertension is deleterious to the brain. Starling's law describes the manner in which fluid is exchanged across membranes according to hydrostatic and osmotic forces. Elevated systemic blood pressure results in increased intracerebral hydrostatic pressure, but normal autoregulatory mechanisms within the brain exist at the arteriolar level to maintain relatively constant blood flow, blood volume, and blood pressures within the cerebral capillaries. As a result, capillary endothelial integrity is preserved. The "blood-brain" barrier is protected. In the injured brain, the process of autoregulation is impaired because compensatory constriction of the arterioles within the brain does not occur. The result is a direct transfer of systemic hypertension to capillary beds in the brain, which causes an increase in cerebral blood flow and blood volume and is heralded by brain swelling. Systemic arterial hypertension following acute brain injury results in brain swelling and elevated ICP.[79–81]

Deciding the most appropriate range of systemic arterial blood pressure for any given patient with brain injury is very difficult. Clearly, both hypertension and hypotension adversely affect cerebral blood flow and precipitate secondary brain injury by inducing relative cerebral ischemia. Cerebral perfusion pressure (CPP; MAP – ICP) has classically been used to optimize intracranial hemodynamics. However, basing treatment upon simplified assumptions about cerebral blood flow and its relationship to CPP and ICP may be erroneous and can result in incorrect therapies, since not all patients exhibit loss of cerebral vascular autoregulation.[82] It may be more appropriate to use measurements of cerebral oxygen consumption with continuous cerebral oxymetric catheters placed in the internal jugular vein. However, these catheters aid in determining global cerebral oxygen utilization and may appear to be normal even in the face of significant areas of localized ischemia and increased oxygen utilization. Despite these limitations, treatment of systemic arterial hypertension should be initiated if systolic blood pressures exceed 200 mm Hg[83] or to maintain CPP in the range of 80 to 100 mm Hg.[84] If CPP is low, then ICP should be treated first if this is elevated. To maintain systolic blood pressure below 200 mm Hg, beta-adrenergic blocking agents such as propranolol or labetalol may be used, which also partially act via alpha-adrenergic blockade and may ameliorate other cardiovascular effects of the excessive catecholamine state. These agents have a relatively long half-life, however, and if intravascular volume has not first been restored before their use, hypotension may result and can persist. Esmolol, another beta-adrenergic blocking agent, has a very short half-life, is given by continuous intravenous infusion, and can be turned off, with relatively rapid return to baseline blood pressure, if profound hypotension results from its use. Vasodilating agents such as nitroprusside, hydralazine, nitroglycerin, diazoxide, and calcium channel blockers should be avoided in the management of systemic hypertension in patients with traumatic brain injury because they may cause cerebrovascular dilatation, resulting in increased cerebral blood flow and subsequent edema.[85]

Myocardial Injury

Myocardial damage, manifested as subendocardial hemorrhage, was found in an autopsy study of 50 patients who died as a result of severe brain injury.[86] The cardiotoxic effects of catecholamines have been recognized since the early 1900s and have been characterized by myocarditis, myocardial necrosis, and myocardial fibrosis, without any evidence of coronary artery disease.[87,88] These changes are strikingly similar to those seen in association with myocardial infarction and pheochromocytoma. A direct correlation between myocardial damage and norepinephrine levels was shown in a prospective study of 114 patients with severe traumatic brain injury.[89] Treatment with atenolol, a selective beta-blocking agent, resulted in fewer injury-related electrocardiographic (ECG) changes and less cardiac necrosis at autopsy and should be considered in potential organ donor patients in order to limit catecholamine-induced cardiac injury to the donor heart. ECG changes such as significant ST-segment depression and T-wave inversion have been described both with and without concomitant evidence of myocardial damage.[90,91] These cardiac effects of acute traumatic brain injury may explain unexpected deaths in patients who might otherwise be expected to survive their injury.

Arrhythmias

The incidence of rhythm disturbances following acute brain injury has been reported in the past to range from approximately 30% to 40%.[92] Sinus tachycardia with episodes of rates of 150 beats per minute or greater is common,[90] but supraventricular tachycardia is the most common arrhythmia seen.[89] Ventricular tachycardia and accelerated idioventricular rhythm, however, are rare.[89,90] Like cardiac necrosis, ECG changes, and hypertension, the tachyarrhythmias are also caused by excessive catecholamine secretion. Clonidine, which is a specific alpha-2 agonist, can suppress central and peripheral norepinephrine activity and has been associated in a direct causal fashion with diminished plasma catecholamine levels in a small group of patients who had severe traumatic brain injury.[93]

NOSOCOMIAL INFECTIONS: EXTRACRANIAL AND INTRACRANIAL

The most common cause of late death following an injury is sepsis. Risk factors usually associated with infection leading to sepsis are massive transfusion, hypotension, prolonged ventilatory support, and nutritional insufficiency.[94] The patient with a severe brain injury, with or without multiple trauma, can suffer from the additional risk of immunologic depression. There is mounting evidence that trauma can result in host defense abnormalities.

In brief, the immune system is a system of surveillance. This response can be both a benefit and a detriment to the host. Normal immune system function is strategic to both modulation and eventual termination of the inflammatory response. Cytokines are an example of an inflammatory mediator system. Dysregulation of appropriate inflammatory controls is thought to result in prolonged inflammation, which has been associated with septic shock, systemic inflammatory response syndrome, and acute respiratory distress syndrome.[95–97]

The normal host defense against bacterial infection has classically been divided into nonspecific and specific factors. An example of a nonspecific factor involved in host defense is phagocytosis. The steps of phagocytosis are chemotaxis (migration of white cells to an area of bacterial infection), opsinization (making bacteria more susceptible to ingestion), ingestion of bacteria by neutrophils, and killing of bacteria.[98,99] Another example of a nonspecific factor is interferon, which is derived from T lymphocytes. Interferon promotes monocyte differentiation while inhibiting its proliferation. Fibronectin, a complex glycoprotein, is important in the normal functioning of phagocytes.[100] Levels of fibronectin, which have a direct correlation with survival, are depressed in patients with trauma.[101] The complement system is a complex series of proteins and glycoproteins capable of generating a broad series of inflammatory actions, such as lysis, chemotaxis, opsinization, and anti-inflammatory effects.[102] The activation of the complement system may be accomplished by the classic pathway through antigen-antibody complexes or by the alternate pathway, which is initiated by protein aggregates, endotoxin, and insoluble compounds with appropriate surface compounds.

Examples of specific immune factors are B cells, which are primarily responsible for the production of immunoglobulins or antibody, and T cells, which are responsible for cell-mediated interactions between macrophages and B cells. Additional cellular elements, including lymphocytes, polymorphonuclear leukocytes, eosinophils, basophils, mast cells, and macrophages, produce an extremely complex array of humoral components and diffuse cellular reactions.

White cell migration is compromised in patients with major trauma.[103] Trauma patients requiring massive transfusions have lower T-cell or lymphocyte counts.[104] The total lymphocyte count can decrease as early as 24 hours post injury, a deficit that can last up to 10 days.[105] Phagocytic function and neutrophil chemotaxis is depressed following major trauma.[106,107] Normally, activation of complement leads to increased bacterial phagocytosis by increasing leukocyte adherence and stimulating chemotaxis of monocytes, macrophages, and neutrophils. Alternate complement pathway titers are markedly decreased post injury.[108]

The person with brain injury who may or may not have multisystem trauma is at substantial risk of developing an impaired immune system. It is essential to be aware of the risk and of potential infections, both extracranially and intracranially. Aggressive system support and bacterial surveillance are surely the order of business in care of the neurologically impaired.

Urinary Tract Infections

The rapid introduction of invasive therapeutic interventions or monitoring devices done in the resuscitation bay or ICU provides pathways for bacterial entry into body areas that are normally sterile. Urinary tract infections (UTIs) are the most common nosocomial infections in the hospital. The vast majority of UTIs, 80%, are due to the placement of an indwelling catheter.[109,110] Organisms may be directly inserted into the bladder, or the catheter may precipite a nidus for bacteremia or upward migration of meatal flora through the thin periurethral space. The risk of bacteremia and the development of infection increases 5% to 10% each day a urinary catheter is left in place.[111] Factors that increase risk for UTI are the duration of catherization, the duration of systemic antibiotics, urinary stasis promoting colonization, elevated serum creatine, and unsealed collection junctions.[112,113]

Criteria for diagnosis begin with a urinalysis demonstrating a large number of bacteria per high-powered field and a leukocytosis. Following a urinalysis, a colony culture count of the urine should be completed (10^5 organisms define a UTI) and antibiotic sensitivities done.[114]

The most common bacteria cultured are gram-negative rods (*Escherichia coli, Proteus, Klebsiella, Enterobacter,* and *Serratia*.[110,112,115] The more common gram-positive organisms seen are enterococci, coagulase-negative staphylococci, and *Staphylococcus aureus*.[110,115,116] Between 1% and 4% of patients will develop a bacteremia.[95,100,101] In the neurologically impaired, fever or changes in urine characteristics may be the only apparent clinically significant findings. Fever, pain, dysuria, and frequent urination are common symptoms in patients whose level of consciousness is not impaired.

Appropriate antibiotic therapy is based on urine cultures and sensitivities in the presence of clinical signs consistent with bacteremia. Removal of the indwelling catheter is warranted if the clinical situation allows. Prophylactic antibiotics have not been useful.[117] The prevention of UTIs begins with maintaining an aseptic technique during insertion, maintaining a closed drainage system whenever possible, hanging drainage bags below the level of the bladder and off the floor, and keeping the perineum cleansed.

Pulmonary Infections

After UTIs, the second most common cause of ICU infections is pneumonia. Pneumonia is the most common significant infection in the ICU setting, and it has the highest mortality rate of the nosocomial infections. A detailed discussion of pulmonary infections is in Chapter 9.

Catheter-Related Infections

Overall, catheter-related bacteremia occurs in less than 1% of hospitalized patients. However, catheter-related infections occur mainly in the ICU.[118] Surgical patients in the ICU for more than three days can develop some form of nosocomial bacteremia (10%), often a catheter-related infection.[119] True catheter-related infections are defined by the presence of fever, leukocytosis, physical signs of purulence, and local inflammation. A more accurate diagnosis for catheter-related bacteremia or septicemia is made when more than 15 colonies of bacteria are cultured from the catheter itself and there is a positive peripheral blood culture of the same organism.[119]

There are three hypotheses to explain the pathogenesis of cather-related infections. The major hypothesis is that the bacteria advance and multiply distally on the external catheter surface within the subcutaneous tract. Thus they gain access to the venous circulation, resulting in a bacteremia.[120] The most common source for catheter-related infection is the skin. The organisms commonly isolated are coagulase-negative staphylococci and *Staphylococcus aureus*, both of which originate from the skin.[121,122] It is felt that infections beginning at the insertion site are the most common sources of catheter-related bacteremia.[123]

The second hypothesis suggests that the hub of the catheter may be the source of catheter-related bacteremia. The basis of this theory is that due to catheter manipulation, bacteria are introduced and migrate down the lumen of the catheter into the venous circulation.[124]

An equally plausible third theory is an occult infection of the host, leading to catheter seeding. This pathogenesis is particularly possible in the septic patient. Risk factors for facilitating catheter seeding are the type of organism, the clinical status of the patient, and the duration of bacteremia and catheter use.[125]

It is most probable that all three theories have merit. Multiple factors either separately or interactively are contributory. The key factors are the status of the host, the organisms isolated, and the environment (the integrity of the skin, the technique of sterility, the frequency and type of dressings). Surgical cutdowns carry a much greater risk of catheter-related infections than a percutaneous catheter insertion.[126] Other important considerations are duration of catheter site and length of hospitalization.[118,125]

Some investigators have suggested that the catheter type plays a role in infection. For example, the use of multilumen catheters was once thought to be a risk factor for catheter-related infections.[127] However, more recent studies have found no correlation between the use of multilumen catheters and catheter-related infections.[128] Triple-lumen catheters used for an average of three weeks had a 2.1% incidence of catheter-related sepsis or bacteremia. The common link between catheter types, whether triple- or single-lumen or pulmonary artery (PA) or arterial (A-line) catheters, is the duration of insertion site and the severity of illness.[129,130] Critically ill patients who require a PA catheter and an A-line have catheter-related septicemia or bacteremia incidence rates of 10% and 9.5%, respectively.[130,131] As duration lengthens, the risk of catheter-related infections climbs.

When a critically ill or injured patient becomes febrile, bacteremic, or septic, a major part of discovering the source is the close examination of catheter sites. Clinical infection of the insertion site mandates the removal of the catheter and the administration of antimicrobials. Surgically implanted catheters, not easily removed or replaced, can remain if abscess formation is not present. The patient should be on antibiotics.[132] Percutaneous catheters that are found to be infected should be removed. When the source of fever and leukocytosis is not clear, patients with a recently inserted central venous catheter should have their sites thoroughly assessed. An infected site should necessitate removal followed by initiation of antibiotics. If the site is clean and the catheter is in place for less than a few days, yet the patient has signs of sepsis and no obvious source, the catheter should be changed over a guidewire and the tip cultured. If the tip cultures positive, removal of the catheter is necessary. This is particularly important when tip and blood cultures are identical. A new site should then be chosen. Obviously, if the tip of the catheter is negative, no further catheter-related maneuvers are necessary. As previously stated, PA catheter or A-line catheter placements of long duration are associated with a significant risk of catheter-related infections. If the site has signs of infection or if there is any suspicion of catheter-related sepsis or bacteremia, the line should be removed and replaced only if absolutely necessary.

The prevention of catheter-related infection begins with routine hand washing by medical personnel, along with proper site care. Clipping of hair, not shaving, is important, and liberal scrubbing of the site with iodine-containing disinfectants is needed.[133] An alternative ointment, polymyxin-neomycin-bacitracin, has been found to have better results than iodophor ointment.[134] Minimizing the manipulation of the catheter, along with diminishing the need for tube changes and decreasing the number of piggyback infusions, can only help in decreasing the incidence of catheter-related infections. It is probable that the best dressing is simple dry gauze and tape.[135] Guidewire exchange is an effective and safe tool for diagnosing catheter-related infection and prolonging the usage of the insertion site. Proper insertion techniques and dressing of insertion sites may prevent infection.[136,137] The application of the Vita Cuff, a biodegradable collagen matrix impregnated with bacteriocidal silver, helps inhibit the propagation of skin flora through the catheter site. The Vita Cuff is secured subcutaneously. The use of the Vita Cuff in the ICU results in a decrease in catheter-related bacteremia from 3.7% to 1%. These catheters were in place from 1 to 73 days,[138] suggesting that the Vita Cuff may actually prolong usage of the insertion site.

Wound Infections

The person with severe brain injury who has associated injuries requiring surgical intervention is at risk for developing a surgical wound infection. Surgical wounds are generally classified as clean wounds (no involvement of the gastrointestinal or respiratory tract), clean-contaminated (elective surgery on the gastrointestinal or respiratory tract), contaminated (inflamed wounds or gross gastrointestinal spillage), and dirty wounds (pus is present). Clean wounds carry an infection rate of 2%, while the rates for clean-contaminated, contaminated, and dirty wounds are 10%, 20%, and 40%, respectively.[139]

Besides one's immune status, several factors can place the critically injured patient at risk for wound infections: (1) misuse or overuse of antibiotics, (2) length of stay in the ICU,[140] (3) duration of operation,[141] and (4) presence of surgical drains.[142,143] Most wound infections involve skin and subcutaneous tissue. The common signs and symptoms are fever, pain, erythema, warmth, and swelling. Drainage, local wound care, and limited use of antibiotics are the essential features in treatment of uncomplicated surgical wounds.

Fortunately, the more serious wound infections are not often seen. Infections occurring within 48 hours following an operation are characteristically caused by clostridia or ß-hemolytic streptococci. They can cause a profound toxicity, resulting in a significant risk of death. Rapid diagnosis, surgical debridement of infected tissue, and antibiotics will diminish the risk of death. The dreaded gas gangrene is caused by *Clostridium perfringens*, a gram-positive, spine-forming obligate anaerobe found in the gastrointestinal and female genital tracts. The infection, which has an incubation period between 8 and 48 hours, can result in myonecrosis. The patient will present with sudden pain and an edematous foul-smelling wound. Hemorrhagic bullae can be present. Rapid diagnosis by Gram's stain and X-ray of the wound demonstrating gas must be followed by extensive debridement and antibiotics. Poor outcomes are seen in patients who have leukopenia, thrombocytopenia, intravascular hemolysis, and liver and renal impairment. Aerobic ß-streptococci can have a similar presentation, although the muscle layer is usually spared, but such cases are rarely seen.

A relatively uncommon infection involving the subcutaneous tissues is necrotizing fasciitis, an insidious process in the early phase. Gram s stain of the wound's exudate can show pathogens such as ß-hemolytic *Streptococcus pyogenes*, *Staphylococcus aureus*, *Peplostreptococcus*, *Bacteroides*, and mixed anaerobic-aerobic bacteria.

With gastrointestinal tract injuries, there is always a risk of developing an intra-abdominal abscess following surgical exploration. The upper intestinal tract harbors a small amount of bacteria. The distal intestinal tract begins to concentrate a great number of bacteria, mostly anaerobes, such as *Bacteroides fragilis*, with the largest concentration being in the colon. The most common aerobe seen is *Escherichia coli*. Sepsis due to an intestinal injury is usually more severe when it involves the colon. Fortunately, colonic injuries are not common in blunt trauma. Patients can present with peritonitis, fever, and leukocytosis. Treatment is surgical drainage, along with the appropriate antibiotics.

Decubitus Ulcer

Decubitus ulcers are sores caused by pressure exerted on subcutaneous tissues and skin compressed between the weight of the body and a fixed object. This compression results in a lack of blood supply, capillary leakage, and edema from increased capillary pressure, which lead to localized ischemia and autolysis.[144] The removal of cellular waste is impeded due to compression of local lymphatics. The toxic metabolic waste affects the immediate area of involvement and propagates injury to the surrounding tissue.

Decubitis ulcers are usually associated with long-term facilities, which demonstrate an incidence of 45%.[145] The incidence of decubitus ulcers in acute care facilities is 3%.[145] Other factors that predispose the critically ill or injured patient to decubitus ulcer are physical and mental debilitation, malnutrition, immune dysfunction, and protein waste, seen in patients with major trauma. Additional predisposing factors are age, obesity, and associated diseases, such as peripheral vascular disease and diabetes.

The classification of decubitus ulcer is based on whether it is superficial or deep.[146] The skin of a superficial ulcer may or may not be intact. If the skin is not intact, there can be involvement of the dermis, the subcutaneous tissue, and the fascia. A deep decubitus ulcer can involve all layers of the skin and may present first as a blister, later changing to an eschar, with involvement of not only subcutaneous tissue and fascia but also muscle, bone, and joints. With deep decubitus ulcers, there can be possible soft tissue infection or osteomyelitis.

The majority of decubitus ulcers occur on the lower body (87%).[147] Most of the lower-body decubiti develop on the hip-buttock area (67%).[147] Prevention of these decubitus ulcers includes optimizing nutritional status, avoiding immune dysfunction, and attending to wound surveillance and good body hygiene. Deep decubiti tend to occur in response to shearing and friction forces.[148] Shearing forces occur across bony prominences and result in stretching and distorting of soft tissue. When the patient is elevated, areas at risk are the sacral and coccygeal areas. Friction forces are characterized by skin abrasions caused by sliding or dragging a patient across a bed or stretcher. These abrasions predispose the underlying soft tissues to infections. Pathogenic organisms localize at these sites of abrasion or tissue necrosis. There can be a significant degree of cross-contamination between infected decubiti and urinary or respiratory tracts.[149] The more common organisms are *Staphylococcus aureus* and *Bacteroides fragilis*.[150] An important aspect of prevention is pressure dispersion. For example, rolling the patient every two hours is a simple method of dispersing pressure. Technological methods that address issues of shearing and friction forces and pressure dispersion include the use of specialized beds. Examples are low–air loss beds (columns of air injected to support the patient), mud beds (viscous medium imparting greater stability than air or water beds), and air-fluidized beds (fine silicone beads dispersed with the use of air).

Nosocomial Sinusitis

Since the latter part of the 1980s, acute paranasal sinusitis has been recognized as a potentially significant source of infection or septicemia in the ICU.[151] The incidence of nosocomial sinusitis is 8% of all ICU admissions.[151] The normal paranasal sinuses are air-filled cavities lined with nasal mucosa. Factors that contribute to the development of sinusitis are decreased ostial patency and impaired sinus mucociliary clearance.[152] The inflammatory process of sinusitis produces changes in the mucosa of the sinus. As a result, secretions from the sinuses drain through the ducts into the nasal meatus. Any clinical situation that blocks these routes may cause secretions to back up into the sinuses and cause infection (Figure 10–8).

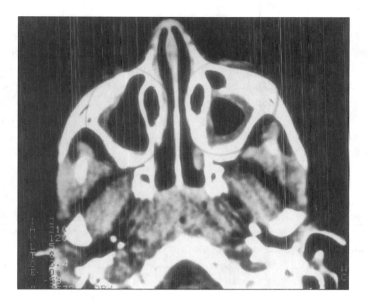

Figure 10–8 Mucoperiosteal thickening due to chronic sinusitis.

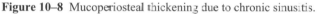

Within the ICU, many factors predispose the patient with craniocerebral injury to acute paranasal sinusitis. Bony or soft tissue injuries to the face resulting in hematomas can predispose the person with brain injury to paranasal sinus suppurations. Persons with brain injury invariably require some form of invasive instrumentation, particularly if they have a Glasgow Coma Score lower than 8.[153] These patients usually require prolonged ventilatory support. Nasal intubation, either singly or in concert with maxillofacial injury or hematoma, can become the genesis of a nosocomial sinusitis. The nasotracheal tube causes a mechanical obstruction of the sinus ostia, resulting in impaired drainage, which allows normal sinus flora to proliferate and become pathogenic.[154,155] In fact, it is not uncommon for the tracheobronchial tree to be colonized with the same organisms found in the sinuses.[151,156,157]

Another predisposing factor for nosocomial sinusitis is the use of nasogastric tubes. These stiff catheters are commonly used for the decompression of the stomach and occasionally as methods of feeding. Like the nasotracheal tubes, these catheters can impede sinus drainage.[158]

The most commonly involved sinus is the maxillary sinus. The ethmoid or sphenoid sinus may also be affected. Persistent fever of unknown source and/or persistent purulent nasal discharge are early diagnostic signs. When the diagnosis is in question, sinus X-rays and a computed tomography (CT) scan should be completed. If signs of opacification or air fluid levels on X-ray or CT scans are apparent, attempts should be made to aspirate fluid from the involved sinuses. Depending upon location of the material, aspirations can be performed under local anesthesia for clinically suspected maxillary sinus infections. General anesthesia is necessary when performing an open ethmoidectomy or sphenoidectomy approach. These procedures can be both diagnostic and therapeutic. The predominant organisms isolated are gram-negative organisms.[151,157,159] The most common organisms implicated are *Pseudomonas aeruginosa*, *Staphylococcus aureus*, and *Staphylococcus epidermidis*. Along with drainage, the patient should be placed on the appropriate antibiotics.

The complications of nosocomial sinusitis are uncommon but are potentially fatal.[160] Complications can be divided into extracranial and intracranial.[161] The potential extracranial sequelae are cellulitis, abscess formation, and cavernous sinus thrombosis. Abscess and cavernous sinus thrombosis tend to be the most severe, carrying a 50% morbidity and a 20% mortality.[162] The intracranial complications seen are meningitis, subdural empyema, and brain abscess. The mortality of intracranial complications is 40%.[163] The management of these complications includes surgical drainage and antibiotics.

Meningitis

The incidence of posttraumatic infections of the CNS is quite low. However, if defense mechanisms are weakened, the person with brain injury becomes unusually susceptible to an intracranial infectious process. The natural defenses that protect the CNS are the blood-brain barrier and the blood–cerebrospinal fluid barrier. If bacteria invade the barriers, then these same barriers impede host defense. Cerebrospinal fluid (CSF), in particular, is not equipped for bacterial clearance. In normal CSF, the levels of opsonic proteins, complement, and specific antibodies are either low or nonexistent.[164,165] Since intracranial defense mechanisms are not particularly efficient, an infection like meningitis can prove to be a potentially lethal complication.

Meningitis is an inflammation of the meninges covering the brain or spinal cord. The pathogenesis for this meningeal inflammation is infection. Infections of the CNS commonly occur as a result of septicemia. In persons who have sustained brain injury, there can be a loss of protective barriers due to the weakened integrity of the dura. Patients sustaining a basilar skull fracture or paranasal sinusitis are at risk for intracranial bacterial invasion.

Meningitis following brain injury is a rare complication whose incidence is 1%.[166] Interuption of the dura can result in CSF leakage or fistula. Posttraumatic CSF rhinorrhea and otorrhea are reported to occur in 17% of patients incurring skull fractures.[167] The incidence of meningitis as a consequence of rhinorrhea or otorrhea is 9% and 18% respectively.[168] The mortality rate for meningitis in persons sustaining craniocerebral trauma varies from 29% to 57.9%.[169–171]

ICP monitoring for greater than 72 hours has been thought to be a contributing factor in the development of infection.[172–174] However, the literature has been somewhat mixed. Some investigations have shown no correlation between duration of ICP monitoring and the incidence of infection.[175–178] Many patients require more than five days of monitoring, and in contrast to duration as a factor of infection, it has been shown that catheter manipulation and flushes with antibiotics increase the rate of monitor-related infections.[179,180]

The clinical presentations in the conscious patient may be headaches, photophobia, vomiting, and chills. Signs of meningeal irritation can be present, such as nuchal rigidity. Additional evidence of meningeal inflammation includes the presence of Kernig's sign, elicited by raising the leg at a 90-degree angle with the hips. Brudzinski's sign can be tested by flexing the neck forward and observing for hip and knee flexion. Persons with brain injury who have a depressed level of consciousness will not present with signs that are particularly unique to meningitis. In the unconscious patient, there can be a worsening of neurological-deficit, fever, seizures, cranial nerve deficits, and motor abnormalities. The presence of CSF leak or fistula can heighten the clinical suspicion of meningitis.[181]

Bacterial meningitis in persons who have sustained a basilar skull fracture, CSF fistula, or paranasal sinusitis caused by craniocerebral injury is due mostly to *Streptococcus pneumoniae*, followed by *Haemophilus influenzae*[181] (non–type B in the adult, type B consistently seen in children). In patients whose mechanism of injury is of the penetrating variety, the more common organisms are *Staphylococcus aureus* or gram-negative rods.[182,183]

The diagnosis of meningitis is based on positive blood cultures and a positive CSF culture via lumbar puncture. The classic CSF findings include a white count between 100 and 15,000 cells with a predominance of polymorphonuclear leukocytes, a reduced level of CSF glucose, and an increased level of CSF protein. Gram's stain of CSF will identify the causative organism in 75% of the cases.[184] In at least 90% of cases, a positive CSF culture will be present when there is purulent CSF.[185]

Prompt initiation of antibiotic therapy is essential in the treatment of bacterial meningitis. The most important consideration in choosing an antibiotic or antibiotics is the ability to penetrate the blood-brain barrier. In the initial phase of treatment, the presence of inflammation can assist the penetration of antimicrobials. The antibiotic of choice for *Streptococcus pneumoniae* is penicillin G; for *Haemophilus influenzae*, ceftriaxone or chloramphenicol; for *Staphylococcus aureus*, nafcillin or vancomycin; and for the gram-negatives, ceftriaxone or trimethoprim-sulfamethoxazole. The duration of therapy is dependent on the infectious organism. If the organism is either *Streptococcus* or *Haemophilus*, patients should be treated for 10 to 14 days. *Staphylococcus* disease with bacteremia is treated for four to six weeks, and gram-negatives require approximately three weeks of therapy.

The role of prophylactic antibiotics for open or basilar skull fractures has always been unclear. Many centers advise against antibiotics with or without an associated CSF leak.[186,187] The theoretical reasons for discouraging the prophylactic use of antibiotics are the risk of superinfection and the development of resistant strains. To date, there are only two prospective randomized studies assessing the role of prophylactic antibiotics for basilar or open skull fractures. Their conclusions were that antibiotic prophylaxis has a role in the management of basilar and open skull fractures.[188,189] The antibiotics should probably be used on a short-term basis.[188] The potential benefits include fewer complications and decreased cost of treatment.

Brain Abscess

A brain abscess is a localized collection of pus within the parenchyma of the brain or meninges (Figure 10–9). The development of brain abscess secondary to penetrating brain injury is well established,[190,191] although brain abscess occurring after blunt injury is quite uncommon.[192,193] Regardless, the overall incidence for brain abscess specifically related to craniocerebral trauma ranges from 3% to 15%,[190–193] with a mortality rate of 33% to 50%.[190,191,194]

The pathophysiology of abscess formation is the entry of bacteria into the brain. The proliferation of bacteria leads to inflammation, petechial hemorrhage, edema, and necrosis. Liquification of the necrotic tissue leads to areas of pus. Abscess formation takes approximately 14 days, and the presence of multiple abscesses is possible but rare.[195] The etiology of the abscess is most commonly *Staphylococcus aureus*, followed by gram-negatives.[196]

The clinical manifestations are variable, occurring 50% of the time, and are dependent on location of abscess.[195] The course can be rapidly deteriorating or benign. When signs and symptoms are present, they can include fever, headaches, altered level of consciousness, nausea/vomiting, seizures, hemiparesis, papilledema, pupillary changes, increased sedimentation rate, and leukocytosis.

The diagnosis of brain abscess should begin with a CT scan. The technique, with the use of contrast, can readily identify the location of the abscess and demonstrate the appearance of multiloculated abscesses. Abscesses usually appear as elliptical formations of low density surrounded by a capsule of heightened density. An area of edema will be displayed as low density, usually surrounding the loculated abscess (Figure 10–10). Laboratory tests may not be useful if there is no systemic infection. Lumbar puncture (LP) is usually contraindicated in the presence of brain abscess due to the possibility of intracranial hypertension, particu-

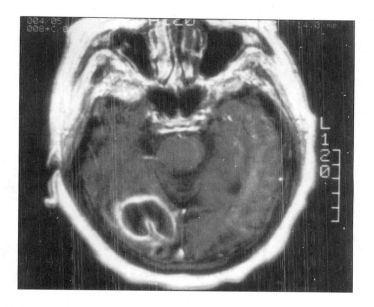

Figure 10–9 Magnetic resonance imaging view of a right occipital abscess.

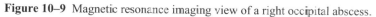

larly when the CT picture demonstrates a midline shift. An LP can precipitate a herniation, resulting in brainstem compression and death. The mortality rate can be as high as 8%.[191] Electroencephalography can assist in the diagnosis of brain abscess by identifying hemispheric location of the abscess and demonstrating slowing of delta waves over the affected area. It cannot detect multiple abscesses or locate a posterior fossa abscess.[195]

The optimal treatment of brain abscess remains somewhat controversial. Modes of treatment include craniotomy with excision and needle catheter drainage or aspiration. Therapy decisions are based upon location. If a lesion is easily accessible, then craniotomy with excision is appropriate. If the abscess is deep or is in a crucial area of the brain, then needle drainage or aspiration, using stereotactic technique under CT control, would be the best course of action. However, if aspiration fails, then excision of the abscess is required.

An additional crucial treatment is antibiotic therapy. Patients with brain abscess should be placed on parenteral antibiotics for one month. A common cause of treatment failure is inadequate antibiotic therapy. The antibiotics chosen must be culture and sensitivity specific and must be able to cross the blood-brain barrier (ie, penicillin G, chloramphenicol, third-generation cephalosporins, and metronidazole). An adjunctive therapy may be steroids, but steroids can interfere with the body's normal immune response and can impede capsule formation.[194] Steroids

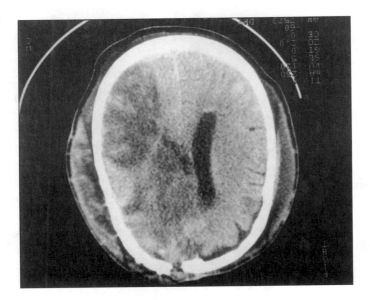

Figure 10–10 Left parietal lobe abscess post craniectomy, with associated edema anteriorly. Study done without contrast.

can reduce cerebral edema[195] and potential herniation and brainstem compression, but they remain a controversial mode of treatment.

Empyema

Empyema is a collection of pus either below the dura (subdural empyema) or above the dura (epidural empyema). Subdural empyema is most commonly caused by paranasal sinus infection. Subdural empyemas account for approximately 25% of all intracranial infections.[196] Persons with brain injury who have a maxillofacial injury or frontal skull fracture or compound depressed skull fracture have an increased risk of developing a subdural empyema,[193,197,198] which carries a mortality rate between 23% and 66%.[198,199]

The pathogenesis of subdural empyema is the organism's ability to gain access to the subdural space following injury to the facial or cranial regions. The most common causative organisms are *Staphylococcus aureus*, *Staphylococcus epidermidis,* and gram-negatives. Most subdural empyemas are acute in onset. Symptoms consistent with subdural empyema are fever, headache, vomiting, lethargy leading to coma, signs of meningeal irritation, and leukocytosis. Focal signs may be present due to a mass effect of the subdural collection. Focal signs, such as hemiparesis, seizure, aphasia, pupillary dilatation, and ocular palsy, tend to occur later, following the development of subdural empyema. The diagnosis may be suspected when the patient has clinical features of a subdural empyema. However, the definitive diagnosis is made by contrast-enhanced CT or magnetic resonance imaging (MRI). Treatment should be aggressive and prompt. The best results are achieved by craniotomy with evacuation of the empyema, debridement, and irrigation. Prolonged antibiotics for several weeks are the other mainstay of treatment.

Epidural empyema is quite uncommon. The cause is usually a penetrating wound to the skull, due to either surgical intervention or missile injury, usually occurring a few weeks following the injury. The clinical symptoms can be fever, headaches, altered level of consciousness, localizing signs, and intracranial hypertension. The most common organism is *Staphylococcus aureus*. The diagnosis is made by either CT scan or MRI. The treatment is surgical evacuation, wound irrigation, and systemic antibiotics.

CONCLUSION

The response to severe acute traumatic brain injury is characterized primarily by hypermetabolism and hypercatabolism. The physiologic changes caused by this response result in complications of nutritional state, electrolyte balance, cardiovascular response, and immune function. The impairment of nutritional status following traumatic brain injury can be severe and persistent and may result in increased risk of infection. Nutritional supplementation should be initiated early following injury to minimize the adverse effects of the induced hypercatabolic state. An expert in nutrition for critically ill patients such as a dietitian, nutritional nurse specialist, or a physician with special interest in nutrition should be called in early to assist in the nutritional management of these critically ill patients. These personnel can become an integral part of the team approach to the care of critically ill patients with acute traumatic brain injury.

Derangement in nutritional status or immune function can compromise the body's natural response to infection. The most significant infection is pneumonia. However, additional extracranial and intracranial infections can occur as a result of invasive monitoring techniques, prolonged ICU stays, and instrumentation of the ICU patient. Prevention, awareness of potential infectious complications, and aggressive treatment are paramount in improving the survivability and functional recovery of persons with brain injury.

Several authors have recently associated improved outcome with early rehabilitation when it is applied to patients with traumatic brain injury while they are still in the ICU.[200,201] Earlier, more aggressive acute rehabilitation beginning in the ICU is becoming the norm for many patients with severe traumatic brain injury. This exposes the members of the rehabilitation team to many of the complications and physiologic derangements that occur early in the course of acute brain injury. It becomes imperative, then, that all health care personnel involved in the care of these patients become familiar with all potential complications and physiologic responses known to occur in patients with acute traumatic brain injury.

REFERENCES

1. Rapp RP, Young B, Twyman D, et al. The favorable effect of early parenteral feeding on survival in head-injured patients. *J Neurosurg.* 1983;58:906–912.

2. Clifton GL, Robertson CS, Choi SC. Assessment of nutritional requirements of head-injured patients. *J Neurosurg.* 1986;64:895–901.

3. Bivins BA, Twyman DL, Young B. Failure of nonprotein calories to mediate protein conservation in brain-injured patients. *J Trauma.* 1986;26:980–986.

4. Ott L, McClain C, Young B. Nutrition and severe brain injury. *Nutrition.* 1989;5:75–79.

5. Sunderland PM, Heilbrun MP. Estimating energy expenditure in traumatic brain injury: comparison of indirect calorimetry with predictive formulas. *Neurosurgery.* 1992;31:246–253.

6. Young B, Ott L, Yingling B, McClain C. Nutrition and brain injury. *J Neurotrauma.* 1992; 9(suppl 1):S375–S385.

7. Petersen SR, Jeevanandam M, Harrington T. Is the metabolic response to injury different with or without severe head injury? Significance of plasma glutamine levels. *J Trauma.* 1993;34:653–661.

8. Robertson CS, Clifton GL, Grossman RG. Oxygen utilization and cardiovascular function in head-injured patients. *Neurosurgery.* 1984;15:307–314.

9. Weissman C, Kemper M, Askanazi J, et al. Resting metabolic rate of the critically ill patient: measured versus predicted. *Anaesthesiology.* 1986;64:673–679.

10. Weekes E, Elia M. Observations on the patterns of 24-hour energy expenditure changes in body composition and gastric emptying in head-injured patients receiving nasogastric tube feedings. *JPEN.* 1996;20:31–37.

11. Ford EG, Jennings LM, Andrassy RJ. Steroid treatment of head injuries in children: the nutritional consequences. *Curr Surg.* 1987;44:311–313.

12. Robertson CS, Clifton GL, Goodman JC. Steroid administration and nitrogen excretion in the head injured patient. *J Neurosurg.* 1985;63:714–718.

13. Young B, Ott L, Phillips R, McClain C. Metabolic management of the patient with head injury. *Neurosurg Clin North Am.* 1991;2:301–320.

14. Robertson CS. Inflammatory cells and the hypermetabolism of head injury. *J Lab Clin Med.* 1991;118:205.

15. Chiolero R, Schutz Y, Lemerch T, et al. Hormonal and metabolic changes following severe head injury or non-cranial injury. *JPEN.* 1989;13:5–12.

16. Clifton GL, Ziegler MG, Grossman RG. Circulating catecholamines and sympathetic activity after head injury. *Neurosurgery.* 1991;8:10–14.

17. Inoue M, McHugh M, Pappius HM. The effect of alpha-adrenergic blockers prazosin and yohimbine on cerebral metabolism and biogenic amine content of the traumatized brain. *J Cereb Blood Flow Metab.* 1991;11:242–252.

18. Chiolero RL, Breitenstein E, Thorin D, et al. Effects of propranolol on resting metabolic rate after severe head injury. *Crit Care Med.* 1989;17:328–334.

19. Haider W, Lackner F, Schlick W, et al. Metabolic changes in the course of severe acute brain damage. *Eur J Intensive Care Med.* 1975;1:19.

20. Deutschman CS, Konstantinides FN, Raup S, et al. Physiological and metabolic response to isolated closed-head injury. Part 1. *J Neurosurg.* 1986;64:89–98.

21. Deutschman CS, Konstantinides FN, Raup S, et al. Physiological and metabolic response to isolated closed-head injury. Part 2. *J Neurosurg.* 1987;66:388–395.

22. Twyman D, Young AB, Ott L, et al. High protein enteral feedings: a means of achieving positive nitrogen balance in head-injured patients. *JPEN.* 1985;9:679–684.

23. Van Way CW. Nutritional support in the injured patient. *Surg Clin North Am.* 1991;71:537–548.

24. McClain CJ, Twyman DL, Ott LG, et al. Serum and urine zinc response in head-injured patients. *J Neurosurg.* 1986;64:224–230.

25. Ranseen JD, Schmitt FA, Holt K, et al. Zinc supplementation and early outcome following severe brain injury. *J Clin Exp Neuropsychol.* 1990.12:34. Abstract.

26. Helling TS, Evans LL, Fowler DL, et al. Infectious complications in patients with severe head injury. *J Trauma.* 1988;28:1575–1577.

27. Miller CH, Quattrocchi KB, Frank EH, et al. Humoral and cellular immunity following severe head injury: review and current investigations. *Neurol Res.* 1991;13:117–124.

28. Quattrocchi KB, Frank EH, Miller CH, et al. Suppression of cellular immune activity following severe head injury. *J Neurotrauma.* 1990;7:77–87.

29. Quattrocchi KB, Frank EH, Miller CH, et al. Impairment of helper T-cell function and lymphokine-activated killer cytotoxicity following severe head injury. *J Neurosurg.* 1991;75:766–773.

30. Ott L, Young B, Phillips R, et al. Brain injury and nutrition. *Nutr Clin Pract.* 1990;5:68–73.

31. Kudsk KA, Mowatt-Larssen C, Bukar J, et al. Effect of a recombinant human insulin-like growth factor 1 and early total parenteral nutrition on immune depression following severe head injury. *Arch Surg.* 1994;129:66–71.

32. Young B, Ott L, Dempsey R, et al. Relationship between admission hyperglycemia and neurologic outcome of severely brain-injured patients. *Ann Surg.* 1989.210:466–473.

33. Sieber FE, Traystman RJ. Special issues: glucose and the brain. *Crit Care Med.* 1992;20:104–114.

34. Young B, Ott L, Twyman D, et al. The effect of nutritional support on outcome from severe head injury. *J Neurosurg.* 1987;67:668–676.

35. Young B, Ott L, Haack D, et al. Effect of total parenteral nutrition upon intracranial pressure in severe head injury. *J Neurosurg.* 1987;67:76–80.

36. Babineau TJ, Pomposelli J, Forse RA, Blackburn GL. Lipids. In: Zaloga GP, ed. *Nutrition in Critical Care.* Saint Louis, Mo: Mosby-Year Book; 1994:191–204.

37. Daly JM, Lieberman MD, Goldfine MS, et al. Enteral nutrition with supplemental arginine, RNA, and omega fatty acids in patients after operation: immunologic, metabolic, and clinical outcome. *Surgery.* 1992;112:56–67.

38. Bower RH, Cerra FE, Bershadsky B, et al. Early enteral administration of a formula (Impact) supplemented with arginine, nucleotides, and fish oil in intensive care unit patients: results of a multicenter, prospective, randomized, clinical trial. *Crit Care Med.* 1995;23:436–449.

39. Kalimo H, Rehncrona S, Soderfeldt B, et al. Brain lactic acidosis and ischemic cell damage: 2. Histopathology. *J Cereb Blood Flow Metab.* 1981;1:313–327.

40. Clifton GL, Robertson CS, Contant CF. Enteral hyperalimentation in head injury. *J Neurosurg.* 1985;62:186–193.

41. Flowers JF, Ryan JA, Gough JA. Catheter-related complications of total parenteral nutrition. In: Fischer J, ed. *Total Parenteral Nutrition.* 2nd ed. Boston, Mass: Little, Brown and Co; 1991: 25–45.

42. Goldmann DA, Maki DG. Infection control in total parenteral nutrition. *JAMA.* 1973;223: 1360–1364.

43. Veterans Affairs Total Parenteral Nutrition Cooperative Study Group. Perioperative total parenteral nutrition in surgical patients: a VA Cooperative study. *N Engl J Med.* 1991;325: 525–532.

44. Kudsk KA, Croce MA, Fabian TC, et al. Enteral versus parenteral feeding: effects on septic morbidity after blunt and penetrating abdominal trauma. *Ann Surg.* 1992;215:503–513.

45. Moore FA, Feliciano DV, Andrassy RJ, et al. Early enteral feeding, compared with parenteral, reduces postoperative septic complications: the results of a meta-analysis. *Ann Surg.* 1992;216:172–183.

46. Kalaferentzos F, Alivazatos V, Panagopoulous K, et al. Nasoduodenal intubation with the use of metoclopromide. *Nutr Supp Serv.* 1987;7:11–13.

47. Wolf DC, Stern MA. Erythromycin elixir facilitates transpyloric passage of enteral feeding tubes: results of a prospective randomized controlled trial. *Am J Gastroenterol.* 1992;87:1278. Abstract.

48. Spapen HD, Duinslaeger L, Diltoer M, Gillet R, Bossuyt A, Huyghens LP. Gastric emptying in critically ill patients is accelerated by adding cisapride to a standard enteral feeding protocol: results of a prospective, randomized, controlled trial. *Crit Care Med.* 1995;23:481–485.

49. Mittal RK, Stewart WR, Schirmer BD. Effect of a catheter in the pharynx on the frequency of transient lower oesophageal sphincter relaxations. *Gastroenterology.* 1992;103:1236–1240.

50. Saxe JM, Ledgerwood AM, Lucas CE, et al. Lower oesophageal sphincter dysfunction preludes gastric feeding after head injury. *J Trauma.* 1994;37:581–586.

51. Vane DW, Shiffler M, Grosfeld JL, et al. Reduced lower esophageal sphincter (LES) pressure after acute and chronic brain injury. *J Pediatr Surg.* 1982;17:960–964.

52. Gauderer MW, Ponsky JL, Izant RJ Jr. Gastrostomy without laparotomy: a percutaneous endoscopic technique. *J Pediatr Surg.* 1980;15:872–875.

53. Meehan SE, Wood RA, Cuschieri A. Percutaneous cervical pharyngostomy: a comfortable and convenient alternative to protracted nasogastric intubation. *Amer J Surg.* 1984;148:325–330.

54. Norton JA, Ott LG, McClain C, et al. Intolerance to enteral feeding in the brain-injured patient. *J Neurosurg.* 1988;68:62–66.

55. Spain DA, DeWeese RC, Reynolds MA, Richardson JD. Transpyloric passage of feeding tubes in patients with head injury does not decrease complications. *J Trauma.* 1995;39:1100–1102.

56. Strong RM, Condon SC, Solinger MR, et al. Equal aspiration rates from postpylorus and intragastric-placed small-bore nasoenteric feeding tubes: a randomized prospective study. *JPEN.* 1992;16:59–63.

57. Lazarus BA, Murphy JB, Culpepper L. Aspiration associated with long-term gastric versus jejunal feeding: a critical analysis of the literature. *Arch Phys Med Rehabil.* 1990;71:46–53.

58. Cech AC, Morris JB, Mullen JL, Crooks GW. Long-term enteral access in aspiration-prone patients. *J Intensive Care Med.* 1995;10:179–186.

59. Hadley MN, Grahm TW. Harrington T, et al. Nutritional support and neurotrauma: a critical review of early nutrition in forty-five acute head injury patients. *Neurosurgery.* 1986;19:367–373.

60. Waters DC, Dechert R, Bartlett R. Metabolic studies in head injury patients: a preliminary report. *Surgery.* 1986;100:531–534.

61. Balzola F, Boggio Bertinet D, Solerio A, et al. Dietetic treatment with hypercaloric and hyperprotein intake in patients following severe brain injury. *J Neurosurg Sci.* 1980;24:131–140.

62. Borzotta AP, Penrings J, Papasdero B, et al. Enteral versus parenteral nutrition after severe closed head injury. *J Trauma.* 1994;37:459–468.

63. Chestnut RM, Marshall LF. Management of severe head injury. In: Ropper AH, ed. *Neurological and Neurosurgical Intensive Care.* New York, NY: Raven Press 1993:203–246.

64. Nelson PB. Fluid and electrolyte physiology, pathophysiology and management. In: Wirth FP, Ratcheson RA, eds. *Neurosurgical Critical Care. Vol 1: Concepts in Neurosurgery.* Baltimore, Md: Williams & Wilkins; 1987:69–80.

65. Nelson PB, Seif SM, Marcon JC, Robinson AG. Hyponatremia in intracranial disease: perhaps not the syndrome of inappropriate secretion of antidiuretic hormone (SIADH). *J Neurosurg.* 1981;55:938–941.

66. Oh MS, Carroll HJ. Disorders of sodium metabolism: hypenatremia and hyponatremia. *Crit Care Med.* 1992;20:94–103.

67. Halimi P, Sigal R, Doyon D, et al. Post-traumatic diabetes insipidus: MR demonstration of pituitary stalk rupture. *J Comput Assist Tomogr.* 1988;12:135–137.

68. Leramo OB, Rao AB. Diplopia and diabetes insipidus secondary to type II fracture of the sella turcica: case report. *Can J Surg.* 1987;30:53–54.

69. Piek J, Chesnut RM, Marshall LF, et al. Extracranial complications of severe head injury. *J Neurosurg.* 1992;77 901–907.

70. Woolf PD, Hamill RW, Lee LA, et al. The predictive value of catecholamines in assessing outcome in traumatic brain injury. *J Neurosurg.* 1987;66:875–882.

71. Hamill RW, Woolf PD, McDonald JV, et al. Catecholamines predict outcome in traumatic brain injury. *Ann Neurol.* 1987;21:438–443.

72. Jennett B, Teasdale G. *Management of Head Injuries.* Philadelphia, Pa: FA Davis; 1981:111–151.

73. Labi ML, Horn LJ. Hypertension in traumatic brain injury. *Brain Inj.* 1990;4:365–370.

74. Clifton GL, Robertson CS, Kype K, et al. Cardiovascular response to severe head injury. *J Neurosurg.* 1983;59:447–454.

75. Kalisky Z, Morrison DP, Meyers CA, Von Laufen A. Medical problems encountered during rehabilitation of patients with head injury. *Arch Phys Med Rehabil.* 1985;66:25–29.

76. Mysiw WJ, Jackson RD. Relationship of new-onset systemic hypertension and normal pressure hydrocephalus. *Brain Inj.* 1990;4:233–238.

77. Talman WT. Cardiovascular regulation and lesions of the central nervous system. *Ann Neurol.* 1985;18:1–13.

78. Shiozaki T, Taneda M, Kishikawa A, et al. Transient and repetitive rises in blood pressure synchronized with plasma catecholamine increases after head injury. *J Neurosurg.* 1993;78:501–504.

79. Schutta HS, Kassell NF, Langfitt TW. Brain swelling produced by injury and aggravated by arterial hypertension: a light and electron microscopic study. *Brain* 1968;91:281–294.

80. Marshall WJ, Jackson JL, Langfitt TW. Brain swelling caused by trauma and arterial hypertension: hemodynamic aspects. *Arch Neurol.* 1969;21:545–553.

81. Langfitt TW, Weinstein JD, Kassell NF. Cerebral vasomotor paralysis produced by intracranial hypertension. *Neurology.* 1965;15:622–641.

82. Bouma GJ, Muizelaar JP, Bandoh K, Marrnarou A. Blood pressure and intracranial pressure-volume dynamics in severe head injury: relationship with cerebral blood flow. *J Neurosurg.* 1992;77:15–19.

83. Kaufman HH, Timberlake G, Voelker J, Pait TG. Medical complications of head injury. *Med Clin North Am.* 1993;77:43–60.

84. Rosner MJ, Daughton S. Cerebral perfusion pressure management in head injury. *J Trauma.* 1990;30:933–941.

85. Robertson CS, Clifton GL, Taylor AA, Grossman RG. Treatment of hypertension associated with head injury. *J Neurosurg.* 1983;59:455–460.

86. Clifton GL, McCorrnick WF, Grossman RG. Neuropathology of early and late deaths after head injury. *Neurosurgery.* 1981;8:309–314.

87. Haft JI. Cardiovascular injury induced by sympathetic catecholamines. *Prog Cardiovasc Dis.* 1974;17:73–86.

88. Rajs J. Relationship between craniocerebral injury and subsequent myocardial fibrosis and heart failure: report of 3 cases. *Br Heart J.* 1976;38:396–402.

89. Cruickshank JM, Neil-Dwyer G, Hayes Y, et al. Reduction of stress/catecholamine induced cardiac necrosis by beta-selective blockage. *Lancet.* September 12, 1987:585–589.

90. McLeod AA, Neil-Dwyer G, Meyer CH, et al. Cardiac sequelae of acute head injury. *Br Heart J.* 1982;47:221–226.

91. Greenspahn BR, Barzilai B, Denes P. Electrocardiographic changes in concussion. *Chest.* 1978;74:468–469.

92. Evans DE, Alter WA, Shatsky SA, Gunby N. Cardiac arrythmias resulting from experimental head injury. *J Neurosurg.* 1976;45:609–616.

93. Payen D, Quintin L, Plaisance P, et al. Head injury: clonidine decreases plasma catecholamines. *Crit Care Med.*1990;18:392–395.

94. Morgan AS. Risk factors for infection in the trauma patient. *J Natl Med Assoc.* 1992;84:1019–1023.

95. Le J, Vilcek J. Tumor necrosis factor and interleukin I: cytokines with multiple overlapping biological activities. *Lab Invest.* 1987;56:234–248.

96. Tracey KJ, Beutler B, Lowry SF, et al. Shock and tissue injury induced by recombinant human cachectin. *Science.* 1986;234:470–474.

97. Barton R, Cerra FB. The hypermetabolism: multiple organ failure syndrome. *Chest.* 1989; 96:1153–1160.

98. Cates KL. Host factors in bacteremia. *Am J Med.* 1983;75(1B):19–25.

99. Johnston RB Jr, Stroud RM. Complement and host defense against infection. *J Pediatr.* 1977;90:169–179.

100. Saba TM. Fibronectin: relevance to phagocytic post response to injury. *Circ Shock.* 1989; 29:257–278.

101. Saba TM. Plasma fibronectin (opsonil glycoprotein): its synthesis by vascular endothelial cells and role in cardiopulmonary integrity after trauma as related to reticuloendothelial function. *Am J Med.* 1980;68:577–594.

102. Frank MM. Complement in the pathophysiology of human disease. *N Engl J Med.* 1987; 316:1525–1530.

103. Meakins JL, Christou NU, Shizgal HM, et al. Therapeutic approaches to anergy in surgical patients. *Ann Surg.* 1979;190:286–296.

104. Polk HC Jr, George CD, Wellhausen SR, et al. A systematic study of host defense process in badly injured patients. *Ann Surg.* 1986;204:282–299.

105. O'Mahony JB, Wood JJ, Rodrick ML Mannick JA. Changes in T lymphocyte subsets following injury: assessment by flow cytometry and relationships in sepsis. *Ann Surg.* 1985;202:580–586.

106. Maderazo EG, Albano SD, Woronick CL, et al. Polymorphonuclear leukocyte migration abnormalities and their significance in severely traumatized patients. *Ann Surg.* 1983;198:736–742.

107. Palder SB, O'Mahony JB, Rodrick M, et al. Alteration of polymorphonuclear leukocyte function in the trauma patient. *J Trauma.* 1983.23:655.

108. Gelfand JA, Donelan M, Burke JF. Preferential activation and depletion of the alternative complement pathway by burn injury. *Ann Surg.* 1983;198:58–62.

109. Kunin CM. *Detection, Prevention and Management of Urinary Tract Infections.* 4th ed. Philadelphia, Pa: Lea & Febiger; 1987.

110. Stamm WE, Martin SM, Bennett JV. Epidemiology of nosocomial infections due to gram-negative bacilli: aspects relevant to development and use of vaccines. *J Infect Dis.* 1977; 136(suppl):S151–S160

111. Valenti W, Reese R. Genitourinary tract infections. In: Reese R, Douglas R, eds. *A Practical Approach to Infectious Disease.* Boston, Mass: Little, Brown and Co; 1986:227–258.

112. Platt R, Polk BF, Murdock B, Rosner B. Risk factors for nosocomial urinary tract infection. *Am J Epidemiol.* 1986;124:977–985.

113. Wong ES. Guideline for the prevention of catheter-associated urinary tract infections. *Am J Infect Control.* 1983;11:28–36.

114. Allgower M, Durig M, Wolff G. Infection and trauma. *Surg Clin North Am.* 1980;60:133–144.

115. Krieger JN, Kaiser DL, Wenzel RP. Urinary tract etiology of bloodstream infections in hospitalized patients. *J Infect Dis.* 1983;148:57–62.

116. Bryan CS, Reynolds KL. Hospital acquired bacteremic urinary tract infection: epidemiology and outcome. *J Urol.* 1984;132:494–498.

117. Hopkins CC. Infection pathogenesis, prevention and treatment. In: Ropper AH, Kennedy SK, Zervas NJ, eds. *Neurologic and Neurosurgical Intensive Care.* Baltimore, Md: University Park Press; 1983:107–117.

118. Hampton AA, Sheretz RJ. Vascular access infections in hospitalized patient. *Surg Clin North Am.* 1988;68:57–71.

119. Maki DG. Risk factors for nosocomial infection in intensive care. *Arch Intern Med.* 1989;149:30–35.

120. Beam TR. Vascular access catheters and infections. *Infect Surg.* 1989;5:156–158.

121. Martin MA, Pfaller MA, Wenzel RP. Coagulase-negative staphylococcal bacteremia. *Ann Intern Med.* 1989;110:9–16

122. Bjornson HS, Colley R, Bower RH, et al. Association between microorganism growth at the catheter insertion site and colonization of the catheter in patients receiving total parenteral nutrition. *Surgery.* 1982;92:720–727.

123. Francesch D, Gerding RL, Phillips G, et al. Risk factors associated with intravascular catheter infections in burned patients: a prospective randomized study. *J Trauma.* 1989;29:811–816.

124. Linares J, Sitges-Serra A, Garau J, et al. Pathogenesis of catheter sepsis: a prospective study with quantitative and semiquantitative cultures of catheter hub and segments. *J Clin Microbiol.* 1985;21:357–360.

125. Henderson DK. Intravascular device-associated infection: current concepts and controversies. *Infect Surg.* 1988;7:365.

126. Moran JM, Atwood RP, Rowe MI. A clinical and bacteriologic study of infections associated with venous cutdown. *N Engl J Med.* 1965;272:554.

127. Hilton E, Haslett TM, Borenstein MT, et al. Central catheter infections: single versus triple lumen catheters. *Am J Med.* 1988;86:667–672.

128. Norwood S, Jenkins G. An evaluation of triple-lumen catheter infections using a guidewire exchange technique. *J Trauma.* 1990;30:706–712.

129. Civetta JM, Hudson-Civetta JA, Dion L. Duration of illness affects catheter-related infection and bacteremia. In: *Program and Abstracts of the 27th Interscience Conference on Antimicrobial Agents and Chemotherapy.* 1987;69:1141.

130. Norwood SH, Cormier B, McMahon NG, et al. Prospective study of catheter-related infection during prolonged arterial catheterization. *Crit Care Med.* 1988;16:836–839.

131. Hudson-Civetta JA, Civetta JM, Martinez OV, Hoffman TA. Risk and detection of pulmonary artery catheter-related infection in septic surgical patients. *Crit Care Med.* 1987;15:29–34.

132. Benezra D, Kiehn TE, Gold JW, et al. Prospective study of infections in indwelling central venous catheters using quantitative blood cultures. *Am J Med.* 1988;85:495–498.

133. King TC, Price PB. An evaluation of iodophors as skin antiseptics. *Surg Gynecol Obstet.* 1963;105:361.

134. Maki DE, Band JD. A comparative study of polyantibiotic and iodophor ointments in prevention of vascular catheter-related infection. *Am J Med.* 1981;70:739–744.

135. Conly JM, Grieves K, Peters B. A prospective randomized study comparing transparent and dry gauze dressing for central venous catheters. *J Infect Dis.* 1989;159:310–319.

136. Snyder RH, Archer FJ, Endy T, et al. Catheter infection: a comparison of two catheter maintenance techniques. *Ann Surg.* 1988;208:651–653.

137. Pettigrew RA, Lang SD, Haydock DA, et al. Catheter-related sepsis in patients on intravenous nutrition: a prospective study of quantitative catheter cultures and guidewire changes for suspected sepsis. *Br J Surg.* 1985;72:52–55.

138. Maki DG, Cobb L, Garman JK, et al. An attachable silver-impregnated cuff for prevention of infection with central venous catheters: a prospective randomized multicenter trial. *Am J Med.* 1988;85:307–314.

139. Wenzel RP, Hunting KJ, Osterman CA. Postoperative wound infection rates. *Surg Gynecol Obstet.* 1977;144:749–752.

140. Northey D. Microbial surveillance in a surgical intensive care unit. *Surg Gynecol Obstet.* 1974;139:321–325.

141. Cruse PJ, Foord R. A five year prospective study of 23,649 surgical wounds. *Arch Surg.* 1973;107:206–210.

142. Nora PF, Vanecko RM, Bransfield JJ. Prophylactic abdominal drains. *Arch Surg.* 1972;105:173–176.

143. Magee C, Rodeheaver GT, Golden GT, et al. Potentiation of wound infection by surgical drains. *Am J Surg.* 1976;131:547–549.

144. Guyton AC, Granger HJ, Taylor AE. Interstial fluid pressure. *Physiol Rev.* 1971;51:527–563.

145. Kenedi RM, Cowden JM, Scales JT, eds. *Bedsore Biomechanics.* Baltimore, Md: University Park Press; 1976.

146. Shea JD. Pressure sores: classification and management. *Clin Orthop.* 1975;112:89–100.

147. Dansereau JG, Conway H. Closure of decubiti in paraplegias. *Plast Reconstr Surg.* 1964;33:474.

148. Dinsdale SM. Decubitus ulcers: role of pressure and friction in causation. *Arch Phys Med Rehabil.* 1974;55:147–152.

149. Sugarman B, Brown D, Musher D. Fever and infection in spinal cord injury patients. *JAMA.* 1982;248:66–70.

150. Rissing JP, Crowder JG, Dunfee T. White A. Bacteroides bacteremia from decubitus ulcer *South Med J.* 1974;67:1179–1182.

151. Caplan ES, Hoyt NJ. Nosocomial sinusitis. *JAMA.* 1982;247:639–641.

152. Rohr AS, Spector SL. Paranasal sinus anatomy and pathophysiology. *Clin Rev Allergy.* 1984;2:387–395.

153. Grindlinger GA, Niehoff J, Hughes SL, et al. Acute paranasal sinusitis related to nasotracheal intubation of the head injured patient. *Crit Care Med.* 1987;15:214–217.

154. Frederick J, Braude AI. Anaerobic infection of the paranasal sinuses. *N Engl J Med.* 1974;290:135–137.

155. Stauffer JL, Olson DE, Petty TL. Complications and consequences of endotracheal intubation and tracheotomy. *Am J Med.* 1981;70:65–76.

156. Sottile FD, Marrie TJ, Prough DS, et al. Nosocomial pulmonary infection: possible etiologic significance of the bacterial adhesion to endotracheal tubes. *Crit Care Med.* 1986;14:265–270.

157. Humphrey MA, Simpson GT, Grindlinger GA. Clinical characteristics of nosocomial sinusitis. *Ann Otol Rhinol Laryngol.* 1987;96:687–690.

158. Chaffee JS. Complications of gastrointestinal intubation. *Ann Surg.* 1949;130:113–123.

159. Evans FO Jr, Sydnor JB, Moore WE, et al. Sinusitis of the maxillary antrum. *N Engl J Med.* 1975;293:735–739.

160. Chandler JR, Langenbrunner DJ, Stevens ER. The pathogenesis of orbital complications in acute sinusitis. *Laryngoscope.* 1970;80 1414–1428.

161. Carter BL, Bankoff MS, Fisk JD Computed tomographic detection of sinusitis responsible for intracranial and extracranial infections. *Radiology.* 1983;147:739–742.

162. Shahin J, Gullane PJ, Dayal VS. Orbital complications of acute sinusitis. *J Otolaryngol.* 1987;16:23–27.

163. Parker GS, Tami TA, Wilson JF, et al. Intracranial complications of sinusitis. *South Med J.* 1989;82:563–569.

164. Simberkoff MS, Moldover NH, Rahal J Jr. Absence of detectable bactericidal and opsonic activities in normal and infected human cerebrospinal fluids: a regional host defense deficiency. *J Lab Clin Med.* 1980;95:362–372.

165. Zwahlen A, Nydegger UE, Vaudaux P, et al. Complement-mediated opsonic activity in normal and infected human cerebrospinal fluid: early response during bacterial meningitis. *J Infect Dis.* 1982;145:635–646.

166. Baltas I, Tsoulfa S, Sakellariou P, et al. Posttraumatic meningitis: bacteriology, hydrocephalus and outcome. *Neurosurgery* 1994 35:422–427.

167. Raaf. Posttraumatic cerebrospinal fluid leaks. *Arch Surg.* 1967;95:648–651.

168. Leech PJ, Paterson A. Conservative and operative mangement of cerebrospinal-fluid leakage after closed head injury. *Lancet.* 1973;1:1013–1016.

169. Buckwold FJ, Hand R, Hansebout RR. Hospital-acquired bacterial meningitis in neurosurgical patients. *J Neurosurg.* 1977;46:494–500.

170. Lau YL, Kenna AP. Post-traumatic meningitis in children. *Injury.* 1986;17:407–409.

171. McCracken GH Jr, Mize SG, Threlkeld N. Intraventricular gentamicin therapy in gram-negative bacillary meningitis of infancy. *Lancet.* 1980;1:787–791.

172. Aucoin PJ, Kotilainen HR, Gantz NM, et al. Intracranial pressure monitors: epidemiologic study of risk factors and infections. *Am J Med.* 1986;80:369–376.

173. Mayhall CG, Archer NH, Lamb VA, et al. Ventriculostomy-related infections: a prospective epidemiologic study. *N Engl J Med.* 1984;310:553–559.

174. Rosner MJ, Becker DP. ICP monitoring: complications and associated factors. *Clin Neurosurg.* 1976;23:494–519.

175. Winfield JA, Rosenthal P, Kanter RK, Casella G. Duration of intracranial pressure monitoring does not predict daily risk of infectious complications. *Neurosurgery.* 1993;33:424–431.

176. Chan KH, Mann KS. Prolonged therapeutic external ventricular drainage: a prospective study. *Neurosurgery.* 1988;23:436–438.

177. Kanter RK, Weiner LB, Patti AM, Robson LK. Infectious complications and duration of intracranial pressure monitoring. *Crit Care Med.* 1985;13:837–839.

178. Smith RW, Alksne JF. Infections complicating the use of external ventriculostomy. *J Neurosurg.* 1976;44:567–570.

179. Stenager E, Gerner-Smidt P, Kock-Jensen C. Ventriculostomy-related infections: an epidemiological study. *Acta Neurochir (Wien).* 1986;83:20–23.

180. Wyler AR, Kelly WA. Use of antibiotics with external ventriculostomies. *J Neurosurg.* 1972;37:185–187.

181. Hand WL, Sandford JP. Posttraumatic bacterial meningitis. *Ann Intern Med.* 1970;72:869–874.

182. Taha JM, Haddad FS, Brown JA. Intracranial infection after missile injuries to the brain: report of 30 cases from the Lebanese conflict. *Neurosurgery.* 1991;29:864–868.

183. Carey ME, Young H, Mathis JL, Forsythe J. A bacteriological study of craniocerebral missile wounds from Vietnam. *J Neurosurg.* 1971;34:145–154.

184. Swartz MN, Dodge PR. Bacterial meningitis: a review of selected aspects. General clinical features, special problems and unusual meningeal reactions mimicking bacterial meningitis. *N Engl J Med.* 1965;272:725.

185. Feigin RD, Dodge PR. Bacterial meningitis: newer concepts of pathophysiology and neurologic sequelae. *Pediatr Clin North Am.* 1976;23:541–556.

186. Hoff JT, Brewin A, Usang HS. Antibiotics for basilar skull fractures. *J Neurosurg.* 1976;44:649.

187. Ignelzi RJ, VanderArk GD. Analysis of the treatment of basilar skull fracture with and without antibiotics. 1975;43:721–726.

188. Demetriades D, Charalambides D, Lakhoo M, Pantanowitz D. Role of prophylactic antibiotics in open and basilar fractures of the skull: a randomized study. 1992;23:377–380.

189. Klastersky J, Sadeghi M, Brihaye J. Antimicrobial prophylaxis in patients with rhinorrhea or otorrhea: a double-blind study. *Surg Neurol.* 1976;6:111–114.

190. Morgan H, Wood MW, Murphy F. Experience with 88 consecutive cases of brain abscess. *J Neurosurg.* 1973;38:698–704.

191. Carey ME, Chom SN, French LA. Experience with brain abscesses. *J Neurosurg.* 1972;36:1–9.

192. Patir R, Sood S, Bhatia R. Post-traumatic brain abscesses: experience of 36 patients. *Br J Neurosurg.* 1995;9:29–35.

193. Jennett B, Miller JD. Infection after depressed fracture: implications for management of non-missile injuries. *J Neurosurg.* 1972;36:333–339.

194. Alderson D, Strong AJ, Ingham HR, Selkon JB. Fifteen year review of the mortality of brain abscess. *Neurosurgery.* 1981;8:1–6.

195. McKinney AS. Brain abscess. *Hosp Med.* 1983;19:13–15.

196. Kaufman DM, Miller MH, Steigbigel MH. Subdural empyema analysis of 17 recent cases and review of the literature. *Medicine (Baltimore).* 1975;54:485–493.

197. Osgood CP, DuJovny M, Holm E, Postic B. Delayed post-traumatic subdural empyema. *J Trauma.* 1975;15:916–921.

198. Bhandari YS, Sarkari NB. Subdural empyema. *J Neurosurg.* 1970;32:35–39.

199. LeBeau J, Creissard P, Harispe L, et al. Surgical treatment of brain abscess and subdural empyema. *J Neurosurg.* 1973;38:198–203.

200. Mackay LE, Bernstein BA, Chapman PE, Morgan AS, Milazzo LS. Early intervention in severe head injury: long-term benefits of a formalized program. *Arch Phys Rehabil.* 1992;73:635–641.

201. Cowley RS, Swanson B, Chapman P, Kitik BA, Mackay LE. The role of rehabilitation in the intensive care unit. *J Head Trauma Rehabil.* 1994;9:32–42.

CHAPTER 11

The Contributions of Speech/Language Pathology in Critical Care

The speech/language pathologist plays an integral role in the critical care rehabilitative needs of patients with severe brain injury. Interventions from this discipline should be initiated within 24 hours of admission. The speech/language pathologist establishes a functional communication system for the patient and assesses and treats cognitive/linguistic impairments. Cognitive-linguistic impairments are a major deficit for these patients, manifesting as reduced responsiveness and level of alertness, decreased attention, and difficulties with auditory comprehension, orientation, and memory. Education is provided to staff and family regarding effective ways to interact with the patient and environmental modifications that can be made to optimize communication and safety.

Speech/language pathology intervention in the intensive care unit (ICU) also includes assessment and treatment of vocal cord function and dysphagia because patients with severe brain injury are at increased risk for aspiration and pneumonia.[1-3] Assessment and treatment of dysphagia include recommendations for initiation of oral feedings or use of nonoral nutrition and for compensation techniques to facilitate safe swallowing.

Adequate vocal cord function protects the airway, thereby decreasing the risk of aspiration and pneumonia. Activities to maintain vocal cord integrity, such as the use of specialized tracheostomy tubes and/or speaking valves, are facilitated by the speech/language pathologist.

Following a thorough chart review, the speech/language pathologist should discuss the patient's condition, stability, present neurologic status, and precautions with the primary care nurse or intensivist. Other relevant information includes respiratory status, amount and consistency of secretions, and cough and gag reflex. Medications, their side effects, and administration schedule should also be identified. This information may provide the rationale for specific patient behaviors, or lack of them, and may determine when a particular session must be deferred.

PATIENT EQUIPMENT AND MONITORING DEVICES

Upon entering the patient's room, the speech/language pathologist should identify the equipment being used. The therapist should observe whether the patient is orally or nasally intubated (Figures 11–1 and 11–2) or whether ventilatory support is delivered via a tracheostomy. The brand, size, and features of the tracheostomy tube should be noted. The type of ventilatory support the patient is receiving should also be identified. Ventilatory support is discussed in Chapter 9.

The therapist should be aware of the vital signs displayed on the monitor. The heart rate should be identified and characterized as fast, normal, or slow and as regular or irregular. The therapist should document if the blood pressure (BP) is high, low, or within normal range and if the mean arterial pressure (MAP) (normal range 60–150 mm Hg) is sufficient to maintain adequate cerebral perfusion. When MAP is too low (<60 mm Hg) or too high (>160 mm Hg), disruption in the autoregulation of blood flow to the brain occurs.[4–10] Minimum and maximum ranges for oxygen saturation, pulse, BP, and MAP are programmed into the monitor. An alarm will sound when these ranges have been exceeded. The therapist should also note where the oxygen saturation reader is clipped on the patient (eg, finger, toe, earlobe). The therapist may need to adjust or replace the clip, since it is easily dislodged with movement.

The therapist should note the presence of other patient equipment, including fixation and traction devices, chest tubes, intravenous (IV) lines, feeding tubes, and restraints. Many of these devices limit movement or cause discomfort, thereby interfering with patient responses.

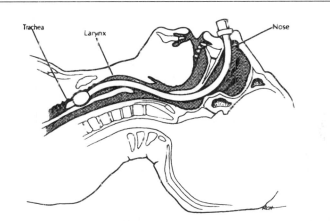

Figure 11–1 Nasotracheal tube in place. *Source:* Reprinted with permission from D. Eubanks and R.C. Bone, *Comprehensive Respiratory Care: A Learning System,* 2nd edition, p. 549, © 1990, Mosby-YearBook, Inc.

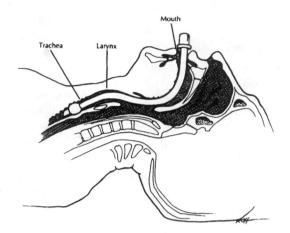

Figure 11–2 Orotracheal tube in place. *Source:* Reprinted with permission from D. Eubanks and R.C. Bone, *Comprehensive Respiratory Care: A Learning System,* 2nd edition, p. 549, © 1990, Mosby-Year Book, Inc.

PATIENT OBSERVATION

The speech/language pathologist should observe the patient at rest before any stimulation. Baseline vital signs should be recorded. These measures provide a reference point for future comparison. Observations made at the bedside include

- presence of random or purposeful movements
- decerebrate or decorticate posturing
- presence of agitated movements or behaviors (eg, thrashing, biting on intubation tube)
- spontaneous or purposeful eye opening
- eye movements (ie, random, fixation, tracking) and gaze preference (ie, left or right)
- conjugate or dysconjugate gaze
- oral-motor movements, including chewing or swallowing
- symmetry or asymmetry of facial, labial, and lingual structures
- symmetrical or asymmetrical movement of upper versus lower extremities or right versus left side

Depending upon the patient's neurologic stability, the initial evaluation may be limited to observing the patient during nursing care, rather than completing a thorough hands-on evaluation. The speech/language pathologist should observe the patient's reactions to routine nursing procedures, such as washing, moving, rolling, or neurologic checks. Noxious stimulation from activities such as placing IVs, arterial lines, or Dobhoff tubes, suctioning, or changing dressings may elicit patient responses. Viewing the patient from different positions (including the head and foot of the bed) may reveal responses that are difficult to view from the standard side-of-the-bed position.

ASSESSMENT

Universal precautions must be routinely used at all times. Gloves should be donned before handling patients who have sustained trauma, since blood and bodily fluids are frequently present. Abrasions, lacerations, surgical incisions, or external fixators may bleed or ooze. Oral secretions may pool in the mouth of an intubated patient. Movement of the patient may dislodge ventilator tubing, necessitating reconnection. Tears may be present when the eyes are opened or the head is repositioned.

Patients who are agitated because of a brain injury, alcohol withdrawal (ie, delirium tremens [DT]), or elevated intracranial pressure (ICP) that is refractory to conventional methods of control may require intermittent or even continuous sedation.[11-13] Optimally, assessment and treatment should be provided when the patient is least sedated and most responsive. Patients who require ongoing sedation may be observed or assessed when neurologic examination is performed. This examination, performed by the nurse or physician, occurs after regular doses of sedation are withheld to observe changes in a patient's neurologic status. Behaviors such as pupillary reactions, response to painful stimulation, and movement are assessed.

Cognition/Alertness/Arousal

The range of potential patient responses to auditory and other types of stimulation includes no response, physiologic changes (ie, heart rate, respiratory rate, temperature, ICP, BP), generalized responses, and localized responses. Generalized responses include a startle, a nonspecific movement of the torso or extremity, posturing, and random eye movements. Localized responses include eye opening following a stimulus, motor or visual localization toward the stimuli, or extremity withdrawal to pain.

The evaluation should begin by calling the patient's name and observing the response. The therapist should avoid using tactile or other cues. The therapist should continue talking to the patient, observing other behaviors such as restlessness or agitation. A strong, yet calm voice should be used, especially when agitation is present. Next, tactile input should be provided to both sides of the body to increase arousal and responses. Tactile stimulation includes light touch, deep pressure, and temperature and should be provided to all extremities and oral/facial areas. The therapist should document responses in terms of abnormality, consistency, and delay in response.

If the patient does not arouse to touch, mobilization can be used. Painful or noxious stimuli may be applied if arousal has not been achieved by other means and if vital signs remain stable. Painful stimulation is given to all four extremities unless prohibited by injuries (ie, burns, wounds, orthopaedic injuries). The preferred method of delivering painful stimulation is to apply pressure to the nailbed of a finger or toe on each extremity. Variations between right and left sides and upper and lower extremities should be recorded, as well as briskness or delays in response. If a concomitant spinal cord injury (SCI) is present, the therapist must be aware of the level of injury and anticipated paralysis. Painful stimulation should be limited to assessment only. If excessive posturing, increased ICP, or elevated BP, heart rate, and other vital sign changes result, then stimulation should be ceased. Combining treatment sessions with the physical and/or occupational therapist is beneficial when mobilization or more noxious stimuli are needed to arouse the patient.

Posturing may occur following painful stimulation. The type of posturing and variations per extremity should be noted. Decorticate posturing generally indicates damage of the corticospinal pathways in the cerebrum. Decerebrate posturing indicates damage of the corticospinal tract at the level of the diencephalon and portions of the upper brainstem.[14,15] The type of posturing observed can provide the speech/language pathologist with indications of possible cortical or brainstem involvement. Identification of injury level then provides some insight into other potential deficits, such as dysphagia or future difficulties with speech production. Chapter 7 defines and illustrates posturing and its implications.

If arousal and responsiveness are achieved, the speech/language pathologist can progress to assessment of auditory comprehension. The patient's primary language should be identified. When English is spoken as a second language, assessment of auditory comprehension should be completed in both the primary and secondary languages. Patients may revert to their primary language following a significant brain injury, regardless of their premorbid command of the English language. In choosing verbal commands, one must consider the physical limitations or abilities of the patient and use a hierarchical progression from basic to multistep commands. The amount of delay observed, the consistency of the response, the number of repetitions or cues needed, and the presence of perseveration should be documented.

Visual Responses

The occupational therapist completes a detailed examination of a patient's visual system. However, a baseline assessment of certain visual responses, coupled with input from the occupational therapist, will aid the speech/language pathologist in developing an appropriate treatment program and may provide information about cranial nerve or brainstem impairment. The therapist should identify if eye opening is spontaneous or elicited by stimulation. The degree and consistency of eye opening and type of stimulus needed (eg, verbal, tactile, noxious) should be noted. If eye opening cannot be elicited and eye injuries do not contraindicate, the eyes should be opened manually by the therapist. Lack of eye opening may also be secondary to ecchymosis from facial injuries or fractures.

Once the eyes are opened, pupil symmetry, reactiveness, and movement should be noted. The eyes should be observed for conjugate gaze (eyes moving together) or dysconjugate gaze (eyes not moving together) and eye gaze preference. Dysconjugate gaze may result in double vision, interfering with visual stimuli (eg, photographs, written words) for orientation or communication activities.

The therapist should also document any evidence of fixation or tracking. Visual responses should be evaluated from both sides of the patient, noting ability or inability to cross midline and move eyes laterally. Information regarding preinjury visual status should be sought. Glasses may be used during assessment and treatment activities if they are available and are not contraindicated by open head, face, or ear wounds or cromaxillary facial fixation devices. The therapist should be aware that glasses meant to maximize premorbid eyesight may be ineffective with new visual deficits that occurred secondary to brain injury.

Oral-Motor Responses

Spontaneous oral-motor and facial movements should be observed for range of motion (ROM), symmetry, speed, precision, strength, intent, and normalcy of movement. These observations help identify cranial nerve impairment. Facial injuries, fractures, and intraoral lacerations may affect oral or facial movements even in the absence of cranial nerve injury, however. Spontaneous swallows and the effectiveness of reflexive and voluntary coughs should be documented. These reflexes provide insight into laryngeal function and the integrity of the swallowing mechanism.

Observation of spontaneous movements may be the only means of assessing patients who are orally intubated. With nasal intubation or tracheostomy, the patient can perform more varied oral-motor movements spontaneously or on command. Even when patients do not follow motor commands, they should be assessed for oral-motor responses to requests, such as requests to open the mouth, swallow, move the tongue, stick out the tongue, close the mouth, pucker the lips, or cough. These skills should be assessed through imitation also, especially if verbal requests were unsuccessful. Tactile stimulation may also be helpful in eliciting oral/facial movements.

Cranial nerves VII (facial nerve) and IX (glossopharyngeal nerve) are responsible for the sense of taste. The facial nerve innervates taste from the anterior two thirds of the tongue, whereas the glossopharyngeal nerve is responsible for the taste receptors in the posterior third of the tongue.[16] Assessment of response to gustatory stimulation is not feasible for orally intubated patients. Although an exchange of air through the nasal passages is necessary for adequate smell and taste sensation, limited assessment can be performed on patients who are nasally intubated or intubated via a tracheostomy.

The only true tastes are salty, sour, sweet, and bitter.[17] Stimulation, pairing tastes that are most different, should incorporate a variety of flavors. Flavors should include those familiar to the patient, eliciting both positive and negative responses. Lemon flavoring, which assists with initiation of the pharyngeal swallow, can also be used.[18] During stimulation, the therapist should identify abnormal oral reflexes; hyper- or hyposensitivity; triggering of the swallowing reflex; facilitation of oral-motor movements, such as lingual movements or chewing; and generalized or localized body responses. Responses such as withdrawal or grimacing should also be noted. Stimulation should be discontinued if increased posturing or agitation is noted.

Movement

Observations of physical movement and motor control will help determine the feasibility of using an extremity or other body part for communication purposes. Brain injury, fractures, and SCI may affect limb movement or control. The physical therapist (PT) and occupational therapist (OT) should assist the speech/language pathologist with this assessment, providing additional detail on the functionality of movement.

Spontaneous movement should be observed, as well as movement secondary to stimulation and imitation. Insight into cognition and language can be provided by observing how performance varies with request versus imitation and how patients are able to alter movement on command or sustain attention for repetitive movements. Weakness or paresis on one side, in the absence of computed tomography (CT) findings, may be the only indicator of contralateral brain injury. These clinical manifestations provide insight into potential speech/language/cognitive deficits.

FORMAL ASSESSMENT TOOLS

A limited number of relevant formalized assessment tools are available. Those tools most relevant in the ICU are descriptive behavioral/cognitive scales.

The Rancho Los Amigos Scale of Cognitive Functioning[19] (RLA) describes a patient's cognitive/behavioral status. It is a descriptive rather than predictive scale that identifies and defines all stages of cognitive/behavioral recovery secondary to brain injury (Exhibit 11–1). The scale uses eight levels, ranging from I (No Response) to VIII (Purposeful-Appropriate). Levels I, II, and III, most frequently seen in the ICU, describe varying levels of coma. This scale can be used to help the family understand the recovery process and future anticipated behaviors (eg, agitation). Using RLA levels to describe patient functioning facilitates consistency within the team.

Several assessment tools, such as the Coma/Near Coma Scale,[20] are designed to detect changes in responsiveness and neurobehavioral function in comatose or "slow-to-recover" patients. Other tools assist in prediction of cognition gains and outcomes, including the Disability Rating Scale,[21-24] the Western NeuroSensory Stimulation Profile,[25] and the Coma Recovery Scale.[26] These scales, however, were normed on patients with brain injury between 43 days and 8.9 months post injury.

The Clinical Neurological Assessment Tool[27] is one exception. This tool detects subtle changes in the comatose state and detects early recovery or deterioration in neurologic functioning. Twenty-one assessment items are rated on varying scales and include response to verbal and tactile stimulation, ability to follow commands, status of muscle tone and body position, and presence of verbalizations, movement, chewing, and yawning. Normative data for this assessment tool were collected on 187 patients with brain injury. Forty-five percent of all patients were assessed within two days of admission to the acute medical hospital. Test validity was established by comparing results to Glasgow Coma Scale[28] findings. Reliability coefficients for mild, moderate, and severe brain injuries were .85, .83, and .87, respectively.

TREATMENT

The contributions of the speech/language pathologist in the ICU, as with other rehabilitation therapies, extend beyond assessment to include goal-oriented treatment and staff/family education. The primary focus of intervention with patients with severe brain injury is to

1. improve responsiveness and interaction with the environment

Exhibit 11–1 Rancho Los Amigos Scale of Cognitive Functioning

I. No Response

Patient unresponsive to all stimuli.

II. Generalized Response

Patient reacts inconsistently and nonpurposefully to stimuli. Responses are limited and often delayed.

III. Localized Response

Patient reacts specifically but inconsistently to stimuli. Responses are related to type of stimulus presented, such as focusing on an object visually or responding to sounds.

IV. Confused, Agitated

Patient is extremely agitated and in a high state of confusion. Shows nonpurposeful and aggressive behavior. Unable to fully cooperate with treatments due to short attention span. Maximal assistance with self-care skills is needed.

V. Confused, Inappropriate, Nonagitated

Patient is alert and can respond to simple commands on a more consistent basis. Highly distractible and needs constant cueing to attend to an activity. Memory is impaired with confusion regarding past and present. The patient can perform self-care activities with assistance. Patient may wander and needs to be watched carefully.

VI. Confused, Appropriate

Patient shows goal-directed behavior, but still needs direction from staff. Follows simple tasks consistently and shows carryover for relearned tasks. The patient is more aware of own deficits and has increased awareness of self, family, and basic needs.

VII. Automatic, Appropriate

Patient appears oriented to home and hospital and goes through daily routine automatically. Shows carryover for new learning but still requires structure and supervision to ensure safety and good judgment. Able to initiate tasks in which he or she has an interest.

VIII. Purposeful, Appropriate

Patient is totally alert, oriented, and shows good recall of past and recent events. Independent in the home and community. Shows a decreased ability in certain areas but has learned to compensate for these deficits.

2. improve cognition/language, including attention, orientation, and comprehension
3. develop and implement a functional communication system
4. facilitate vocal cord integrity through participation in tracheostomy management
5. facilitate oral feeding using compensation techniques necessary for safe swallowing

For the speech/language pathologist, cotreatments with other rehabilitation therapists can be useful. Physical movement can facilitate arousal and potentially improve patient responsiveness. Coordinating speech/language therapy with physical or occupational therapy (PT or OT) provides that opportunity. Input from the PT or OT on the use of specific movements or on functional extremity usage is vital when establishing a means of communication (Figure 11–3).

Interventions with the patient in the ICU should be scheduled to provide periodic sessions of stimulation throughout the day. Adequate rest periods must be

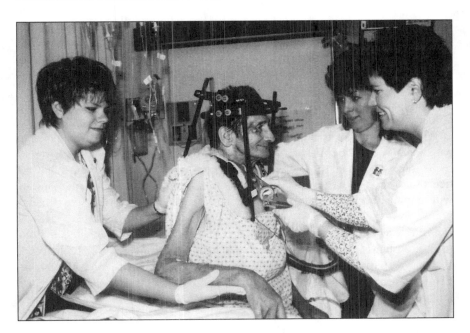

Figure 11–3 Joint rehabilitation treatment sessions facilitate input on positioning and movement to maximize use and carryover of a communication system. This is especially important when concomitant injuries are present, such as spinal cord injury.

permitted. The patient will benefit most from two (or even three) sessions spaced throughout the day. Sessions may be limited initially to 15 to 20 minutes, depending upon arousal, fatigue, and attending factors. When daily treatment schedules are developed, the nurse can be instrumental in providing input to the therapists regarding medication schedule, timing of nursing care, and scheduled medical procedures. Each ICU unit develops its own routines and schedules (eg, when bedside X-rays, operating room procedures, nursing procedures, and family meetings are commonly scheduled). Effective scheduling is based upon good communication with the nursing staff and ongoing experience in the unit. Most important, rehabilitation staff must be flexible and must recognize the hierarchy of individual patient priorities.

The therapist must monitor vital signs during therapy sessions. A brief rest period may be needed if vital signs fluctuate too frequently beyond acceptable levels. Calming the patient and removing the stimulus may be adequate to restore normal vital signs. If stabilization does not occur, cessation of treatment may be warranted.

Responsiveness/Interaction with the Environment

Improving purposeful and appropriate responses is one area of focus for patients functioning at RLA II and III. The therapist should control the type of stimulation provided, using single and multisensory input (eg, verbal, tactile, visual). All cues should be provided in a clear, concise manner. Treatment should attempt to increase the consistency of a response while reducing the amount of cues and the number of repetitions. The time delay from stimulus to response should be reduced over a period of time.

When assessing or treating arousal and responsiveness, the speech/language pathologist should be cognizant of the potential for long delays between the verbal request and the patient response. Much stimulation may be needed with some patients to elicit any level of response. Patients with brainstem or thalamic injuries will be more difficult to arouse, often requiring longer or more aggressive stimulation.

Therapy activities to increase responsiveness and interaction with the environment are often similar to those used to increase attending and comprehension. When an activity is presented, the therapist is able to glean a great deal of information from the patient's response. The information one is able to surmise is more important than the activity itself.

Cognition/Language

Attention is initially fleeting with patients with brain injury. Tasks must first focus on familiar and relevant stimuli, even incorporating family members into sessions. Once a patient is able to attend to stationary stimuli or persons, attending can be expanded by incorporating visual tracking. Again, familiar persons, photographs, and personal items can be used.

Orientation should be provided throughout treatment sessions. Family members, nurses, and other care providers should be instructed to provide orientation during their interactions as well. The therapist should first greet the patient, introduce himself or herself, and orient the patient to place, date, reason for hospitalization, and length of stay. Other information, such as time of day and family updates, may also be added. Negative information should be avoided at this stage of recovery, especially with restless, agitated, or posturing patients. During recovery, orientation to person improves first, followed by place, situation, and then time. Orientation to time improves later because it is a continuum that requires encoding and decoding of new information.[29]

Environmental cues can be used to increase orientation. Posters of family pictures, audiotapes of familiar voices, calendars, and pictures of the hospital and treating therapists must be strategically placed in the patient's visual environment, although overstimulation and distraction must be avoided.

Auditory comprehension is best treated once the therapist has information on patient responsiveness, physical capabilities and limitations, and visual skills. Verbal requests should progress from simple one-part commands to multistep commands. Verbal commands should incorporate requests requiring physical motor, oral-motor, and visual responses. At lower RLA levels, it may be difficult to diagnose differentially auditory comprehension deficits from motor or oral apraxia.

Communicative Intent

One of the primary functions of the speech/language pathologist in the early stages of recovery is to establish a functional and consistent means of communication for the patient. A functional communication system is developed after assessing communicative intent, cognition, comprehension, vision, and motor control. Communicative intent includes all verbal, gestural, graphic, motor, and/or behavioral actions that are used to communicate thoughts, emotions, or responses (Figure 11–4). Patients with severe brain injury will exhibit communicative intent on one of three levels. The most basic level of communicative intent involves generalized responses to stimulation in the immediate environment. Examples include posturing, withdrawal and/or facial grimacing, and pulling of tubes. Higher responses are stimulus bound. Second-level responses include avoiding stimulation by turning the face away from stimuli, closing the eyes when a person enters the room, or resisting manual eye opening. On the third level, patients actively seek out an individual with a definite intention to communicate. The patient may use

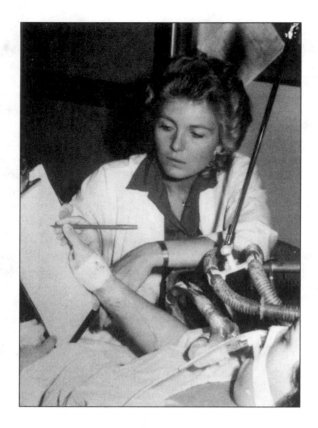

Figure 11–4 An intubated patient with a severe brain injury is able to use writing to improve communication of basic needs and wants.

various forms of communication (eg, gestures, mouthing, yes/no responses) and may try to express communication that spans the spectrum from basic needs to more involved thoughts or questions.

Communication ability may be impaired by many factors, including cognitive deficits, multiple injuries, intubation, and use of physical restraints. Communication systems help overcome obstacles to effective communication. The most common basic communication system uses eye movements, hand squeezes, or movements of the fingers or feet. Head shaking, mouthing of words, and picture boards are generally more successful at higher levels of functioning. Eye movements may include direct eye gaze or a basic eye-blink system, which can convey yes/no responses as well as more complex messages if appropriate. The speech/language pathologist should determine if eye blinks, eye gaze, hand squeezes, and extremity movements are reflexive or purposeful. Certain positions or individuals (eg, family) may enhance the consistency of responses. Initial trials should focus on functional and meaningful needs (eg, pain, hot, cold, sick, thirsty). When a functional system has been identified, family and staff must use the same system consistently.

Electronic technology plays a limited role with patients at RLA levels II to III. Appropriate systems for these patients are considered training devices by the augmentative communication community. They include single-switch activation devices with common objects, lights, or rotary and other scanners (Figure 11–5). Single-switch scanning of two colored lights can be used to facilitate yes/no responses. Switch activation can also initiate recordings of family voices or familiar music. Simple rotary scanning, paired with auditory and visual cues, can be used to communicate basic needs. The application of these devices for communication purposes depends on the patient's level of functioning.

Regardless of the system, certain basic principles must be applied if an alternative communication system is used:

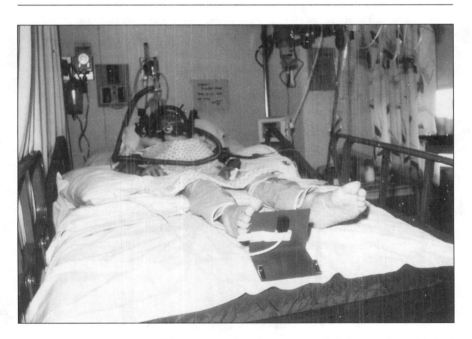

Figure 11–5 The nursing call button was adapted as a foot switch for a patient with dual diagnoses of brain injury and spinal cord injury.

1. Systems must be kept functional with limited stimuli.
2. Systems must be used consistently by all staff and family members.
3. The stimuli, position of the patient, and mode of response must remain consistent with each use.
4. Reinforcement (eg, obtaining item requested) must be provided immediately.
5. The patient must be given adequate time to process information and provide a response.
6. Staff and family members must receive clear instructions for use.
7. Instructions should be posted at the bedside, since it is impossible to train each staff member who will come into contact with the patient.

At times, with an extended ICU length of stay, application of more sophisticated (nonbasic) electronic devices may be appropriate. Several factors may interfere with attempts to use electronic equipment in the ICU environment:

- *Electrical.* The application of electronic equipment must be minimized, since it may produce electrical interference with monitors and diagnostic procedures.
- *Auditory.* The auditory output from many electronic devices may be difficult to hear in the ICU or difficult to distinguish from sounds produced by monitors, ventilators, and other patient care equipment.
- *Visual.* LED displays on electronic communication devices can be difficult for patients to see. Patients with visual field cuts, impaired visual acuity, and decreased sustained attention are especially affected.
- *Behavior.* The presence of aggressive and agitated behavior poses a risk of damage to delicate electronic systems.
- *Placement.* Placement issues are one of the primary sources of nonapplicability of electronic equipment. The most functional placement of a device is directly in front of the patient. Most patients in the ICU, however, are often supine in bed. Specialty beds may limit attachment of devices, as well as the ability to position the patient upright or near 90 degrees. The therapist must avoid placement of equipment in areas that would impede access to medical intervention in an emergency situation.

VOCAL CORD INTEGRITY

Maintaining the integrity of the vocal cords has an ABC effect on the patient with a brain injury:

- *Airway protection:* Adequate adduction of the vocal cords provides a valving mechanism to protect the airway from secretions, food, and liquid. Secretions are a potential nidus of aspiration pneumonia, which occurs frequently in this population.[1,3]
- *Behavior:* Facilitating the ability to speak can potentially reduce the frustration and agitation that patients experience when attempting to express basic wants and needs.
- *Communication:* An effective communication system reduces a patient's overall level of confusion. The inability to speak has been identified as a primary source of insecurity, fear, anxiety, and panic for ventilator-dependent patients.[30]

Clinically, it is easier to maintain vocal cord function than to restore function secondary to disuse. The speech/language pathologist therefore takes an active and aggressive role in facilitating voice restoration. This approach involves the cooperative efforts of the physician, respiratory therapist, and speech/language pathologist. Primary and secondary injuries can affect a patient's functional use of speech. The major source of primary injury is neurologic, including cranial nerve injury and cortical injury. Cranial nerve injury affects the movement and coordination of the laryngeal musculature. Cortical injury results in motor speech disorders, such as apraxia and dysarthria. Other kinds of primary injury include direct-impact or penetrating injuries to the laryngeal or oral area. Facial fractures, intraoral lacerations, and laryngeal fractures are examples of impact and penetrating injuries. Secondary injuries occur as a result of medical intervention or postinjury complications, such as those seen following endotracheal intubation or prolonged tracheostomy usage. The speech/language pathologist should be alerted to the presence of multiple intubations, traumatic intubations, emergent cricothyroidotomy, or self-extubation.[31-37]

Intubation may cause temporary inflammation and minor mucosal ulcerations of the vocal cords and posterior laryngeal commissure.[38-40] These immediate temporary changes occur in approximately 88% to 94% of patients.[41,42] When pressure from the endotracheal tube exceeds mucosal capillary pressure, ischemia occurs, producing irritation first, followed by congestion, edema, and ulceration.[43,44] Healing of these mucosal ulcers occurs through primary reepithelialization (with a 78% occurrence) or secondary granuloma formation (with a 7% occurrence).[40] Granulation tissue proliferates at the margins of the injured area, persisting even after the tube is removed. Occasionally, extensive changes promote formation of new collagen that matures to fibrous scar tissue.[45-47] Laryngeal healing by way of granuloma or scar formation leads to more serious complications. Those complications include laryngospasm, tracheomalacia, fibrosis, laryngeal and tracheal stenosis, vocal cord immobility, tracheoesophageal fistula, or even respiratory failure.[38,45,48–63] The frequency of these serious complications is as low as 3% and as high as 76%.[31,33–41,44,46–49,52–57,60,61,64–68] These complications can affect swallowing and speech skills. Secondary vocal dysfunction includes stridor, hoarseness, breathiness, decreased pitch range, and sore throat or pain and discomfort during speaking and swallowing.

Many factors contribute to the increased risk of complications following intubation.[42,45,50,52,57,69–73] Risk factors include

- size of the tracheal tube relative to the larynx and trachea
- shape and composition of the tube
- inflation pressure of the cuff
- presence of a nasogastric tube
- movement of the tube within the trachea
- intubation trauma
- multiple extubations and reintubation
- depth of insertion of the endotracheal tube (eg, between T-1 and T-4)
- duration of endotracheal intubation

Higher incidences of long-term sequelae have been reported in patients with seizure disorders (25%) and severe brain injury (19%).[41,45] It must be remembered that the larynges of adults are more rigid and therefore less tolerant of intubation trauma.

In the ICU, patients with brain injury requiring speech/language services will be ventilator dependent via either an endotracheal or a tracheostomy tube. Therefore, the speech/language pathologist must have theoretical and clinical knowledge of ventilatory modes, endotracheal intubation, and tracheostomies. An inexperienced and unknowledgeable therapist can make incorrect recommendations that negatively affect a patient's medical condition.

Tracheostomy Tubes

A *tracheotomy* (the term describing the surgical operation) is performed on patients experiencing respiratory insufficiency who are thought to require prolonged ventilatory support. The *tracheostomy site* (the term describing the artificial opening) is between the second, third, and fourth tracheal rings (Figure 11–6). A tracheostomy tube is inserted in the opening, preventing normal air exchange through the vocal cords.

Tracheostomy tubes may be made of metal, polyvinyl chloride, or other synthetic materials (eg, silicone). Polyvinyl chloride tubes are more flexible than metal or silicone tubes. The type of injury (eg, penetrating or blunt), the estimated

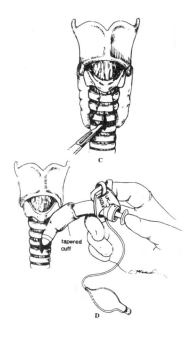

Figure 11–6 Surgical incision through the second, third, and fourth tracheal rings during a tracheotomy with subsequent insertion of the tracheostomy tube into the anterior tracheal wall (with obturator in place). *Source:* Reprinted with permission from Mallinckrodt Medical, St. Louis, Mo.

length of time that ventilatory support will be needed, and the presence of agitation or posturing determine which type of tube is needed.

Tracheostomy tubes have a variety of features and options: they may have disposable or nondisposable inner cannulas and may be cuffed or cuffless and single- or double-fenestrated (Figure 11–7) or nonfenestrated. Figure 11–8 and Exhibit 11–2 identify and define standard features of tracheostomy tubes. A tracheostomy interferes with normal function and may result in

- absent or reduced vocalizations
- reduced ability to cough
- reduced oral/pharyngeal sensation
- increased risk of infection
- decreased gas exchange
- decreased olfaction (smell) and gustation (taste)
- decreased laryngeal elevation and swallowing[74]

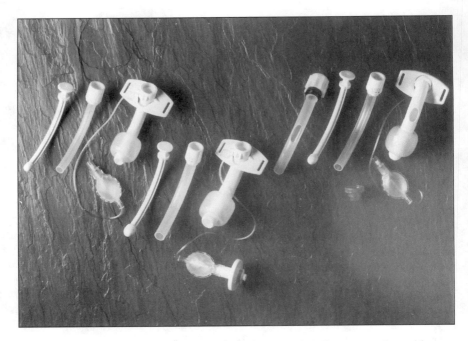

Figure 11–7 Shiley cuffed nonfenestrated and fenestrated tracheostomy tubes with components. Components include obturator and standard or fenestrated inner cannulas. Courtesy of Mallinckrodt Medical, St. Louis, Missouri.

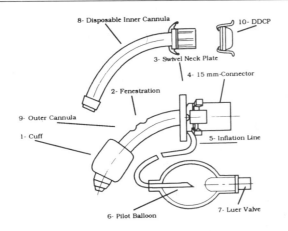

Figure 11–8 Standard parts and features of a tracheostomy tube. DCCP = decannulation plug or cap. Courtesy of Mallinckrodt Medical, St. Louis, Missouri.

Exhibit 11–2 Definitions of Standard Parts and Features of a Tracheostomy Tube

1. The **cuff** is an optional feature that separates the upper and lower airways when inflated, redirecting airflow of the mouth and nose through the tracheostomy tube. Cuffs are usually filled with air, although silicone foam–filled cuffs are also available.

2. **Fenestration(s)** are holes in the outer and/or inner cannula that allow air passage through the vocal cords up to the mouth and the nose. Fenestrations may be single or multiple.

3. The **swivel neck plate (flange)** helps to position and secure the tracheostomy tube to the patient's neck. Information regarding the size and specific features of the tracheostomy tube may be displayed on the neck plate.

4. A **15-mm hub connector** constitutes the end portion of many inner cannulas and is sized to connect with most standard respiratory equipment. Separate 15-mm hub adaptors are available for metal tracheostomy tubes that do not have this feature.

5. The **inflation line** is the thin plastic piece that attaches the pilot balloon to the cuff and inflates or deflates it.

6. The **pilot balloon**, found on cuffed tracheostomy tubes, indicates the amount of air pressure present within the cuff. The balloon hangs from the outer cannula.

7. A **Luer syringe** is used to inflate or deflate the cuff when attached to the Luer valve.

8. The **inner cannula** is the removable tube that is inserted into the outer cannula. It acts as a passageway for airflow and allows for the removal of secretions by suctioning or coughing. Several brands use disposable inner cannulas.

9. The **outer cannula** is the tube that is inserted through the surgical opening, providing an artificial passage for breathing and acting as a pulmonary toilet. The outer tube may or may not house an inner tube. The inner tube may be removable, depending on the brand.

10. The **decannulation plug** or **cap** attached to the outer cannula when the inner cannula is removed. It directs airflow through the nose and mouth while impeding airflow through the tracheostomy tube. The plug may be used during the weaning process before removal of the tracheostomy tube.

Courtesy of Mallinckrodt Medical, St. Louis, Missouri.

Serious complications may include tracheal stenosis and necrosis, tracheoesophageal fistula, granulation formation, tracheomalacia, tracheal erosion, bacterial infection, and upper-airway abnormalities.[75–77] These complications, which can lead to dysphonia, dysphagia, and aspiration pneumonia, can be the result of inappropriate cuff inflation (Figure 11–9) [75,78]

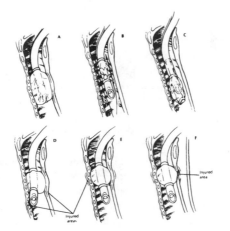

Figure 11–9 Complications secondary to inappropriate cuff inflation. (A) Overinflation of cuff and distension over tube end; (B) rupture of the cuff; (C) slippage of the cuff; (D) uneven inflation of the cuff; (E) overinflation of the cuff, resulting in tracheal stenosis and necrosis; (F) overinflation of the cuff, resulting in tracheoesophageal fistula. Courtesy of Mallinckrodt Medical, St. Louis, Missouri.

Vocal Communication Options

Talking Tracheostomy Tubes

Vocal communication options for ventilator-dependent patients are available only to those who have tracheostomies. Oral and nasal intubation prevents voicing because the endotracheal tube passes through the vocal cords, preventing adduction. Talking tracheostomy tubes, inserted by a physician, are especially suited for patients who can tolerate cuff deflation because of aspiration risks or compromise of adequate ventilation. Talking tracheostomy tubes facilitate communication while maintaining vocal cord integrity and increase smell and taste. These tubes are connected to an alternate air source (eg, wall oxygen) via an air port, separating the functions of speech and breathing. Air is funneled through the tube's fenestration site toward the vocal cords. The CommuniTrach I, the Portex Trach-Talk Tube, and the Bivona tracheostomy tube with talk attachment are examples of talking tracheostomy tubes (Figure 11–10).[79–81]

Functional use of these tubes may require troubleshooting and problem solving. Laryngeal spasms brought on by continual air passage may result in strained voicing. Alterations in airflow volume may reduce this occurrence. Inconsistent voicing may result when secretions plug fenestration sites. Adequate suctioning and

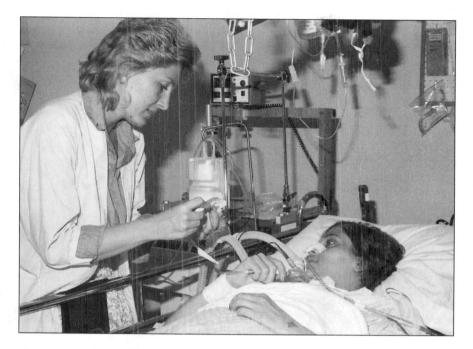

Figure 11–10 A speech/language pathologist teaches a patient how to use CommuniTrach for speaking.

irrigation reduce this risk. The CommuniTrach's air port is located at the 6 o'clock position. Maintaining airflow can be difficult when the tube becomes kinked.[82] Halo traction, neck collars, neck swelling, and even slightly flexed head positions may result in kinking. Patients can experience discomfort secondary to the unfamiliar flow of air from the trachea to the oral cavity. Motor or behavioral impairments may prohibit the patient from occluding the air port. Reduced cognition also makes it difficult for a patient to understand the correlation between occlusion and speech production.

Tracheostomy Speaking Valves

Tracheostomy speaking valves allow the patient to inhale through the tracheostomy opening but exhale through the trachea and nasal and oral cavities. These one-way valves easily attach to the 15-mm hub of a tracheostomy tube (Figure 11–11). They are contraindicated for patients with severe upper-airway obstruction or stenosis. They can, however, produce substantial benefits to the patient, including

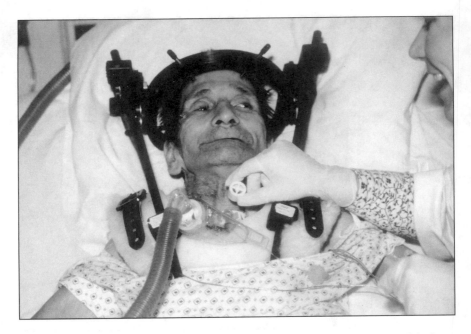

Figure 11–11 A Passy-Muir speaking valve attaches easily to the 15-mm hub of the inner cannula.

- more normal vocalizations at increased volume
- reduction in oral and nasal secretions
- increased smell and taste
- improved swallowing
- decreased risk of infection from finger occlusion
- assistance in the decannulation process
- increased effectiveness of the cough reflex
- increased ability to blow the nose
- decreased frustration with communication attempts[74,83–93]

The Passy-Muir speaking valve uses a positive closure design, maintaining an airtight seal until opening during inspiration. This positive closure design increases back pressure in the lungs, thereby improving pulmonary function. It has also been shown to reduce aspiration.[94] The Passy-Muir speaking valve is the only valve that is Food and Drug Administration registered for use with ventilator-assisted patients. Other tracheostomy speaking valves, such as the Montgomery, Hood, and Kistner, can be used only with extubated patients.

The Passy-Muir speaking valve, positioned on the 15-mm tracheostomy tube hub, attaches directly to the ventilator tubing. The tracheostomy tube cuff must be deflated before or simultaneous with placement on the tracheostomy tube (Figure 11–12). Joint sessions with the speech/language pathologist and respiratory therapist can facilitate coordination of these tasks. One or more staff members must be present to monitor the patient's vital signs, silence ventilator alarms that are triggered secondary to the deflated cuff, and provide additional ventilator breaths if needed. The therapist must be prepared to provide immediate suctioning when secretions pool in the posterior oral cavity. Patients must then adjust to the passage of air through the oral cavity. Vocalizations can be produced only during the ventilator's exhalation cycle. Patients with cognitive deficits, including decreased insight and memory, may find coordination of exhalation and voicing difficult. A connection between cognitive functioning and initiation of verbal speech exists. At lower RLA levels, the patient may lack the cognitive skills to initiate verbal

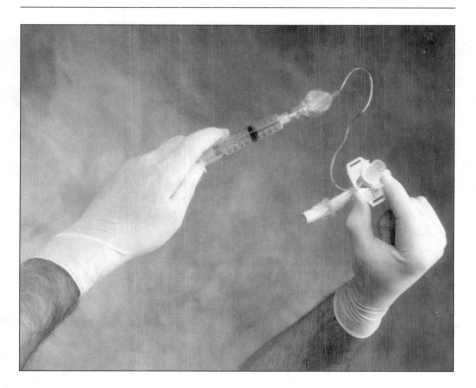

Figure 11–12 Removal of air from the tracheostomy tube cuff. Courtesy of Mallinckrodt Medical, St. Louis, Missouri.

speech. The understanding of how to "turn on" the voice is impaired, especially in a patient who relies on mouthing words. The use of automatic tasks, such as coughing, clearing the throat, or spontaneous social greetings, may be helpful when initiating voicing with talking tracheostomy tubes or speaking valves.

With any of these devices, voicing is not guaranteed and is affected by the condition of the vocal cords. Prolonged disuse or injury can interfere with voicing. Treatment begins by establishing audible voice and progresses to production of single words and phrases.

SWALLOWING

Adequate nutrition and hydration are vital for optimal recovery from brain injury. Patients with brain injury have significant increases in resting metabolic expenditure due to abnormal posturing and increased tone.[95] Deficits that affect nutritional intake must be addressed early to ensure adequate caloric intake and reduce the risk of pulmonary complications. Patients with brain injury are at risk for pulmonary complications secondary to difficulties mobilizing secretions[96] and have increased incidence of pneumonia,[3,97-99] which negatively affects morbidity and mortality.[100,101]

The bulk of studies researching swallowing disorders within the brain-injured population focus on a later phase of recovery (the rehabilitation hospital).[102-104] However, patients within the trauma center exhibit a high incidence of dysphagia and aspiration.[1,105] The occurrence rate of dysphagia within the brain-injured population ranges from 27% to 82%, with aspiration rates ranging from 38% to 45% (Figure 11–13).[1,102-105]

Yorkston et al[104] studied the prevalence and severity of speech and swallowing disorders in three different populations of patients with brain injuries (trauma center, acute rehabilitation, and outpatient rehabilitation). The severity of brain injury for patients in the trauma center ranged from mild to severe. Swallowing disorders were exhibited in 77.5% of these patients, with 45% of those exhibiting an inability to meet their nutritional needs orally.

Mackay and Morgan[105] investigated the prevalence of swallowing disorders and relationship between cognition and oral intake in 54 patients with severe brain injuries in a trauma center. Videofluoroscopic evaluations were completed an average of 17.6 days post injury. The occurrence rate of swallowing disorders was 61%, with a 41% incidence rate for aspiration. The most common deficits were loss of bolus control, reduced lingual control, decreased tongue base retraction, delay in the trigger of the swallow reflex, and reduced laryngeal closure. Patients with normal swallowing averaged 8.2 days from initiation to achievement of total oral feeding, compared with 29.3 days for patients with swallowing disorders. All patients averaged RLA IV at initiation of oral feeding. Total oral feeding was

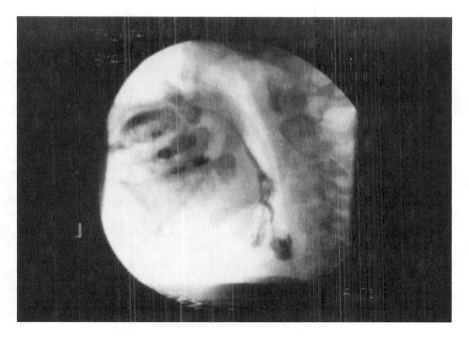

Figure 11–13 Demonstration of aspiration of thickened liquids during and after the swallow with a patient with a severe brain injury.

achieved for more than 89% of all patients when cognitive levels equivalent to RLA V/VI and VI/VII were achieved. Decreased attending, increased agitation, and short-term memory deficits interfered with oral intake of food.

Nature of Dysphagia

Patients with swallowing disorders secondary to brain injury may exhibit a variety of oropharyngeal abnormalities, including

- abnormal oral reflexes
- reductions in lingual range of motion or coordination of lingual movement
- increases in muscle tone of the oral musculature
- reductions in labial strength
- delay in triggering the pharyngeal swallow
- reductions in velopharyngeal closure
- reductions in strength of the base of the tongue
- abnormal pharyngeal constrictor activity
- reductions in laryngeal elevation

These patients are also at risk for physical injuries to the head and neck secondary to the traumatic event. These injuries, which can further impair the swallowing function, include

- facial fractures, which may restrict jaw opening and affect rotary chewing movements
- laryngeal fractures, which may affect laryngeal closure and elevation
- damaged, loose, or missing teeth, which may affect mastication of more solid items
- intraoral lacerations and damage, which may affect oral manipulation of food or liquids
- puncture wounds to the neck, which may reduce pharyngeal wall constriction, resulting in pharyngeal residue after the swallow
- vocal cord damage, which may impact laryngeal closure and an effective cough
- damage to the lungs or pulmonary system, which may affect tolerance of aspiration
- wounds to the chest, which may cause esophageal perforation
- spinal cord injury, which may restrict movement of pharyngeal walls and effective cough, affecting bolus transit and swallowing

A significant percentage of these patients will undergo tracheotomy. Studies have demonstrated that the presence of a tracheostomy can induce or increase aspiration. As many as 69% of patients with tracheostomies will demonstrate aspiration.[106–113] The presence of aspiration has also been documented in ventilated patients.[114–117] Silent aspiration is known to occur more frequently in neurologically impaired populations. This type of aspiration, characterized by the lack of physical or physiologic symptoms, occurs at a rate of 10% to 15% in patients with brain injury.[118] Reduced levels of consciousness also predispose to aspiration.[1,119] The symptoms of developing pneumonia may not surface in a premorbidly healthy young individual as readily as in an elderly, ill patient. Development of aspiration pneumonia can have a significant effect on the recovery process.[1,100,101]

The pathophysiology of aspiration in tracheotomized patients is multifactorial. Some factors that predispose to aspiration include reduced laryngeal elevation, desensitization of the larynx, discoordination of the swallowing musculature, and disruption of normal glottic closure.[110,113–117,120] The duration of vocal cord closure during swallowing is shorter in patients with tracheostomies, further increasing the risk of aspiration.[108,120,121]

These patients may also sustain injuries secondary to medical procedures and surgeries, including emergent cricothyroidotomy performed at the scene of the injury, prolonged endotracheal intubation, traumatic intubation, multiple intubations, and self-extubation attempts.[122] Such injuries, including paralysis or paresis of the vocal cords and tracheoesophageal fistula, can interfere with and even prevent oral feeding.

Timing of the Swallowing Assessment

The timely initiation of a bedside swallowing assessment is based on the patient's medical stability, level of alertness, and ability to participate. Results of this early assessment provide valuable information to physicians in developing a nutritional plan of care. The speech/language pathologist recommends the need for short-term versus long-term nutritional support (eg, total parenteral nutrition [TPN] versus gastrostomy [J-tube] or percutaneous endoscopic jejunostomy [PEG]). Ongoing intervention focuses on reducing the risk of aspiration, and thus the possibility of medical complications, such as aspiration pneumonia. Depending on the patient's level, evaluation may identify the safest food consistencies, best patient positioning, and most effective swallowing strategies to ensure safe swallowing.

Initiation of oral feeding versus alternative forms of nutrition must consider the patient's cognitive and behavioral status. Cognitive impairments affect oral intake throughout the recovery period.[102,105,123] Decreased attention and level of alertness and increased distractibility and agitation commonly affect oral intake during the early stages of recovery. These deficits can increase the likelihood of aspiration and increase time spent on meals. Impulsivity, judgment, memory, and organization may also affect oral intake as the patient recovers.

Bedside Assessment and Observation

The bedside dysphagia evaluation incorporates information gleaned from the oral-motor assessment and combines this with the observation of oral and pharyngeal dysphagia symptoms. Those symptoms include

- coughing or "choking" episodes during swallowing of liquids or foods
- increases in labored breathing during or after swallowing, observed at the bedside, reported by the patient, or noted via physiological parameter changes in respiratory or heart rate, or oxygen saturation levels
- gurgly or wet-sounding vocal quality, especially after swallowing food or liquid
- changes in the amount or type of secretions during or after eating
- occurrences of weak unproductive cough
- decreases in oral manipulation of food or liquid, including loss of food anteriorly from the mouth

- decreases in mastication or movement of food anteriorly to posteriorly in the oral cavity
- decreases in laryngeal elevation or coordination of movement
- perceived delays or inconsistency with triggering the pharyngeal swallow
- spiking of temperature within two hours after a meal
- history of pneumonia

Videofluoroscopic studies, helpful in assessing the nature of pharyngeal swallowing impairments, including aspiration, are not practical for patients in the ICU. Reduced neurologic functioning at this stage of recovery, paired with the difficulty in transporting ventilator-dependent patients, generally precludes use of this assessment technique.

Tracheostomy

When completing a dysphagia evaluation on a tracheotomized patient, the nurse or respiratory therapist should suction secretions from the patient before administering any food or liquid. The speech/language pathologist should take note of the patient's baseline respiratory and oxygen saturation level status, as well as the color, amount, and viscosity of the patient's secretions. If a cuff is present, it should be optimally deflated to limit its effect on swallowing. Mechanical tethering due to the tracheostomy tube can occur, resulting in decreased laryngeal elevation, especially when the cuff is overinflated.[108,124–126] Decreased laryngeal elevation may result in residue in the pyriform sinus or reduction in airway protection. Diminished laryngeal sensation may also occur secondary to decreased airflow through the laryngeal, pharyngeal, and oral cavity areas in patients with tracheostomies and may affect swallowing and increase the risk of silent aspiration.

For patients tolerating cuff deflation and using speaking valves, assessment includes swallowing trials with the speaking valve in place. Alternately, finger occlusion of the tracheostomy tube during swallowing trials should be attempted. Occlusion increases subglottic pressure, facilitating the swallow. Comparing vocal quality before and after feeding trials can help identify aspiration. Vocalizations, however, may be observed only during spontaneous activities, such as throat clearing or coughing or during suctioning.

Cuff inflation is recommended for patients with increased risk of aspiration and/or multiple pulmonary complications (Figure 11–14). Suctioning before and immediately after initial cuff deflation clears secretions situated above the cuff. The risk of aspiration is reduced again by adequate reinflation. The therapist, however, should be cognizant that aspiration is still possible if leakage occurs around the cuff.

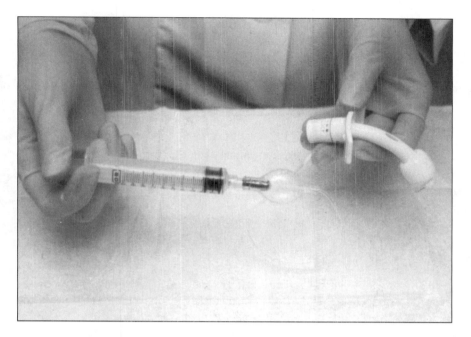

Figure 11–14 Technique used for cuff inflation. Courtesy of Mallinckrodt Medical, St. Louis, Missouri.

Food coloring, methylene blue dye, or food or liquid consistencies with distinct colors (eg, chocolate pudding and grape juice) can be employed to assist with identification of aspiration. If tinted tube feedings are used to assess reflux, distinguishable colors should be used during the dysphagia evaluation. Suctioning should occur immediately following a series of swallows of a particular food or liquid consistency. Following a brief delay, suctioning may be used to assess aspiration due to pooled material. The therapist should communicate all consistencies and colors used. The nurse can continue to monitor for aspiration after the evaluation is completed.

Ventilator-Dependent Patients

Evaluation and initiation of oral feeding are not appropriate with patients who are orally or nasally intubated. Once a patient is tracheotomized, however, continued ventilator dependency does not preclude evaluation or initiation of oral feeding. With only minor adjustments, the general assessment parameters used with tracheotomized patients can be applied to ventilator-dependent patients. Four areas should be considered prior to assessment:

1. The mode of ventilatory support should be identified. This information provides input to the speech/language pathologist regarding the speed of presentation of food and liquid and identifies whether ventilator alarms will be triggered secondary to spontaneous breaths during and after swallowing.
2. Evaluation of vocal cord movement should be completed via a speaking valve or "talking" tracheostomy tube prior to the dysphagia evaluation. The results identify whether the valving mechanism is intact so that airway protection can be maximized.
3. A patient's tolerance for cuff deflation should be identified. Deflation will be necessary to clear secretions above the cuff during the evaluation process. If tolerated, cuff deflation may be incorporated into recommendations.
4. The therapist should identify cuff pressure necessary for adequate ventilation and whether that pressure results in an adequate seal. The presence of an adequate seal will minimize aspiration during feeding trials.

Speaking valve usage is not recommended during swallowing assessment for ventilator-dependent patients. Reduced subglottic pressure is not relative within a closed system (eg, ventilator dependency) as it is within an open system (eg, nonventilator tracheostomy). Tracheal and oral suctioning and feeding trials should follow similar patterns to those outlined for tracheotomized patients. Safe swallowing is maximized when initiation of the swallow is coordinated with the start of the expiratory phase of respiration.[127]

Initiation of Oral Feeding

Results of the dysphagia evaluation, the cognitive/behavioral status of the patient, effects of medication, and the pulmonary and medical status must be considered in determining recommendations regarding initiation of oral feedings. Tolerance of aspiration in the early stages of recovery is often reduced. If evaluation results suggest inconsistent aspiration or if uncertainty regarding tolerance for small amounts of aspiration exists, decisions regarding initiation of oral feedings should be made in concert with the physician.

Trial oral feedings are more commonly used in the ICU because of decreased level of functioning and decreased ability to use precautionary strategies. For some patients, the use of small periodic feedings may be appropriate. It is the responsibility of the speech/language pathologist to educate staff and family regarding the safest postures or techniques for swallowing.

In summary, the following are examples of options that can be used with patients in the ICU:

1. prefeeding trials by the speech/language pathologist only (for patients not able to tolerate ongoing oral feeding secondary to aspiration risk, fatigue, and cognitive/behavioral issues)
2. initiation of ongoing oral feeding, using restricted consistencies (eg, pureed foods, thick liquids)
3. continued use of food coloring for ongoing monitoring of aspiration
4. use of compensatory strategies to minimize the risk of aspiration. The use of more complex techniques (eg, Mendehlson maneuver, supraglottic swallow) is not appropriate because of reduced cognition and carryover.
5. cuff inflation during feeding to minimize the amount of aspiration

The active involvement of the speech/language pathologist continues throughout the patient's recovery until adequate, safe, and independent oral feeding is accomplished.

FAMILY INVOLVEMENT

The speech/language pathologist's interactions with the family begin in the ICU. This therapist assumes a primary role in the family's education on brain injury sequelae. The family's initial concerns are the patient's survival and the extent and severity of the injury. The family looks to the physicians to provide this information.

It is appropriate, as early as the ICU, to educate the family on general stages of recovery and predicted deficits based on location and/or type of injury. The therapist must inform families that prediction of exact deficits and time frames are not possible, especially during early stages of recovery. Explanations and review of the Rancho Los Amigos Scale of Cognitive Functioning[19] is appropriate. This information allows families to anticipate future skills and deficits during recovery. One area where this is especially helpful is agitation. Providing families with appropriate interaction techniques maximizes patient/family contact. Families need to understand the source of the agitation and recognize the presence of posttraumatic amnesia during this phase. In some situations, an educated family's interactions can reduce the frequency of sedating medications or need for restraints.

Observation and/or participation in therapy reduce the anxiety and helplessness felt by the family. These interactions help facilitate "reconnection" between a family member and the patient. For patients using talking tracheostomy tubes or speaking valves, family participation in therapy allows an opportunity for verbal interaction. Family members, because of their long-term emotional ties to the patient, can be valuable to the therapist by stimulating patient responses.

Within the ICU setting, families begin to develop trusting relationships with rehabilitation professionals. The positive outlook and rehabilitation's focus on patient ability versus disability become motivating factors that many families come to rely on. Ideally, consistency with rehabilitation therapists should be maintained during the entire trauma center course. Changes in nursing staff and potentially physicians (eg, residents, critical care physicians) occur as the patient moves from critical care to step-down unit to medical/surgical floors. A consistent rehabilitation team therefore becomes a stable support for the family.

CONCLUSION

The contributions of the speech/language pathologist within the ICU setting are preventive and rehabilitative. Involvement with patients with brain injuries should include assessment as well as active treatment with patients at RLA II and above. The speech/language pathologist facilitates improved cognition and language, including arousal, responsiveness, and orientation. This team member potentially develops and fosters a means for functional communication, even at its most primitive level. Improving communication and orientation can facilitate reduced patient frustration, confusion, and agitation.

Involvement with tracheostomy management and dysphagia is preventive, reducing the risk of secondary medical complications that can thwart the recovery process. Maintaining the integrity of the vocal cords affects airway protection, communication, and potentially behavior. The use of talking tracheostomy tubes or speaking valves can reduce or eliminate secondary laryngeal or vocal complications. With a high incidence of respiratory complications such as pneumonia, maximizing airway protection and minimizing aspiration become vitally important.

The speech/language pathologist is part of the critical care team contributing to the overall plan of care. That plan includes ongoing education of staff and family. Information and terminology must be appropriate to the needs of the family. Clinical knowledge and experience must be appropriate to communicate effectively with physicians and staff. The therapist must be well trained in relevant areas of medical speech pathology and brain injury to maximize contributions and minimize complications.

REFERENCES

1. Woratyla SP, Morgan AS, Mackay L, et al. Factors associated with early onset pneumonia in the severely brain-injured patient. *Conn Med.* 1995;59:643–647.

2. Piek J, Chesnut RM, Marshall LF, et al. Extracranial complications of severe head injury. *J Neurosurg.* 1992;77:901–907.

3. Hsieh AH, Bishop MJ, Kubilis PS, Newell DW. Pneumonia following closed head injury. *Am Rev Respir Dis.* 1992;146:290–294.

4. Bouma GJ, Muizelaar JP. Relationship between cardiac output and cerebral blood flow in patients with intact and with impaired autoregulation. *J Neurosurg.* 1990;73:368–374.

5. Bouma GJ, Muizelaar JP, Bandoh K. Marmarou A. Blood pressure and intracranial pressure-volume dynamics in severe head injury: relationship with cerebral blood flow. *J Neurosurg.* 1992;77:15–19.

6. Bruce DA, Langfitt TW, Miller JD, et al. Regional cerebral blood flow, intracranial pressure, and brain metabolism in comatose patients. *J Neurosurg.* 1973;38:131–144.

7. Jaggi JL, Obrist WD, Gennarelli TA, Langfitt TW. Relationship of early cerebral blood flow and metabolism to outcome in acute head injury. *J Neurosurg.* 1990;72:176–182.

8. Marion DW, Darby J, Yonas H. Acute regional cerebral blood flow changes caused by severe head injuries. *J Neurosurg.* 1991;74:407–414.

9. Robertson CS, Contant CF, Narayan RK, Grossman RG. Cerebral blood flow, AVDO2, and neurologic outcome in head-injured patients. *J Neurotrauma.* 1992;9:S349–S358.

10. Rosner MJ, Daughton S. Cerebral perfusion pressure management in head injury. *J Trauma.* 1990;30:933–941.

11. Rea GL, Rockswold GL. Barbiturate therapy in uncontrolled intracranial hypertension. *Neurosurgery.* 1983;12:401–405.

12. Rockoff MA, Marshall LF, Shapiro HM. High-dose barbiturate therapy in humans: a clinical review of 60 patients. *Ann Neurol.* 1979;6:194–199.

13. Shapiro HM, Wyte SR, Loeser J. Barbiturate augmented hypothermia for reduction of persistent intracranial hypertension. *J Neurosurg.* 1974;40:90–100.

14. Scherer P. Assessment: the logic of coma. *J Nurs.* May 1986;86:542–549.

15. Leahy NM. *Quick Reference to Neurological Critical Care Nursing.* Gaithersburg, Md: Aspen Publishers, Inc; 1990.

16. Liebman M, Tadmore R. *Neuroanatomy Made Easy and Understandable.* 4th ed. Gaithersburg, Md: Aspen Publishers, Inc; 1991.

17. Mitchell PH, Cammermeyer M, Ozura J, Woods NF. *Neurological Assessment for Nursing Practice.* Reston, Va: Reston Publishing Co; 1984.

18. Logemann J. Swallowing disorders diagnosis and treatment strategies. Presented at Continuing Education Seminar, Introductory and Advanced Swallowing Disorders; February 3–5, 1995; Fort Lauderdale, Fla.

19. Hagen C. Language disorders secondary to closed head injury: diagnosis and management. *Top Lang Disord.* 1981;1:73–87.

20. Rappaport M, Dougherty AM, Kelting DL. Evaluation of coma and vegetative states. *Arch Phys Med Rehabil.* 1992;73:628–634.

21. Rappaport M, Hall KM, Hopkins K, et al. Disability Rating Scale for severe head trauma patients: coma to community. *Arch Phys Med Rehabil.* 1982;63:118–123.

22. Hall K, Cope DN, Rappaport M. Glasgow Outcome Scale and Disability Rating Scale: comparative usefulness in following recovery in traumatic head injury. *Arch Phys Med Rehabil.* 1985;66:35–37.

23. Fleming JM, Mass F. Prognosis of rehabilitation outcome in head injury using the Disability Rating Scale. *Arch Phys Med Rehabil.* 1994;75:156–163.

24. Gouvier WD, Blanton PD, LaPorte KK, Nepomuceno C. Reliability and validity of Disability Rating Scale and Levels of Cognitive Functioning Scale in monitoring recovery from severe head injury. *Arch Phys Med Rehabil.* 1987;68:94–97.

25. Ansell BJ, Keenan JE. The Western Neuro Sensory Stimulation Profile: a tool for assessing slow-to-recover head-injured patients. *Arch Phys Med Rehabil.* 1989;70:104–108.

26. Giacino JT, Kezmarsky MA, DeLuca J, Cicerone KD. Monitoring rate of recovery to predict outcome in minimally responsive patients. *Arch Phys Med Rehabil.* 1991;72:897–901.

27. Crosby L, Parsons LC. Clinical neurologic assessment tool: development and testing of an instrument to index neurologic status. *Heart Lung.* 1989;18:121–129.

28. Teasdale G, Jennet B. Assessment of coma and impaired consciousness: a practical scale. *Lancet.* 1974;2:81–84.

29. Sohlberg MM, Mateer CA. *Introduction to Cognitive Rehabilitation Theory and Practice.* New York, NY: Guilford Press; 1989.

30. Bergbom-Engberg I, Haljamae H. Assessment of patients' experience of discomforts during respiratory therapy. *Crit Care Med.* 1989;17:1068–1072.

31. Grap MJ, Glass C, Lindamood MO. Factors related to unplanned extubation of endotracheal tubes. *Crit Care Nurs.* 1995;15:57–65.

32. Maguire GP, LeLorenzo LJ, Moggio RA. Unplanned extubation in the intensive care unit: a quality-of-care concern. *Crit Care Nurs Q.* 1994;17:40–47.

33. Tindol GA, DiBenedetto RJ, Kosciuk L. Unplanned extubations. *Chest.* 1994;105:1804–1807.

34. Seudeal I, Garner CV, Kaye W. Accidental extubation in the ICU. *Chest.* 1992;102:184S. Abstract.

35. Coppolo DP, May JJ. Self-extubations: a 12-month experience. *Chest.* 1990;98:165–169.

36. Vassal T, Anh NG, Gabillet JM, et al. Prospective evaluation of self-extubations in a medical intensive care unit. *Intensive Care Med.* 1993;19:340–342.

37. Lowy FD, Carlisle PS, Adams A, Feiner C. The incidence of nosocomial pneumonia following urgent endotracheal intubation. *Infect Control.* 1987;8:245–248.

38. Colice GL. Resolution of laryngeal injury following translaryngeal intubation. *Am Rev Respir Dis.* 1992;145:361–364.

39. Colice GL, Stukel TA, Dain B. Laryngeal complications of prolonged intubation. *Chest.* 1989;96:877–884.

40. Lindholm CE. Prolonged endotracheal intubation. *Acta Anaesthesiol Scand.* 1969;33(suppl): 1–131.

41. Thomas R, Kumar EV, Kameswaran M, et al. Post intubation laryngeal sequelae in an intensive care unit. *J Laryngol Otol.* 1995;109:313–316.

42. Santos PM, Afrassiabi A, Weymuller EA Jr. Risk factors associated with prolonged intubation and laryngeal injury. *Otolaryngol Head Neck Surg.* 1994;111:453–459.

43. Gaynor EB, Greenberg SB. Untoward sequelae of prolonged intubation. *Laryngoscope.* 1985;95:1461–1467.

44. Weymuller EA Jr. Laryngeal injury from prolonged endotracheal intubation. *Laryngoscope.* 1988;98(suppl 45) 1–15.

45. Benjamin B. Prolonged intubation injuries of the larynx: endoscopic diagnosis, classification, and treatment. Presented at American Broncho-Esophagological Association; April 13–14, 1992; Palm Desert, Calif.

46. Whited RE. Posterior commissure stenosis post long-term intubation. *Laryngoscope.* 1983; 93:1314–1318.

47. Whited RE. A prospective study of laryngotracheal sequelae in longer-term intubation. *Laryngoscope.* 1984;94:367–377.

48. Keane WM, Denneny JC, Rowe LD, Atkins JP Jr. Complications of intubation. *Ann Otol Rhinol Laryngol.* 1982;91:584–587.

49. Jones MW, Catling S, Evans E, et al. Hoarseness after tracheal intubation. *Anaesthesia.* 1992;47:213–216.

50. Hartley M, Vaughan RS. Problems associated with tracheal intubation. *Br J Anaesth.* 1993;71:561–568.

51. Berkowitz, RG. The management of posterior glottic stenosis following endotracheal intubation. *Aust NZ J Med.* 1994;64:621–625.

52. Yang KL. Tracheal stenosis after a brief intubation. *Anesth Analg.* 1995;80:625–627.

53. McCulloch TM, Bishop MJ. Complications of translaryngeal intubation. *Clin Chest Med.* 1991;12:507–521.

54. Heffner JE. Timing of tracheotomy in ventilator-dependent patients. *Clin Chest Med.* 1991;12:611–625.

55. Stauffer JL, Olson DE, Petty TL. Complications and consequences of endotracheal intubation and tracheotomy: a prospective study of 150 critically ill adult patients. *Am J Med.* 1981;70: 65–76.

56. Whited RE. Laryngeal dysfunction following prolonged intubation. *Ann Otol Rhinol Laryngol.* 1979;88:474–478.

57. Kastanos N, Estopa Miro R, Marin Perez A, et al. Laryngotracheal injury due to endotracheal intubation: incidence, evolution and predisposing factors. *Crit Care Med.* 1983;11:362–367.

58. Burns HP, Dayal VS, Scott A, et al. Laryngotracheal trauma: observations on its pathogenesis and its prevention following prolonged orotracheal intubation in the adult. *Laryngoscope.* 1979;89:1316–1325.

59. Stone DJ, Bogdonoff DL. Airway considerations in the management of patients requiring long term endotracheal intubation. *Anesth Analg.* 1992;74:276–287.

60. Bishop MJ, Weymuller EA Jr, Fink BR. Laryngeal effects of prolonged intubation. *Anesth Analg.* 1984;63:335–342.

61. Holdgaard HO, Pedersen J, Schurizen BA, et al. Complications and late sequelae following nasotracheal intubation. *Acta Anaesthesiol Scand.* 1993;37:475–480.

62. Cheong KF, Chan MYP, Sin-Fai-Lam KN. Bilateral vocal cord paralysis following endotracheal intubation. *Anaesth Intensive Care.* 1994;22:206–208.

63. Dalton C. Bilateral vocal cord paralysis following endotracheal intubation. *Anaesth Intensive Care*. 1995;23:350–351.

64. Kark AE, Kissin MW, Auerback R, Meikle M. Voice changes after thyroidectomy: role of the external laryngeal nerve. *Br Med J.* 1984;289:1412–1415.

65. Dunham CM, LaMonica C. Prolonged tracheal intubation in the trauma patient. *J Trauma*. 1984;24:120–124.

66. Peppard SB, Dickens JH. Laryngeal injury following short-term intubation. *Ann Otol Rhinol Laryngol.* 1983;92:327–330.

67. Kambic V, Radsel Z. Intubation lesions of the larynx. *Brit J Anaesth.* 1978;50:587–589.

68. Jones GO, Hale DE, Wasmuth CE, et al. A survey of acute complications associated with endotracheal intubation. *Cleveland Clin Q.* 1968;35:23–31.

69. Charter SP, Mannar R, Jones AS. Laryngotracheal stenosis after percutaneous tracheostomy. *Anaesthesia.* 1994:825–826.

70. Iqbal S, Zuleika M. Eighty-seven days of orotracheal intubation. *Anaesthesia.* 1995;50:343–344.

71. Dubick MN, Wright BD. Comparison of laryngeal pathology following long term oral and nasal endotracheal intubations. *Anesth Analg.* 1978;57:663–668.

72. Ellis PDM, Bennett J. Laryngeal trauma after prolonged endotracheal intubation. *J Laryngol Otol.* 1977;91:69–74.

73. Hawkins DB. Pathogenesis of subglottic stenosis from endotracheal intubation. *Ann Otol Rhinol Laryngol.* 1987;96:116–117.

74. Mason MF. Vocal treatment strategies. In: Mason MF, ed. *Speech Pathology for Tracheostomized and Ventilator Dependent Patients*. Newport Beach, Calif: Voicing Inc; 1993:337–381.

75. Mason MF, Meehan K, Holinger LD. Tracheostomy and tracheostomy tubes. In: Mason MF, ed. *Speech Pathology for Tracheostomized and Ventilator Dependent Patients*. Newport Beach, Calif: Voicing Inc; 1993:127–183.

76. Akers SM, Barther TC, Pratter MR. Respiratory care. In: Sandel ME, Ellis DW, eds. *The Coma-Emerging Patient*. Philadelphia, Pa: Hanley & Belfus, Inc; 1990:527–542.

77. Law JH, Barnhart K, Rowlett W, et al. Increased frequency of obstructive airway abnormalities with long-term tracheostomy. *Chest.* 1993;104:136–138.

78. Snowberger P. Decreasing tracheal damage due to excessive cuff pressures. *Dimens Crit Care Nurs.* 1986;5:136–143.

79. Leder SB. Importance of verbal communication for the ventilatory dependent patient. *Chest.* 1990;98:792–793.

80. Leder SB. Verbal communication for the ventilator dependent patient: voice intensity with the Portex talk tracheostomy tube. *Laryngoscope.* 1990;100:1116–1120.

81. Leder SB, Traquina DN. Voice intensity of patients using a CommuniTrach I cuffed speaking tracheostomy tube. *Laryngoscope.* 1989;99:744–746.

82. Leder SB, Astrachan DI. Stomal complications and airflow line problems of the CommuniTrach I cuffed talking tracheotomy tube. *Laryngoscope.* 1989:99:194–196.

83. Eggleston G, Stanek GA, McCauley MD, et al. Utilization of Passy-Muir tracheostomy speaking valve with acute CHI patients. Presented at 6th National Traumatic Brain Injury Symposium; March 13–15, 1991; Baltimore, Md.

84. Manzano JL, Lubillo S, Henriquez D, Martin JC. Verbal communication of ventilator-dependent patients. *Crit Care Med.* 1993;21:512–517.

85. Nodell RE, Singletary T. Procedures for the Passy-Muir tracheostomy speaking valve. Presented at 3rd International Conference, Respiratory Care and Speech Pathology; October 1990; Knoxville, Tenn.

86. Frey JA, Wood S. Weaning from mechanical ventilation augmented by the Passy-Muir speaking valve. Presented at American Lung Association/American Thoracic Society International Conference; May 12, 1991; Anaheim Calif.

87. Coppola L, Milleori P. Case studies with Passy-Muir tracheostomy speaking valve. April 1989; Presented at Columbia-Presbyterian Medical Center Respiratory Conference, New York, NY.

88. Zirlen DM, Hadcad LN. Using Passy-Muir tracheostomy speaking valves with brain injured adults. Presented at 8th Annual Symposium of the National Head Injury Foundation; December 1989; Chicago, Ill.

89. Light RW, Aten JL, Fischer C, Chiang JT. Decannulation procedures for patients with chronic tracheostomies. Presented at American College of Chest Physicians 16th World Congress on Diseases of the Chest; October 1989; Boston, Mass.

90. Boylan M. Communication approaches for tracheostomized and ventilator dependent patients. Presented at American Speech-Language-Hearing Association Annual Convention; November 17–20, 1989; Saint Louis, Mo.

91. Fornataro LM, Swanik NJ, Sturm P. Use of the Passy-Muir tracheostomy speaking valve in tracheostomized patients. Presented at American Speech-Language-Hearing Association Annual Convention; November 1988; Boston, Mass.

92. Prentice W, Baydur A, Passy V. Passy-Muir tracheostomy speaking valve on ventilator dependent patients. Presented at Annual Meeting of American Lung Association/American Thoracic Society; May 14–17, 1989; Cincinnati, Ohio.

93. Passy V. Passy-Muir tracheostomy speaking valve. *Otolaryngol Head Neck Surg.* 1986;95:247–248.

94. Dettelbach MA, Gross RD, Mallmann J, Eibling DE. Effect of the Passy-Muir valve on aspiration in patients with tracheostomy. *Head Neck.* 1995;17:297–302.

95. Gadisseux P, Ward JD. Nutritional support of head-injured patients. In: Becker DP, Gudeman SK, eds. *Textbook of Head Injury.* Philadelphia, Pa: WB Saunders Co; 1989:241–254.

96. Cooper KR. Respiratory complications in patients with serious head injuries. In: Becker DP, Gudeman SK, eds. *Textbook of Head Injury.* Philadelphia, Pa: WB Saunders Co; 1989:255–264.

97. Frost EA. Respiratory problems associated with head trauma. *Neurosurgery.* 1977;1:300–306.

98. Rodriguez JL, Gibbons KJ, Bitzer LG. et al. Pneumonia: incidence, risk factors, and outcome in injured patients. *J Trauma.* 1991;31:907–912.

99. Helling TS, Evans LL, Fowler DL, et al. Infectious complications in patients with severe head injury. *J Trauma.* 1988;28:1575–1577.

100. Mosconi P, Langer M, Cigada M, Mandelli M. Epidemiology and risk factors of pneumonia in critically ill patients. *Eur J Epidemiol.* 1991;7:320–327.

101. Frost EA. Respiratory problems associated with head trauma. *Neurosurgery.* 1977;1:300–306.

102. Winstein CJ. Neurogenic dysphagia: frequency, progression and outcome in adults following head injury. *Phys Ther.* 1983;63 1992–1997.

103. Lazarus C, Logemann JA. Swallowing disorders in closed head trauma patients. *Arch Phys Med Rehabil.* 1987;68:79–84.

104. Yorkston KM, Honsingeer MJ, Mitsuca PM, Hammen V. The relationship between speech and swallowing disorders in head injured patients. *J Head Trauma Rehabil.* 1989;4:1–16.

105. Mackay L, Morgan AS. Early swallowing disorders with severe head injuries: relationships between RLA and the progression of oral intake. *Dysphagia.* 1993;8:161.

106. Muz JM, Mathog RH, Nelson R, Jones JA. Aspiration in patients with head and neck cancer and tracheostomy. *Am J Otolaryngol.* 1989;10:282–286.

107. Cameron JL, Reynolds J, Zuidema GD. Aspiration in patients with tracheostomies. *Surg Gynecol Obstet.* 1973;136:68–70.

108. Nash M. Swallowing problems in the tracheotomized patient. *Otolaryngol Clin North Am.* 1988;21:701–709.

109. Eibling DE, Bacon G, Synderman CH. Surgical management of chronic aspiration. In: *Advances in Otolaryngology: Head and Neck Surgery.* Chicago, Ill: Mosby-Year Book; 1993;7:93–113.

110. Feldman SA, Deal CW, Urquhart W. Disturbance of swallowing after tracheostomy. *Lancet.* 1966;11:954–955.

111. Betts R. Posttracheostomy aspiration. *N Engl J Med.* 1965;273:155.

112. DeVita MA, Spierer-Rundback L. Swallowing disorders in patients with prolonged orotracheal intubation or tracheostomy tubes. *Crit Care Med.* 1990;18:1328–1330.

113. Sasaki CT, Suzuki M, Horiuchi M, Kirchner JA. The effect of tracheostomy on the laryngeal closure reflex. *Laryngoscope.* 1977;87:1428–1433.

114. Elpern EH, Scott MG, Petro L, Ries MH. Pulmonary aspiration in mechanically ventilated patients with tracheostomies. *Chest.* 1994;105:563–566.

115. Treloar DM, Stechmiller J. Pulmonary aspiration in tube fed patients with artificial airways. *Heart Lung.* 1984;13:667–670.

116. Elpern EH, Jacobs ER, Bone RC. Incidence of aspiration in tracheally intubated adults. *Heart Lung.* 1987;16:527–531.

117. Spray SB, Zuidema GD, Cameron JL. Aspiration pneumonia: incidence of aspiration with endotracheal tubes. *Am J Surg.* 1976;131:701–703.

118. Logeman JA, Pepe J, Mackay LE. Disorders of nutrition and swallowing: intervention strategies in the trauma center. *J Head Trauma Rehabil.* 1994;9:43–56.

119. Finegold SM. Aspiration pneumonia. *Rev Infect Dis.* 1991;13(suppl 9):S737–S742.

120. Shaker R, Milbrath M, Ren J, et al. Deglutitive aspiration in patients with tracheostomy: effect of tracheostomy on the duration of vocal cord closure. *Gastroenterology.* 1995;108:1357–1360.

121. Feldman SA, Deal CW, Urquhart W. Disturbance of swallowing after tracheotomy. *Lancet.* 1966;1:954–955.

122. Buckwalter JA, Sasaki CT. Effect of tracheotomy on laryngeal function. *Otolaryngol Clin North Am.* 1984;17:41–48.

123. Cherney LR, Halper AS. Recovery of oral nutrition after head injury in adults. *J Head Trauma Rehabil.* 1989;4:42–50.

124. Butcher RB II. Treatment of chronic aspiration as a complication of cerebrovascular accident. *Laryngoscope.* 1982;92:681–685.

125. Arms RA, Dines DE, Tinstman TC. Aspiration pneumonia. *Chest.* 1974;65:136–139.

126. Bonanno PC. Swallowing dysfunction after tracheostomy. *Ann Surg.* 1971;174:29–33.

127. Swanson BL, Schwartz-Cowley R, Dininny DH. Safe and effective oral feeding of ventilator-assisted trauma patients. *Panam J Trauma.* 1991;2:81–87.

CHAPTER 12

Audiological Issues in Critical Care

Traumatic injury to the brain is frequently accompanied by injury to the peripheral and central mechanisms that control hearing and auditory perception. Therefore, the patient with brain injury must be assessed for risk factors suggesting damage to the auditory mechanical structures, sense organs, and pathways. Ideally, all patients admitted with a diagnosis of traumatic brain injury should undergo some type of risk assessment screening to establish the likelihood of damage to auditory structures. After risk assessment, the patient is placed in one of several categories regarding the type of assessment required and appropriate timing for intervention. The audiologist then establishes the presence, type, and degree of hearing loss, to whatever extent possible. In conjunction with other trauma team members, the audiologist establishes an appropriate ongoing evaluation and/or treatment plan to alleviate or compensate for discovered losses. In addition, the audiologist provides the patient's family with information, support, and help with long-term follow-up when permanent hearing loss is discovered. Audiologists in many institutions may also perform, interpret, or assist with auditory evoked-potential testing for the purposes of establishing the physiologic functioning status of neural pathways.

MECHANISMS OF DAMAGE TO THE EAR AND APPROPRIATE PATIENT SELECTION

The appropriate selection of patients requiring audiologic care can be difficult in the intensive care unit (ICU) environment. In the general practice of audiology, patients typically present for testing when they or those around them notice communication difficulty. Patients with moderate or severe traumatic brain injury are unable to indicate that a loss of hearing has occurred. Additionally, the lowered states of consciousness that accompany brain injury make it difficult for those around the patient to suspect decreased hearing. Trauma team members must therefore rely on characteristic constellations of injuries that suggest damage to auditory structures in order to select appropriately patients in need of audiologic care.

Literature references report that approximately 30% to 80% of all blunt injuries to the head result in some type of minor or significant hearing loss.[1–11] Fractures of the skull vault in the temporal or basilar regions are particularly associated with auditory trauma and are highly correlated with hearing loss.[6–13] Therefore, all patients experiencing such fractures should be referred for audiologic assessment at some point in the hospital course. Consultation with an otolaryngologist should also be considered for these patients. Audiology and otolaryngology involvement ensures that appropriate medical/surgical intervention or auditory rehabilitative therapy can be instituted at the earliest appropriate point. Figure 12–1 illustrates a logical flowchart describing appropriate audiologic referral of patients with traumatic brain injury by major diagnostic category.

The type and severity of hearing loss occurring after skull vault fracture are related to the force of the injury and the location of the fracture.[2,3,5–9,11,14–16] Fractures of the temporal bone usually occur along a longitudinal or a transverse axis. Such classification may be somewhat arbitrary, however, because many fractures contain both longitudinal and transverse elements.[2,13] Longitudinal fractures of the temporal bone result from blows to the side of the head and run parallel to the petrous ridge. The line of fracture typically extends along an axis posterior and superior to the plane of the ear canal, along the roof of the middle ear, into the carotid canal. Bleeding into the middle-ear space results in hemotympanum, perforated tympanic membrane, and otorrhea of blood or cerebrospinal fluid.[2,4,8,10] In some cases, shearing forces will cause subluxation or complete fracture of the ossicular chain, usually at the incudostapedial joint or at some point along the incus, which is the only ossicle not firmly anchored to an adjacent structure.[4] Approximately 60% to 80% of patients with longitudinal temporal bone fracture will experience mild to moderate conductive hearing loss.[2,6,7,16] Conductive hearing loss is defined as the hearing loss occurring from a decreased ability of the outer and/or middle ear to transmit sound energy through the middle-ear structures. Because the line of fracture is anterior to the cochlea, sensorineural damage occurs less often. Sensorineural hearing loss is defined as the loss of perception occurring secondary to damage to the inner hair cells of the cochlea.

Transverse temporal bone fractures run perpendicular to the petrous ridge and arise from blows to the frontal or occipital area. The fracture line begins at the foramen magnum, extends from the posterior fossa through the petrous pyramid to the middle cranial fossa, and usually runs directly through the cochlea and vestibular labyrinth.[2,6] The seventh and eighth cranial nerves may be torn or stretched. Occasionally, the medial wall of the middle ear may also be involved.[4,6] Trans-

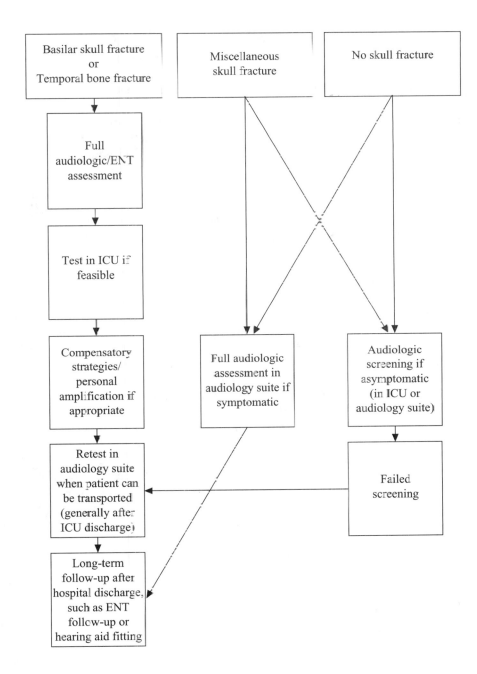

Figure 12–1 Audiologic referral flowchart.

verse temporal bone fracture results in severe to profound unilateral sensorineural hearing loss in 95% to 100% of cases.[2,6,7,16] Additional sequelae are vertigo, nystagmus, severe tinnitus, and facial nerve paralysis.

Less common late complications of transverse temporal bone fracture include cholesteatoma and meningitis.[17,18] The otic capsule consists partly of fibrous bone, which does not heal with normal calcification. Thus, the fracture line remains a fibrous gap through which invagination of middle-ear epithelium may occur, providing a substrate for cholesteatoma formation or a route of entry for pathogens. Children with transverse temporal bone fracture are especially at risk for meningitis due to the higher incidence of otitis media.[7,11,12,15]

Blows to the head may also result in hearing loss even when no evidence of temporal bone fracture exists.[1,3,5,19] Studies show that half of patients with skull fracture in areas other than the temporal bone will experience some type of minor or significant hearing loss.[5,6,16] The resultant hearing loss may be of conductive or sensorineural etiology, although high-frequency sensorineural loss is the most prevalent hearing loss that occurs in the absence of temporal bone fracture. This high-frequency loss is thought to result from concussive forces transmitting high-intensity vibratory energy to the inner ear.[6] This vibratory energy acts as an internal source of intense "noise" exposure and results in a characteristic notch at 4 kHz. Interruption of the blood supply to the cochlea may also contribute to the damage.[6,8,16]

Another mechanism of injury can be explained by describing the forces that occur when a freely movable head is struck with blunt force. Because the brain and skull differ in composition and weight, they accelerate with different velocities. Therefore, the movement of the brain will lag behind the movement of the skull due to the differences in inertia. The brain continues to accelerate after the forward motion of the skull has ceased, causing significant collision with the skull. Severe deceleration of the skull also produces angular deceleration of the brain. This rotary displacement forces the brainstem to act as a pivot about which the rest of the brain turns. Eighth-nerve laceration and hemorrhage appear to be common occurrences in this scenario. Because the incidence of hearing loss exceeds the occurrence of skull fracture, one may assume that all survivors of traumatic brain injury should receive audiologic assessment or screening at some point in the hospital course or in outpatient follow-up.

CHART REVIEW

The audiologist should gather pertinent information regarding the patient's injuries and current status, as well as any preinjury problems that may affect the audiologic outcome. This information is useful in determining the appropriate time for intervention and appropriate test methodology. If the patient's family are available, they may provide information to the audiologist or other team members regarding previous hearing aid use or prior hearing problems.

The audiologist should note the presence of fractures and other injuries that may relate to decreased central auditory functioning, such as subdural hematomas, infarcts, herniations, or other brain injuries. Such lesions may affect central audition processes if they occur in the brainstem or cortical auditory regions. The audiologist should be particularly diligent about ascertaining whether cerebrospinal fluid otorrhea has been noted. In such cases, insertion of ear canal transducers or probe tips is contraindicated, because a significant risk of meningitis is present.

TEST RATIONALE AND METHODOLOGY

Rationale for Audiologic Testing in the ICU

Peripheral or central hearing loss negatively affects the ability of therapists and other trauma team members to communicate with patients who have suffered traumatic brain injury. Because early initiation of rehabilitation therapy has been shown to reduce overall length of stay and to increase functional outcomes, efforts should be made to maximize the quality of interactions between therapists and patients.[20,2] Patients also benefit when they are able to hear and understand medical and nursing staff, other members of the hospital team, and family members. Early diagnosis of hearing loss and implementation of an intervention or monitoring plan afford patients a head start in recovery, as well as a connection to those who care most deeply about them.

Ideally, all patients at risk for hearing loss secondary to trauma should be evaluated audiologically as soon as feasible. The ICU environment and the nature of severe traumatic injury impede the ability to test hearing quickly and accurately in this population. Identifying patients with hearing loss in the ICU may not be a wise use of resources for many institutions. Institutions that do have the resources should target patients at significant risk for assessment either in the ICU or after transfer to intermediate care or the regular nursing unit when the ability to transport to the audiology department becomes feasible. Those patients at low risk of hearing impairment may be assessed at some point before discharge from the hospital or on an outpatient basis. For patients assessed in the ICU, appropriate intervention and/or monitoring can be implemented quickly to help accomplish the goals of early rehabilitation. The knowledge that hearing loss exists may also help the trauma team members understand and interpret the patient's responsiveness or lack of responsiveness.

If hearing loss is identified, the audiologist may suggest intervention strategies to help compensate for the loss during the hospitalization. For instance, if a patient is found to have a unilateral hearing loss of any type or degree, therapists and medical personnel should be told to speak to the patient on his or her unaffected side. If a patient is found to have bilateral hearing loss of significant degree, a personnel amplification system such as the Williams Pocket-Talker may be used in therapy sessions. In cases in which eventual surgical intervention or hearing aid fitting is appropriate, the audiologist may educate and prepare the family regarding these matters. In all cases, the audiologist serves as the resource person for provision of information and coordination of follow-up services.

Early identification of hearing loss may not be feasible or cost-effective for all trauma/critical care units. Facilities that do not have the resources to commit to early audiologic evaluation of patients with brain injury should ensure that otolaryngologic referrals are made for patients with suspected hearing loss and that audiologic assessment occurs at the earliest appropriate point.

Test Methodology

The audiologist must formulate a patient-specific plan for testing that includes choice of appropriate test methodology and equipment. Unlike traditional testing, audiologic testing in the ICU environment is complicated by many factors. These factors may be described in three separate categories: organizational, environmental, and patient specific.

Organizational Issues

The audiologist must be familiar with the roles of all ICU team members, the overall flow of events in the ICU, priorities in patient care issues, and complications that may arise during the typical ICU stay. Thorough preparation before venturing into the ICU and appropriate communication with nursing and medical personnel during testing will help the audiologist make the maximum contribution possible to the patient and the ICU team.

The audiologist should communicate with the nurse or intensivist to ensure that the patient will be available for testing, that the proposed time is convenient for testing, and that there are no contraindications to any audiologic procedures. In addition, the nurse or physician can provide the most recent update on the patient's condition, medication schedule, and other pertinent data.

Environmental Issues

The ICU environment typically presents the audiologist with a myriad of acoustical and electrical noise sources that pose a significant challenge to accurate hearing assessment. The audiologist must contend with noise generated by conversations and movement of people and equipment and from the different monitoring devices used in the ICU that rely on audible displays and alarms. Some noise sources can be controlled by asking visitors to leave during testing, drawing the privacy curtain around the patient's bed, or closing the room door if the room is separated from the rest of the ICU. The volume on some monitor alarms may be lowered if nursing personnel are available to watch the patient or if there is a central monitor at the nursing station desk. All reasonable steps should be taken to remove or decrease noise levels before testing.

Because noise reduction in the ICU cannot approach the noise reduction available in a sound-treated booth, the audiologist should perform a "biologic calibration" of equipment prior to testing to establish correction factors for the background noise. The audiologist begins by collecting his or her own thresholds for test stimuli in a sound treated booth, using a properly calibrated portable audiometer. The audiologist then brings the portable audiometer to the patient's bedside in the ICU. When background noise has been minimized, the audiologist rechecks his or her own thresholds. Each frequency threshold obtained in the sound treated booth is subtracted from the corresponding threshold obtained in the ICU. The decibel differences represent rough correction factors that are then subtracted from corresponding thresholds obtained from the patient.

Ventilators, intravenous (IV) pumps, pulse oximeters, intracranial pressure (ICP) monitors, electric beds, video display terminals, televisions, portable X-ray equipment, and other miscellaneous items contribute to an electrically noisy environment. Electrical noise produces interference in physiologic auditory tests such as auditory evoked-potential tests. Many of these sources of interference cannot be removed. Communication with nursing personnel is essential in determining what pieces of equipment can be safely disconnected. In general, electric beds and televisions may be safely disconnected, as well as some video display terminals, if central monitors are available at the nursing station.

Strategies for dealing with electrical noise during evoked-potential testing include manipulating test parameters and methods, in addition to decreasing the external noise. For example, using shorter braided electrode wires will decrease electrical noise because the antenna effect is diminished. Carefully placing the physiologic amplifier and the electrode intake wires away from fluid lines, electric cords, stimulus generators, and video monitors will also counteract electric noise. Notch filters centered at power line frequencies should be enabled. Using a single-channel recording technique with the inverting electrode opposite the ground electrode will help phase-cancel ambient electrical noise. Averaging over long periods of time may also reduce variable noise in the test tracings. When electrical noise factors cannot be controlled by using the above methods, evoked-potential testing may need to be discontinued.

Patient Factors

The patient's level of consciousness is the single most important factor in determining which test methodology to use. Physiologic test methods such as auditory evoked-potential testing, tympanometry and acoustic reflex assessment, or otoacoustic emissions testing may be necessary to assess patients with a Rancho Los Amigos Scale of Cognitive Functioning (RLA) level of less than or equal to III. For patients functioning at RLA level IV, it may be necessary to defer testing secondary to agitation, decreased attending, and reduced reliability of responses. However, if auditory evoked-potential testing is needed for these patients, sedation and/or paralytic medications may be used during testing. The audiologist performing the test should confer with the intensivist to see if postponing or canceling the test session is preferable to medicating the patient.

Because it is not uncommon for injuries and/or complications to extend a patient's length of stay in the ICU, patients at RLA level V or higher may require testing in that environment. Many are able to complete a routine audiogram if they can consistently use a motor response to indicate that the auditory stimulus has been heard. The audiologist should confer with other members of the rehabilitation team to help establish a response system.

Physical limitations to audiologic testing include interference from head and neck stabilization devices, bandages, sutures, and ICP bolts or other monitoring devices. Many of these items limit the ability to place earphones, probe tips, or electrode wires on the patient. If the patient has had severe injury to the face or external ears, swelling and laceration may also interfere with the ability to place audiologic transducers or probes. The audiologist should be prepared to use alternative methods when possible. For instance, properly calibrated insert earphones may be used if halo devices prevent the placement of circumaural earphones. If a bone conduction headband cannot be placed on the head secondary to halo device or because of swelling or bandages, the bone vibrator can be held in place with a long strip of elasticized Velcro. Electrode positions may be moved slightly if sutures are on the preferred site. The audiologist may also inquire about the feasibility of partially removing bandages so that electrode sites can be accessed.

ASSESSMENT OF HEARING ACUITY

Pure Tone Audiogram

Table 12–1 lists the main behavioral and physiologic components of the audiologic test battery. The pure tone audiogram, the single most important test within the battery, gives an elemental description of the patient's peripheral hearing acuity. The audiologist presents a series of tones at octave intervals from 0.25 to 8 kHz sequentially to one ear and then to the other. The intensity is lowered in 10-dB steps from a clearly audible signal until the patient no longer responds to the stimulus. The audiologist then uses a bracketing procedure to establish the hearing threshold for each frequency.

Table 12–1 Audiologic Test Battery

Behavioral Methods	Physiologic Methods
Pure Tone Air Conduction Assessment • Assesses peripheral acuity for pure tones • Status of middle-ear and inner-ear acuity determines outcome	Tympanometry • Assesses ease or difficulty with which the middle ear transforms sound energy to the inner ear • Provides description of middle-ear status but does not directly indicate hearing acuity
Pure Tone Bone Conduction Assessment • Assesses cochlear acuity for pure tones • Difference between air conduction and bone conduction determines middle-ear component	Acoustic Reflex Assessment • Assesses status of the stapedial reflex, which reduces transmission of sound energy to the inner ear when loud stimuli are presented • Does not directly assess hearing acuity • May be abnormal in middle- and inner-ear disorders, as well as in retrocochlear pathology
Speech Reception Threshold Assessment • Assesses peripheral threshold for speech perception • Generally not done in ICU setting	Otoacoustic Emissions Assessment • Assesses status of cochlear echoes present in normal-hearing ears • Separates normal from abnormal ears • Does not directly measure hearing loss
Word Recognition Performance Assessment • Assesses ability to recognize and repeat speech stimuli (monosyllabic words) at a suprathreshold level • Generally not done in ICU setting	BAEP Latency-Intensity Function Assessment • Assesses threshold of the brainstem response to auditory stimulation • Indirectly measures hearing acuity

By comparing thresholds obtained with air conduction circumaural or insert transducers to thresholds obtained with a bone conduction transducer, the audiologist can determine whether hearing loss is conductive, sensorineural, or mixed in nature. When air conduction thresholds roughly equal bone conduction thresholds, any hearing loss present is considered sensorineural. When bone conduction thresholds are significantly better than air conduction thresholds (an "air-bone gap"), the hearing loss is considered conductive. Elevated air conduction thresholds combined with an air-bone gap signify a mixed hearing loss. The pure tone audiogram best describes the patient's hearing acuity and is the preferred method of testing when reasonable levels of cooperation can be obtained from the patient.

In all cases, early identification of hearing loss is the first step in determining a case management plan. Patients with suspected hearing loss should be retested in an acoustically isolated sound suite when they have recovered sufficiently for transportation. The case management plan may change if hearing loss abates or if the patient's increased ability to cooperate for testing indicates that a previously suspected hearing loss is not present.

Tympanometry

Tympanometry is an assessment of middle-ear function that describes the ease or difficulty with which the tympanic membrane and middle-ear ossicles transmit vibratory energy to the cochlea. During tympanometric testing, a probe tip is inserted into the outer ear canal. After a hermetic seal is obtained, a tone is introduced into the canal while the canal is pressurized over a small negative to positive range. The variations in sound pressure level are measured and translated into graphic and numeric descriptions of middle-ear motion. A healthy middle ear will display a particular pattern and range of numerical values. A diseased or injured middle ear will show distinct variations from those normal patterns and values.

Middle-ear pathology is a common complication of injury to the skull and can be easily confirmed by tympanometric testing.[22] Perforated tympanic membranes will display unusually large tympanometric volume measures. Hemotympanum will show up as a markedly lowered static admittance value with a characteristic flat tracing. Ossicular discontinuity or subluxation may result in extremely high static admittance values with or without large notching patterns evident in the tracings. Monomeric tympanic membranes may also result in tympanometric patterns and admittance values that are similar to those seen with ossicular discontinuity and subluxation; therefore, other tests must be done to provide the differential diagnosis.

The presence of a large air-bone gap and intact acoustic reflex arc coupled with high static admittance and notching tympanometric pattern suggests an ossicular discontinuity medial to the stapedial connection. A large air-bone gap combined with absent acoustic reflexes, high static admittance, and notching pattern may indicate ossicular discontinuity lateral to the stapedial muscle connection or may be indicative of a monomeric tympanic membrane, combined with large amounts of blood or other fluid within the middle-ear space. In this scenario, otoscopic examination may hold clues to the differential diagnosis, as will the passage of time. Middle-ear effusion secondary to injury tends to resolve eventually, whereas ossicular discontinuity tends to persist. High static admittance and/or notched tympanometric pattern in the absence of a significant air-bone gap suggests a monomeric tympanic membrane without significant ossicular damage or middle-ear effusion.

Acoustic Reflex Testing

Acoustic reflex testing can be considered an extension of tympanometric testing. In an effort to protect the inner ear from hair cell damage, the acoustic admittance of the middle ear changes slightly when intense noise causes the stapedial muscle to contract. With muscle contraction, the ossicular chain stiffens slightly to lessen the amount of vibratory energy being transmitted to the cochlea. This change in middle-ear admittance can be measured following tympanometry.

The acoustic reflex may be absent if damage to the seventh and/or eighth cranial nerve is present, if damage to the central relay mechanisms in the brainstem is present, or if hearing loss is great enough to cause significant attenuation of intense noise. It may be present but not measurable when hemotympanum or ossicular discontinuity causes admittance changes so great that they easily mask the presence of the small change seen with muscle contracture. Acoustic reflex assessment helps in the differential diagnosis of hearing loss when it is used in the test battery approach. The advantages of both tympanometric and acoustic reflex testing are that the tests are based on physiologic phenomena and do not require a behavioral response from the patient. Although neither test directly assesses hearing acuity, both offer insight into injury to the structures of the ear.

Otoacoustic Emissions Testing

Otoacoustic emissions (OAEs) are physiologic phenomena associated with the normal hearing process.[23,24] These emissions of sound energy are produced by the hair cells in the inner ear and can be measured with sensitive low-noise microphones placed in the ear canal. Otoacoustic emissions may occur spontaneously or may be evoked by certain stimuli. Otoacoustic emissions produced by broadband click stimuli have proved to be a reliable indicator of healthy, normally functioning cochleae and are thought to be a positive-feedback mechanism by which the cochlea improves sensitivity and frequency specificity.[23,24]

An expanding body of research on OAEs is establishing this technique as a mainstay in audiologic assessment.[23–27] Otoacoustic emission testing is being used in neonatal screening programs with good results.[25,27] More research is needed to assess the application of OAE testing to patients with traumatic brain injury. Because OAEs are a physiologic phenomenon, the patient's state of consciousness does not interfere with the ability to obtain results. The test requires minimal preparation of the patient and can be completed in relatively short periods of time. The major drawback of attempting OAE testing in the ICU, however, is that it is sensitive to moderate or higher levels of extraneous noise.

During OAE testing, a small probe tip is inserted into the ear. A broadband click is presented to the ear canal and monitored by an ultrasensitive microphone. The receiving microphone measures the sound pressure level in the ear canal and subtracts the combined response of the signal, the ear canal resonance, and the background noise from the entire sample. The otoacoustic emission from the cochlea is then amplified, filtered, and graphically illustrated on a computer screen.

Click-evoked otoacoustic emissions will be absent in patients with hearing loss greater than approximately 25- to 30-dB hearing level (HL), normal hearing being defined as a threshold up to 25 dB HL.[24,26] The emissions will also be absent if a significant conductive component is present. Therefore, testing on a large-scale basis should easily separate patients with normal peripheral hearing from patients with abnormal peripheral hearing. Sensitivity and specificity data obtained in experiments involving neonatal screening appear to be high.[25,27]

Brainstem Auditory Evoked-Potential Testing

Brainstem auditory evoked-potential (BAEP) testing may be used to establish hearing acuity in patients who are unable to respond for behavioral audiologic testing. The response of the auditory pathway in the brainstem is generally unaffected by the depth of coma and is not altered by most medications. Using BAEP testing for the purpose of establishing hearing acuity is, however, time consuming and technically complicated by the ICU environment, as previously explained.

During BAEP testing, approximately three to five surface electrodes are placed on the patient's head on conventionally accepted 10 to 20 system sites. Insert, circumaural, or bone conduction transducers may be placed in, on, or around the patient's ears. Stimuli are then introduced at varying intensity levels sequentially to the ears. The physiologic data received from the surface electrodes are then amplified, filtered through a specified band-pass, and analyzed over a 10- to 20-millisecond time window. Characteristic wave patterns are discerned from the test tracings. The intensity level at which these characteristic wave patterns disappear is designated as the BAEP threshold. This threshold is then converted to an estimate of the pure tone threshold for the frequency region represented by the test stimulus.

The technical difficulties inherent in BAEP testing center mostly on the fact that the auditory brainstem response is extremely small in comparison to ongoing electroencephalography (EEG) and myogenic activity. In conventional BAEP techniques, a broadband click stimulus is typically used because it elicits the largest and most reliable brainstem response. The broadband click is used not for its frequency content but for its relatively instantaneous onset time. This instantaneous onset allows for maximum synchronous firing of cochlear and eighth nerve fibers and results in a response large enough to measure. The bulk of the response comes from the basilar end of the cochlea and the outer wrapping of the eighth-nerve fibers because these are the most numerous fibers and the most proximal. The basilar end of the cochlea and the outer wrapping of the eighth nerve contain mostly high-frequency fibers centered somewhere on the 2- to 4-kHz range of the frequency spectrum. Therefore, the audiologic information obtained from the test is limited to that narrow range.

Frequency-specific stimuli can be used to describe hearing acuity over a larger range. The easiest and most reliable stimuli to use in frequency-specific BAEP testing are Blackman filtered tone pips. These specially filtered tone pips afford a reasonable compromise between frequency specificity and onset times that are quick enough to elicit a measurable response. Latency-intensity functions must be run for tone pips centered at several frequencies covering a broad portion of the frequency region in order to accurately describe the patient's hearing acuity. Consequently, the test session may become quite lengthy. In many, if not most, cases, it may be more appropriate to postpone audiologic evaluation until the patient is able to respond to behavioral methods of assessment. For patients with brain injury, evoked-potential testing is more often used to assess the integrity of the brainstem and central auditory pathways.[28–49] However, threshold testing can provide information on the hearing acuity of patients who are undergoing evoked-potential testing for neurologic assessment.

Evoked-Potential Testing for Assessment of Neurologic Integrity

Because evoked-potential tests are tests of function, they can augment the information garnered from the neurologic examination and from measures of anatomical structure, such as radiographic and magnetic resonance imaging studies.[28,30,39,49–52] Evoked-potential testing may be especially illuminating when neurologic examination is limited because of the administration of sedative or paralytic drugs.

The objective of BAEP testing is to describe the ability of the auditory brainstem to transmit auditory information through its pathways. Auditory brainstem function has been shown to be a good indicator of brainstem function in general and can be a sensitive measure of brainstem dysfunction arising from diffuse severe cerebral injury.[38,53] Because of these associations, the information obtained can be correlated with other clinical studies and the physical assessment to obtain a judgment regarding the patient's prognosis.[30,39,40,47,50,52,54-58] Studies indicate that a normal BAEP test result is generally associated with a good neurologic outcome and that a poor test result is generally associated with a poor outcome or death.[40,47,52,55,56]

The role of the examiner and interpreter in evoked-potential testing may vary between institutions. Audiologists are educated and certified to perform and interpret these studies for the assessment of peripheral hearing acuity and neurologic function. Some institutions use EEG technicians to obtain tracings that are subsequently interpreted by neurologists. Because peripheral hearing loss interferes with the ability to obtain information regarding the neurologic function of the brainstem, audiologic assessment of the patient should precede the assessment of neurologic integrity of the auditory brainstem. Audiologic assessment will generally consist of BAEP threshold testing using brief-duration click stimuli at least and tympanometry if indicated by history, physical examination, or threshold tests.

The characteristic waveforms present in a normal BAEP response consist of five peaks occurring at regular 1-millisecond intervals following onset of the auditory stimulus. These waveforms, labeled I through V, represent the transmission of impulses through the relay nuclei in the brainstem. In abnormal auditory brainstem function, these waveforms may be delayed in latency from stimulus onset, reduced in amplitude, or absent. Traumatic brain injury may cause multiple abnormalities in the BAEP response or may result in no abnormality at all if the injury is limited to areas above the brainstem level.

Comparison of results obtained with right-ear stimulation to those obtained with left-ear stimulation is diagnostic in determining the presence of brainstem herniation or unilateral influences such as subdural hematoma or other focal lesions.[37,39,49] Bilaterally symmetric reduced or absent responses are indicative of diffuse injury to the brainstem if peripheral hearing loss is ruled out.[28,29,32,33,38,44,46,57] Brainstem injury may be primary, occurring from focal hemorrhagic lesions or shearing and tearing of brainstem fibers, or may be secondary to cerebral insult.[33,34,45] Severe diffuse cerebral injury may cause secondary brainstem injury by virtue of retrograde damage to nerve fibers from hemorrhage, swelling, or metabolic changes.[38,59] Focal and diffuse cerebral lesions can also exert pressure on the lateral ventricles, forcing excess cerebrospinal fluid into the third and fourth ventricles, elevating pressure to levels that cause damage to the nuclei beneath the floor of the ventricles.[38]

When somatosensory evoked-potential (SEP) testing is coupled with auditory evoked-potential testing, outcome prognostication increases.[29,30,41,46,47,56,57,60-62] One prospective study showed that 93% of patients with brain injury had a good outcome when SEP and BAEP were normal, whereas 100% had poor outcomes when both SEP and BAEP responses were absent.[40] Serial multimodality evoked-potential testing contributes to the description of severity and the focal versus diffuse nature of the brain injury by virtue of its ability to describe damage to different sensory systems and its ability to document changes over time.[54,62]

Other auditory evoked-potential tests may be used to assess the integrity of central auditory pathways. Middle latency response (MLR) and P300 response represent the activity of the auditory midbrain and auditory cerebral cortex, respectively. Although less widely used, these tests can potentially describe activity above the brainstem level and increase knowledge of the patient's condition.[36,43,58,63-67] The main drawbacks of central evoked-potential testing are the increased normal variability of these tests when compared to BAEP, increased length of test time, and increased level of expertise necessary to perform and interpret the test. In addition, P300 testing is significantly affected by the level of consciousness and consequently is more difficult to interpret when the patient is at RLA level III or below.[43,65,66]

Patients who may benefit from BAEP, MLR, P300, or SEP testing include those that are receiving sedative or paralytic medication to reduce intracranial-cranial pressure, patients that are at RLA level III or below and whose course appears unclear, and patients whose condition appears to be deteriorating without obvious cause. Serial testing may be necessary if the patient's condition is discordant with the initial test results or if questions remain regarding the clinical status of the patient. Results obtained over several days will usually give clues as to which direction the patient is headed clinically.

The use of BAEP and SEP testing has had a role in determining brain death among the profoundly brain injured.[60,68-70] If peripheral hearing loss is confidently ruled out, a diagnosis of brain death can be made when an absent BAEP response is coupled with absent SEP responses and other commonly accepted signs of irreversible coma, including prolonged serial isoelectric EEG results, absence of all spontaneous muscle activity, and absolute unresponsiveness to all stimuli, all in the absence of hypothermia or intoxication by central nervous system depressants.

CONCLUSION

Injury to the skull and brain results in significant hearing deficits in a large number of patients. Peripheral hearing, the first step in the communicative chain, is frequently affected. Damage to brainstem level and central elements of the auditory system is also common. Audiologic referral for high-risk patients at some point in the hospital or outpatient course is important to diagnose hearing loss adequately and to initiate a referral or treatment plan. The effectiveness of rehabilitation and intensive care therapy is intimately related to the patient's ability to hear.

Early identification of hearing loss while the patient is still in the ICU setting may be possible for some patients in some facilities. Such identification allows for initiation of a treatment or monitoring plan at a much earlier point in the patient's recovery. If partial compensation for the identified hearing loss is made, then physical, occupational, and speech/language therapy may be more effective. Additionally, the patient benefits from an enhanced ability to hear his or her physicians, nurses, other medical personnel, and family members.

Audiologic testing in the ICU itself may include a series of behavioral and physiologic tests designed to assess various elements of the auditory system. Behavioral testing generally involves the assessment of hearing acuity by means of the pure tone audiogram. The pure tone audiogram requires that the patient have a reasonable level of consciousness and ability to cooperate; therefore, its use is limited to those patients at RLA level V or above who can use some type of consistent motor response to indicate that test signals have been heard.

Various physiologically based tests are available to assess patients who are unable to complete a pure tone audiogram. Tympanometry and acoustic reflex testing assess the status of the middle ear and acoustic reflex arcs. Although these tests do not assess hearing, they do offer insight into the extent of damage to the auditory system. Brainstem auditory evoked-potential testing is a physiologically based test that can assess the integrity of the auditory brainstem pathways. Peripheral hearing can be measured with this technique by decreasing the stimulus levels until the response is extinguished. Assessment of the neurologic function of the auditory brainstem can also offer insights into the nature of the brain injury and the prognosis for the patient's recovery. Otoacoustic emissions analysis is a relatively new physiologically based test that can assess the status of peripheral hearing. More research is needed in this new method to establish its utility in the brain-injured population.

All audiologic testing performed in the ICU environment is plagued by significant technical difficulty. Assessments that occur in the ICU should always be considered rough estimates of the patient's condition. Testing in an acoustically isolated sound suite should be attempted when the patient has recovered sufficiently for transportation or at some point in the hospital or outpatient course. When hearing loss is suspected during the acute phase of the patient's course, compensatory strategies should be used by medical and rehabilitative personnel. These strategies may include (1) directing conversations to the unaffected side when unilateral hearing loss is present, (2) decreasing background noise whenever possible, (3) speaking to the patient face to face, using clear pronunciation, (4) repeating and rephrasing important points, and (5) using a temporary personal amplification system when bilateral hearing loss appears likely.

The audiologist as a member of the rehabilitation team serves as a consultant to other rehabilitation and ICU team members, assesses hearing in appropriate patients, establishes a monitoring or treatment and referral plan, and provides education and support for the patient's family members. The development of a protocol plan for audiologic intervention in trauma cases should be considered in facilities that seek to maintain high levels of quality care in the ICU. Audiologists in facilities with trauma programs should offer their services in helping to establish such protocols.

REFERENCES

1. Abd Al-hady MR, Shehata O, E.-Mously M, Sallam FS. Audiologic findings following head trauma. *J Laryngol Otol.* 1990;104: 927–936.

2. Cannon CR, Jahrsdoerfer RA. Temporal bone fractures. *Arch Otolaryngol.* 1983;109:285–286.

3. Hall JW III, Huang-fu M, Gennarelli TA. Auditory function in acute severe head injury. *Laryngoscope.* 1982;92:883–889.

4. Hough JVD, Stuart WD. Middle ear injuries in skull trauma. *Laryngoscope.* 1968;78:899–937.

5. Kochhar LK, Deka RC, Kacker SK, Raman EV. Hearing loss after head injury. *Ear Nose Throat J.* 1990;69:537–542.

6. Makashima K, Snow JB. Pathogenesis of hearing loss in head injury. *Arch Otolaryngol.* 1975; 101:426-432.

7. McGuirt WF, Stool SE. Temporal bone fractures in children: a review with emphasis on long-term sequelae. *Clin Pediatr.* 1992;31:12–18.

8. Pearson BW, Barber HO. Head injury: some otoneurologic sequelae. *Arch Otolaryngol.* 1973;97:81–84.

9. Podoshon L, Fradis M. Hearing loss after head injury. *Arch Otolaryngol.* 1975;101:15–18.

10. Wennmo C, Svensson C. Temporal bone fractures: vestibular and other related ear sequelae. *Acta Otolaryngol.* 1989;468:379–383.

11. Zimmerman WD, Ganzel TM, Windmill IM, Nazar GB, et al. Peripheral hearing loss following head trauma in children. *Laryngoscope.* 1993;103:87–91.

12. Glarner H, Meuli M, Hof E, Gallati V, et al. Management of temporal bone fractures in children: analysis of 127 cases. *J Trauma.* 1994;36:198–201.

13. Waldron J, Hurley SEJ. Temporal bone fractures: a clinical diagnosis. *Arch Emerg Med.* 1988,5:146–150.

14. Makishima K, Sobel SF, Snow JB. Histopathologic correlates of otoneurologic manifestations following head trauma. *Laryngoscope* 1976;86:1303–1314.

15. Williams WT, Ghorayeb BY, Yeakley JW. Pediatric temporal bone fractures. *Laryngoscope.* 1992;102:600–603.

16. Momose KJ, Davis KR, Rhea JT. Hearing loss in skull fractures. *Amer J Neuroradiol.* 1983;4:781–785.

17. Botrill ID. Post-traumatic cholesteatoma. *J Laryngol Otol.* 1991;105:367–369.

18. Ghorayeo BY, Yeakley JW, Hall JW III, Jones BE. Unusual complications of temporal bone fractures. *Arch Otolaryngol Head Neck Surg.* 1987;113:749–753.

19. Koefoed-Nielsen B, Tos M. Posttraumatic sensorineural hearing loss: a prospective long-term study. *Otorhinolaryngol.* 1982;44:206–215.

20. Cope DN, Hall K. Head injury rehabilitation: benefits of early intervention. *Arch Phys Med Rehabil.* 1982;63:433–437.

21. Mackay LE, Bernstein BA, Chapman PE, et al. Early intervention in severe head injury: long term benefits of a formalized program. *Arch Phys Med Rehabil.* 1992;73:635–641.

22. Cavaliere F, Masieri S, Liberini L, et al. Tympanometry for middle ear effusion in unconscious ICU patients. *Eur J Anaesthesiol.* 1992;9:71–75.

23. Smurzynski J, Kim DO. Distortion-product and click-evoked emissions of normally hearing adults. *Hear Res.* 1992;58:227–240.

24. Probst R, Harris FP. Transiently evoked and distortion product otoacoustic emissions: comparison of results from normally hearing and hearing-impaired human ears. *Arch Otolaryngol.* 1993; 119:858–860.

25. Bonfils P, Avan P, Francois M, et al. Distortion product otoacoustic emissions in neonates: normative data. *Acta Otolaryngol.* 1992;112:739–744.

26. Gorga MP, Neely ST, Bergman BM, et al. A comparison of transient-evoked and distortion product otoacoustic emissions in normal-hearing and hearing-impaired subjects. *J Acoust Soc Am.* 1993;994:2639–2648.

27. Lafreniere D, Smurzynsk J, Jung M, Leonard G. Otoacoustic emissions in full term newborns at risk for hearing loss. *Laryngoscope.* 1993;103:1334–1341.

28. Aguilar EA, Hall JW, Mackey-Hargadine J. Neuro-otologic evaluation of the patient with acute, severe head injuries: correlations among physical findings, auditory evoked responses, and computerized tomography. *Otolaryngol Head Neck Surg.* 1986;94:211–219.

29. Cant BR, Hume AL, Judson JA, Shaw NH. The assessment of severe head injury by short-latency somatosensory and brain-stem auditory evoked potentials. *Electroencephalogr Clin Neurophysiol.* 1986;65:188–195.

30. Cusumano S, Paolin A, DiPaoli F, et al. Assessing brain function in post-traumatic coma by means of bit-mapped SEPs, BAEPs, CT, SPET and clinical scores: prognostic implications. *Electroencephalogr Clin Neurophysiol.* 1992;84:499–514.

31. Facco E, Martini A, Zuccarello M, et al. Is the auditory brain-stem response (ABR) effective in the assessment of post-traumatic coma? *Electroencephalogr Clin Neurophysiol.* 1985;62:332–337.

32. Ganes T, Lundar T. EEG and evoked potentials in comatose patients with severe brain injury. *Electroencephalogr Clin Neurophysiol.* 1988;69:6–13.

33. Hall JW III, Mackey-Hargadine J. Auditory evoked responses in severe head injury. *Semin Hear.* 1984;5:313–336.

34. Hall JW III, Speilman G, Gennarelli TA. Auditory evoked responses in acute severe head injury. *Am Assoc Neurosurg Nurs.* 1982;14:225–231.

35. Hansotia PL. Persistent vegetative state: review and report of electrodiagnostic studies in eight cases. *Arch Neurol.* 1985;42:1048–1052.

36. Kaga K, Nagal T, Takamori A, Marsh RR. Auditory short, middle, and long latency responses in acutely comatose patients. *Laryngoscope.* 1985;95:321–325.

37. Karnaze DS, Marshall LF, McCarthy CS, et al. Localizing and prognostic value of auditory evoked responses in coma after closed head injury. *Neurology.* 1982;32:299–302.

38. Kawahara N, Sasaki M, Mii K, et al. Sequential changes of auditory brain stem responses in relation to intracranial and cerebral perfusion pressure and initiation of secondary brain stem damage. *Acta Neurochir.* 1989;100:142–149.

39. Krieger D, Adams HP, Schwarz S, et al. Prognostic and clinical relevance of pupillary responses, intracranial pressure monitoring, and brainstem auditory evoked potentials in comatose patients with acute supratentorial mass lesions. *Crit Care Med.* 1993;21:1944–1993.

40. Mahapatra AK. Evoked potentials in severe head injuries: a prospective study of 40 cases. *J Ind Med Assoc.* 1990;88:217–220.

41. Newlon PG, Greenberg RP. Evoked potentials in severe head injury. *J Trauma* 1984;24:61–66.

42. Noseworthy JH, Miller J, Murray TJ, Regan D. Auditory brainstem responses in post concussion syndrome. *Arch Neurol.* 1981;38:275–278.

43. Rappaport M, Hemmerle AV, Rappaport ML. Short and long latency auditory evoked potentials in traumatic brain injury patients. *Clin Electroencephalogr.* 1991;22:199–202.

44. Scherg M, von Cramon D, Elton M. Brainstem auditory-evoked potentials in post-comatose patients after severe closed head injury. *J Neurol.* 1984;231:1–5.

45. Tsubokawa T, Nishimoto H, Yamamoto T, et al. Assessment of brainstem damage by the auditory brainstem response in acute severe head injury. *J Neurol Neurosurg Psychiatry.* 1980;43: 1005–1011.

46. de Weerd AW, Groeneveld C. The use of evoked potentials in the management of patients with severe cerebral trauma. *Acta Neurol Scand.* 1985;72:489–494.

47. Yongche Shin D, Ehrenberg B, Whyte J, et al. Evoked potential assessment: utility in prognosis of chronic head injury. *Arch Phys Med Rehabil.* 1989;70:189–193.

48. Hall JW III. Auditory brain stem response spectral content in comatose head-injured patients. *Ear Hear.* 1986;7:383–389.

49. Zuccarello M, Fiore DL, Pardatscher K, et al. Importance of auditory brainstem responses in the CT diagnosis of traumatic brainstem lesions. *Am J Neurol Radiol.* 1983;4:481–483.

50. Alster J, Pratt H, Feinsod M. Density spectral array, evoked potentials, and temperature rhythms in the evaluation and prognosis of the comatose patient. *Brain Inj.* 1993;7:191–208.

51. Garcia-Larrea L, Artru F, Bertrand O, et al. The combined monitoring of brain stem auditory evoked potential and intracranial pressure in coma: a study of 57 patients. *J Neurol Neurosurg Psychiatry.* 1992;55:792–798.

52. Narayan RK, Greenberg RP, Miller JD, et al. Improved confidence of outcome prediction in severe head injury: a comparative analysis of the clinical examination, multimodality evoked potentials, CT scanning, and intracranial pressure. *J Neurosurg.* 1981;54:751–762.

53. Harris DP, Hall JW III. Feasibility of auditory event-related potential measurement in brain injury rehabilitation. *Electrophysiol Tech Audiol Otol.* 1990;11:340–350.

54. Facco E, Munari M, Casartelli Liviero M, et al. Serial recordings of auditory brainstem responses in severe head injury: relationship between test timing and prognostic power. *Intensive Care Med.* 1988;14:422–428.

55. Karnaze DS, Weiner JM, Marshall LF. Auditory evoked potential in coma after closed head injury: a clinical-neurophysiologic coma scale for predicting outcome. *Neurology.* 1985;35:1122–1126.

56. Lindsay K, Pasaoglu A, Hirst D, et al. Somatosensory and auditory brainstem conduction after head injury: a comparison with clinical features in prediction outcome. *Neurosurgery.* 1990; 26:278–285.

57. Newlon PG, Greenberg RP, Hyatt MS, et al. The dynamics of neuronal dsyfunction and recovery following severe head injury assessed with serial multimodality evoked potentials. *J Neurosurg.* 1982;57:168–177.

58. Ottoviani F, Almadori G, Calderazzo AB, et al. Auditory brain-stem (ABRs) and middle latency auditory responses (MLRs) in the prognosis of severely head-injured patients. *Electroencephalogr Clin Neurophysiol.* 1986;65:196–202.

59. Mahapatra AK, Tandon PN. Brainstem auditory evoked response and vestibulo-ocular reflex in severe head injury patients: a prospective study of 60 cases. *Acta Neurochir.* 1987;87:40–43.

60. Goldie W, Chiappa KH, Young RR, Brooks EB. Brainstem auditory and short latency somatosensory evoked responses in brain death. *Neurology.* 1981;31:248–256.

61. Hall JW III, Tucker DA. Sensory evoked responses in the intensive care unit. *Ear Hear.* 1986;7:220–232.

62. Hilz MJ, Litscher G, Weis M, et al. Continuous multivariable monitoring in neurological intensive care patients: preliminary report on four cases. *Intensive Care Med.* 1991;17:87–93.

63. Firsching R, Luther J, Eidelberg E, et al. 40-Hz: middle latency auditory evoked response in comatose patients. *Electroencephalogr Clin Neurophysiol.* 1987; 67:213–216.

64. Kileny P, Paccioretti D, Wilson AF. Effects of cortical lesions on middle-latency auditory evoked response (MLR). *Electroencephalogr Clin Neurophysiol.* 1987;66:108–120.

65. Pratap-Chand R, Sinniah M, Salem FA. Cognitive evoked potential (P300): a metric for cerebral concussion. *Acta Neurol Scand.* 1988;78:185–189.

66. Rappaport M, McCandless KL, Pond W, Krafft MC. Passure P300 response in traumatic brain injury patients. *J Neuropsych Clin Neurosci.* 1991;3:180–185.

67. Serafini G, Acra W, Scuteri F, et al. Auditory evoked potentials at 40 Hz (SSR 40 Hz) in post-trauma coma patients. *Laryngoscope.* 1994;104:182–184.

68. Firsching R, Frowein RA, Wilhelms S, Buchholz F. Brain death: practicability of evoked potentials. *Neurosurg Rev.* 1992;15:249–254 .

69. Hall JW III, Mackey-Hargadine J, Kim EE. Auditory brain-stem response in determination of brain death. *Arch Otolaryngol.* 1985;111:613–620.

70. Machado C. Multimodality evoked potentials and electroretinography in a test battery for an early diagnosis of brain death. *J Neurol Sci.* 1993;37:125–130.

CHAPTER 13

Pharmacologic Management of Persons with Severe Brain Injury

The problem of drug-induced sedation in comatose and obtunded patients with brain injuries is more serious than generally appreciated, and it deserves special attention. The critical care team should bear in mind that sedative side effects can be magnified in the injured brain, primarily because of disruption of the blood-brain barrier, and that even small changes in arousal can affect the patient's responsiveness. The use of inappropriate sedating medications can lead to an increased length of stay, the development of medical complications, and, in some instances, slowed neurologic recovery. Some medications such as neuroleptics can even have irreversible side effects such as tardive dyskinesia. Medications given to the unconscious patient should be carefully reviewed with the pharmacist on a regular basis. Unnecessary medications should be discontinued if possible. Necessary drugs should be replaced with ones that are less sedating (Table 13–1).

Management of agitated behavior with environmental and behavioral techniques can often be enhanced with medications. Commonly used medications such as neuroleptics and anxiolytics increase confusion and add to the patient's memory deficits. In the intensive care unit (ICU), intravenous administration of propofol (Diprivan) is favored. Once the patient is capable of ingesting enteric medication, the use of carbamazepine, lithium, beta blockers, and newer serotoninergics is recommended.

The use of seizure prophylaxis with phenytoin after the first week is no longer the standard of care. Physiatrists are waiting until a patient has a posttraumatic seizure before starting carbamazepine or valproic acid, drugs that appear to have fewer cognitive and behavioral side effects in patients with brain injuries. Even the use of gastrointestinal medications, such as H_2-receptor antagonists like cimetidine, can have untoward cognitive and behavioral side effects. Metoclopramide can have significant effects on the dopaminergic system. Thus, cisapride is the preferred drug to increase gastric emptying. Sucralfate, for a variety of rea-

Table 13–1 Less Sedating Drug Options for Patients with Severe Brain Injury

Sedating Drugs To Be Avoided	Less Sedating Alternatives
ANTICONVULSANT	
Phenytoin	Carbamazepine
Phenobarbital	Valproic acid
ANTIHYPERTENSIVE	
Propranolol	Clonidine
Metoprolol	Verapamil
Methyldopa	Diuretics
ANTISPASTICITY MEDICATIONS	
Baclofen	Dantrolene sodium
Amitriptyline	Carbamazepine
Doxepin	Paroxetine
Imipramine	Methylphenidate
Trazodone	Fluoxetine
	Levodopa/carbidopa
	Sertraline
GASTROINTESTINAL MEDICATIONS	
Cimetidine	Sucralfate
Metoclopramide	Antacids
	Cisapride
	Erythromycin

sons, including its lack of sedative properties, is the preferred medication for the prevention of gastric ulceration.

The trend in the treatment of spasticity is to avoid the use of medications that can have profound sedative effects. Nerve and motor point blocks and the use of botulism toxin injected into spastic muscles combined with the use of inhibitive casting are the preferred methods of spasticity control and contracture prevention for patients with brain injuries.

THE ROLE OF NEUROTRANSMITTERS

Acute Stage of Recovery

Neurotransmitters are the chemical messengers that allow the nerve cells to communicate with each other across the synaptic cleft. It is postulated that an excess of excitatory and inhibitory neurotransmitters (eg, glutamate and acetyl-choline) is released immediately following a traumatic brain injury. This release of excessive neurotransmitters initiates a cascade of events that cause the opening of multiple cellular access channels to various molecules, especially calcium. Usually, the concentration of calcium is higher extracellularly than intracellularly.[1] The massive influx of the extracellular calcium into the cells reaches neurotoxic levels (more than 10 times normal), and it is more than the cell can actively pump out.[2–4] The subsequent formation of certain radical compounds causes the cell to lyse and therefore die.[5–8] Unfortunately, most of this damage occurs within 30 minutes following an injury, when treatment is extremely difficult.[4,6] Recently, there have been studies to indicate that some degeneration is slower in certain regions of the brain, such as the hippocampus, where the damage may occur within hours or days.[9,10]

Two mechanisms have been noted to prevent the entry of excessive calcium into the cell: one is voltage activated and the other is receptor activated.[1,11] The receptor-activated channels, which open when excitatory neurotransmitters are released, can perhaps be blocked with antagonists to glutamate, acetylcholine, or aspartate.[6,12] Acute interventions that would prevent the flow of calcium into the cells have been postulated, but to be therapeutically effective, they must be performed so close to the event that they are not therapeutically feasible. However, preventing the influx of calcium into the cells of certain areas that may be affected later, such as the hippocampus, may prevent further cell damage and death and lead to better functional outcomes.[9,10]

It is also thought that the release of excitatory neurotransmitters is the cause for hypermetabolism in the acute post-trauma state. The hypermetabolic state can itself lead to further tissue damage and death. Studies by Miner indicate that damage of the cardiac neuromuscular junction by this excess of neurotransmitters may be the cause of the postinjury cardiomyopathy seen in young adults who have sustained brain injuries.[13]

It is also postulated that free radical formation leads to cell damage and death. Prevention of the formation of free radicals is dependent on appropriate levels of vitamins E, C, and A and of glutathione.[14–19] One possible partial explanation for the less-than-favorable outcomes seen in the elderly may be the lack of these anti-oxidants in the elderly and nutritional insufficiency.[20,21] The low levels of these antioxidants may explain the greater degree of excitotoxic damage seen after a brain injury in these populations—another reason that the maintenance of good nutrition following brain injury is important.

After the calcium enters the cell, the calcium ions bind to the mitochondria and block electron transfer. The calcium ions also cause the release of excessive hydrogen into the acidic cytoplasm. The greater-than-normal amounts of oxygen are reduced to superoxides and are eventually converted into peroxide.[22,23] Excessive amounts of radicals that are released in the cytosol (due to the paucity of regulatory mitochondrial enzymes) cause damage to the cell membrane.[22] In the presence of additional superoxide and/or iron, hydrogen peroxide forms -OH.[24] The formation of the free radicals through the breakdown of hydrogen peroxide or reduction of oxygen destroys the cell membrane. It is therefore thought that the administration of greater-than-normal amounts of mitochondrial enzymes may help with cell survival and perhaps improve functional recovery.[7,8,19] Superoxide dismutase removes the superoxide radical, and glutathione peroxidase and catalase remove peroxide.[20,25–29] Several studies have noted that the free radical scavengers have demonstrated some efficacy in reducing cell loss and improving functional outcome.[25,27,30,31]

Postacute Stage of Recovery

There appears to be a deficiency or paucity of neurotransmitters in the postacute phase of recovery, and this lack of neurotransmitters in the presence of intact neural tissue is postulated to be one cause of decreased functional ability. Feeney and coworkers have done much of the preliminary animal work in which the roles of neurotransmitters on functional recovery have been studied.[32–35] Recent research indicates that the rate of recovery following traumatic brain injury is significantly affected by various medications given days, weeks, and months after the injury.[32,35–44]

MEDICATIONS THAT FACILITATE OR HINDER RECOVERY

Cholinergic and Anticholinergic Drugs

In 1957, Sachs noted that high levels of acetylcholine were associated with higher magnitudes of injury, suggesting that acute excitation of cholinergic receptors may contribute to the pathophysiology of brain injury through excitotoxic mechanisms.[45] Several studies indicate that preinjury treatment or immediate postinjury treatment with an anticholinergic agent such as scopolamine decreases behavioral deficits after brain injury. This is probably due to the modulation of the excessive neuronal excitation seen immediately postinjury.[46–50] The fact that the anticholinergic medication must be available immediately upon the time of injury decreases the usefulness of such a regimen. For example, treatment with scopolamine 15 minutes after injury significantly reduced motor deficits associated with fluid percussion brain injury in rats. However, treatment with the same drug 30 or 60 minutes after injury had no beneficial effect.[48]

Just days after injury, acetylcholine levels decrease below normal, and the administration of cholinergic agonists may be somewhat beneficial.[46] In 1934,

Sciclounoff found that use of acetylcholine, a cholinergic agonist, 30 to 40 days after a stroke had beneficial effects on the recovery of function.[51] Eight years later, a study using primates that was done in 1942 by Ward and Kennard also noted the positive effects of cholinergic agonists on motor recovery.[52]

Many medications given to patients with brain injury are given in an attempt to alter the central nervous system and act at the synapse. Often medications are used to modify the amount of neurotransmitters within the synaptic cleft and improve the exchange of information between neurons.

Gamma-Aminobutyric Acid (GABA) and Benzodiazepines

Studies in rats indicate that chronic administration of the benzodiazepine diazepam (Valium) enhances subcortical degeneration produced by unilateral lesions of the anteromedial cortex.[53] The rats with unilateral anteromedial cortex lesions suffered from transient behavioral deficits (their recovery from somatosensorimotor asymmetries occurred within two weeks), whereas the rats with direct damage to the subcortical tissue developed chronic deficits.[54] Although benzodiazepines' causing permanent sensory deficits in humans has been neither studied nor reported, cautious use is warranted until their use has been investigated thoroughly. Regardless, their use should be limited, since they can have profound sedative effects and cause memory impairment, attentional deficits, and other cognitive difficulties for patients with brain injuries.

Catecholaminergic and Anticatecholaminergic Drugs

Norepinephrine, epinephrine, and dopamine are all catecholamines. Dopamine was originally thought to be just a precursor to both epinephrine and norepinephrine, but it is now known to function independently of its precursor role. Catecholamines play significant roles in learning, memory, motivation, sleep-wake cycles, and arousal. The catecholamine hypothesis of affective disorders postulates that a relative deficiency of catecholamines, primarily norepinephrine, is causative in the development of depression and that excesses of catecholamines play a role in the development of mania. A relative excess of central dopaminergic activity is related to the development of schizophrenia.[55]

The first research as to the beneficial effects of the catechol dopamine in patients with brain injury was done in patients with Parkinson's disease, who showed enhanced motor function after they received levodopa (L-dopa).[55,56] The work of Feeney et al suggests that it is possible to facilitate motor recovery after brain injury in rats by the administration of a single injection of a catecholamine agonist such as amphetamine. It is possible to retard motor recovery by the administration of a catecholamine antagonist such as haloperidol, which inhibits alpha-adrenergic activity. Amphetamine was effective when given early post injury, concurrently with appropriate motor experiences (rehabilitation).[43,57-60]

Studies were carried out to determine which catechol, norepinephrine (NE) or dopamine (DA), was responsible for the facilitation of recovery process. Intraventricular infusions of both neurotransmitters were carried out, and only NE facilitated motor recovery in animals similar to that caused by amphetamine.[35,57,61,62] Further studies showed that NE antagonists or the depletion of NE not only slowed the recovery of function after brain injury but also caused the reappearance of the same motor deficits in animals that had long since recovered from brain injury.[41,42,58,59,61,63-66] Recently, another study confirmed that norepinephrine, rather than dopamine, is the critical neurotransmitter in the facilitation of motor recovery. Animals given a surplus of dopamine failed to demonstrate an accelerated recovery of motor deficits when the synthesis of norepinephrine was blocked by the coadministration of the inhibiting enzyme dopamine ß-hydroxylase (which blocks the synthesis of norepinephrine).[62]

Apparently, the cerebellum contralateral to the cortical injury may also be involved in the manifestation of hemiparesis after injury. Cerebellar ablation results in a permanent motor deficit similar to that seen with sensorimotor cortex injury. In this type of cerebellar injury, catecholamine agonists interfere with recovery.[61] The cerebellum appears to be able to compensate for injury to the sensorimotor cortex. The reverse does not appear to be true, in that the sensorimotor cortex is not able to compensate for injuries in the cerebellum.[67]

A single injection of NE into the contralateral, but not ipsilateral, cerebellum 24 hours after injury to the sensorimotor cortex facilitates functional recovery.[68,69] The cerebellum appears to be involved in the maintenance of functional recovery once it occurs. Infusion of phenoxybenzamine (an alpha-adrenergic antagonist) into the contralateral, but not the ipsilateral, cerebellum reinstates a unilateral motor deficit in recovered animals.[63] In addition, peripheral administration of clonidine (an alpha-2-adrenergic agonist) reinstates a unilateral deficit in recovered animals.[66]

In addition to the facilitation or retardation of sensorimotor function, the NE system appears to be involved in other areas of the brain. Therefore, it may be possible to facilitate recovery of function from a host of other behavioral deficits in addition to motor deficits. Some reports in the literature suggest that it is possible to facilitate the recovery from visual deficits in animals by giving amphetamines combined with visual experiences. Dopamine agonists have been successfully used to treat akinetic mutism.[70] Stroke patients given a single dose of amphetamine in addition to physical therapy were reported to demonstrate accelerated motor recovery.[71] Dextroamphetamine improved speech in aphasic patients[72] and improved cognitive function in patients with brain injuries.[73,74]

Amantadine improved arousal and responsiveness in the coma-emerging population in two reports.[75,76] Bromocriptine has been reported to improve initiation in patients with akinetic mutism.[77,78] The use of Sinemet (levodopa/carbidopa) helped a patient recover after being in a vegetative state for six months.[79]

Although early (10 to 30 days) administration of an NE agonist may be useful after most cortical injuries in humans, such drugs may have deleterious effects in patients with damage to the cerebellum or brainstem when hemorrhage is a potential problem.[71,73,80] In addition, many psychostimulant drugs (which generally affect NE) may prove clinically beneficial, especially if they are specific NE agonists, such as desipramine, that do not appear to be "addictive."[81-83]

Dopaminergic drugs, such as levodopa (L-dopa), combined with carbidopa (Sinemet), may also have some beneficial effect on depressed NE systems because dopamine is taken up by noradrenergic cells before its conversion to NE within the vesicle (Figure 13–1).[84] Moreover, it appears that when rehabilitative techniques are used in conjunction with the dopaminergic agents, the results for both the drug and the therapy are enhanced. The combined effect of rehabilitation and stimulatory medications has been observed in animal studies by Feeney and colleagues[57,58] and a study of the recovery vision in falcons done by Fox et al.[85]

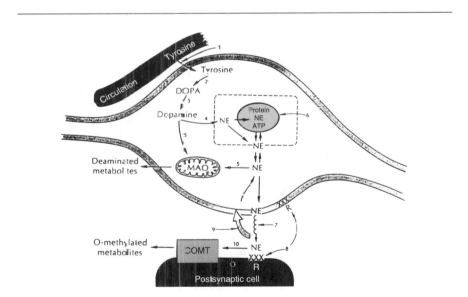

Figure 13–1 Schematic model of noradrenergic neuron. *Source:* From *The Biochemical Basis of Neuropharmacology,* 7/E by Jack R. Cooper Floyd E. Bloom Robert H. Roth. Copyright 1986. Used by permission of Oxford University Press, Inc.

Clinically, pharmacologic intervention in minimally responsive patients usually involves the use of the direct dopamine agonist bromocriptine (Parlodel) and the indirect agonist levodopa with carbidopa (Sinemet). In addition, amantadine (Symmetrel) and drugs such as dextroamphetamine, methylphenidate (Ritalin), and pemoline (Cylert) can be used in this regard. Physicians often use combinations of these medications to increase arousal and facilitate recovery of consciousness in minimally responsive patients.[86] Stimulatory medications are best used with patients who demonstrate inconsistent ability to follow commands. This should be coupled with the discontinuation of all sedating medications, or at least substitution of less sedating medications.[86–88] These medications are unlikely to "stimulate" a patient to begin to follow commands; they are more likely to help a patient who is intermittently following commands to become more consistent. Certainly, the possibility of increasing arousal through accentuation of NE and DA neurotransmitters' activity can be considered once the patient is out of danger from increased intracranial pressure.[88] It has also been suggested that anti-Parkinson drugs, such as levodopa or L-dopa, bromocriptine, and amantadine, may benefit some patients by increasing dopaminergic activity.[39,84,89,90] One advantage of using some of the anti-Parkinsonian drugs in the minimally responsive patient is that they may also help with central fever.[86,87]

The combination of levodopa and carbidopa (Sinemet) minimizes the peripheral side effects of the drug and increases the amount available for use within the central nervous system, since the carbidopa acts as a carrier across the blood-brain barrier. Levodopa acts presynaptically and is an antagonist at the DA receptor site, thus keeping the DA in the synaptic cleft. Side effects include dyskinesias, bradykinetic episodes (the "on-off" phenomenon), hallucinations, gastrointestinal disturbances (nausea, vomiting, anorexia, and slowing of gastric motility), and orthostatic hypotension. Sinemet is a combination drug that is available in ratios of 1:10 (100 mg of levodopa to 10 mg of carbidopa) and 1:4 (100 mg of levodopa to 25 mg of carbidopa). The typical starting dose is usually the 1:25 combination tablet given three or four times a day. This is increased by one tablet every 2 to 3 days until a maximum of six tablets per day is reached. Some clinicians advocate, in addition to the carbidopa, the use of other enzyme inhibitors such as L-deprenyl (a monoamine oxidase inhibitor).[55]

Amantadine is theorized to act both pre- and postsynaptically. It is thought to increase both cholinergic and gabaminergic activity. The usual starting dose is 50 mg to 100 mg/d, and the maximum dose is 400 mg/d. Since amantadine is excreted unchanged in the urine, the dosage should be decreased in patients with impaired renal function. Side effects are usually not a problem but may include peripheral edema, light-headedness, orthostatic hypotension, hot and dry skin, livedo reticularis, confusion, and hallucinations.[55]

Bromocriptine is in the ergot-alkaloid class of drugs and is a direct dopamine receptor–stimulating agent. Bromocriptine is generally well tolerated, but patients may experience gastrointestinal distress and orthostasis. Starting doses are usually 2.5 mg/d, and if that dose is tolerated, it can be increased quickly to the same 2.5-mg dose given three to four times per day. Once the daily dose is at 10 mg/d, it can be increased by 2.5 mg every four days until the desired effect is achieved. Dosages higher than 40 mg/d are rarely necessary in patients with brain injury. However, the manufacturer notes a maximum daily dose of 100 mg/d.[55]

Classic psychostimulants such as dextroamphetamine, methylphenidate, and pemoline have been theorized to have mixed noradrenergic and dopaminergic agonist activity. Noted cardiac side effects of tachycardia and hypertension limit the clinical usefulness of dextroamphetamine. However, others have reported that it is useful for patients with brain injury and recommend a starting dose of 4 mg once or twice a day. The maximum dose recommended is 60 mg/d. To avoid problems with insomnia with dextroamphetamine and methylphenidate, the last dose of the day should be given at least six hours before bedtime. Other side effects at higher doses can include anxiety, dysphoria, increased irritability, headache, palilalia, stereotypical thoughts or actions, hallucinations, insomnia, and motor disturbances, including dyskinesias, tics, and worsening of spasticity. Methylphenidate is generally better tolerated, although it shares the side-effect profile of dextroamphetamine. The usual dose is 5 mg once or twice a day until a maximum daily dose of 60 mg/d is reached. Pemoline is another dopaminergic agonist that is very much like methylphenidate and dextroamphetamine. It is typically started at 37.5 mg/d and increased by 18.75 mg/wk until a maximum dose of 75 mg/d is reached. The most frequent side effects of insomnia and anorexia are dose related. In addition to their use in the minimally responsive patient, these psychostimulants can often be used to alleviate some of the residuals of acquired brain injury in which patients exhibit frontal lobe apathy, "psychomotor retardation," attentional deficits, and slowed reaction time in the postacute stage of recovery.[55]

Serotonergic Drugs

Serotonergic drugs such as trazodone (Desyrel) have been reported to produce some transient effects on the motor recovery following brain injury.[81,91–94] An infusion of serotonin shortly after injury into the ventricle only transiently disrupts motor function: within one hour, and as serotonin levels return to normal, motor function returns to normal.[91] Nevertheless, there are some reports of therapeutic use of the serotonin precursor L-tryptophan in the treatment of cerebellar ataxia,[95,96] methysergide in the treatment of stroke,[97] and mianserin in the treatment of appetite disorders following brain injury.[98] In addition, the use of trazodone had been particularly helpful for the acutely agitated patient with altered sleep/wake cycles. Cognitive effects attributed to serotonin include the mediation of arousal and enhancing both memory and learning. The role of serotonin in the regulation of mood and behavior has been reported extensively in the literature.[55]

Typical starting dose for trazodone is 50 mg/d at bedtime with tube feeding (which enhances absorption), and the dose can be increased by 25 mg to 50 mg every three to four days. The maximum dose of 400 mg/d is rarely necessary for patients with brain injury.[55] Furthermore, the use of a morning dose of a dopaminergic agonist such as methylphenidate combined with a nighttime dose of trazodone may help a low-level patient with an out-of-sync sleep/wake cycle stay awake during the day and sleep at night. Moreover, certain serotonergically acting drugs, such as fluoxetine (Prozac), may have a role in increasing arousal. Usual starting dose for fluoxetine is 20 mg/d as a morning dose. Typically, 40 mg can be given once or twice a day. A maximum dose of 80 mg/d is rarely indicated.[55] Sertraline (Zoloft) is a newer antidepressant that acts by inhibiting the reuptake of serotonin that can be given at any time of the day. The starting dose is 50 mg/d, up to a maximum of 200 mg/d.[91]

Although rare, the excessive use of serotonergic medications may lead to the development of agitation as part of the "serotonin syndrome." This syndrome is characterized by various combinations of myoclonus, rigidity, hyperreflexia, shivering, confusion, agitation, restlessness, autonomic instability, fever, nausea, diaphoresis, flushing, rhabdomyolysis, coma, and even death. The syndrome typically develops after serotonergic medications are started or the dose is increased.[99]

TREATMENT OF SPECIFIC MEDICAL PROBLEMS IN THE ICU

Agitation and Restlessness

Sedating a patient with traumatic brain injury as he or she begins to arouse is often very difficult, since the patient can be quite confused. Agitation can cause additional injury with withdrawal of tubes and catheters and dislodging of all kinds of paraphernalia meant to protect and provide for the patient's well-being. It is felt that restraints may not be effective, can be dangerous, may cause even more agitation, and in some patients may even be fatal.[87,88]

Any change in a patient's behavior warrants a complete examination, with emphasis on noxious stimuli such as occult fractures, yet-to-be diagnosed peripheral nerve injuries, and skin lesions and decubiti. Close inspection of the tracheostomy, gastrostomy, or jejunostomy sites should be carried out. Stools, gastric contents, and any emesis should be tested for occult blood to rule out the possibility of a gastrointestinal bleed as a noxious stimulus. Other medical complications such as seizures, especially partial complex seizures that arise from temporal lobe injury, infections of the central nervous system, and the development of a space-occupying mass within the cranium, such as hydrocephalus or a late subdural hematoma, should be considered as possible etiologies for a change in the patient's behavior. A thorough review of the patient's cardiopulmonary status, endocrine, hepatic, renal, and metabolic status should be done. The past medical history should be reviewed for indications of alcohol or other substance withdrawal. All pharmacologic interventions should be reviewed for adverse effects and toxicity. Many medications that have been traditionally recommended for use in the agitated patient have been noted to cause an increase in confusion and thus may make the agitation worse.[87,100–102]

Environmental management strategies typically used to treat agitated patients include one-to-one nursing care and video monitoring, as well as environmental modifications such as the use of fully padded side rails, subdued lighting, decreased noise, and the use of calming music and taped voices. The use of Posey vests and mitts instead of four-point leather restraints is advocated whenever possible (Exhibit 13–1). In nonambulatory patients, the removal of all restraints and the use of a floor or Craig bed may be helpful.[103–105] In today's era of managed care and significantly shortened stays, the prompt resolution of agitation becomes increasingly important to avoid interference with other treatment goals. Therefore, pharmacologic intervention has become increasingly important in the treatment of agitation.

There is a wide variation in the pharmacologic strategies used by physicians to treat agitation. Medications that are typically tried include stimulating agents, such as amantadine or methylphenidate; antidepressants, such as low-dose amitriptyline or trazodone; and agents that reduce the excitatory or augment inhibitory effects, such as propranolol and other beta blockers, lithium, carbamazepine, and buspirone.[106] During episodes of extreme agitation in which the patient is a danger to himself or herself or others, the use of a parenteral, short-acting sedative such as lorazepam with and without the addition of haloperidol may be indicated. Injections (intramuscularly or intravenously) of 5 mg of haloperidol and 2 mg of lorazepam (Ativan) every 20 minutes are recommended for emergency situations in which the patient is a danger to himself or herself or others. This is an acute management recommendation only and should not be used for prolonged management.[55,84,87,88]

Whatever method is used to decrease the agitated behavior, objective measures, such as the Overt Agitation Scale (OAS),[107] should be used to determine if the interventions are effective. The OAS is a 16-item scale developed by Yudofsky et al that assesses four categories of behavior: verbal aggression, physical aggression against objects, physical aggression against self, and physical aggression against others. Typically, patients are agitated during the phase of posttraumatic amnesia (PTA); thus, the use of assessment tools, such as the Galveston Orientation and Amnesia Test (GOAT),[108] may be helpful. GOAT is a brief structured interview that quantifies the patient's orientation and recall of recent events. The GOAT

Exhibit 13–1 Nonpharmacologic Environmental Management Strategies for Agitated Patients with Brain Injury

1. Reduce the level of stimulation in the environment:
   - Place patient in a quiet, private room.
   - Remove noxious stimuli if possible—for example, tubes, catheters, restraints, and traction.
   - Limit unnecessary sounds—for example, TV, radio, and background conversations.
   - Limit number of visitors.
   - Instruct staff to behave in a calm and reassuring manner.
   - Limit number and length of therapy sessions.
   - Provide therapies in patient's room.
2. Protect patient from harming self or others:
   - Place patient in a floor bed with padded side panels (Craig bed).
   - Assign 1:1 or 1:2 sitter to observe patient and ensure safety.
   - Avoid taking patient off unit.
   - Place patient in locked ward.
3. Reduce patient's cognitive confusion:
   - Have one person speak to patient at a time.
   - Maintain same staff to work with patient.
   - Minimize contact with unfamiliar staff.
   - Communicate to patient briefly and simply—for example, one idea at a time.
   - Reorient patient to place and time repeatedly.
4. Tolerate restlessness when possible:
   - Allow patient to thrash about in floor bed.
   - Allow patient to pace around unit, with 1:1 supervision.
   - Allow confused patient to be verbally inappropriate.

score can range from 0 to 100, with a score of 75 or better defined as emergence from PTA.

In the intensive care unit, propofol (2,6,di-isopropylphenol; Diprivan) has been noted to be useful for the sedation of patients with a variety of diagnoses. It is easily given intravenously, and sedation is easily maintained with little alteration in the infusion rate.[109,110] It has also been found to be effective in reducing intracranial pressure and providing anesthesia and sedation in critically ill patients.[111,112] One of the major advantages is that it allows rapid change in the level of sedation and requires less recovery time when compared to midazolam (Versed).[113] Midazolam, a short-acting benzodiazepine that is commonly used for sedation in the ICU, has another disadvantage in that it can adversely affect brain-injured patients' respiratory centers and suppress spontaneous respiration. Studies suggest that administration of less propofol by continuous infusion, both for the induction and maintenance of anesthesia and for better control of left ventricular filling pressures, may minimize hemodynamic changes and maintain cerebral perfusion pressure (CPP) above the safe lower limit of 50 mm Hg.[114–121]

Seizure Prophylaxis

It is estimated that approximately 5% of all patients with traumatic brain injuries who are hospitalized will develop posttraumatic epilepsy (PTE). Posttraumatic epilepsy has been described in greater detail by Jennett.[122,123] PTE may be early-onset epilepsy, which occurs in the first week, and late posttraumatic epilepsy, which occurs after the first week. Goddard first described the "kindling" model of posttraumatic epileptogenesis from research in which brief trains of weak electrical stimulation were applied to susceptible areas of animal brains until a seizure appeared.[124] When the kindling stimulations were continued for a prolonged period of time, less stimulation was required to induce the seizures, and spontaneous seizures eventually appeared, thus suggesting that electrical activity "sparks" a seizure and that continued electrical activity causes a seizure focus or scarred area. Moreover, this model also has been used to explain the prophylactic use of antiseizure medication, in which early treatment suppresses seizures over the short term and prevents the evolution of newly developing seizures into chronic epilepsy.[125–129]

An alternative model of posttraumatic epileptogenesis involves cortical deposits of hemosiderin and its components of iron and ferric chloride.[130] Patients with focal cerebral injuries, such as subdural hematomas and penetrating head injuries that involve the contact of blood with cerebral tissue, show an increased incidence of posttraumatic seizures.[131] Contusion or cortical laceration causes an extravasation of red blood cells, followed by hemolysis and deposition of hemoglobin. Iron liberated from hemoglobin is then sequestered as hemosiderin, which is often found in patients with posttraumatic epilepsy.[132] Willmore et al demonstrated that recurrent focal epileptiform discharges may result from the cortical injection of ferrous or ferric chloride.[130,133] The iron salts and hemoglobin in neural tissue may contribute to epileptogenesis by initiating lipid peroxidation, damaging cell membranes, and inhibiting neuronal Na-K adenosine triphosphatase.[125]

The incidence of development of late PTE is greater following those injuries in which dura has been penetrated, such as depressed skull fractures and gunshot wounds in which fragments of bone are driven into the brain parenchyma. Approximately 35% to 50% of patients with this type of penetrating brain injury develop PTE.[122,123,134] As has been noted, blood appears to have an irritating effect on the brain, and patients with acute intracranial hemorrhage, particularly subdural hemorrhage, are more prone to development of PTE.[122,123,134] Patients who have evidence of focal injury, such as aphasia or hemiparesis, are also thought to be apt to have more of a chance of developing PTE because they are more apt to develop seizure foci in the area of the damage.[122,123,134]

Determining seizure risk on an individual patient is very difficult. In 1979, Feeney and Walker devised a mathematical model to estimate seizure risk based on a combination of risk factors.[135] However, this has not proved to be helpful in most clinical situations.[136] Until recently, patients were frequently placed on seizure prophylaxis in the acute neurosurgical setting. Neurosurgeons traditionally prescribed phenytoin or phenobarbital because these could be administered parenterally and had been in use the longest.

During the past decade, several randomized, controlled, prospective studies have been published that have failed to show efficacy of anticonvulsant prophylaxis in the development of late PTE.[131,137–140] In four out of the five studies, the incidence of PTE was actually higher in the phenytoin-treated group.[137–140] In addition, one trial using carbamazepine as the primary seizure prophylaxis failed to show any efficacy.[131] Although the recent studies have shown that using phenytoin beyond the first week following a brain injury does not prevent the development of late posttraumatic brain epilepsy, it does appear to have effect on the incidence of early PTE. Temkin et al noted that 3.6% of the phenytoin-treated group developed early seizures compared with 14.2% of the patients in the placebo group.[139]

Additionally, the neurobehavioral side effects of phenytoin and other sedating anticonvulsants, such as phenobarbital, can be detrimental to the patient who already has slowed thinking or memory loss.[57] In the study by Temkin et al, among the patients with severe brain injury who received phenytoin prophylaxis, 78% were unable to undergo cognitive testing because their cognitive impairment was too severe. In contrast, only 47% of the placebo-treated patients were unable to be tested due to the severity of their cognitive impairment.[139] Clinical experience supports the conclusion that these drugs appear to hamper the patient's overall recovery.[141]

It should be noted that these medications can have a profound effect on a patient's ability to follow commands. It is not unusual for a comatose patient being maintained on phenytoin (Dilantin) or phenobarbital within therapeutic range to begin to arouse and start following commands once these medications are discontinued.[86,141]

Most posttraumatic epilepsy is thought to be of the partial variety, either simple partial or complex partial, which is secondarily generalized.[122,123] Carbamazepine (Tegretol) has shown to be as effective as phenytoin and phenobarbital for generalized tonic-clonic seizures and to be more effective in the control of partial seizures.[142] Carbamazepine is well-tolerated and has few side effects, which are usually ameliorated by starting with a low dose and gradually building up to therapeutic range. In the comatose patient, some of these side effects, such as gastrointestinal distress, headaches, dizziness, and diplopia, are not evident. The most limiting side effect of carbamazepine is bone marrow suppression. The transient leukopenia can be monitored as long as the white blood cell count is above 4,000 cells per mm[3], with 50% of the white blood cells being neutrophils.[87,143] A major disadvantage of carbamazepine is its relatively short half-life, which makes three-times-a-day dosing mandatory.

Another medication that can be used, valproic acid (Depakote), although initially sedating, has been shown to have fewer cognitive and behavioral side effects. Gabapentin (Neurontin), another new antiepileptic medication, may prove to be helpful in patients with PTE, and studies are currently under way.[87,141]

Most physiatrists specializing in brain injury rehabilitation are no longer using seizure prophylaxis in patients who have not had seizures beyond the first week. Most now wait for the patient to have the first documented seizure and then choose the most appropriate anticonvulsant for the patient.[87,136,141] Carbamazepine appears to be the drug of choice for seizure management because of its decreased number of behavioral and cognitive side effects.[87,144,145]

Gastrointestinal Disturbances

A medication that is frequently used in the ICU for gastrointestinal disturbances but that causes significant arousal problems for patients with traumatic brain injury is metoclopramide (Reglan). Metoclopramide is similar to the phenothiazines, and while it can help initially with reflux by increasing gastric emptying in a small percentage of patients, it is not particularly useful over the long term and has been known to cause significant cognitive difficulties, especially in those regaining consciousness. Metoclopramide has indirect cholinergic effects that increase peristalsis and decrease reflux at the gastroesophageal sphincter. Potential side effects of extrapyramidal movements and even permanent tardive dyskinesia are the result of its antidopaminergic activity. In addition to impeding cognitive recovery, patients have developed swallowing difficulties as the result of the use of metoclopramide. If the patient has to be on metoclopramide for any reason, administration should be limited to two weeks or less.[86,87,136,146] If reflux leading to aspiration is of concern, the head of the bed should be elevated, and the patient should be tried on various formulas or smaller feedings. Clinically, the use of blue food coloring or methylene blue to dye tube feedings helps identify tracheal aspirations of feedings as opposed to mouth secretions.[87]

A newer medication, cisapride (Propulsid), also acts in an indirect cholinergic manner. Unlike metoclopramide, cisapride has direct antiemetic properties, and, more important, since it has no effect on the dopaminergic system, it is a good choice of medication for patients with brain injuries and significant reflux. Alternatively, erythromycin may be useful in increasing gastric emptying. Like cisapride, it has no known sedative side effects and may be useful for patients with cognitive deficits as long as its potential for interaction with carbamazepine is kept in mind.

Moreover, using a small jejunostomy tube will prevent the potential problem of aspiration by avoiding the patient's cardiac sphincter between the esophagus and the stomach, as well as the pyloric sphincter between the stomach and duodenum. However, a gastrostomy is preferred once the patient is in an active therapy program in order to give the patient bolus feedings and eliminate the need for a continuous feeding pump. Thus, a jejunostomy tube threaded through a primarily placed gastrostomy tube is the favored method.[86,87]

As with most patients with polytrauma, the patient with brain injury has an increased risk of gastrointestinal bleeding secondary to stress ulceration during the acute neurosurgical care phase.[147] It is not unusual for patients to be placed on H_2-receptor antagonist prophylaxis with medication such as cimetidine or ranitidine.[148] Since cognitive and behavioral disturbances have been noted in patients with H_2 antagonists, these medications should be withdrawn once the risk of gastrointestinal bleeding is past. A very good alternative is sucralfate (Carafate), which prevents ulceration of the gastric mucosa by coating the mucosa of the stomach and providing an effective barrier against the harmful effects of hyperacidity. Sucralfate does not decrease the acidic content of the gastrointestinal tract, nor does it affect cognition. It appears to have several clinical advantages over the other methods of decreasing gastric acidity in patients with brain injury. Alternatively, antacids such as Mylanta and Maalox can be given at regular intervals through the feeding tube to increase the alkalinity of the stomach without affecting cognition; however, this decrease in acidity can allow bacterial overgrowth. Patients aspirating gastric contents containing bacteria are at increased risk for developing aspiration pneumonia. Therefore, sucralfate is the preferred medication for gastric ulcer prophylaxis in the acute patient with a brain injury in the ICU.

Autonomic Disturbances

Autonomic disturbances, such as hypertension, are frequently the result of high intracranial pressure and catecholamine release with increased cardiac output and tachycardia.[13,149] Focal brain injuries with lesions near the hypothalamus can also cause hypertension.[150] Treatment with beta blockers may be necessary, especially if the patient is in a hyperdynamic state. The use of beta blockers, such as propranolol, should be limited to the period of time when they are essential, since most hypertension secondary to brain injury is self-limited. Beta blockers can cause significant sedation. The least cognitively sedating drugs, such as diuretics or clonidine (Catapres), would be better choices.

Temperature instability infrequently occurs but can present as either central fever or hypothermia. Patients with prolonged febrile illness without a documented source can have a central fever.[151] Central fever is usually secondary to lesions in the anterior hypothalamus or to generalized decerebration. Patients with central fever usually do not have temperatures that exceed 101°F or 38°C unless they have an accompanying infection that will add to their temperature. In addition, febrile episodes can occasionally result from medications or from malignant neuroleptic syndrome secondary to phenothiazines. Temperature elevation as a result of brain injury can be treated with physical modalities such as cooling blankets and tepid baths or pharmacologically with morphine or neuroleptic-type medications, as well as dopamine agonists, dantrolene sodium, propranolol, and prostaglandin inhibitors such as indomethacin.[86,87,136,152,153] The mechanism of action for these medications is not yet known.

Spasticity Management

Medications given to decrease spasticity can have profound effects on a patient's arousal and cognition. Typical medications that have been used for spasticity, such as baclofen (Lioresal) and diazepam (Valium), are particularly well suited to spasticity due to spinal cord injury but are not necessarily helpful in patients with spasticity due to brain injury.[154]

It appears that spasticity resulting from brain injury is more heavily influenced by such factors as postural changes, body positioning, and labyrinthian and tonic neck reflexes than is the case in spinal cord injury. Moreover, spasticity can be a source of extreme discomfort in patients with brain injury who have intact sensation and thus can lead to increased agitation. Spasticity can have some beneficial effects, such as maintaining muscle bulk, preventing deep-vein thrombosis or osteoporosis, and allowing patients with marginal motor strength to stand and transfer. It can, at times, interfere with function, cause pain or disfigurement, interfere with nursing care, and contribute to the formation of contractures that mandate treatment. In the ICU, maintenance of range of motion is particularly important to prevent further disability. Interestingly, most patients (greater than 75%) with severe brain injury will eventually become ambulatory if contracture formation is prevented.

The trend is away from pharmacologic intervention and toward the use of various physical modalities (Figure 13–2). These include the application of heat or cold; stretch; splinting; casting, including inhibitive casting; proper positioning; functional electrical stimulation; vibration; relaxation techniques; muscle reeducation; and biofeedback. In the ICU, complications from fisting can be minimized by inserting rolled terry-cloth washcloths into the fisted hand; this is usually better tolerated than the use of rigid cones, at least at first. As the patient improves,

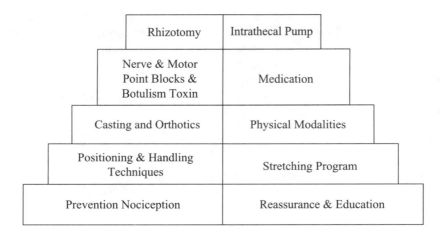

Rhizotomy	Intrathecal Pump
Nerve & Motor Point Blocks & Botulism Toxin	Medication
Casting and Orthotics	Physical Modalities
Positioning & Handling Techniques	Stretching Program
Prevention Nociception	Reassurance & Education

Figure 13–2 Physical modalities for spasticity treatment.

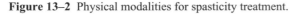

antispasticity ball splints with the thumb held in abduction can be used. However, if the palmar splints cause an increase in the grasp reflex, then the use of a dorsal splint with thumb abduction may be better. For the lower extremities, positioning the hips and knees in flexion by using pillows and sandbags is far superior to using footboards and positioning splints in breaking up trunk and lower-extremity extensor posturing.[155] If these measures, combined with the use of ankle splints, do not adequately control the extensor tone, and if side-lying is either not effective or not practical, then the use of inhibitive casts is warranted. To prevent skin breakdown, inhibitive casts must be applied by trained, skilled therapists. The casts are made out of plaster or the more costly fiberglass and are changed every three to five days. Soft contractures are worked out by combining the inhibitory casting with serial casting, in which the joint is stretched several degrees with each successive application.

Combined with inhibitive casting, chemical neurolysis using nerve blocks and motor point blocks can be administered before drug therapy is begun. The nerve blocks can even be temporary, using short-acting agents such as Marcaine or more "permanent" blocks with phenol or alcohol.[156–160] Studies have shown that multimodality treatment without the use of medication not only is useful in the acute care setting in preventing contractures but can be effective for many months following their withdrawal.[161]

A newer modality is botulism toxin (BoTox). It has been used successfully in some centers for the control of spasticity as well. Botulism toxin has strong neuromuscular blocking properties that inhibit the release of acetylcholine and cause flaccid paralysis. Originally, it was approved by the Food and Drug Administration for the treatment of blepharospasm, facial spasm, strabismus, and torticollis. A minute amount of the toxin is injected directly into the hyperactive muscle, using needle electrodes that confirm needle placement, and the toxin diffuses through the muscle. Clinical effect does not become evident until 3 days later, and the full effect is not seen until one week to ten days after the injection. The procedure is usually well tolerated, with few to no systemic side effects reported by the patients. The effect on the muscle usually lasts four to six months, during which time the patient with a brain injury hopefully is gaining some volitional control. The biggest drawback in the use of BoTox is the expense, and because large amounts can exert systemic effects by systemic migration, no more than 400 units can be administered in a single sitting. Repeated injections may not be as effective in controlling spasticity due to the development of antibodies and for other unknown reasons. Clinical studies currently under way will hopefully answer some of the outstanding questions.[1-2]

When drug therapy is indicated, it is usually not in the acute phase of recovery. Dantrolene sodium (Dantrium) is usually the preferred drug, since it appears to have the fewest cognitive or sedating side effects.[86,154] Dantrolene sodium acts by influencing the amount of calcium from the sarcoplasmic reticulum, thus decreasing the force of the muscle contraction, which in turn reduces the tension in spastic muscles.

CONCLUSION

Many medications can have deleterious effects on the patient's arousal and general recovery, and appropriate substitutions should be used whenever possible. In addition, there is now a handful of identified "stimulatory" medications that enhance patients' arousal and perhaps their general recovery. Whatever medication is tried, objective measures of its efficacy should be used, and medications found to have no or little beneficial effect should be discontinued. In addition, regular review of the medications with a pharmacist is recommended to enhance patients' recovery by the educated selection of appropriate medications for a wide range of complications.

REFERENCES

1. Kostyuk PG, Tepikin AV. Calcium signals in nerve cells. *Physiol Sci.* 1991;6:6-10.
2. Lipton P, Lobner D. Mechanisms of intracellular calcium accumulation in the CA1 region of rat hippocampus during anoxia in vitro. *Stroke.* 1990;21(suppl 11):III60–64.
3. Manev H, Favaron M, Guidotti A, Costa E. Delayed increase in Ca2+ influx elicited by glutamate: role in neuronal death. *Mol Pharmacol.* 1989;36:379–387.

4. Manev H, Favaron M, De Erausquin G, Guidotti A, et al. Destabilization of ionized Ca2+ homeostasis in excitatory amino acid neurotoxicity: antagonism by glycosphingolipids. *Cell Biol Int Rep.* 1990;14:3–14.

5. Choi DW. Glutamate neurotoxicity and diseases of the nervous system. *Neuron.* 1988;1:623–634.

6. Choi DW. Glutamate neurotoxicity in cortical cell culture is calcium dependent. *Neurosci Lett.* 1985;58:293–297.

7. Tyler DD. Role of superoxide radicals in the lipid peroxidation of cellular membranes. *FEBS Lett.* 1975;51:180–183.

8. Yu BP, Suescun EA, Yang SY. Effect of age-related lipid peroxidation on membrane fluidity and phospholipase A2: modulation by dietary restriction. *Mech Ageing Dev.* 1992;65:17–33.

9. Petito CK, Feldman E, Pulsinelli WA, Plum F. Delayed hippocampal damage in humans following cardiorespiratory arrest. *Neurology.* 1987;37:1281–1286.

10. Pulsinelli WA, Brierley JB, Plum F. Temporal profile of neuronal damage in a model of transient forebrain ischemia. *Ann Neurol.* 1982;11:491–498.

11. Triggle DJ. Calcium antagonists: history and perspective. *Stroke.* 1990;21(suppl 12):IV49–IV58.

12. Young W. The post-injury responses in trauma and ischemia: secondary injury or protective mechanisms? *Cent Nerv Sys Trauma.* 1987;4:27–51.

13. Miner ME. Systemic effects of brain injury. *J Trauma.* 1985;2:75.

14. Bendich A, Machlin AJ, Scandurra O. The antioxidant role of vitamin C. *Adv Free Radic Biol Med.* 1986;2:419-444.

15. Bendich A, D'Apolito P, Gabriel E, Machlin LJ. Interaction of dietary vitamin C and vitamin E on guinea pig immune responses to mitogens. *J Nutr.* 1984;114:1588–1593.

16. Beuttner GR. Ascorbate autoxidation in the presence of iron and copper chelates. *Free Radic Res Commun.* 1986;1:349–353.

17. Aust SD, Svingen BA. The role of iron in enzymatic lipid peroxidation. In: Pryor WA, ed. *Free Radicals in Biology.* Vol 5. New York, NY: Academic Press; 1982:1–28.

18. Aust SD, Morehouse LA, Thomas CE. Role of metals in oxygen radical reactions. *J Free Radic Biol Med.* 1985;1:3-25.

19. Girotti AW. Mechanisms of lipid perioxidation. *J Free Radic Biol Med.* 1985;1:87–95.

20. Al-Turk WA, Stohs SJ, el-Rashidy FH, Othman S, et al. Changes in glutathione, glutathione reductase, and glutathione-S-transferase as a function of cell concentration and age. *Pharmacology.* 1987;34:1–8.

21. Al-Turk WA, Stohs SJ. Hepatic glutathione content and aryl hydrocarbon hydroxylase activity of acetaminophen-treated mice as a function of age. *Drug Chem Toxicol.* 1981;4:37–48.

22. Chance B. The energy-linked reaction of calcium with mitochondria. *J Biol Chem.* 1965;240:2729–2748.

23. Siesjo BK, Bendek G, Koide T, Westerberg E, et al. Influence of acidosis on lipid peroxidation in brain tissues in vitro. *J Cereb Blood Flow Metab.* 1985;5:253–258.

24. Haber F, Weiss JJ. The catalytic decomposition of hydrogen peroxide by iron salts. *Proc R Soc Lond Ser.* 1934;A147:332–351.

25. Liu TH, Beckman JS, Freeman BA, Hogan EL, et al. Polyethylene glycol-conjugated superoxide dismutase and catalase reduce ischemic brain injury. *Am J Physiol.* 1989;256:H589–H593.

26. Crapo JD, Tierney DF. Superoxide dismutase and pulmonary oxygen toxicity. *Am J Physiol.* 1974;226:1401–1507.

27. Forsman M, Fleischer JE, Milde JH, Steen PA, et al. Superoxide dismutase and catalase failed to improve neurologic outcome after complete cerebral ischemia in the dog. *Acta Anaesthesiol Scand.* 1988;32:152–155.

28. Gregory EM, Fridovich I. Oxygen toxicity and superoxide dismutase. *J Bacteriol.* 1973; 114:1193–1197.

29. Gregory EM, Yost FJ Jr, Fridovich I. Superoxide dismutases of *Escherichia coli*: Intracellular localization and functions. *J Bacteriol.* 1973;115:987–991.

30. Chan PH, Longar S, Fishman RA. Protective effects of liposome-entrapped superoxide dismutase on posttraumatic brain edema. *Ann Neurol.* 1987;21:540-547.

31. Kontos HA, Wei EP. Superoxide production in experimental brain injury. *J Neurosurg.* 1986;64:803–807.

32. Feeney DM, Sutton RL. Pharmacotherapy for recovery of function after brain injury. *CRC Crit Rev Neurol.* 1987;3:135–197.

33. Feeney DM, Sutton RL, Boyeson MG, et al. The locus coeruleus and cerebral metabolism: recovery of function after cortical injury. *Physiol Psychol.* 1985;13:197–203.

34. Feeney DM, Weisand MP, Kline AE. Noradrenergic pharmacotherapy, intracerebral infusions and adrenal transplantation promote functional recovery after cortical damage. *J Neural Transplant Plast.* 1993;4:199–213.

35. Feeney DM, Westerberg VS. Norepinephrine and brain damage: alpha noradrenergic pharmacology alters functional recovery after cortical trauma. *Can J Psychol.* 1990;44:233–252.

36. Boyeson MG. Neurotransmitter aspects of traumatic brain injury. In: Bach-y-Rita P, ed. *Traumatic Brain Injury.* New York, NY: Demos Publications; 1989:97–104.

37. Boyeson MG. Neurochemical alterations after brain injury: clinical implications for pharmacologic rehabilitation. *Neurorehabilitation.* 1991;1:33–43.

38. Boyeson MG, Jones JL, Harmon RL. Sparing of motor function after cortical injury: a new perspective on underlying mechanisms. *Arch Neurol.* 1994;51:405–414.

39. Feeney DM. Pharmacologic modulation of recovery after brain injury: a reconsideration of diaschisis. *J Neurol Rehabil.* 1991;5:113–128.

40. Goldstein LB, Matchar DB, Morgenlander JC, et al. Drugs influence the recovery of function after stroke. *Stroke.* 1990;21:179.

41. Goldstein LB, Coviello A, Miller GD, et al. Norepinephrine depletion impairs motor recovery following sensorimotor cortex injury in the rat. *Restor Neurosci.* 1991;3:41–47.

42. Goldstein LB, Davis JN. Clonidine impairs recovery of beam walking after a sensorimotor cortex lesion in the rat. *Brain Res.* 1990;508:305–309.

43. Goldstein LB, Davis JN. Post-lesion practice and amphetamine-facilitated recovery of beam-walking in the rat. *Restor Neurol Neurosci.* 1990;1:311–314.

44. Sutton RL, Feeney DM. Alpha-adrenergic agonists and antagonists affect recovery and maintenance of beam-walking ability after sensorimotor cortex ablation in the rat. *Restor Neurol Neurosci.* 1992;4:1–11.

45. Sachs E Jr. Acetylcholine and serotonin in the spinal fluid. *J Neurosurg.* 1957;14:22–27.

46. Hayes RL, Jenkins LW, Lyeth BG. Neuro-transmitter-mediated mechanisms of traumatic brain injury: acetylcholine and excitatory amino acids. *J Neurotrauma.* 1992;9:173–187.

47. Lyeth BG, Dixon CE, Jenkins LW, et al. Effects of scopolamine treatment on long-term behavioral deficits following concussive brain injury to the rat. *Brain Res.* 1988;452:39–48.

48. Lyeth BG, Ray M, Hamm RJ, et al. Post-injury scopolamine administration in experimental traumatic brain injury. *Brain Res.* 1992;569:281–286.

49. Robinson SE, Fox SD, Posner MG, et al. The effect of MI muscarinic blockade on behavior following traumatic brain injury in the rat. *Brain Res.* 1990;511:141–148.

50. Saija A, Robinson SE, Lyeth BG, Dixon CE, et al. The effects of scopolamine and traumatic brain injury on central cholinergic neurons. *J Neurotrauma.* 1988;5:161–170.

51. Sciclounoff S. L'acetylcholine dans le traitment de l'ictus hemiplegique. *Presse Med.* 1934;56:1140–1142.

52. Ward AA, Kennard MA. The effect of cholinergic drugs on recovery of function following lesions of the central nervous system. *Yale J Biol Med.* 1942;15:189–228.

53. Sims JS, Jones TA, Fulton RL, et al. Benzodiazepine effects on recovery of function linked to trans-neuronal morphological events. *Soc Neurosci Abstr.* 1990;16:342.

54. Hernandez TD, Jones GH, Schallert T. Co-administration of Ro 15-1788 prevents diazepam-induced retardation of recovery of function. *Brain Res.* 1989;487:89–95.

55. Zasler, ND. Advances in neuropharmacological rehabilitation for brain dysfunction. *Brain Inj.* 1992;6:1–14.

56. Koller WC, Wong GF, Lang A. Post-traumatic movement disorders: a review. *Movement Disord.* 1989;4:20–36.

57. Feeney DM, Gonzalez A, Law WA. Amphetamine, haloperidol, and experience interact to affect rate of recovery after motor cortex injury. *Science.* 1982;217:855–857.

58. Hovda DA, Feeney DM. Amphetamine with experience promotes recovery of locomotor function after unilateral frontal cortex injury in the cat. *Brain Res.* 1984;298:358–361.

59. Hovda DA, Feeney DM. Haloperidol blocks amphetamine-induced recovery of binocular depth perception after bilateral visual cortex ablation in the cat. *Proc West Pharmacol Soc.* 1985;28:209–211.

60. Hovda DA, Feeney DM, Salo AA, et al. Phenoxy-benzamine but not haloperidol reinstates all motor and sensory deficits in cats fully recovered from sensorimotor cortex ablations. *Soc Neurosci Abstr.* 1983;9:1001.

61. Boyeson MG, Feeney DM. Adverse effects of catecholaminergic drugs following unilateral cerebellar ablations. *Restor Neurol Neurosci.* 1991;3:227–233.

62. Boyeson MG, Feeney DM. Intraventricular norepinephrine facilitates motor recovery following sensorimotor cortex injury. *Pharmacol Biochem Behav.* 1990;35:497–501.

63. Boyeson MG, Krobert KA, Grade CM, Scherer PJ. Unilateral, but not bilateral, locus coeruleus lesions facilitate recovery from sensorimotor cortex injury. *Pharmacol Biochem Behav.* 1992;43:771–777.

64. Boyeson MG, Krobert KA, Scherer PJ, et al. Reinstatement of motor deficits in brain-injured animals: the role of cerebellar norepinephrine. *Restor Neurol Neurosci.* 1193;5:283–290.

65. Porch B, Wyckes J, Feeney DM. Haloperidol, thiazides and some antihypertensives slow recovery from aphasia. *Soc Neurosci Abstr.* 1985;11:52.

66. Stephens J, Goldberg G, Demospoulos JT. Clonidine reinstates deficits following recovery from sensorimotor cortex lesion in rats. *Arch Phys Med Rehabil.* 1986;67:666–667.

67. Yu J, Eidelber E. Recovery of locomotor function in cats after localized cerebellar lesions. *Brain Res.* 1983;273:121–131.

68. Boyeson MG, Krobert KA. Cerebellar norepinephrine infusions facilitate recovery after sensorimotor cortex injury. *Brain Res Bull.* 1992;29:435–439.

69. Boyeson MG, Scherer PJ, Grade CM, Krobert KA. Unilateral locus cceruleus lesions facilitate motor recovery from cortical injury through supersensitivity mechanisms. *Pharmacol Biochem Behav*. 1993;44:297–305.

70. Ross ED, Stewart MD. Akinetic mutism from hypothalamic damage: successful treatment with dopamine agonists. *Neurology*. 1981;31:1435-1439.

71. Crisostomo EA, Duncan PW, Propst M, Dawson DV, et al. Evidence that amphetamine with physical therapy promotes recovery of motor function in stroke patients. *Ann Neurol*. 1988; 23:94–97.

72. Homan R, Panksepp J, McSweeny J, et al. d-Amphetamine effects on language and motor behaviors in a chronic stroke patient. *Soc Neurosci Abstr*. 1990;16:439.

73. Walker-Batson D, Unwin H, Curtis S, et al. Use of amphetamine in the treatment of aphasia. *Restor Neurol Neurosci*. 1992;4:47–50.

74. Bleiberg J, Barmo VM, Cederquist J, Reeves D, et al. Effects of Dexedrine on performance consistency following brain injury. *Neuropsychiatry, Neuropsychol, Behav Neurol*. 1993;6:245–248.

75. Nickels JL, Schneider WN, Dombovy ML, Wong TM. Clinical use of amantadine in brain injury rehabilitation. *Brain Inj*. 1994;8:709–718.

76. Horiguchi J, Imnai Y, Shoda T. Effects of long term amantadine on clinical symptoms and EEG of a patient in a vegetative state. *Clin Neuropharmacol*. 1990;12:84–88.

77. Campagnolo DI, Katz RT. Successful treatment of akinetic mutism with post synaptic dopamine agonist. *Arch Phys Med Rehabil*. 1992;73:975.

78. Crismon ML, Childs A, Wilcox RE, Barrow N. The effect of bromocriptine on speech dysfunction in patients with diffuse brain injury (akinetic mutism). *Clin Neuropharmacol*. 1988;11:462–466.

79. Haig AJ, Ruess JM. Recovery from vegetative state of six months' duration associated with Sinemet (levodopa/carbidopa). *Arch Phys Med Rehabil*. 1990;71:1081–1083.

80. Walker-Batson D, Devous MD, Curtis SS, et al. Response to amphetamine to facilitate recovery from aphasia subsequent to stroke. In: Prescott TE, ed. *Clinical Aphasiology*. Austin, Tex: Pro-Ed; 1991:20.

81. Boyeson MG, Harmon RL. Effects of trazadone and desipramine on motor recovery in brain-injured rats. *Am J Phys Med Rehabil*. 1993;72:286–293.

82. Gustafson I, Westerberg E, Wieloch T. Protection against ischemia-induced neuronal damage by the alpha 2-adrenoceptor antagonist idazoxan: influence of time of administration and possible mechanisms of action. *J Cereb Blood Flow Metabol*. 1990;10:885–894.

83. Gustafson I, Westerberg E, Weiloch T. Extracellular brain cortical levels of noradrenaline in ischemia: effects of desipramine and postischemic administration of idazoxan. *Exp Brain Res*. 1991;86:555–561.

84. Zasler ND. Acute neurochemical alterations following traumatic brain injury: research implications for clinical treatment. *J Head Trauma Rehabil*. 1992;7:102–105.

85. Fox R, Lehmkuhle SW, Bush RC. Stereopsis in the falcon. *Science*. 1977;197:79–81.

86. Bontke, CF, Baize CM, Boake C. Coma management and sensory stimulation. *Phys Med Rehabil Clin*. 1992;3:259–272.

87. Bontke CF, Boake C. Principles of brain injury rehabilitation. In: Braddom R, ed. *Textbook of PM&R*. Philadelphia, Pa: WB Saunders Co; 1995:1027–1052.

88. Bontke CF, Zasler ND, Boake C. Rehabilitation of the head injured patient. *Neurotrauma*. In press.

89. Lal S, Merbitz CP, Grip JC. Modification of function in head-injured patients with Sinemet. *Brain Inj*. 1988;2:225–233.

90. Wroblewski BA, Glenn MB. Pharmacological treatment of arousal and cognitive deficits. *J Head Trauma Rehabil*. 1994;9:19–42.

91. Boyeson MG, Harmon RL, Jones JL. Differential effects of fluoxetine, amitriptyline, and serotonin on functional motor recovery after sensorimotor cortex injury. *Am J Phys Med Rehabil*. 1994;73:76–83.

92. Costa JL, Ito U, Spatz M, Klatzo I, et al. 5-hydroxytryptamine accumulation in cerebrovascular injury. *Nature*. 1974;2489:135–136.

93. Nakayama H, Ginsberg MD, Deitrich WD. (S)-emopamil, a novel calcium channel blocker and serotonin S2 antagonist, markedly reduces infarct size following middle cerebral artery occlusion in the rat. *Neurology*. 1988;38:1667–1673.

94. Osterholm JL, Bell J, Meyer R, Pyenson J. Experimental effects of free serotonin on the brain and its relationship to brain injury. *J Neurosurg*. 1969;31:408–412.

95. Sandyk R, Iacona RP, Fisher H. Post-traumatic cerebellar syndrome: response to l-tryptophan. *Int J Neurosci*. 1989;47:301–302.

96. Trouillas P, Brudon F, Adeleine P. Improvement of cerebellar ataxia with levoratory form of 5-hydroxy tryptophan: a double-blind study with quantified data processing. *Arch Neurol*. 1988;45:1217–1222.

97. Weintraub MI. Methysergide (Sansert) treatment in acute stroke: community pilot study. *Angiology*. 1985;36:137–142.

98. Morley JE. An approach to the development of drugs for appetite disorders. *Neuropsychobiology*. 1989;21:22–30.

99. Bodnar RA, Lynch T, Lewis L, Kahn D. Serotonin syndrome. *Neurology*. 1995;45:219–223.

100. Cope DN. Neuropharmacology and brain damage. In: Christiansen AL, Uzzel BP, eds. *Neuropsychological Rehabilitation: Current Knowledge and Future Direction*. Boston, Mass: Kluwer; 1987:19–39.

101. Gualtieri CT. Pharmacotherapy and the neurobehavioral sequelae of traumatic brain injury. *Brain Inj*. 1988;2:101–129.

102. Sutton RL, Weaver MS, Feeney DM. Drug-induced modifications of behavioral recovery following cortical trauma. *J Head Trauma Rehabil*. 1987;2:50–58.

103. Brigman C, Dickey C, Zeeger LJ. Agitated aggressive patient during recovery from a head injury. *Am J Nurs*. 1983;83:1408–1412.

104. Herbel K, Schermerhorn L, Howard J. Management of agitated head-injured patients: a survey of current techniques. *Rehabil Nurs*. 1990;15:66–69.

105. Patterson TS, Sargent M. Behavioral management of the agitated head trauma client. *Rehabil Nurs*. 1990;15:248–249.

106. Yudofsky SC, Silver JM, Schneider SE. Pharmacologic treatment of aggression. *Psychiatr Ann*. 1987;17:397–404.

107. Yudofsky SC, Silver JM, Jackson W, Endicott J, et al. The Overt Aggression Scale for the objective rating of verbal and physical aggression. *Am J Psychiatry*. 1986;143:35–39.

108. Levin HS, Benton AL, Grossman RG. *Neurobehavioral Consequences of Closed Head Injury*. New York, NY: Oxford University Press; 1982.

109. Kay NH, Uppington J, Sear JW, Douglas EJ, et al. Pharmacokinetics of propofol ("Diprivan") as an induction agent. *Postgrad Med J*. 1985;61(suppl 3):55–57.

110. Newman LH, McDonald JC, Wallace PG, Ledingham IM. Propofol infusion for sedation in intensive care. *Anaesthesia.* 1987;42:929–937.

111. Beller JP, Pottecher T, Lugnier A, Mangin P, et al. Prolonged sedation with propofol in ICU patients: recovery and blood concentration changes during periodic interruptions in infusion. *Br J Anaesth.* 1988;61:583–588.

112. Grounds RM, Lalor JM, Lumley J, Royston D, et al. Propofol infusion for sedation in the intensive care unit: preliminary report. *Br Med J.* 1987;294:397–400.

113. Aitkenhead AR, Pepperman ML, Willatts SM, Coates PD, et al. Comparison of propofol and midazolam for sedation in critically ill patients. *Lancet.* 1989;2:704–709.

114. Ravussin P, Guinard JP, Ralley F, Thorin D. Effect of propofol on cerebrospinal fluid pressure and cerebral perfusion pressure in patients undergoing craniotomy. *Anaesthesia.* 1988; 43(suppl):37–41.

115. Ravussin P, Thorin D, Guinard JP, Freeman J. Effect of propofol on cerebrospinal fluid pressure in patients with and without intracranial hypertension. *Anesthesiology.* 1989;71:A120.

116. Herregods L, Verbeke J, Rolly G, Colardyn F. Effects of propofol on elevated intracranial pressure: preliminary results. *Anaesthesia.* 1988;43:107–109.

117. Vandesteene A, Trempont V, Engelman E, Deloof T, et al. Effect of propofol on cerebral blood flow and metabolism in man. *Anaesthesia.* 1988;43(Suppl):42–43.

118. Bruce DA, Langfitt TW, Miller JD, Schutz H, et al. Regional cerebral blood flow, intracranial pressure, and brain metabolism in comatose patients. *J Neurosurg.* 1973;38:131–144.

119. Messetter K, Nordstrom CH, Sundbarg G, Algotsson L, et al. Cerebral hemodynamics in patients with acute severe head trauma. *J Neurosurg.* 1986;64:231–237

120. Pinaud M, Lelausque JN, Chetanneau A, Fauchoux N, et al. Effects of propofol on cerebral hemodynamics and metabolism in patients with brain trauma. *Anesthesiology.* 1990;73:404–409.

121. Nordstrom CH, Messeter K, Sundbarg G, Schalen W, et al. Cerebral blood flow, vasoreactivity, and oxygen consumption during barbiturate therapy in severe traumatic brain lesions. *J Neurosurg.* 1988;68:424–431.

122. Jennett B. Posttraumatic epilepsy. In: Rosenthal M, Griffith ER, Bond MR, Miller JD, eds. *Rehabilitation of the Adult and Child with Traumatic Brain Injury.* 2nd ed. Philadelphia, Pa: FA Davis Co; 1990:89-93.

123. Jennett B. *Epilepsy after Nonmissile Head Injuries.* 2nd ed. Chicago, Ill: William Heinemann; 1975.

124. Goddard GV. Development of epileptic seizures through brain stimulation at low intensity. *Nature.* 1967;214:1020–1021.

125. Willmore LJ. Post traumatic epilepsy: cellular mechanisms and implications for treatment. *Epilepsia.* 1990;31(suppl 3):S67–S73.

126. McNamara JO, Rigsbee LC, Butler LS, Shin C. Intravenous phenytoin is an effective anticonvulsant in the kindling model. *Ann Neurol.* 1989;26:675–678.

127. Wada JA. Pharmacological prophylaxis in the kindling model of epilepsy. *Arch Neurol.* 1977;34:389–395.

128. Goldenshon ES. The relevance of secondary epileptogenesis to the treatment of epilepsy: kindling and the mirror focus. *Epilepsia.* 1984;25(suppl 2):S156–S173.

129. Hauser WA. Prevention of posttraumatic epilepsy. *N Engl J Med* 1990;323:540–542.

130. Willmore LJ, Sypert GW, Munson JB. Recurrent seizures induced by cortical iron injection: a model of posttraumatic epilepsy. *Ann Neurol.* 1978;4:329–336.

131. Glotzner FL, Haubitz I, Miltner F, Kapp G, et al. Seizure prevention using carbamazepine following severe brain injuries. *Neurochirurgia.* 1983;26:66–79.

132. Payan H, Toga M, Berard-Badier M. The pathology of posttraumatic epilepsies. *Epilepsia.* 1970;11:81–94.

133. Hammond EJ, Ramsay RE, Villareal HJ, Wilder BJ. Effects of intracortical injection of blood and blood components of the electrocorticogram. *Epilepsia.* 1980:21:3–14.

134. Annegers JF, Grabow JD, Broover RV, Laws ER Jr, et al. Seizures after head trauma: a population study. *Neurology.* 1980;30:683–689.

135. Feeney DM, Walker AE. The prediction of posttraumatic epilepsy: a mathematical approach. *Arch Neurol.* 1979;36:8–12.

136. Bontke CF. Medical complications related to traumatic brain injury. *Phys Med Rehabil State Art Rev.* 1989;3:43–52.

137. McQueen JK, Blackwood DH, Harris P, Kalbag RM, et al. Low risk of late post traumatic seizures following severe head injury: implications for clinical trials of prophylaxis. *J Neurol Neurosurg Psychiatry.* 1983;46:899–904.

138. Penry JK, White BG, Brackett CE. A controlled prospective study of the pharmacologic prophylaxis of post traumatic epilepsy. *Neurology.* 1979;29:600–601. Abstract.

139. Temkin NR, Dikemen SS, Wilensky AJ, Keihm J, et al. A randomized, double-blind study of phenytoin for the prevention of posttraumatic seizures. *New Engl J Med.* 1990;323:497–502.

140. Young B, Rapp RP, Norton JA, Haack D, et al. Failure of prophylactically administered phenytoin to prevent late posttraumatic seizures. *J Neurosurg.* 1983;58:236–241.

141. Yablon SA. Posttraumatic seizures. *Arch Phys Med Rehabil.* 1993;74:983–1001.

142. Mattson RH, Cramer JA, Collins JF, Smith DB, et al. Comparison of carbamazepine, phenobarbital, phenytoin, and primidone in partial and secondarily generalized tonic-clonic seizures. *N Engl J Med.* 1985;313:145–151.

143. Pisciotta AV. Carbamazepine: hematological toxicity. In: Woodbury DM, Penry JK, Pippenger CE, eds. *Antiepileptic Drugs.* 2nd ed. New York, NY: Raven Press; 1982:533–541.

144. Glenn MB, Wroblewski B. Anticonvulsants for the prophylaxis of post traumatic seizures. *J Head Trauma Rehabil.* 1986;1:73–74.

145. Ramsey RE. Advances in pharmacotherapy of epilepsy. *Epilepsia.* 1993;34(suppl 5):S9–S16.

146. Bonfiglio RL, Costa JL, Bonfiglio RP. Awakenings II: pharmacologic roles of metoclopramide and Sinemet in akinetic mutism. *Arch Phys Med Rehabil.* 1991;72:817. Abstract.

147. Chesnut RM. Medical complications of the head injured patient. In: Cooper PR, ed. *Head Injury.* 3rd ed. Philadelphia, Pa: Williams & Wilkins; 1993.

148. Halloran LG, Zfass AM, Gayle WE, Wheeler CB, et al. Prevention of acute gastrointestinal complications after severe head injury: a controlled trial of cimetidine prophylaxis. *Am J Surg.* 1980;139:44–48.

149. Sandel ME, Abrahms PL, Horn LJ. Hypertension after brain injury: case report. *Arch Phys Med Rehabil.* 1986;67:469–472.

150. Rossitch E Jr, Bullard DE. The autonomic dysfunction syndrome: aetiology and treatment. *Br J Neurosurg.* 1988;2:471–478.

151. vanHilten JJ, Roos RA. Posttraumatic hyperthermia: a possible result of fronto-diencephalic dysfunction. *Clin Neurol Neurosurg.* 1991;93:223–225.

152. Benedeck G, Toth-Daru P, Janaky J, Hortobagyi A, et al. Indomethacin is effective against neurogenic hyperthermia following cranial trauma or brain surgery. *Can J Neurol Sci.* 1987;14:145–148.

153. Meythaler JM, Stinson AM. Fever of central origin in traumatic brain injury controlled with propranolol. *Arch Phys Med Rehabil.* 1994;75:816–818.

154. Weintraub AH, Opat CA. Motor and sensory dysfunction in the brain injured adult. *Arch Phys Med Rehabil.* 1989;3:59.

155. Cowley RS, Swanson B, Chapman P, Kitik BA, et al. The role of the rehabilitation in the intensive care unit. *J Head Trauma Rehabil.* 1994;9:32–42.

156. Glenn MB. Nerve blocks. In: Glenn MB, Whyte J, eds. *The Practical Management of Spasticity in Children and Adults.* Philadelphia, Pa: Lea & Febiger. 1990 227–258.

157. Khalili AA, Betts HB. Peripheral nerve block with phenol in the management of spasticity: indications and complications. *JAMA.* 1967;200:1155–1157.

158. Loubser PG, Bontke CF, Baize CM. Quadruple motor neurolysis for shoulder and elbow flexor hypertonicity. *Arch Phys Med Rehabil* 1991;72:826.

159. Loubser PG, Bontke CF, Baize CM. Intramuscular neurolytic blocks for upper extremity spasticity in head injury. *Anesthesiology.* 1989;71:A763.

160. Loubser PG, Bontke CF, Vandeventer J. Selective epidural phenol rhizolysis for hip flexor spasticity. *Arch Phys Med Rehabil.* 1989;70:A38.

161. Lehmkuhl LD, Thoi LL, Baize C, Kelley CJ, et al. Multimodality treatment of joint contractures in patients with severe brain injuries: cost, effectiveness, and integration of therapies in the application of serial/inhibitive casts. *J Head Trauma Rehabil.* 1990;5:23–42.

162. Borg-Stein J, Stein J. Pharmacology of botulism toxin and implications for use in disorders of muscle tone. *J Head Trauma Rehabil.* 1990;5:23–42.

CHAPTER 14

Crisis Intervention: Care and Involvement of the Family

The Chinese symbol for *crisis* (Figure 14–1) captures the word's essential elements, for it combines the pictographs for the concepts "danger" and for "opportunity." The danger in any crisis is inherent in the event itself and the uncertainty of the outcome. Opportunity provides individuals and families with a window of chance to overcome difficult odds, evoking skills that until that point in time may have remained dormant.

Severe brain injury represents a profound crisis for the patient. During the early stages of recovery, what may be recognized but "often unappreciated is the fact that the family of the patient is also involved in a psychological crisis, the resolution of which has significant consequences on the long-term outcome for the patient and the family unit."[1(p68)] Significant and often unknown challenges lie ahead for these families. Like the individual, no family chooses brain injury; thus, all proceed in emotionally uncharted territory.

Over a life span, members within a family system become psychologically and behaviorally connected to each other. Every family possesses "transactional patterns": unwritten, yet dynamic rules about giving and taking within the system.[2] These rules dictate how members solve problems, meet each other's individual needs, and express differences of opinion.

During a crisis, families bring with them a unique heritage in the form of communication patterns, coping mechanisms, personal and societal values, and cultural and ethnic traditions. When an unexpected injury occurs to a family member, change ensues for the entire family. Previously successful transactional patterns are no longer effective. Members must choose, often unconsciously, to use ineffective patterns or to develop new ones. On the surface, some families appear to incorporate this sudden change with relative ease, whereas others are thrown into utter chaos.[3]

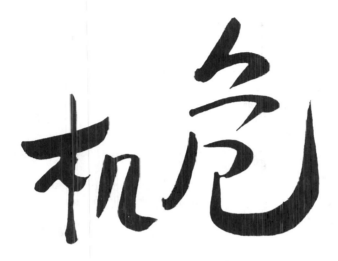

Figure 14–1 The Chinese symbol for crisis, encompassing the two pictographs for danger and opportunity.

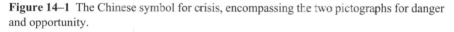

Sudden trauma, as in a traumatic brain injury, calls upon the family to absorb an extreme amount of anxiety. This anxiety is compounded with frustration, helplessness, guilt, anger, and, usually, the novelty of the experience for the family. The sudden nature of the event, which is the hallmark characteristic of trauma, prohibits anticipation or planning. The family generally has no direct experiences on which to draw. Clear rules of behavior no longer exist. Structure around which to organize time or priorities disappears. Reacting to the moment, often inadequately, the family has no sense of when the crisis will be over or what the outcome will be.

Timely assessment of family dynamics and appropriate intervention by health care professionals are crucial to maximizing patient and family outcomes. The family serves as a great source of support for the patient with brain injury.[4,5] Studies have demonstrated that strong support positively affects outcome.[6,7] Thus, the family's responses to the crisis of severe brain injury must be channeled down a path most beneficial for the patient.

ANATOMY OF A CRISIS

Human beings exist in a state of emotional equilibrium, a state of balance or homeostasis. Unique and distinctive coping skills are used to maintain acceptable levels of comfort and adaptation to one's milieu. Individuals are constantly challenged to solve problems in order to maintain that balance.[8] When something disrupts the status quo and a state of disequilibrium occurs, one strives to regain previous levels of equilibrium.[9] In essence, the individual must either solve the problem or adapt to nonsolution. When a problem touches a person at a vulnerable spot, he or she is confronted with an imbalance between the perceived difficulty and his or her own available repertoire of previously successful coping skills, sometimes resulting in decompensation. A person may then move from an emotionally hazardous situation into a crisis state. Tension rises and discomfort is felt as the person becomes less able to find a solution. Associated feelings of anxiety, fear, guilt, shame, and helplessness ensue.

If the situation is experienced primarily as a threat, extreme anxiety may be the dominant reaction. If the crisis is experienced primarily in terms of a loss, depression and mourning will predominate.[10]

"Crisis is not simply the experience of adversity, but embodies the response of the individual, family, or group to that experience."[11(p23)] Crisis is a turning point from which nothing thereafter will ever be the same. Encountering and resolving crisis is a normal process that each person faces many times during life. Potential crises are widely divergent. According to Kercher,[10] crisis can be classified as either situational or maturational (also known as *accidental* or *developmental*, respectively). In both types, the person perceives the stressful event as a threat to his or her equilibrium such that his or her usual adaptive coping mechanisms are not sufficient to resolve the problem.

Maturational crises occur as a result of the normal processes of growth and development; they are the inevitable phase of transition from one stage of psychosocial development to another. These situations are often anticipated throughout the course of human life. It is not the specific developmental stage itself that constitutes the crisis but rather the "period of internal reorganization which renders the individual particularly vulnerable to external hazards."[11(p26)] Such periods include the beginning of school, adolescence, marriage, parenthood, and retirement. Situational crises arise from unexpected or sudden events, such as natural disasters, sudden relocation, or changes in roles that require assumption of new responsibilities, such as the loss of loved ones, separation, severe illness or injury, or hospitalization.

HISTORICAL DEVELOPMENT OF CRISIS THEORY

Crisis theory has developed through the contributions of social psychiatry, ego psychology, and learning theory. Although the first sociopsychologic definition of crisis is attributed to Thomas[12] in 1909, Erich Lindemann and Gerald Caplan, two psychiatrists at the Harvard University School of Public Health, are credited with providing the basis for contemporary crisis theory. The theory developed from

Lindemann's classic study of grief reactions following the 1942 fire at Boston's Coconut Grove nightclub, in which 493 people perished.[13] Lindemann observed that acute grief was a normal and necessary reaction following bereavement. He illustrated a method of early preventive intervention to minimize the development of psychopathology, including depressions, psychosomatic symptomatologies, and phobic behaviors. He provided a theoretical frame of reference on the grief process, exemplifying a series of stages through which an individual passes on the way to accepting and resolving loss.

This frame of reference supported the development of crisis intervention techniques, and in 1946 Lindemann and Caplan established the Wellesley Project, a communitywide program outside of Boston for mental health. The program emphasized the use of preventative intervention.

The contributions of ego psychology stem from theories developed directly from Freud's work[14] on psychoanalysis. Caplan[15] reported that the most important aspects of mental health are the state of the ego, its level of maturity, and the quality of its structure.

Caplan probably provided the most influential contributions to crisis theory[8,15] by defining the theory of emotional homeostasis. He identified patterns by which individuals use specific methods of habitual problem solving and coping. When crisis occurs, equilibrium is disrupted and the individual's coping mechanism fails. According to Caplan,[8] a crisis has four developmental phases:

1. An initial rise in tension occurs when one is confronted with a hazardous situation. The individual responds with habitual problem-coping behaviors.
2. A lack of successful resolution increases discomfort and anxiety.
3. A further increase in tension mobilizes internal and external resources. Unsuccessful problem-solving measures are instituted in a trial-and-error fashion.
4. Tension increases as the problem can be neither solved nor avoided. When the level increases beyond the "breaking point," major disorganization occurs.

Aguilera[9] suggested that several balancing factors can effect a return to equilibrium. The absence of one or more of these balancing factors may block resolution of the problem and precipitate a crisis. This paradigm is illustrated in Figure 14–2.

FACTORS THAT INFLUENCE A CRISIS

Several diverse factors can negatively influence an individual's perception of threat or his or her ability to use adequate coping behaviors. Economic and

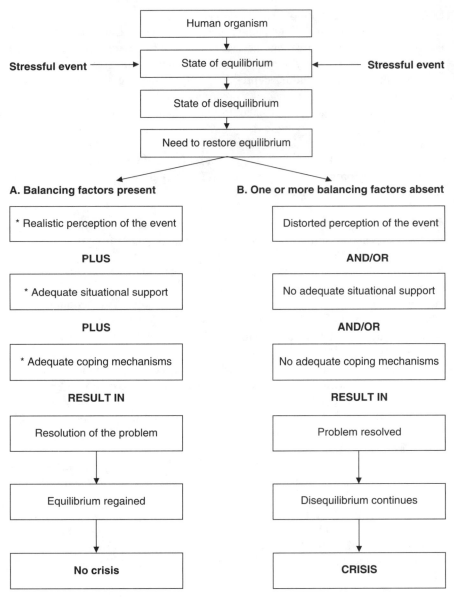

*Balancing factors.

Figure 14–2 Paradigm: the effect of balancing factors in a stressful event. *Source:* Reprinted with permission from D. Aguilera, *Crisis Intervention: Theory & Methodology,* 7th edition, p. 32, © 1994, Mosby-Year Book, Inc.

lifestyle situations in the modern world are vastly different from those of the past. Extended families, family size, and strength of blood ties once fostered intertwined support systems. But our current society is characterized by high mobility in both personal and professional domains. Urban life often requires that people relate to each other on a more superficial rather than personal level. Rising divorce rates often result in single-parent households. Value systems, beliefs, and interests vary greatly and are individualized rather than being community based. As a result, people are more isolated from the emotional support of families and close friends.[16,9(pp1–12)] Certainly, cultural issues influence the perceptions, responses, and behaviors of families. This area is addressed later in the chapter.

A greater sense of isolation and helplessness occurs in medical emergencies because of unfamiliar surroundings and unfamiliar issues. Heightened anxiety contributes to feelings of lack of control and lack of understanding the ramifications of the injury and interventions.

Other factors contributing to vulnerability include coexistent physical or social stresses such as unemployment or premorbid illness. Previous experiences with traumatic injuries may have a positive or a negative impact on present situations.

Factors unique to brain injury set it apart from other causes of crises. In 1967, Fahy et al[17] reported that 46% of patients with brain injuries had evidence of previous social maladjustment, placing their families at additional risk for reduced coping skills.

The age trends for patients with traumatic brain injury uniquely increase the stress upon a family system. Peaks are found bimodally with patients under the age of 29 and over age 65. Patients under 29 usually tend to be male and may be assuming pivotal responsibilities for their often newly established families. The over-age-65 population may place additional responsibilities on their adult children, who may be struggling with young children of their own.

The nature of severe brain injury multiplies the anxiety and other emotions felt by the family. Often uncertainty exists regarding the severity and prognosis of the injury. The families are faced with a sudden long-term injury that will never "go away." Regardless of desire or investment on the part of family members, there may be no expectations that life will return "to normal" following a period of convalescence.

ASSESSMENT

On the way to the hospital, "We do not speak of what is happening inside us; we're trying to stay calm. Underneath my heart, a box forms, its lid tightly sealed, holding in the demon emotions that would pull me into chaos. Panic pushes violently at the closed lid of this box when we are out of the car on our way in to the hospital."[18(p3)]

Interaction with the family often begins in the emergency room. Different staff members may be responsible for different aspects of family assessment and intervention. Specific assignments will vary among institutions. However, the social worker and the nurse bear most of the responsibility for interacting with the family on an ongoing basis. In the early stages, the physician also plays a critical role and is often the medical professional most sought out by the family to provide information on patient status and prognosis. Other team members, including therapists, will also have ongoing contact with the family following the initial resuscitation and transfer to the intensive care unit (ICU).

Because trauma occurs suddenly and because status and intervention may change frequently, crisis intervention for the family must be initiated immediately and must be constantly reassessed. Assessment and intervention often occur concurrently and may be difficult to separate. Braulin et al[19] depict a model for crisis intervention exemplifying the relationship between assessment and intervention (see Figure 14–3). The model incorporates a sequential progression, but it recognizes the potential for multiple stressful situations during the recovery period. Thus, the opposing arrows allow family members to move forward or backward within the model.

The overall goal in assessment is to derive a global and accurate picture of the family and the patient and to relate it to the present situation. Special focus should be placed on four areas: (1) defining the family's perception of the traumatic event, (2) identifying the problem, (3) identifying the family's coping abilities, and (4) identifying available support systems for the family and patient.

When a family arrives at the emergency department (ED), obtaining information is the most pressing concern. A designated staff member should discern, as quickly and as completely as possible, the circumstances surrounding the trauma. Information regarding the patient's status and mechanism of injury will help one anticipate the family's responses and questions.[20] Areas that should be addressed include the following:

1. What is the primary area of concern for the trauma team (eg, brain injury, shock, spinal cord injury, bleeding)?
2. What is the initial plan of care (eg, computerized tomography (CT) scan, other diagnostic tests, operating room)?
3. What events precipitated the trauma (eg, accident, suicide attempt, assault, crime, argument)?
4. Was anyone else involved in the accident, and if so, who was at fault? Guilt and blame can further exacerbate a crisis situation and must be dealt with early in the intervention.

The crisis counselor (eg, social worker or nurse) should communicate briefly the initial reactions of the family to the attending physician before his or her inter-

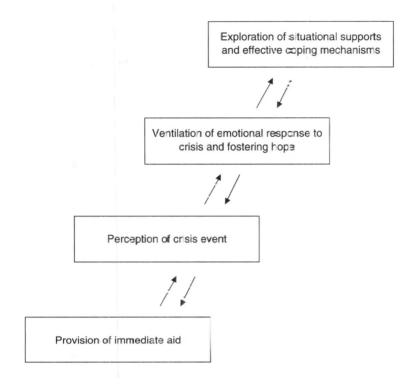

Figure 14–3 A model for crisis intervention in trauma. *Source:* Reprinted from *Critical Care Quarterly,* © 1982, Aspen Publishers, Inc.

action with the family. The physician will then be better prepared for questions and interpersonal dynamics he or she will encounter. Coordination between the crisis counselor and the physician reduces redundancy, maintains consistency with the family, and facilitates timely intervention. "A little help, rationally directed and purposely focused at a strategic time, is more effective than more extensive help given at a period of less emotional accessibility."[10(p229)]

The crisis counselor can then begin the interview process by developing an overall sense of the family system. What are the roles of the various family members, and how do members relate to each other? Information provided by the family about the patient should be included. What are the present life circumstances of the patient and pertinent family members, including work status, education, and social involvement? Are any active stressors present? What are the social, cultural, and spiritual customs of the family?

The counselor must also begin to identify coping abilities and support systems. Has the family had similar experiences previously? How has it coped with high-anxiety situations in the past? How does the family respond to problems that it cannot solve? What is the extent of the geographic mobility within the family? Are there other family members and friends who can be called upon to help? With whom do family members have the closest ties?

Finally, direct questions regarding the family's response to the crisis are essential. What are the family's current reactions? Are they overwhelmed, angry, mistrustful? What is their understanding of the current situation and status of the patient? Although families are often overwhelmed with the suddenness and severity of the injury, they are generally open to receiving information and providing opinions regarding their needs.

Because communication is the cornerstone of crisis intervention, much can be gained from listening to what the family say, as well as how they say it. An effective interviewer will take note of the suprasegmentals of communication, including facial expressions, body language, eye contact, and rate of speech. The manner in which family members answer questions, their interactions, and their ability to organize and remember information reveals a great deal about their ego functioning and their present mental states. History taking in and of itself can be therapeutic for the family.

Numerous studies spanning over 17 years have researched the needs of families of critically ill patients.[21-41] Some studies questioned families regarding their needs, using scales such as the Critical Care Family Needs Inventory[28] (CCFNI). Others explored who was responsible for meeting the families' needs and whether these needs were met. Other variables included the timing of assessment and the patients' diagnoses. Some studies are available that specifically addressed the needs of families of critically ill patients with brain injuries. Table 14–1 outlines the 10 most important needs from each study, and the frequency with which each need is mentioned across studies.

In the 13 studies reviewed, only one need was consistently identified: to know specific facts regarding the patient's diagnoses and prognosis. This need occurred in more than 90% of studies and included the need to have questions answered honestly and the need to be called at home about changes in the patient's condition. To know the prognosis/outcome/chance for recovery, to receive information in understandable explanations, and to believe that hospital personnel care about the patient were identified among the 10 most important needs in more than 80% of the studies.

INTERVENTION

As previously described, habitual problem-solving measures are generally unsuccessful when one is confronted with a hazardous situation. This lack of success, coupled with increasing tension, culminates in crisis. However, rather than abandoning the use of problem-solving techniques, classic crisis intervention incorporates it into treatment. John Dewey[42] in 1910 outlined the classic steps within a problem-solving approach: (1) a difficulty is felt; (2) the difficulty is located and defined; (3) possible solutions are suggested; (4) consequences are considered; and (5) a solution is accepted.

To initiate intervention, the therapist helps the family define the problem from available information and focus on issues in a logical sequence. Because persons under stress often do not "hear" what is initially said to them, restating and reinforcing information will help families assimilate data.

The problem-solving approach follows a structured, logical sequence, whereby each step depends on the preceding ones. Most people are not consciously aware that their decisions follow a defined, logical sequence of reasoning; what they see is that some solutions are more easily reached than others.

Classic crisis models follow the assumption that most crisis situations are abated within six weeks.[43] With crisis intervention, the ultimate goal for the family is to establish a level of emotional equilibrium equal to or better than the precrisis level. When dealing with brain injury, these goals must be modified because a total restitution of the patient's emotional and cognitive functions to pretrauma levels is seldom realistic.[44] Recovery from a brain injury far exceeds six weeks; therefore, far more resilience and resourcefulness on the part of the family is required. The therapeutic task still focuses on redefining the stressful situation, but strong emphasis is placed on mobilizing the family's resources for its resolution. The family must become active participants from the onset rather than passive recipients. The long-term nature of recovery from brain injury necessitates that interventions be initiated at the earliest possible moment in order to optimize the family's ability to provide the necessary support. In the absence of a natural support system, hospital personnel, as well as state and local agencies and support groups, may need to be used as surrogates.

Phases of Recovery

Families experiencing a traumatic crisis appear to go through six distinct phases before they are able to reorganize, reintegrate, and regain their homeostatic state.[45] This progression is similar to the stages of recovery from brain injury (ie, Rancho Los Amigos Scale of Cognitive Functioning [RLA] levels),[46] in that families can also follow a distinct predictable pattern of recovery but can differ in how long they stay within each stage. Similarly, not all family members pass equally through all stages or use the same exact sequence of phases. Each family member, like each family group, retains individual patterns of adaptation. The first and last phases, however, signify the initiation and culmination of the crisis. Despite individual variation, a systematic method of recovery is present (Figure 14–4).

Table 14–1 Review of the 10 Most Important Needs of Families of Critically Ill Patients in Published Studies from 1979 to 1993

Need	Molter[21] 1979	Rodgers[22] 1983	Mathis[23] 1984 With TBI	Mathis[23] 1984 Without TBI	Daley[24] 1984	Bouman[25] 1984 36 h after Admission	Bouman[25] 1984 96 h after Admission	Spatt et al[27] 1986
To know specific facts re: what is wrong with patient and progress	X	X	X	X	X	X	X	X
To have questions answered honestly	X	X	X	X	X[a]	X	X	X
To be called at home about changes	X	X	X	X	X[a]	X	X	X
To know prognosis/ chance for recovery	X	X		X	X	X	X	X
To receive information in understandable explanations	X	X		X		X	X	X[b]
To believe that hospital personnel care about patient	X	X	X	X			X	X
To have reassurance that best possible care is being given to patient		X	X	X	X	X	X	X
To have hope	X	X	X	X				X
To know exactly what/why things are being done for patient		X	X	X		X	X[a]	X[b]
To receive information once a day	X	X	X	X		X		X[b]
To know how patient is being treated medically			X			X	X	X
To see patient frequently	X				X	X		X
To have a specific person to call at hospital								
To talk to a physician					X			X
To have a waiting room nearby	X							
To be reassured patient is all right					X			
To talk to a nurse each day								
To have a telephone near waiting room								
To feel accepted by hospital personnel			X					
To have someone be concerned with relative's health								
To know which staff would give what type of information								

a. Identified twice with slight variations in description.
b. Three-way tie.

Leske[28] 1986	O'Neill-Norris & Grove[29] 1986	Jaconio et al[31] 1990	Forrester et al[32] 1990	Price et al[34] 1991	Freichels[35] 1991 <72 h	Freichels[35] 1991 7–10 d	Engl[39] 1993 With BI	Engl[39] 1993 Without BI	Frequency	%
X	X	X	X	X	X	X	X	X	17	100
X	X	X	X	X	X	X	X		16	94
X		X	X	X	X	X	X	X	16	94
X	X	X	X	X	X	X	X		15	88
X	X	X	X	X	X	X	X	X	15	88
X	X	X	X	X	X		X	X	14	82
		X	X	X	X	X	X		13	76
X	X	X	X	X	X	X			12	71
X		X	X	X	X			X	12	71
X	X				X			X	10	59
		X	X	X		X	X	X	10	59
X						X	X	X	8	47
	X					X	X		3	18
									2	12
									1	6
									1	6
	X								1	6
	X								1	6
									1	6
								X	1	6
								X	1	6

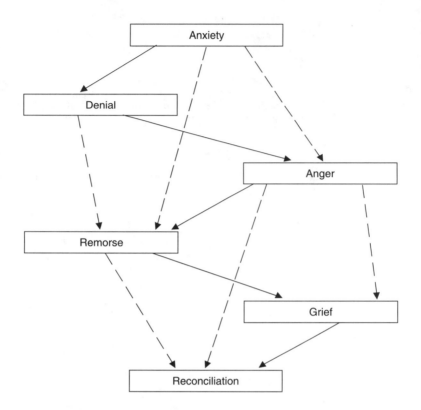

Figure 14–4 Six phases of a crisis that families experience in regaining a homeostatic state. The solid arrows depict the more commonly seen progression. The dotted-line arrows depict other possible sequences of phases.

Anxiety

Often the first phase a family experiences is a period of high anxiety. Persons under severe stress typically experience physical manifestations that may include high-pitched voice, tight neck and shoulder muscles, fainting, nausea, and diarrhea.

Providing brief and explicit information is the most valuable help that can be offered to family members during this phase. One should state exactly where the patient is, reassure the family that the most modern and sophisticated lifesaving technologies are being used, and inform them that the physician will provide a complete report as soon as it is safe to leave the patient. Information should be repeated frequently. The counselor should ask the family to reiterate the information and include their interpretation of its meaning. Families should also be encouraged to vent their feelings about this new catastrophic event.

Denial

Denial is the refusal to grant the truth of a statement. However, in the face of a crisis, denial serves to buy the family time: time necessary to adapt and adjust to the reality of what has happened.[3] The denial phase, otherwise known as the "everything will be all right" phase, allows the family time to gather support and strength. Denial acts as a psychologic preparation for any further bad news the family encounters.

An essential element of this phase is hope. Except when death is inevitable, hope should never be totally removed. A family's ability to maintain hope is a key factor in its ability to maintain coping skills.

The counselor interacting with the family should seek to confirm the reality of the situation without negating their denial. An example is "From what you've told me, Todd seems like a very strong and active man. It must be hard for you to believe he's had a brain injury." The therapist must balance the two factors: the need for denial and the need for the family to deal with the reality of the situation.

Providing support means giving information in a climate of hope.[47] Hope can be fostered through physical contact and verbal communication at the bedside. "These manifestations of hoping generate a sense of energy within the family, which allows the family to better utilize resources to confront the myriad of problems."[19(p44)] Often, the transition out of the denial phase occurs after the family is able to spend time with the patient. However, some family members may hold on to their denial for longer periods of time. Special attention through follow-up sessions must be made to help these individuals deal with the reality of the situation.

Anger

The anger phase is like the agitated stage of brain injury recovery (RLA IV) in that it manifests itself with varying severity and with different behaviors. Anger can be directed toward oneself, another family member, a physician, police, or prehospital personnel in an attempt to place blame. Family members may generalize anger by blaming society for allowing such things as high speeds, lack of gun control, and lenient drunk-driving laws. Anger is another defense mechanism that safeguards individuals from feeling pain.

Families must be free to ventilate angry feelings, and counselors must focus on helping the family define the real cause of their anger. When family members are able "to hear what they are thinking," they begin to recognize the illegitimacy of their blame. They come to understand that they are in actuality blaming the patient for disrupting their lives and causing such stress and turmoil. These families need reassurance that such feelings are not "bad."

Remorse

Remorse uniquely combines elements of both guilt and sorrow. This period is appropriately coined the "if only" stage. The family members judge themselves on the part they played in contributing to the crisis, whether emotionally ("If only I didn't argue with him"; "If only I'd been more understanding") or physically ("If only I hadn't let him go"; "If only I'd been there earlier").

During conversations, the counselor must listen and provide a realistic perception as to how much blame family members can assume. Encouraging conversation and providing reassurance helps families reason out thoughts, fears, and misperceptions.

Grief

Grief is a natural process and a primitive emotion—a combination of sadness and anger over the loss of a person. The grieving phase is often the time when the family's sense of loss becomes almost overwhelming. The intense pain involved makes this the most difficult stage to witness or to experience. Yet grief cannot be erased; it must be allowed to run its course. "The ability to engage in the painful but effective process of depression and mourning allows the family to say goodbye to the 'lost' family member and prepare for the 'new' member the patient has become."[1(p70)] Tears and sobbing are a natural way for families to experience relief. "Unvented grief has undesirable consequences: a persistent constriction of all emotions, a loss of spontaneity, enduring somberness."[48(p144)]

The grieving process can be facilitated by encouraging families to vent their feelings. These feelings must be recognized by family members in terms of both their own emotions and the emotions of those around them who are also living through this event. This stage can persist for long periods. Grieving for a significant person can last about a year.

Reconciliation

Reconciliation is not necessarily accepting what has happened, but rather putting things into perspective. Family members are reconciled to the fact that something terrible has happened and that it will not soon go away. This stage usually occurs after the previous stages. Most often, the reality of the situation is clear, and anger, guilt, and sorrow have usually been expressed.

At this stage, family solidarity emerges and family members use each other for strength. The sense of hope does not diminish but becomes more realistic. The family does not deny or underestimate the tragedy but comes to the realization that no matter what, they will survive. The counselor, along with other team members, may now begin to develop a realistic, feasible plan for the coming weeks and months.

Coping

Throughout these stages, the family is confronted with the need and desire to cope effectively with this life-changing crisis. Coping is an adjustive reaction made in response to actual or imagined stress in order to maintain psychologic integrity.[45] Humans respond to stress by one of three reactions: fight, flight, or compromise. Attack reactions usually involve overcoming the stress-inducing obstacles. Flight reactions simply involve physically removing the threat from the environment or removing oneself from the threatening situation. Compromise, which is unique to humans, involves accepting substitute goals or changing values and standards and is utilized when both fight and flight from the threatening situation are impossible or unrealistic. Normally, defense mechanisms are used constructively in the process of coping and are seen as extremely important for survival.

Through the process of daily living, people learn to use many methods to reduce tension and cope with anxiety. Coping mechanisms are reinforced through problem solving. Lifestyles are developed around patterns of response, which in turn are established to cope with stressful situations.

Cognition plays an important role in determining both the nature and degree of an individual's coping responses. Differences in one's cognitive perception of the injury's threat to an important life goal or value account for large differences in coping behaviors. Cognitive style[50] is therefore individualistic in the way a person assimilates and uses information from the environment.

Not all families have within their repertoire of past experiences adequate coping mechanisms to adapt to a crisis. Families are, however, generally more receptive in a crisis, since they may be aware that past coping mechanisms are not working. Staff and family members must therefore explore alternative methods of coping.

The crisis counselor works with the family to identify the perceived outcome of the event in relation to its future goals and values. A secondary appraisal then identifies the scope of coping alternatives available. Once new coping skills have been identified and applied, the counselor affirms the process so that the family may generalize it for future planning. Since coping behaviors are not static, new responses may occur whenever a new significance is attached to a situation.

KEY FAMILY NEEDS

Families have five key needs during crisis. All health care professionals must understand and remember these needs in their acute interactions with the family.

Thy are: (1) maintaining hope, (2) garnering information, (3) being with the patient, (4) feeling helpful and needed, and (5) recognizing personal needs. The concept of hope, so vital to a family's ability to deal with a catastrophic situation, was discussed in the section on denial. The remaining four areas will be discussed in this section.

Garnering Information

"We have gradually moved into an era of consumerism that has come to include patient and family rights, one of the biggest of these being access . . . to extensive and full information . . . [regarding] the critically injured family member."[51(p24)] Families need and want consistent and frequent information. Often the desire for information exceeds what information is available. The combination of providing medical information and defining the involvement and role of the family helps to decrease confusion and gives structure to a potentially unpredictable situation. Information itself is supportive in that it helps families cope better with the situation.

Early contact with the family is the starting point for helping them understand brain injury and often sets the stage for accepting more education during the recovery process. All team members must be cognizant of their use of technical terminology and must gear their discussions to a level appropriate for that individual family.

Once the intensivist and rehabilitation therapist initiate intervention in the ICU, family education begins to encompass a more global and consistent perspective. An initial family meeting should be scheduled once these clinicians and therapists have completed their assessments. This meeting should occur after the first week of admission. All team members, including the physician(s), nurse, social worker, and rehabilitation therapists, should participate. Results of assessments, the plan of care, anticipated disposition, and the need for continued rehabilitation should be reviewed.

One of the primary focuses of early rehabilitation is education. Family education should be provided in verbal and written formats. An organized family packet is a valuable resource because families may have difficulty assimilating and remembering information given to them, especially in the early stages. The packet reinforces information that may have been forgotten, was unclear, or needs further explanation. Family packets allow individuals to assimilate information at their own pace and can help ease the long hours usually spent in the waiting room.

Family members should be encouraged to write down information, including terminology that needs further explanation, names of pertinent staff, and potential questions for physicians and staff. Physicians may see the patient when the family is not available. When updates are given, families may be attempting to assimilate new information rather than asking questions regarding previous concerns.

During the course of acute hospitalization, family members will come into contact with many different professionals. Families who are only beginning to face this crisis may be confused as to roles and identities. The form in Exhibit 14–1 may help families record the names and telephone numbers of those professionals who have contact with their loved ones. An information sheet describing the basic functions of potential team members is shown in Exhibit 14–2.

Other types of written information may be helpful to families. The RLA Scale of Cognitive Functioning[46] should be provided and explained to families, since this tool is used throughout the recovery course. Although RLA levels are only general descriptions of function and behavior, they provide a means for families to identify progress and anticipate future behaviors (eg, agitation). During the acute phase, additional information should be provided regarding brain injury recovery patterns. Resources that more specifically describe deficits and abilities along the continuum of recovery are helpful. However, families must be told that a loved one's course of recovery is unknown and that exact patterns and extent of recovery cannot be prognosticated. These unknowns do not represent a lack of experience or knowledge, but rather a truer, more accurate and honest appraisal of brain injury recovery. The family will come to appreciate this aspect better when they are farther down the recovery path. "In the very beginning, . . . professionals who spoke with us would have been wise to avoid predictions. They gave us the false impression they knew a lot more than we did."[18(p159)]

A diagram to identify various patient equipment is also helpful. Not all families are comfortable constantly asking nurses the names and functions of various equipment, lines, and tubes. This diagram can provide the basis for understanding which pieces of equipment can be touched and what to do when alarms sound. Although understanding equipment may seem like a small unimportant issue, it helps keep the family informed and "in touch" with their loved one.

All families should be provided information regarding support groups and advocacy associations. Many states have brain injury associations whose role is to provide information, support, and advocacy for all persons with brain injuries and their families. Not all families will choose to contact these agencies, especially during the early critical stages. However, all families deserve to be informed of their existence. The judgment as to whether a family is ready for this information can be made only by the family members themselves.[18] A list of state associations is included in Appendix 14–A.

Being with the Patient

Wanting to see the patient is a very natural spontaneous reaction of the family. While the patient is still in the ED, the nature of injuries and the need for tests, procedures, or surgery may prevent visits from the family until the patient has arrived in the ICU. However, if at all possible, requests to visit should be granted

Exhibit 14–1 Information Sheet Provided to Families To Organize the Names and Phone Numbers for Team Members

Traumatic Brain Injury Team

The following members of the TBI Team are concerned with providing the best care for your relative. They are available to answer any questions you may have regarding their assessment of your family member and the specialized services we provide.

Team Member	Name	Phone/Beeper
Surgical Resident	_____	_____
Attending Physician	_____	_____
Primary Nurse	_____	_____
Physical Therapist	_____	_____
Occupational Therapist	_____	_____
Speech/Language Therapist	_____	_____
Social Worker	_____	_____
Continuing Care/ Discharge Planner	_____	_____
Dietitian	_____	_____
Other Physician(s) (and area of specialty)	_____	_____
	_____	_____
	_____	_____
	_____	_____
	_____	_____
Others	_____	_____
	_____	_____
	_____	_____

Source: Courtesy of Saint Francis Hospital and Medical Center, Department of Rehabilitation Medicine, Hartford, Connecticut.

at the earliest appropriate time. Obviously, the social worker and/or nurse prepares the family by drawing a mental picture of what the patient will look like in an attempt to desensitize them to the changes that have occurred in their loved one's appearance.

At times, it may be difficult for family members to show affection because of uncertainty about what is safe or appropriate. The nurse can be especially helpful

Exhibit 14–2 Information Sheet Provided to Families To Describe the Roles of Team Members

---

TBI TEAM MEMBERS

AUDIOLOGIST—The professional who evaluates and provides rehabilitation for hearing disorders. The audiologist evaluates multifaceted disorders, provides ongoing monitoring and counseling, and makes recommendations to the family and staff that will improve communication ability, thereby fostering the rehabilitation process.

CONTINUING CARE/DISCHARGE PLANNER—A nurse or social worker who coordinates with families regarding posthospital placement, community resources, and legal and financial issues, including insurance coverage, conservatorship, and other legal decisions.

DIETITIAN—The professional who determines the nutritional status and needs of a patient. The dietitian works with the physician and other team members, making recommendations on diet and caloric needs based upon method of feeding (IV, tube, oral).

NEUROPSYCHOLOGIST—A psychologist with special training in brain-behavior relationships. The neuropsychologist may be involved in evaluating, defining, and remediating cognitive/behavioral consequences of brain disorders.

NEUROSURGEON—The surgeon who manages central nervous system–injured persons through surgical intervention or directing the care of the patient with a brain injury. The neurosurgeon makes recommendations regarding the acute and chronic care of these patients.

NURSE—The primary provider of care at the bedside 24 hours a day. The nurse monitors changes in patient status, assists in the coordination of interdisciplinary services, and provides family support. The nurse is the primary link between the physician and the family in providing up-to-date information on patient status.

OCCUPATIONAL THERAPIST—This therapist maximizes the patient's ability to function independently and safely. The occupational therapist will evaluate and treat physical, sensory, visual, cognitive, and behavioral skills as they relate to activities of daily living (eg, feeding, bathing, dressing).

ORTHOPAEDIC SURGEON—The surgeon who treats the injured musculoskeletal system, stressing early fixation and mobilization of the trauma patient.

PHYSIATRIST—The doctor of physical medicine and rehabilitation who evaluates and makes recommendations regarding the rehabilitative aspects of care.

PHYSICAL THERAPIST—The therapist who evaluates and treats functional mobility. Therapy focuses upon strengthening, range of motion, and independence as they relate to movement in bed, transfers, use of a wheelchair, and walking.

RESPIRATORY THERAPIST—The therapist responsible for maintaining adequate breathing in patients in coordination with the physician. The respiratory

continues

Exhibit 14–2 continued

therapist assists the patient in weaning off the ventilator while ensuring that the patient receives adequate oxygen throughout the admission.

SOCIAL WORKER—The professional who provides counseling and support to families in dealing with the feelings inherent in a crisis, such as fear, shock, anger, and hope. The social worker helps orient families to the hospital, obtains a psychosocial history, and directs families to resources in the community.

SPEECH/LANGUAGE PATHOLOGIST—This therapist evaluates and treats communication, language, cognitive, and swallowing deficits. He or she also evaluates and provides recommendations for use of specialized tracheostomy tubes and speaking valves. Treatment areas include cognition, language (comprehension, verbal expression, numerical reasoning), and speech production.

TRAUMA/CRITICAL CARE SURGEON—The surgeon specializing in trauma and critical care who treats the multisystem-injured patient. The traumatologist coordinates and oversees the multidisciplinary approach to trauma patients.

Source: Courtesy of Saint Francis Hospital and Medical Center, Department of Rehabilitation Medicine, Hartford, Connecticut.

in assisting families and patients reacquaint themselves by encouraging and demonstrating contact by touching and talking to the patient. Physical and behavioral interactions between the patient and specific family members can also provide insight into decisions that may be made in the future about caretaking roles.

There is an ongoing need for families to be with or see their loved ones frequently. Patient contact is viewed as critical to the overall adaptation of family members to the crisis. Patient/family contacts can be maximized by suggesting ways to interact that include verbal, nonverbal, and tactile modes. Exhibit 14–3 outlines potential guidelines based upon RLA level.

Feeling Helpful and Needed

During the critical phase following brain injury, the opportunities and responsibilities of caring for an individual are taken away from the family. The instinct to nurture a loved one who is sick or has been hurt is innate. This loss of control leaves families feeling helpless. How often we have heard families say, "I just can't sit here doing nothing"?

Tactile and verbal contact with the patient is critical to family adaptation and serves to reduce feelings of helplessness. Involving the family in patient care also serves a useful purpose in that it provides a focus for heightened family energies. Activities may include involvement at the bedside or performing tasks for the pa-

Exhibit 14–3 Guidelines for Interaction with Patients with Brain Injuries

---

GUIDELINES FOR INTERACTION WITH PATIENTS WITH BRAIN INJURIES

Level I. **No Response**   *Level II.* **Generalized Response**
  A. Suggestions for Interacting with the Patient
    1. Talk to the patient in a normal conversational manner. It may seem awkward to carry on a conversation with a nonresponsive patient. Remember though, that hearing is usually the first sense to return and we really never know what the patient is hearing. For this same reason, do not discuss the patient's medical condition in his or her presence and encourage other family members to avoid doing so.
    2. Provide appropriate stimulation for the patient.
      a. Varying the environmental stimuli is important to the patient. Alternate periods of quiet time with periods of radio, TV or conversation.
      b. Avoid stimuli which seem to startle or frighten the patient.
    3. Change the patient's position frequently, as demonstrated by the nurse or physical therapist.

Level III. **Localized Response**
  A. Suggestions for Interacting with the Patient
    1. Continue to talk to the patient in normal conversational tones. Talk about his or her interests in order to focus his or her attention on you.
    2. Use simple 1-part directions. Use 1 or 2 short sentences at a time. Allow delay time for patient to respond before repeating instructions.
    3. Realize that level of awareness fluctuates and that attention span is very diminished.
    4. Encourage patient to verbalize if appropriate.
    5. Provide orientation to person, place, and time frequently.
    6. Remember that the patient needs appropriate rest periods. Do not constantly bombard patient with stimuli or overly fatigue the patient.
    7. Do not expect patient to remember or recall recent events.
    8. Provide the patient with visual orientation cues (examples: large calendar, family pictures).

Level IV. **Confused/Agitated**
  A. Suggestions for Interacting with the Patient
    1. Family members must realize that agitation is due to patient's own confusion, fear, and disorientation and that he or she is not angry with family or staff.
      a. One of the primary concerns is maintaining patient safety. Physical restraints should be used only when patient safety is compromised.

continues

Exhibit 14–3 continued

   b. Avoid contacts to which the patient responds negatively (eg, physical contact, loud noise).
   c. Do not react to outbursts with anger.
   d. Do not stay with the patient alone if you are uncomfortable or fearful. Do not hesitate to call the nurse for assistance or advice.
   e. Adjust your manner of interacting with the patient to produce a calm, soothing, relaxed atmosphere.
   f. Remember that as the patient progresses to higher levels, he or she will not remember his/her behaviors during this stage.
2. Use short, simple directions and repeat them frequently. Allow for delayed response.
3. Simplify vocabulary you use, and slow down your rate of speech.
4. Don't expect the patient to remember recent events or instructions. Memory span is only minutes long.
   a. If the patient provides incorrect information, correct him or her gently. Do not argue with the patient or criticize him or her for forgetfulness.
5. Provide, rather than test, orientation information frequently (date, hospital, city, cause of hospitalization).
   a. Provide pictures of family members, familiar people, and familiar places for frequent reorientation to the past. Key into the patient's previous areas of interests (hobbies, sports).
6. Prepare the patient for tasks he or she is about to perform. Talk him or her through the task.
7. Don't expect attention span of greater than 2 minutes.
8. Build upon success—pick tasks the patient can complete; don't challenge him or her.
9. Be aware that the patient responds to emotional level of others. If you are nervous, the patient will be nervous.
10. Treat the patient as an adult, not a child.

Level V. **Confused/Inappropriate/Nonagitated**
   A. Suggestions for Interacting with the Patient
      1. The patient will perform automatic tasks best but must be supervised to maintain safety.
      2. Don't expect patients to demonstrate memory of recent events or ability to learn new information at this stage.
         a. Patients are not out of posttraumatic amnesia and cannot retain new information or concentrate on specific tasks for over 2 to 3 minutes. You will need to repeat frequently.
         b. Provide ways to support his or her memory, and reinforce these methods regularly. Printed daily schedules to which you direct his or her attention are helpful.

continues

Exhibit 14–3 continued

3. Provide orientation information without quizzing patient.
   a. Use gentle cues such as "Look at the snow outside," "What time of the year is it?" rather than "What season is it?"
   b. The patient may confabulate about current events or past information. Acknowledge his or her belief, then correct gently. Example: "I know it seems like you are in Boston, but you are really in Hartford."
4. Use 1-step directions and concrete simple vocabulary.
5. The patient will not recognize or understand subtle humor, sarcasm, or voice inflection.
6. Take into account that attention span for individual structured tasks is about 2 to 3 minutes. If you provide enough varied tasks, the patient may work 20 to 30 minutes.
7. Talk to him or her in an adult manner.
8. Agitated or hostile behavior at this level is usually caused by demands or pressures that exceed the patient's tolerance at that moment.
   a. Reassure, don't pressure.
   b. Don't react to anger with expressions of anger. Back off if you need a while to cool down.
   c. If the patient does become agitated, change the task or topics, give him or her a brief rest period, and/or calmly and gently repeat the suggestion to relax.
   d. Some patients respond well to a soothing touch as a reminder to relax.

Level VI. **Confused/Appropriate**
A. Suggestions for Interacting with the Patient
   1. The patient is not yet fully out of posttraumatic amnesia but is beginning to remember some new day-to-day information. His or her recall of the past will be shallow and inconsistent.
      a. You can reduce your cueing to elicit information.
      b. A daily journal will be used to make the patient aware that he or she needs help remembering. You will have to assist in the journal writing, perhaps by writing what he or she tells you about the past half hour's activities and quizzing gently for these recollections.
   2. You can use more complex directions (2-step) and normal vocabulary with the patient.
      a. You will have to be quite concrete and specific.
      b. A patient at this level of recovery will still be unaware of the subtle information communicated in humor, sarcasm, vocal inflection, and gestures.
   3. The patient may need a great deal of emotional support at this time but may maintain emotional control while performing routine tasks that are within his or her capabilities.

continues

Exhibit 14–3 continued

> **4.** Unless a patient needs to learn adaptive techniques, you can expect him or her to take responsibility for performance of basic ADL tasks when reminded and to do other brief tasks without direct supervision.
>
> **5.** The patient may acknowledge his or her physical and memory impairments when you mention them, although he or she will not always be able to volunteer this information independently.

Level VII. **Automatic/Appropriate**
  A. Suggestions for Interacting with the Patient
    1. Use normal conversation when talking with the patient.
      a. At this level, vocabulary does not need to be simplified.
      b. Use moderately complex directions when interacting with the patient (2–3 step).
    2. Expect literal interpretation of what is said.
      a. Patient will not catch subtle humor.
      b. Patient may misunderstand the speaker's intent due to lack of recognition of underlying tone and gestures.
    3. Expect general day-to-day carryover for activities.
      a. Frequently discuss daily events with patient to encourage recall of detail.
      b. Patient should use memory notebook independently as a resource if physically able.
    4. Encourage patient to assume responsibility for his or her daily routine.
      a. Patient should bring self to and from therapies independently with assistance of written schedule if physically capable.
      b. Patient should be responsible for total ADL and general upkeep of room if physically able.
    5. Expect denial of future implications of disabilities (cognitive, physical, memory).
      a. Patient may feel he or she is completely normal, even though he or she may acknowledge some problems when questioned.
      b. The need for continued therapy should be strongly supported by all staff.
      c. Help the patient recognize his or her disabilities and abilities by pointing out examples in behaviors as you observe them.
    6. It may be necessary to design tasks or situations so that the patient can control emotional expressions.
      a. Give patient necessary support to undertake more difficult activities.
      b. Allow patient to express fear or anger about his or her disabilities.
      c. If patient's emotional expressions are dangerous or offensive to others, temporarily remove the patient from the situation and explain why you would prefer he or she act differently.

continues

Exhibit 14-3 continued

Level VIII. **Purposeful/Appropriate**
A. Suggestions for Interacting with the Patient
  1. Use normal conversation when talking with the patient.
    a. Vocabulary does not need to be simplified.
    b. Expect understanding of complex directions.
  2. Patient may continue to take things literally but will respond to explanations of meanings of tone and gestures.
    a. Expect beginning comprehension of underlying meanings in conversation.
    b. Clear up any misunderstandings that may occur by providing appropriate explanations.
  3. Expect detailed carryover of daily events.
    a. Patient should continue to use notebook independently to recall new information.
    b. Reinforce the fact that memory problems may be permanent and that the patient must learn ways to compensate.
  4. Expect patient to carry out daily responsibilities independently (eg, getting up and performing morning routine, transporting self to and from therapy).
  5. Patient will make long-range plans and goals at this level.
    a. Expect patient to begin to incorporate present physical and mental abilities and limitations into his or her future planning.
    b. Patient and staff should engage in mutual planning of goals and methods of accomplishing goals. Consider patient's premorbid activities and interests.
  6. Patient's tolerance for frustration is greatly increased; however, certain situations may continue to produce stress and anger.
    a. Do not expect patient's emotional control to be as good as it was before the injury.
    b. Attempt to discover mutually with the patient what situations will provoke emotional outbursts.
    c. Assist the patient in avoiding these situations or learning new ways to cope with them.

Courtesy of Saint Francis Hospital and Medical Center, Department of Rehabilitation Medicine, Hartford, Connecticut.

tient outside the hospital. Nursing and rehabilitation therapists can help the family care for the patient's personal hygiene, and do positioning or basic range-of-motion exercises.

Although families need to feel helpful, specific members may have different comfort levels. Staff must be sensitive to degrees of family participation. Sisters and brothers may be more enthusiastic and comfortable assisting with exercise and hygiene activities than husbands, wives, and parents, who may feel more comfortable observing and asking questions about patient reactions or responses.

Families can provide unique contributions to staff's overall interactions with the patient. They should be encouraged to bring in labeled photographs of the patient, family, friends, special events, and pets. Individual versus group pictures are preferred. Small objects or items of clothing that may be familiar or meaningful to the patient can also be brought in. These items can be incorporated into treatment sessions, facilitating recognition of familiar or long-term memories.

Families can also paint a unique mental picture of the patient for the staff. Understanding the patient's premorbid personality, likes, dislikes, interests, and values assists staff in viewing the patient as a person rather than a patient. Alerting staff to premorbid difficulties with vision and hearing is also important. Other background information, such as that in Exhibit 14–4, can help provide topics for discussion with the patient during therapy or other interactions. Information on food likes and dislikes can be used by the speech/language pathologist during initial trials with oral feeding.

Subtle signs of premorbid personality can often be ascertained from early patient behaviors and responses. Often the family observes these behaviors first. However, loved ones, out of strong desire and love, can sometimes overrationalize patient responses to mean more than they do. Regardless, staff must be sensitive to relatives' observations. Staff should not automatically negate these observations but should observe and discuss them when the family is present.

The unique assistance relatives can provide promotes a feeling of contribution and inclusion in the overall treatment plan. Family members feel helpful rather than helpless, and this empowers them in the role of contributors throughout the recovery process.

Recognizing Personal Needs

Families consistently place little emphasis on their own personal needs during a crisis. In the earliest stages of crisis, experienced professionals recognize that telling family members to rest or go home to sleep is often futile, even though maintaining adequate rest and nutrition is necessary to mobilize energies. The family should be encouraged to establish an organized system for staggering or alternating visitors. Because early stress and fatigue will cause "burnout," the family should be encouraged to reserve its strength for the period after the initial crisis when the patient's neurologic status has improved. Doing so will provide greater benefit to the patient than maintaining a day-and-night vigil in the early stage of hospitalization.

Nurses can reduce stress by assuring family members that they will be called if any changes occur and that they may call during the night or upon waking. Al-

Exhibit 14–4 Patient Information Sheet Completed by Family Members

---

PATIENT INFORMATION SHEET

In order to plan an individualized treatment program, we request as much detailed information as possible. Please complete this form and return it to a therapist or nurse as soon as possible.

PATIENT NAME: _____ NICKNAME: _____
OCCUPATION (If student, area of study): _____
HIGHEST LEVEL OF EDUCATION: _____
IMMEDIATE/SIGNIFICANT FAMILY MEMBERS (List name and
 relationship):

_____
_____

CLOSE FRIENDS: _____
PETS (list name and type): _____
What kind of music does the patient enjoy?

_____
_____

Hobbies/Interests: _____
Prior to this injury, how would friends describe this person?

_____

What achievements, interests, or goals are most important to this person?

_____

Hand Dominance: Left   Right   Glasses: Yes   No
Hearing Problems: Yes   No   **Please bring in glasses or hearing aid**
List Favorite Foods: _____
Does he/she like: oatmeal Yes No   chocolate/vanilla pudding: Yes No
chocolate/vanilla milkshake Yes No   chocolate/vanilla ice cream   Yes No
                     sherbert   Yes No
List foods this person dislikes: _____
List foods this person is allergic to: _____
Other: _____
_____
_____
_____
_____

Courtesy of Saint Francis Hospital and Medical Center, Department of Rehabilitation Medicine, Hartford, Connecticut.

though schedules are difficult to set in the ICU, families should be told approximately when therapy will be provided or when medical procedures and team rounds will occur. Reducing waiting time allows the family an opportunity to schedule activities and meet outside obligations.

Loved ones are frequently concerned with issues affecting major family responsibilities, such as loss of income and the need for financial support or long-term care of children. These concerns may be set aside during the early focus on the patient's prospects for immediate survival. Responsibilities of work, school, and parenting cannot be ignored, however, and the family soon realizes it must continue to perform critical functions. Redefining roles and responsibilities becomes necessary, taxing coping energies, yet also providing a therapeutic avenue for positive action.

SPECIAL NEEDS OF CHILDREN AND SIBLINGS

Children or siblings may have as many or more problems than adult family members. Depending on age, children have difficulties understanding what has happened to their parent or sibling. When a parent has been injured, his or her absence may be associated with desertion or punishment. Consequently, the child may fear that the remaining parent will leave as well. Nightmares and aggressive behaviors may develop. As the uninjured parent spends excessive time at the hospital, younger children remaining at home often feel neglected and insecure.[7]

Parents experience guilt when away from the patient, as well as guilt when away from children at home. Stress bears heavily on parents who return home from the hospital needing to interact and play with children, despite their overwhelming fatigue. Young children may resent an injured parent or sibling because of the attention he or she is receiving.

Negative behaviors are frequently noted, including aggressive interactions with peers, fighting, acting out, emotional outbursts, poor academic performance, and both physical and verbal withdrawal. For these reasons, parents should inform teachers of the ensuing crisis situation. Once the source of the behaviors (ie, the acute injury and crisis) is recognized, adjusting responses, improving parent/child communication, and restructuring and accommodating daily schedules can help reduce these behaviors. Children should be provided a means of participating and contributing to the recovery process. Young children should be encouraged to make cards, pictures, and even audiotapes that can be brought into the hospital. Activities can be coordinated by the uninjured parent and other relatives or in school by the child's teacher.

CULTURAL DIVERSITY IN THE CONTEXT OF CRITICAL CARE

Human beings comprise varied geographic populations called races. Race, however, does not determine how people behave or react. Those responses are inherently cultural. Culture encompasses religious and spiritual dimensions, language and communication patterns, and behavioral roles. Norms, values, and beliefs, family dynamics, economics, diet, and dress are all culturally defined.[52] Ethnic cultural groups have a sense of identity in their roots and historical ancestral ties. Cultural aspects are learned, are passed from one generation to the next, and guide thinking, decision making, and actions in a patterned way.[53] Cultures are not permanently fixed; they are dynamic and ever-evolving. As we enter the close of the 20th century, the United States continues to expand its cultural diversity.

The combination of saving lives and humanizing care is a great challenge and responsibility that falls upon critical care staff. In its own manner, the critical care environment is a subculture. Staff have their own values, beliefs, worldviews, and interpretations, as do their consumers, the patients and families who come to the unit for care. Therefore, health care professionals must consider cultural factors within the context of the medical environment. Changing demographics support the need for understanding and respecting patient and family cultural differences. In times of crisis, people do not put aside but rather rely more heavily on their deeply ingrained cultural ties.

Some cultural dispositions do exist and are not unfounded or erroneous. Expansive literature is available documenting rituals and customary behaviors of many ethnic groups.[52,54-7] Beliefs and behaviors that affect health and illness and death and dying are part of every culture. Within this context, disease and illness are not synonymous; rather, the disease is what the physician treats, and the illness is what the patient experiences. "Disease is malfunction or maladaptation of the biologic or psychophysiologic subsystem of the individual."[52(p64)] Illness, however, involves an individual's personal, interpersonal, and cultural responses to the disease.[72] Illness, therefore, is culturally shaped. Cultural beliefs affect how health problems are identified and discussed, how treatment is pursued, to whom one goes for care, and how that care is evaluated.[73]

Medical advances with ethical implications, such as life-sustaining measures, have revealed variations in cultural responses. For example, substantially fewer minority populations take advantage of advance directives. More African Americans and Hispanics support life-sustaining measures regardless of severity of illness, whereas more whites agree to stop life-sustaining measures in the face of terminal illness.[74,75] Persons of color are also often skeptical of the health care system. With a complex history of limited access to services, individuals within these cultures may not trust physicians to act in the patient's best interest.[76] Patients and families are not likely to disclose much about themselves to staff unless a trusting relationship is established.

"In a sense, because of changing medical technology, death has moved from the realm of nature to that of culture in our society."[77(p247)] Modern bioethics is largely based on the cultural beliefs of white, middle-class, Western philosophy, which emphasizes individual decision making. Yet for many cultures, decision-making styles are largely family centered. Family-centered decision making is especially true for Mexican American and Korean American families.[70] Asians often retain the cultural values of strong familial interdependency. In many Asian subcultures, a patriarchal structure is supported within the family. Responsibility and decisions are passed from fathers to eldest sons.[52] Chinese and Ethiopian families specifically oppose truth telling because they feel it causes the patient to lose hope.[78,79] In many Afro-Caribbean cultures, the extended family structure may be complex, but family influence is strong, often affecting the decision-making process.[59]

Some cultures have strong beliefs regarding medical issues. Jehovah's Witnesses and Rastafarians may reject blood transfusions. Muslims may object to organ transplantation.[64] Some cultures, such as Muslim, Sikh, and Hindu cultures, value modesty highly and prefer female physicians to treat female patients.[62–64]

Caution, however, must be exercised to avoid culturally stereotyping individuals. Negative stereotypes can be fostered when staff are supplied with an atlas of cultural traits common among ethnic groups. Additionally, staff must guard against cultural imposition, the act of imposing one's own philosophy irrespective of an individual's values and beliefs.

The more sound method of interpretation is to read patients, as opposed to judging culture as a demographic variable that predicts specific behaviors. Gender differences should also be approached in a similar fashion. "Considering culture as a predictive variable is inherently limited—that is, simply plugging race or ethnicity into a multiple-regression analysis or, in a clinical context, assuming someone's name, appearance, or national origin is a predictive factor."[77(p245)] The inherent limitation with the concept of common cultural traits is that they disregard or cloud the important intracultural variations that exist in most societies. Culture is constantly evolving and is meaningful only when interpreted within the context of a patient's unique history, family constellation, and socioeconomic status.

Koenig and Gates-Williams[77(p248)] suggest that rather than using a cookbook approach to culture, one should assess each patient and family individually, while following uniquely culturally sensitive guidelines. These guidelines are outlined in Exhibit 14–5.

Individual cultural beliefs should be accommodated as long as the act does not interfere with clinical management or is not dangerous to the patient or others in the environment. A dying Muslim patient may wish to lie with his or her face toward Mecca. Moving the patient's bed or repositioning the head toward the right shoulder can generally be accommodated with relative ease. In direct contrast are those beliefs that create dispute and conflict. Physicians, also, act in accord with deeply held values, since biomedicine has its own set of cultural practices.

Advances in medicine have improved the salvageability of the life, creating new challenges in the areas of death and dying. The use of life support and issues of brain death, for example, confront the physician and family with ethical dilem-

Exhibit 14–5 Culturally Sensitive Guidelines for Family Assessment

1. Assess the language used to discuss the patient's illness and disease, including the degree of openness in discussing the diagnosis, prognosis, and death itself.
2. Determine whether decisions are made by the patient or a large social unit, such as the family.
3. Consider the relevance of religious beliefs, particularly about the meaning of death, the existence of an afterlife, and belief in miracles.
4. Determine who controls access to the body and how the body should be approached after death.
5. Assess how hope for a recovery is negotiated within the family and with health care professionals.
6. Assess the patient's degree of fatalism versus an active desire for the control of events into the future.
7. Consider issues of generation or age, gender, and power relationships, both within the patient's family and in interactions with the health care team.
8. Take into account the political and historical context, particularly poverty, refugee status, past discrimination, and lack of access to care.
9. To aid in the complex task of interpreting the relevance of cultural dimensions in a particular case, make use of available resources, including community or religious leaders, family members, and language translators.

Source: Reprinted with permission of *The Western Journal of Medicine,* Vol. 163, No. 3, p. 248), © 1995, The Western Journal of Medicine.

mas. "The challenge for clinical practice is to allow ethical pluralism—a true engagement with and respect for diverse perspectives—without falling into the trap of absolute ethical relativism."[77(p248)]

CONCLUSION

The family and its support system play a vital role in the continuum of care following severe brain injury. The way in which the family responds to a crisis may drastically affect the outcome for the injured individual. The health care system places expectations on the family to cope appropriately, provide the necessary support for the patient, and follow through on recommendations and suggestions. The family also enters the crisis with expectations of the health care system. It depends on the hospital to provide the best care possible, to be open and honest with information, to be accessible to the family, and to be culturally sensitive to the individual needs of the patient and family. The immediate nature of the crisis does not allow the family to prepare its response or to understand the nature of brain injury. In the initial stages of the crisis, its reactions and responses will be based on its premorbid values, coping mechanisms, cultural and ethnic traditions, support systems, and past experiences. The prophylactic inclusion of family dynamics in the curriculum for health care personnel would facilitate more effective understanding of psychosocial roles and cultural forces and their impact on outcome.[80]

Health care personnel also bear the responsibility of understanding the full continuum of recovery from brain injury. All team members must work together to assist families in understanding the "whole picture" in terms of what has occurred and what is to come. Trauma centers should incorporate a forum to celebrate the successful triumphs of the survivors and their families, inviting health care providers, including physicians, to participate. These gatherings reinforce the perseverance, hard work, and endless potential that these individuals and their families possess.

REFERENCES

1. Cope DN, Wolfson B. Crisis intervention with the family in the trauma setting. *J Head Trauma Rehabil*. 1994;9:67–81.

2. Soderstrom S, Fogelsjoo A, Fugl-Meyer KS, Stensson S. A program for crisis-intervention after traumatic brain injury. *Scand J Rehab Med*. 1988;17(suppl):47–49.

3. Kleeman K. Family systems adaptation. In: Cardona VD, Hurn PD, Mason PJ, Scanlon AM, Verse-Berry SW, et al, eds. *Trauma Nursing from Resuscitation to Rehabilitation*. Philadelphia, Pa: WB Saunders Co; 1988:199–219.

4. Baker J. Family adaptation when one member has a head injury. *J Neurosci Nurs*. 1990;22:232–237.

5. Testani-Dufour L, Chappel-Aiken L, Gueldner S. Traumatic brain injury: a family experience. *J Neurosci Nurs*. 1992;24:317–323.

6. Mauss-Clum N, Ryan MR. Brain injury and the family. *J Neurosurg Nurs*. 1981;13:165–169.

7. Rodgers P, Kreutzer JS. Family crisis following head injury: network intervention strategy. *J Neurosurg Nurs*. 1984;16:343–346.

8. Caplan G. *Principles of Preventive Psychiatry*. New York, NY: Basic Books; 1964.

9. Aguilera DC. *Crisis Intervention: Theory and Methodology*. 7th ed. St Louis, Mo: Mosby; 1994.

10. Kercher EE. Crisis intervention in the emergency department. *Emerg Med Clin North Am*. 1991;9:219–232.

11. Hobbs M. Crisis intervention in theory and practice: a selective review. *Br J Med Psychol*. 1984;57:23–34.

12. Thomas W. *A Sourcebook of Social Origins*. Boston, Mass: R Gadger; 1909.

13. Lindemann E. Symptomatology and management of acute grief. *Am J Psychiatry*. 1944;101:141–148.

14. Freud S. Determinism, belief in chance and superstition: some points of view. In: Strachey JS, ed. *The Standard Edition of the Complete Psychological Works of Sigmund Freud*. Vol 6. London, England: Hogarth Press; 1901.

15. Caplan G. *An Approach to Community Mental Health.* London, England: Tavistock; 1964.

16. Cavanaugh S. Psychiatric emergencies. *Med Clin North Am.* 1986;70:1185–1202.

17. Fahy TJ, Irving MH, Millac P. Severe head injuries: a six-year follow-up. *Lancet.* 1967;2:475–479.

18. Rife JM. *Injured Mind, Shattered Dreams.* Cambridge, Mass: Brookline Books; 1994.

19. Braulin JLD, Rook J, Sillis GM. Families in crisis: the impact of trauma. *Crit Care Q.* 1982;5:38–46.

20. Moonilal JM. Trauma centers: a new dimension for hospital social work. *Soc Work Health Care.* 1982;7:15–25.

21. Molter NC. Needs of relatives of critically ill patients: a descriptive study. *Heart Lung.* 1979;8:332–339.

22. Rodgers CD. Needs of relatives of cardiac surgery patients during the critical care phase. *Focus Crit Care.* 1983;10:50–55.

23. Mathis M. Personal needs of family members of critically ill patients with and without acute brain injury. *J Neurosurg Nurs.* 1984;16:36–44.

24. Daley L. The perceived immediate needs of families with relatives in the intensive care setting. *Heart Lung.* 1984;13:231–237.

25. Bouman CC. Identifying priority concerns of families of ill patients. *Dimens Crit Care Nurs.* 1984;3:313–319.

26. Stillwell SB. Importance of visiting needs as perceived by family members of patients in the intensive care unit. *Heart Lung.* 1984;13 238–242.

27. Spatt L, Ganas E, Hying S, Kirsch E, Koch M. Informational needs of families of intensive care patients. *Qual Rev Bull.* 1986;12:16–21.

28. Leske JS. The needs of relatives of critically ill patients: a follow-up. *Heart Lung.* 1986;15:189–193.

29. O'Neill-Norris L, Grove SK. Investigation of selected psychosocial needs of family members of critically ill patients *Heart Lung.* 1986;15:194–199.

30. Lynn-McHale DJ, Bellinger A. Need satisfaction levels of family members of critical care patients and accuracy of nurses' perceptions. *Heart Lung.* 1988;17:447–453.

31. Jaconio J, Hicks G, Antonioni C, O'Brien K, Rasi M. Comparison of perceived needs of family members between registered nurses and family members of critically ill patients in intensive care and neonatal intensive care units. *Heart Lung.* 1990;19:72–78.

32. Forrester DA, Murphy PA, Price DM, Monaghan JF. Critical care family needs: nurse-family members confederate pairs. *Heart Lung.* 1990;19:655–661.

33. Hickey M. What are the needs of families of critically ill patients? A review of the literature since 1976. *Heart Lung.* 1990; 19:401–415.

34. Price DM, Forrester DA, Murphy PA, Monaghan JF. Critical care family needs in an urban teaching medical center. *Heart Lung.* 1991;20:183–188.

35. Freichels TA. Needs of family members of patients in the intensive care unit over time. *Crit Care Nurs Q.* 1991;14:16–29.

36. Rukholm E, Bailey P, Coutu-Wakulczyk G, Bailey WB. Needs and anxiety levels in relatives of intensive care unit patients. *J Adv Nurs.* 1991;16:920–928.

37. Macey BA, Bouman CC. An evaluation of validity, reliability, and readability of the Critical Care Family Needs Inventory. *Heart Lung.* 1991;20:398–403.

38. Murphy PA, Forrester DA, Price DM, Monaghan JF. Empathy of intensive care nurses and critical care family needs assessment. *Heart Lung.* 1991;21:25–30.

39. Engli M, Kirsivali-Farmer K. Needs of family members of critically ill patients with and without acute brain injury. *J Neurosci Nurs.* 1993;25:78–85.

40. Foss KR, Tenholder MF. Expectations and needs of persons with family members in an intensive care unit as opposed to a general ward. *South Med J.* 1993;86:380–384.

41. Warren NA. Perceived needs of the family members in the critical care waiting room. *Crit Care Nurs Q.* 1993;16:56–63.

42. Dewey J. How We Think. Boston, Mass: DC Heath; 1910.

43. Aguilera DC, Messick JM. *Crisis Intervention: Theory and Methodology.* 4th ed. St Louis, Mo: CV Mosby Co; 1982.

44. Soderstrom S, Fogelsjoo A, Fugl-Meyer KS, Stenson S. Traumatic brain injury crisis intervention and family therapy: management and outcome. *Scand J Rehabil Med.* 1992;26(suppl):132–141.

45. Epperson MM. Families in sudden crisis: process and intervention in a critical care center. *Soc Work Health Care.* 1977;2:265–274.

46. Hagen C. Language disorders secondary to closed head injury: diagnosis and treatment. *Top Lang Disord.* 1981;1:73–87.

47. Grahame L. The family system in acute care and acute rehabilitation. In: Williams JM, Kay T, eds. *Head Injury: A Family Matter.* Baltimore, Md: Paul H Brookes Publishing; 1991.

48. Paul L. Crisis intervention. *Ment Hyg.* 1966;50:141–145.

49. Coleman JC. Abnormal Psychology and Modern Life. Chicago, Ill: Scott, Foresman & Co; 1950.

50. Cropley A, Field T. Achievement in science and intellectual style. *J Appl Psychol.* 1969;53: 132–135.

51. Kleeman KM. Families in crisis due to multiple trauma. *Crit Care Nurs Clin North Am.* 1989; 1:23–31.

52. Germain CP. Cultural concepts in critical care. *Crit Care Q.* 1982:61–77.

53. Leininger M. *Transcultural Nursing: Concepts, Theories, and Practices.* New York, NY: John Wiley & Sons; 1978.

54. Spector R. *Cultural Diversity in Health and Illness.* New York, NY: Appleton-Century-Crofts; 1979.

55. DeGarcia RT. Health care of the American-Asian patient. *Crit Care Update.* 1980;7:16–29.

56. Murillo-Rhode I. Health care for the Hispanic patient. *Crit Care Update.* 1980;7:29–36.

57. Bello TA. The Latino patient in the emergency department. *J Emerg Nurs.* 1980;6:13–26.

58. Shubin S. Nursing patients from different cultures. *Nursing.* 1980;80:78–81.

59. Green J. Death with dignity: the Afro-Caribbean community. *Nurs Times.* 1993;88:50–51.

60. Green J. Death with dignity: Buddhism. *Nurs Times.* 1989;85:40–41.

61. Green J. Death with dignity: Judaism. *Nurs Times.* 1989;85:64–65.

62. Green J. Death with dignity: Sikhism. *Nurs Times.* 1989;85:56–57.

63. Green J. Death with dignity: Hinduism. *Nurs Times.* 1989;85:50–51.

64. Green J. Death with dignity: Islam. *Nurs Times.* 1989;85:56–57.

65. Turner-Weeden P. Death and dying from a Native American perspective. In: Infeld DL, Gordon AK, Harper BC, eds. *Hospice Care and Cultural Diversity.* Binghamton, NY: Haworth Press; 1995:11–13.

66. Zeller C. Cultural vignettes: a multicultural educational teaching strategy. *Nurs Educator*. 1995:20:8–9.

67. Pickett M. Cultural awareness in the context of terminal illness. *Cancer Nurs*. 1993;16:102–106.

68. Talamantes MA, Lawler WR, Espino DV. Hispanic American elders: caregiving norms surrounding dying and the use of hospice services. In: Infeld DL, Gordon AK, Harper BC, eds. *Hospice Care and Cultural Diversity*. Binghamton, NY: Haworth Press; 1995:35–49.

69. Asai A, Fukuhara S. Lo B. Attitudes of Japanese and Japanese-American physicians towards life-sustaining treatment. *Lancet*. 1995;346:356–359.

70. Blackhall LJ, Murphy ST, Frank G. Ichel V, Azen S. Ethnicity and attitudes toward patient autonomy. *JAMA*. 1995;274:820–825.

71. Neubauer BJ, Hamilton CL. Racial differences in attitudes toward hospice care. *Hospice J*. 1990;6:37–48.

72. Kleinman A. Concepts and a model for the comparison of medical systems as cultural systems. *Soc Sci Med*. 1978;12:85–93.

73. Kleinman A. Culture, illness, and care: clinical lessons from anthropologic and cross-cultural research. *Ann Intern Med*. 1978;88:251–258.

74. Garrett J, Harris RP, Norborn JK, Patrick DL, Danis M. Life-sustaining treatments during terminal illness: who wants what? *J Gen Intern Med*. 1993;8:361–368.

75. Caralis PV, Davis B. Wright K, Marcial E. The influence of ethnicity and race on attitudes toward advance directives, life-prolonging treatments, and euthanasia. *J Clin Ethics*. 1993;4:155–165.

76. Adler NE, Boyce WT, Chesney MA, Folkman S, Syme SL. Socioeconomic inequalities in health: no easy solution. *JAMA*. 1993;269:3140–3145.

77. Koenig BA, Gates-Williams J. Understanding cultural difference in caring for dying patients. *West J Med*. 1995;163:244–249.

78. Muller JH, Desmond B. Ethical dilemmas in a cross-cultural context: a Chinese example. *West J Med*. 1992;157:323–327.

79. Beyene Y. Medical disclosure and refugees: telling bad news to Ethiopian patients. *West J Med*. 1992;157:328–332.

80. Craig MC. Copes WS, Champion HR. Psychosocial considerations in health care. *Crit Care Nurs Q*. 1988;11:51–58.

State Brain Injury Associations and Affiliates

ALABAMA Head Injury Foundation
PO Box 550008, Birmingham, AL 35255
(205) 328-3505, (800) 433-8002, FAX (205) 328-2479

ARIZONA Head Injury Foundation
630 North Craycroft Road, Suite 139, Tucson, AZ 85711-1441
(520) 747-7140, (800) 432-3465, FAX (602) 790-4409

Brain Injury Association of ARKANSAS
PO Box 935, North Little Rock, AR 72115-0935
(501) 771-5011, (800) 235-2443

CALIFORNIA Head Injury Foundation
PO Box 160786, Sacramento, CA 95816-0786
(916) 442-1710, (800) 457-CHIF, FAX (916) 442-7305

Brain Injury Association of COLORADO, Inc.
6825 East Tennessee Avenue, Suite 405, Denver, CO 80224
(303) 355-9969, (800) 955-2443, FAX (303) 355-9968

Brain Injury Association of CONNECTICUT, Inc.
1800 Silas Deane Highway, Suite 224, Rocky Hill, CT 06067
(860) 721-8111, (800) 278-8242, FAX (860) 721-9008

DELAWARE Head Injury Foundation
PO Box 9876, Newark, DE 19714
(302) 475-2286, (800) 411-0505

Courtesy of Brain Injury Association, Washington, D.C.

Brain Injury Association of FLORIDA, Inc.
North Broward Medical Center
201 East Sample Road, Pomparo Beach, FL 33064
(954) 786-2400, (800) 992-3442, FAX (954) 786-2437

Brain Injury Association of GEORGIA
1447 Peachtree Street NE, Suite 810, Atlanta, GA 30309
(404) 817-7577, FAX (404) 817-7521

Brain Injury Association of ILLINOIS
1127 South Mannheim Road, Suite 213, Westchester, IL 60154
(708) 344-4646, (800) 699-6443, FAX (708) 344-4680

Brain Injury Association of INDIANA
5506 East 16th Street, Suite B-5, Indianapolis, IN 46218
(317) 356-7722, (800) 407-4246, FAX (317) 356-4241

Brain Injury Association of IOWA, Inc.
2101 Kimball Avenue LL7, Waterloo, IA 50702
(319) 291-3552, (800) 475-4442, FAX (319) 291-3484

Brain Injury Association of KANSAS and Greater Kansas City
1100 Pennsylvania, Suite 305, Kansas City, MO 64105-1336
(816) 842-8607, (800) 783-1356, FAX (816) 842-1531

Brain Injury Association of KENTUCKY
3910 Dupont Square South, Suite D, Louisville, KY 40207-4648
(502) 899-7141, (800) 592-1117, FAX (502) 899-7141

LOUISIANA Head Injury Foundation
217 Buffwood Drive, Baker, LA 70714-3755
(504) 775-2780, FAX (504) 387-6252

Brain Injury Association of MAINE
PO Box 2224, Augusta, ME 04338-2224
(207) 626-0022, (800) 275-1233, FAX (207) 622-6947

Brain Injury Association of MARYLAND Inc
916 South Rolling Road, Baltimore, MD 21228
(410) 747-7758, (800) 221-6443, FAX (410) 747-7759

MASSACHUSETTS Brain Injury Association
Denholm Building, 484 Main Street, Suite 325, Worcester, MA 01608
(508) 795-0244, (800) 242-0030, FAX (508) 757-9109

Brain Injury Association of MICHIGAN Inc
8137 W. Grand River, Suite A, Brighton, MI 48116-9346
(810) 229-5880, (800) 772-4323, FAX (810) 229-8947

Brain Injury Association of MINNESOTA
43 Main Street SE, Suite 135, Minneapolis, MN 55414
(612) 378-2742, (800) 669-6442, FAX (612) 378-2789

MISSISSIPPI Head Injury Association
PO Box 55912, Jackson, MS 39296-5912
(601) 981-1021, (800) 641-6442, FAX (601) 981-5562

Brain Injury Association of MISSOURI
700 Corporate Park Drive, Suite 330, St. Louis, MO 63105
(314) 862-4466, (800) 377-6442, FAX (314) 726-0051

Brain Injury Association of MONTANA
MSU-B Montana Center, Room 147, Billings, MT 59101-0298
(406) 657-2077, FAX (406) 657-2807

Brain Injury Association of NEBRASKA Inc.
PO Box 397, Milford, NE 68405
(402) 761-2781, (800) 743-4781, FAX (402) 761-2219

NEW HAMPSHIRE Brain Injury Foundation
2 1/2 Beacon Street, Suite 17, Concord, NH 03301
(603) 225-8400

NEW JERSEY Head Injury Association Inc.
1090 King George Post Road, Suite 708, Edison, NJ 08837
(908) 738-1002, (800) 669-4323, FAX (908) 738-1132

NEW MEXICO Head Injury Foundation
2819 Richmond NE, Albuquerque, NM 87107
(505) 889-8008, (800) 279-7480, FAX (505) 883-1079

Brain Injury Association of NEW YORK State
10 Colvin Avenue, Albany, NY 12206
(518) 459-7911, (800) 228-8201, FAX (518) 482-5285

Brain Injury Association of NORTH CAROLINA Inc
PO Box 748, 133 Fayetteville Street Mall, Suite 310, Raleigh, NC 27602
(919) 833-9634, (800) 377-1454, FAX (919) 833-5414

Head Injury Association of NORTH DAKOTA
2111 E. Main Avenue, Suite 14, West Fargo, ND 58708
(701) 281-0527, (800) 279-6344, FAX (701) 281-3878

OHIO Head Injury Association
1335 Dublin Road, Suite 50-A, Columbus, OH 43215-1000
(614) 481-7100, (800) 686-9553, FAX (614) 481-7103

Brain Injury Association of OKLAHOMA Inc
PO Box 88, Hillsdale, OK 73743-0088
(405) 635-2237, (800) 765-6809, FAX (405) 635-2238

Brain Injury Association of OREGON
1118 Lancaster Drive NE, Suite 345, Salem, OR 97301
(503) 585-0855, (800) 544-5243

Brain Injury Association of SOUTH CAROLINA
PO Box 1945, Orangeburg, SC 29116
(803) 533-1613, (800) 767-9701, FAX (803) 531-3376

Brain Injury Association of TENNESSEE
699 W. Main Street, Suite 208, Hendersonville, TN 37075
(615) 264-3052, (800) 480-6693

Brain Injury Association of TEXAS
6633 Highway 290 East, Suite 306, Austin, TX 78723
(512) 467-6872, (800) 392-0040, FAX (512) 467-9035

Brain Injury Association of UTAH
1800 S West Temple, Suite 203, Box 22, Salt Lake City, UT 84115
(801) 484-2240, (800) 281-8442, FAX (801) 484-5932

VERMONT Head Injury Foundation
PO Box 1837, Station A, Rutland, VT 05701
(802) 446-3017

Brain Injury Association of VIRGINIA
3212 Cutshaw Avenue, Suite 315, Richmond, VA 23230
(804) 355-5748, (800) 334-8443, FAX (804) 355-6381

Brain Injury Association of WASHINGTON
PO Box 52890, Bellevue, WA 98015-2890
(206) 451-0000, (800) 523-LIFT, FAX (206) 536-0620

Brain Injury Association of WEST VIRGINIA
PO Box 574, Institute, WV 25112-4892
(304) 766-4892, (800) 356-6443, FAX (304) 766-4940

Brain Injury Association of WISCONSIN Inc
735 N. Water Street, Suite 701, Milwaukee, WI 53202
(414) 271-7463, (800) 882-9282, FAX (414) 271-7166

Brain Injury Association of WYOMING
246 South Center, Suite 16, Casper, WY 82601
(307) 473-1767, (800) 643-6457, FAX (307) 237-5222

The following are BIA contacts in the representative states:

ALASKA Head Injury Foundation
8121 E. 18th Avenue, Anchorage, AK 99504
(907) 337-1441

IDAHO Head Injury Association
76 West 100 North, Blackfoot, ID 83221
(208) 785-0685

PACIFIC Head Injury Foundation
1775 S. Beretania, Room 203, Honolulu, HI 96826
(808) 941-0372

SOUTH DAKOTA Brain Injury Association
221 South Central, Suite 32, Pierre, SD 57501

SOUTHERN NEVADA Head Injury Association
4074 Autumn Street, Las Vegas, NV 89120
(702) 452-2674

NORTHERN NEVADA Head Injury Association
Nevada Community Enrichment Program
70 Smithridge Drive, Suite C, Reno, NV 89502
(702) 828-7171

WASHINGTON DC Head Injury Foundation
2100 Mayflower Drive, Lake Ridge, VA 22191
(202) 877-1464

NOVA SCOTIA Head Injury Association
PO Box 499, Dartmouth, NS B2Y 3Y8, CANADA
(902) 425-5060

CHAPTER 15

The Benefits of Combining Rehabilitation with Critical Care: Future Focus in Therapy and Medications

Critically ill patients with severe brain injuries are remaining alive longer and surviving devastating pathophysiologic changes. Increased survival is largely due to recent advances in our understanding of cellular physiology, immunity, nutrition, sepsis, treatment techniques, and technology. Published research involving the basic sciences and clinical therapeutic contributions as they relate to severe brain injury and improved outcomes has increased significantly in the past decade. Studies use different methodologies to demonstrate these facts and can be classified in three categories:

- Class I—Prospective randomized controlled trials; gold standard of clinical trials
- Class II—Prospective data collection and retrospective analysis
- Class III—Retrospective data collection[1]

The focuses of present and future research include increasing understanding of basic science contributions, early pharmacologic intervention, critical care management, and rehabilitation. These areas encompass the most promising future advances in the quest to improve functional outcomes for individuals with severe brain injury.

BENEFITS OF SECONDARY MEDICAL PREVENTION

Reduced morbidity is anticipated when patients receive care in a contained area with specially trained and adequately deployed staff. Secondary prevention involves reducing or eliminating medical or other cascading effects secondary to an incurred brain injury. These benefits, however, are difficult to document. Medical interventions have short- and long-term consequences and can be viewed from an economic or medical perspective.[2] Short-term benefits include acute patient responses to interventions, reduced complications, and reduced lengths of stay (LOSs) in the intensive care unit (ICU). Long-term benefits include decreased mortality, reduced LOSs, and increased functional outcomes after discharge.

The primary goals of management of severe brain injury in the ICU are preventing secondary neurologic injury and reducing complications that develop in other organ systems. Neuromedical concerns include the treatment and monitoring of elevated intracranial pressure (ICP), treatment of respiratory insufficiency and/or failure, and identification and treatment of medical complications, such as electrolyte abnormalities, pneumonia, and sepsis.

Timely initiation of many interventions in the critical care environment can influence neurologic recovery. Promptly recognizing and treating increased ICP, for example, can improve chances for survival and potentially neurologic outcome.[3-11] Other complications, if not prevented with aggressive early interactions, can increase lengths of stay and initiate a cascade of other problems that may delay or impede recovery.[12]

Hypotension and hypoxia have a deleterious effect on patient outcomes.[10,13-19] Several class II studies support this premise. Because early hypotension has been found to significantly increase morbidity and mortality, it should be avoided or quickly corrected.[13,14,20] Suggested guidelines include avoiding systolic blood pressure of less than or equal to 90 mm Hg and a Pao_2 of less than or equal to 60 mm Hg. The association between hypotension and outcome is related to the adequacy of cerebral perfusion. Improved mortality for patients with severe brain injury has been reported in studies in which cerebral perfusion pressure (CPP) was actively maintained above 70 mm Hg[21-25] when compared with mortality rates from the Traumatic Coma Data Bank.[26] It is difficult to isolate CPP management, within these studies, as the sole intervention that improved outcomes. However, no adverse effects have been reported in the maintenance of adequate CPP (>70 mm Hg). Research suggests that maintaining CPP in that range can substantially reduce mortality and improve neurologic outcome.

The use of early prophylactic hyperventilation can also have deleterious effects on outcome for patients with severe brain injury. A recent class I study demonstrated significantly improved three- and six-month outcomes for patients who were not prophylactically hyperventilated.[27] Research suggests that prophylactic hyperventilation should be avoided during the first five days post injury, with specific emphasis on the initial 24 hours.

Metabolic events occur as a result of severe brain injury and have been implicated in secondary neuronal injury. Optimal nutrition can improve these processes and thereby affect the mortality and neurologic recovery rates of patients with severe brain injury. Correlations between mortality and inadequate nutrient intake have been shown.[28] Short-term outcomes are significantly improved in patients receiving early parenteral nutrition as compared to enterally fed patients receiving less calories and protein.[29] Improved neurologic outcomes have also been noted when there is less caloric deficit.[30,31]

Ethical considerations limit the use of nonfed control groups to prove the neurologic benefit of nutritional support. However, the majority of available literature supports the need for early (by day 7) adequate nutritional support to combat the adverse effects of extreme catabolism. Additionally, nutritional support also appears to decrease the incidence of infectious complications.

Different medical interventions have been examined to determine effect on patient outcomes. Unfortunately, many studies assess only short-term outcomes. Certainly, some of these short-term benefits can eliminate or reduce other cascading secondary events or reduce LOS and hospital costs. The present and future challenge is to extend these studies to identify potential impact on long-term and functional outcomes.

FUTURE MEDICAL ADVANCES

New advances in the understanding of the pathophysiology of brain injury are emerging from laboratory research and new monitoring modalities in the ICU. Much of the neurologic dysfunction caused by a brain injury is due not to the initial insult but to the secondary cascade of biochemical events initiated by the injury.[32-35] The knowledge that neuronal damage may be progressive and not complete at the time of insult implies that there are windows of opportunity during which interventions may be implemented that could prevent or significantly reduce secondary damage. A variety of potential therapies are currently being tested in both animal and human models.

Pharmacologic Intervention

Biochemical mediators of secondary brain injury include oxygen free radical toxicity, lipid peroxidation, excitatory amino acids, and autolytic enzymes. Areas of active neuropharmacologic research involve the role of oxygen radical scavengers, N-methyl-D-aspartate (NMDA) antagonists, calcium antagonists, and catecholamines.

Excitatory Amino Acids

A massive release of inhibitory and excitatory neurotransmitters occurs shortly after brain injury. Levels of glutamate, acetylcholine, and aspartate, all excitatory amino acids, increase. These events result in the opening of receptor-activated postsynaptic channels, allowing massive cellular calcium ion influx.[33,36,37] Of the three main receptor sites, the NMDA receptor site exerts greater control over calcium entry and is 70% more permeable to calcium entry than the quisqualate and kainate receptors.[38] High levels of calcium activate phospholipases, which increase arachidonic acid metabolism.[39] As levels continue to increase, a hypermetabolic state ensues.[40-42] Increased metabolism depletes glucose stores, and the injured tissue becomes unable to generate new glucose. This cascade of events ultimately results in cell death.

NMDA antagonists inhibit the effect of excitatory amino acids. Blocking the excitatory amino acid receptor sites limits the amount of metabolic activity occurring at the site of injury and potentially prevents additional tissue trauma and ischemia. Pharmacologically, glutamate toxicity can be reduced by blocking the NMDA receptor. Drug studies have focused on noncompetitive compounds such as dextromethorphan and dizocilpine maleate, also known as MK-801, and competitive antagonists, such as CGS 19775 and d-CPP-ene.[43-49]

Both noncompetitive and competitive NMDA antagonists appear to increase regional cerebral blood flow.[50] MK-801 has been found to be neuroprotective in animals with focal ischemia.[51-53] d-CPP-ene, another NMDA receptor antagonist, is highly potent in binding to receptor sites and has been found to cross the blood-brain barrier more effectively than MK-801.[54] d-CPP-ene also has anticonvulsant properties.[55] Some animal studies on NMDA antagonists suggest trends toward improved neurologic recovery, including reduced motor dysfunction and memory loss,[56-58] but greater improvements occurred when the drug was given prior to or immediately at injury.[59-62] Other studies have noted reductions in lesion size.[52,63] Clinical trials studying the benefits of a competitive NMDA receptor antagonist, SDZ EAA 494, with severe brain injury have recently begun. Expanded trials to identify optimal compounds and the timing of administration are needed in the future.

Since calcium ions may enter the cell by multiple pathways besides receptor-activated channels, blockage of just one channel may be of limited efficacy. Calcium may also enter the cell via voltage-activated channels.[64] Two calcium channel-blocking drugs, nimodipine and nicardipine, have been examined in both animal and human trauma trials. Calcium channel blockers were initially studied as a potential prevention for ischemic deterioration after subarachnoid hemorrhage and have been found to be effective. Some improved outcomes, including decreased morbidity and mortality, have been observed in patients with brain injury.[65-76] The dosage and timing of administration varied among these studies. Because of multiple pathways of calcium entry, there appears to be some credibility in examining outcomes when a combination of calcium channel and receptor blockers is administered. Because the majority of calcium influx occurs within the first 30 minutes post injury, timely administration of any of these medications is vital.[35] Results of a study investigating outcomes secondary to early, aggressive nimodipine use with severe brain injury are pending.[77] Continued investigation regarding the benefit of these medications is needed.

Oxygen Free Radical Formation

Oxygen free radicals, a normal byproduct of aerobic metabolism, can be toxic to normal cells and tissue. In the normal brain, these radicals are broken down to oxygen and water and are harmless to tissue. After brain injury, however, cellular protective mechanisms are impaired, with radicals accumulating within the cell. Infiltrating neutrophils, oxidation of hemoglobin, mitochondrial disruption, and increased arachidonic acid metabolism are all sources of oxygen free radicals following brain injury. The formation of oxygen radicals occurs for at least one hour post injury.[78] Proteins, carbohydrates, nucleic acids, and lipids are destroyed, resulting in alteration of the structural integrity and function of the cell membrane. These alterations increase permeability, allowing extracellular calcium to enter the cell. Although multiple oxygen radical species are involved, damage secondary to the superoxide anion is felt to be significant in that it contributes to the formation of other damaging oxygen radicals.[79]

When administered, oxygen radical scavengers combine with oxygen radicals to form less toxic substances. Oxygen radical scavenger drugs are thought to reduce ischemia and improve ICP control. Studies have shown that the use of superoxide dismutase (SOD) has a beneficial effect on vascular abnormalities that occur secondary to fluid-percussion brain injury.[80–83] The conjunction of SOD with polyethylene glycol (PEG) extends the biological half-life to approximately five days.[79] Phase II clinical testing of PEG-SOD has been initiated in patients with severe brain injury.[79] PEG-SOD has been found to be well tolerated in patients with severe brain injury.[79] Results indicate trends toward easier maintenance of desired ICP levels and improved three- and six-month outcomes.[79–88] Future phase III trials are planned.

Lipid Peroxidation

Lipid peroxidation is a key posttraumatic degenerative mechanism affecting posttraumatic edema, metabolic dysfunction, and ischemia.[89–97] Free radical molecules are highly reactive because of the presence of an unpaired electron in the outer orbit. Following brain injury, free radicals react with phospholipids in the cell membranes to produce lipid peroxides. This reaction destroys the polyunsaturated tails of membrane phospholipids, causing them to lose their normal configuration, and results in damage to the integrity of the cell membrane. Permeability is increased, allowing extracellular calcium to enter the cell. An ischemic cascade that can result in cell death is initiated.

The use of antioxidants may interrupt these processes and prevent some of the neurologic damage following brain injury. Lazaroids, synthetic nonglucocorticoid steroids, inhibit cell membrane breakdown by inhibiting lipid peroxidation.[34] Lazaroids are also thought to function as oxygen free radical scavengers, thereby stabilizing cell membranes and blocking neuronal deterioration. In animal studies, lipid peroxidation has been inhibited through the use of methylprednisolone and tirilazad mesylate (U-74006F), a 21-aminosteroid.[98–101] Some studies have yielded encouraging results from the use of tirilazad,[100–108] whereas others have reported a lack of benefit.[109,110] Phase II clinical trials were completed, focusing on safety and initial efficacy of the drug.[111] Phase III trials, however, involving multiple centers, were suspended by the Upjohn Company in December 1994. Final results are still pending.

Bradykinins

Only recently has laboratory investigation begun to augment our knowledge of the role that bradykinins play in neuronal injury. What is clearly known is that bradykinin is a nine–amino acid peptide formed from kininogen by the action of the enzyme kininogenase. It is one of the first compounds produced at the site of tissue injury. The consequence of bradykinin production is the release of a series of reactions that produce the cardinal manifestations of inflammation.

When there is a tissue injury, a series of biochemical reactions results in the production of bradykinins, one of which is the kinin system interaction with clotting.[112] A component of the clotting system is the activation of factor XII. A fragment of factor XII is called prekallikrein activation. This fragment is converted to an active proteolytic enzyme called kallikrein. From a series of positive-feedback enzymes, bradykinin is produced. Bradykinin initiates the following features of inflammation: (1) dilatation of arterioles, (2) constriction of veins, (3) contraction of smooth muscles, and (4) initiation of edema at the site of injury.[113] Bradykinin is also a potent stimulator of other mediators of inflammation (which are beyond the scope of this chapter).

In the normal function of neurons, various metabolites generated by bradykinin are useful. However, other bradykinin-induced substances, such as oxygen-containing free radicals, are harmful to neuronal cell integrity. These free radicals induce free radical–catalyzed lipid peroxidation. This can result in a loss of cerebral vascular autoregulation, destructive changes in vascular permeability, and cerebral edema.[114] Bradykinin is a known potent stimulator of second messengers, such as calcium. Calcium is a principal second messenger that affects cellular activity. Calcium elevations can be induced by bradykinins from the intracellular stores of Ca^{++} via the action of inositol-trisphosphate.[115] Persistent Ca^{++} elevation results in destroying cellular integrity, ultimately leading to neuronal cell death.

Both the brain and the spinal cord possess all the components necessary for the activation of the kallikrein/kinin system. Several mechanisms are activated that may result in the increased production of bradykinins, including the previously mentioned clotting system. An additional mechanism is cellular destruction, leading to the release of lysosomal enzymes acting on kininogen to release bradykinins. When tissue is injured or becomes ischemic, acidity increases. Acidity inhibits kinase inactivation of bradykinin, causing increased levels of bradykinin. It is now apparent that endogenous kinins play a major role in the pathogenesis of cerebral abnormalities caused by neurotrauma and ischemia.[116]

Current laboratory investigation strongly suggests that bradykinin plays a dominant or direct role in the loss of cerebrovascular autoregulation after severe brain injury and is a potent stimulator of the production of oxygen-containing free radicals and lipid peroxidation productions. Clinical trials are currently under way to study novel bradykinin receptor antagonists, and some in the field suspect that this therapy, used in combination with others (ie, bradykinin antagonists and calcium channel blockers or NMDA antagonists), will achieve the best possible outcome.

Hypothermia

Hypothermia has been used in the management of patients with brain injury since 1943.[117-121] The use of conventional hypothermia (body temperature less than 30°C), however, has been abandoned in the last decade because of inconclusive outcomes, management problems, and the presence of side effects such as cardiac arrhythmias and coagulation abnormalities.[122-128] Moderate hypothermia (32°C to 33°C), however, is not associated with cardiac instability or other side effects.[126,129,130] Moderate hypothermia has the potential to limit secondary brain injury by stabilizing cell membranes, suppressing cerebral metabolism, and preventing toxic levels of extracellular excitatory amino acids.[131-137] The effects of hypothermia on cerebral metabolism have been found to be sustained for at least five days after injury.[138] In recent studies, moderate hypothermia has significantly reduced intracranial pressure and cerebral blood flow during cooling, with no increases in these parameters after patients were rewarmed.[138-140] These studies have demonstrated a trend toward improved survival and improved outcome in hypothermia versus normothermia groups.[138-140] In 1977, Marion and colleagues completed a class I study investigating the long term outcomes of moderate hypothermia. Significantly improved outcomes at three and six months post injury were identified in patients with admission coma scores of 3 or 4. Results also suggested improved outcomes at one year post injury for this same group of patients.[141]

Vulnerability to posttraumatic ischemia is greatest within the first 24 hours. Peak increases in the extracellular amino acid glutamate occur within 1 hour after injury and return to baseline within 2 to 3 hours. Research suggests that if hypothermia is used to treat ischemia and reduce toxic levels of excitatory amino acids, then a 24-hour treatment should be sufficient.[138,141]

Research on the benefits of moderate hypothermia is largely based on animal studies.[122,142-148] A limited number of class I studies exists.[138,139,141] However, these studies have demonstrated that moderate hypothermia has the potential to limit secondary brain injury, increase survival rate, and improve neurologic outcome in individuals sustaining severe brain injury.[138-141] This treatment modality may be an important therapeutic adjunct in the management of these patients and warrants continued investigation.

Pharmacologic Directions

The future development of potential therapies for acute brain injury will be led by methodologically sound outcome-oriented clinical trials on both animals and humans. Measures have already been taken to standardize these research designs for outcome measures in brain injury.[149] Neuropharmacologic intervention advances are emerging secondary to increased understanding and knowledge from the laboratory on the biochemical cascades following brain injury. Optimism exists that these advances will translate into improved functional outcomes.

BENEFITS OF REHABILITATIVE INTERVENTIONS

The rehabilitation component is less recognized by the medical community for its contributions in the ICU. It was in 1982 that Cervelli and Berrol described the ideal model rehabilitation system as incorporating early, aggressive intervention with rehabilitation care beginning in the ICU.[150] "Rehabilitation is the momentum that moves the patient through the [recovery] cycle, although it often is identified as an isolated period within the cycle."[151(p364)]

Rehabilitation should be initiated within 24 to 48 hours of admission. In those instances in which medical stability is questionable or a patient's level of function is rapidly declining, discretion must be taken in the initiation of service. Early, aggressive rehabilitation, for appropriate patients, includes physical and occupational therapy, speech/language pathology, and, at some institutions, physiatry. Early rehabilitation intervention includes assessment and direct treatment to improve a patient's level of function and to prevent secondary complications. Intervention is sensitive to the acute medical needs of the patient and must be altered continuously depending upon those needs. Family training and education are integral components of service provided in the ICU by rehabilitation specialists.

Early rehabilitation intervention is *not synonymous* with traditional coma stimulation or sensory stimulation programs. These programs historically focus upon treatment of the patient in a vegetative state rather than during the early acute phase of recovery. "Most coma stimulation is therefore not coma stimulation at all, but rather, vegetative or low level stimulation."[152(p37)]

Early-intervention programs should follow established protocols and procedures that outline the mission and purpose of the program, identify team members and their scope of practice, and describe specific discipline procedures and the rationale for such procedures. Available scientific evidence and published studies should be included. Physician support is essential in adopting and applying this programmatic approach. The support of the traumatologist, neurosurgeon, and/or critical care intensivist is needed for initiation of services.

Rehabilitation staff should be properly trained before patient treatment and should have an understanding of their professional limitations as well as contributions. Standardized education programs should include training in the following areas:

1. use and application of ICU equipment (eg, monitors, ventilators, specialized beds)
2. purpose and location of patient equipment (eg, lines, tubes, stabilization devices)
3. completion of a thorough chart review
4. purpose and side effects of common medications
5. rationale for initiation, suspension, and discontinuation of treatment
6. assessment of patients
7. appropriate goal writing for a critical care population
8. treatment techniques
9. guidelines for interaction with minimally responsive and cognitively impaired patients

Additional components of the rehabilitation educational program include required readings on select brain injury topics and the use of cotreatment sessions with experienced peers.

There are limited published studies scientifically identifying the benefits of early rehabilitation and the use of brain injury teams in the trauma center. The only pertinent class I studies to demonstrate the benefits of early rehabilitation have been animal studies, most of which were published prior to 1980. In more recent years, class II studies have been published that support the concept of acute rehabilitation intervention, even within the confines of the ICU.

Historically, studies of other types of central nervous system (CNS) injuries, such as spinal cord injuries (SCIs), have clearly identified the benefit of early rehabilitation.[153–156] One study[153] reported on outcomes before and after the establishment of a multidisciplinary acute spinal cord injury team. Results revealed a correlation between establishment of the team and statistically significant reductions in LOSs in the acute care hospital and significant reductions in febrile illness and incidence of tracheostomy. Other studies have identified the principal benefit of early rehabilitation as decreased hospital LOS.[154,155] These decreases were largely a factor of avoidance of pressure sores and other preventable medical complications. Reduced mortality rates have been noted for patients with SCI admitted within one day of injury compared to those not admitted to an organized, multidisciplinary SCI care system.[155]

Animal Studies

Some of the basis of support for early rehabilitation intervention stems from animal research.[157–162] Information extrapolated from these studies suggests correlations between timing of intervention and functional outcomes. The pioneer of this model was a psychologist named Shepard Ivory Franz (1874–1933). His research, dating back to 1902,[157] studied the cerebral mechanisms of behavior and applied the results to rehabilitation. Other investigators followed, using animal models to study how brain lesions affect learning and memory and how training programs can minimize the effects of these lesions.

Yu,[159] in 1976, published a paper reviewing animal studies on functional recovery with and without training following brain damage. The studies cited, using cat and monkey models, reported improved functional recovery through the use of training (rehabilitation). Yu stated that "results of functional recovery with training in animal experiments strongly suggest that rehabilitation can play a much more active and specific role, in fact that rehabilitation is essential for recovery."[159(p40)]

Rosenzweig[160] reviewed extensive experimental findings to justify how animal models contributed to rehabilitation. He cited studies that demonstrated how "enriched" environments and training significantly improved functional outcomes in brain-lesioned animals.

Black et al[161] demonstrated that functional recovery of a hemiplegic limb in experimentally brain-lesioned monkeys was significantly better for those animals placed in an early-treatment program. Black et al assessed outcomes of two groups of brain-injured monkeys, differing only in the timing of initiation of therapy. The "immediate" group began training (therapy) immediately, with training for the "delay" group being postponed for four months. Monkeys receiving immediate treatment improved over a six-month period to 82% of their preoperative performance. The "delay" group progressed to 67% recovery following six months of treatment. "The data suggest that, to be most effective, the training should begin as soon as possible after the insult to the brain has occurred."[161(p66)]

Controversy remains as to the relevance between animal studies and human subjects. Researchers such as Rosenzweig argue that there is a lack of information to make the assumption that animal models are within the same taxon as man. However, Rosenzweig states that investigators who study the problems and challenges of recovery of human function and rehabilitation should be familiar with "the other side," namely, the techniques and resources of research with animal models.

Physical/Motor Skills

The consequences of delayed or absent physical/motor intervention engender less controversy. Decreased mobility is common in the critical care patient with severe brain injury. All body systems can be affected by this immobility, including musculoskeletal, respiratory, cardiovascular, gastrointestinal, urinary, integumentary, and neurological systems.[151,163] Lack of appropriate positioning and adequate range of motion (ROM) can result in the formation of decubiti and contractures.[164,165] Limitations in ROM can occur within the initial phases of recovery, even while the patient is still in coma. These limitations can progress to fixed deformities within a few weeks when therapy is not provided.

Spasticity is a common complication in brain injury that can compromise function. Aggressive physical and occupational therapy immediately post injury can help normalize abnormal tone. Patients receiving physical therapy within 24 hours of injury experience lower percentages of abnormal muscle tone on admission to rehabilitation.[166] Physical outcomes at discharge from inpatient rehabilitation are also affected by early rehabilitation. Statistically significant improvements have been reported in range of motion, muscle tone, balance, and mobility when therapy was initiated 2 days versus 23 days post brain injury.[167]

Within the acute phase of injury, the physical and occupational therapists use mobilization and positioning techniques to minimize the effects of decerebrate and decorticate posturing. Abnormal posturing can adversely affect ROM and alignment of fractures stabilized with skeletal traction.[168] Systems other than the musculoskeletal system can also be affected (Figure 15–1). Posturing is strongly associated with elevated ICP.[169,170] Increased ICP is a major factor influencing morbidity and mortality rates associated with brain injuries. Strategies to reduce acute ICP should focus on control of factors that may aggravate intracranial hypertension, such as posturing.

Normal bone-building activities are dependent upon weight bearing and movement. Increased release of calcium can occur in the immobile patient with brain injury, with bones becoming increasingly porous and fragile. Abnormal calcification over large joints may occur if this process continues, resulting in permanent heterotopic ossification (HO). HO is more commonly identified during the rehabilitation hospital phase of care. However, the delay or absence of proper treatment in the acute care environment contributes to the formation of HO. The reported incidence of HO in adults ranges from 11% to 76%,[171–173] depending upon the method of detection and timing of assessment. The incidence of HO was found to be 22.5% in children with brain injuries, aged 6 to 21 years, who were admitted to a rehabilitation facility.[174] HO was identified as occurring an average of 47 days post injury. Although specific data on the presence, absence, or timeliness of acute therapy are often not noted, patients with HO are reported to have "had sustained

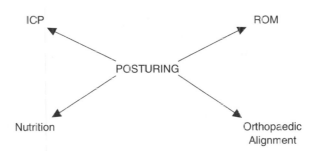

Figure 15–1 Four potential areas adversely affected by abnormal posturing in the patient with a severe brain injury.

a period of immobility" with "increased tone and spasticity in the involved extremity."[174(p259)]

When initiation of treatment is delayed, therapy must focus on reversal of these newly developed deficits.[175–177] Techniques performed at rehabilitation hospitals, including serial casting, surgical tendon release, and Botox injections, can be costly and may not always be successful in restoring ROM or functional mobility. The need for these techniques may have been prevented or reduced by providing therapy in the early postinjury stages. Some institutions use serial casting in the ICU, when significant hypertonicity is present immediately post injury. For appropriate patients, this technique can be effective and has been demonstrated not to significantly increase ICP or decrease CPP in patients with severe brain injuries.[178]

Patients admitted with brain injuries frequently have concomitant fractures or other orthopaedic injuries. In studies completed on patients with various isolated orthopaedic injuries (eg, hip, radius, or pelvic fractures), results support the contention that early mobilization and timely provision of therapy facilitate reduced LOSs, improved physical independence, and earlier return to work.[179–182]

Life-threatening injuries are of primary importance in the emergency and critical care settings. However, other seemingly minor injuries can have significant impact on functional outcome. Interventions by the physical and occupational therapists can result in the identification of injuries unnoticed during the initial resuscitation. These injuries can include clavicle fractures; wrist, hand, ankle, or foot injuries/fractures; and acromioclavicular separations. If not properly treated, these injuries can result in loss of motor function and pain, potentially affecting functional outcome.

Poor outcomes, including nonfunctioning joints, present major problems for survivors of brain injury. Prevention continues to be the most successful form of treatment. Prompt and timely therapy aids in prevention and should occur simultaneously with primary care. Intervention "should start at an early stage when predictable symptoms are still absent."[171(p169)] Rogers, in 1988, stated that "an efficient prophylactic regimen has to be initiated in the acute stage of the head-injury, while the patient is still in coma and in the intensive care unit."[171(p170)]

Medical Benefits

The patient with severe brain injury is in a hypermetabolic state that causes protein breakdown and muscle atrophy. Abnormal tone and spasticity increase energy expenditure. Posturing increases metabolic expenditure and oxidative requirements.[183–185] Prolonged immobilization increases protein and negative nitrogen balance. Team members must work toward reducing those aggravating factors that deplete nutritional sources.

Physical and occupational therapy techniques positively influence a patient's nutritional status. Positioning and ROM techniques reduce tone and posturing, resulting in reduced energy expenditure. These techniques must be initiated early and aggressively to be effective. Carryover of these techniques by nursing is vital.

Early percussion, vibration, and postural drainage mobilize respiratory secretions, reducing the risk of pulmonary infections. Overall mobilization of the patient, including ROM exercises, positioning, sitting (if appropriate), and ambulation, stimulates respiratory function.

Speech/language pathology contributions include the early identification of swallowing disorders, need for nonoral supplementation, and maintenance of vocal cord function. The early identification of swallowing disorders and aspiration is important for a population with a high incidence of pneumonia.[12,186–189] Identifying long-term nutritional needs facilitates timely implementation of appropriate nonoral supplementation (ie, percutaneous endoscopic gastrostomy or jejunostomy or gastrostomy or jejunostomy tube) and eliminates unnecessary extended LOSs. Safe and appropriate initiation of oral feeding reduces the risk of cascading complications, including aspiration pneumonia.

The early use of speaking valves and talking tracheostomy tubes in appropriate patients maintains mobility of the vocal cords. Active mobility of the cords reduces the risk of aspiration by maintaining an effective valving mechanism to protect the airway. The longer the immobility, the greater the risk of prolonged inadequate airway protection.

Improved Cognition and Level of Functioning

Improvements in cognition, behavior, and generalized level of functioning due to early rehabilitation intervention have been demonstrated through a variety of assessment tools and measures. Improvements in these areas have been noted at discharge from acute hospitals as well as inpatient rehabilitation facilities. Several studies have identified cognitive/behavioral changes at acute hospital discharge through the use of the Rancho Los Amigos Scale of Cognitive Functioning (RLA).[190] Patients with severe brain injury demonstrated greater increases in cognition when receiving early rehabilitation intervention.[156,167,191] Increases in RLA level ranged from 0.5 to 1.5. Statistically significant increases were also demonstrated upon discharge from rehabilitation facilities when rehabilitation was initiated within 2 days versus 23 days post injury.[167] Increases of 0.5 to 1 RLA level were noted.

The impact of early rehabilitation affects short-term as well as extended outcomes. Improved long-term outcomes (ie, 30 months post injury) have been noted for patients admitted to rehabilitation earlier (within 35 days post injury) versus later (after 35 days postinjury).[192] Early-admission patients were found to be mildly disabled on the Disability Rating Scale (DRS)[193,194] (DRS 1.79) as compared to late-admission patients (range, 0 [minimal impairment] to 30 [death]) who were moderately disabled (DRS 4.07). Statistically significant differences were also noted between these groups on the Social Status Outcome Scale[195] (0.52 versus 2.30, respectively, on a range from 0 [maximum independence and productivity] to 3 [maximum handicap])

Improvements in specific cognitive/language areas at discharge from inpatient rehabilitation facilities have been noted for patients receiving immediate rehabilitation post injury versus those whose rehabilitation was delayed for over three weeks.[167] Statistically significant improvements were noted in the areas of attention, thought organization (problem solving, categorization, insight), higher-order language (ie, pragmatics, analysis, and inferential thinking), and speech/language skills (dysarthria, aphasia, word finding). Improvements were noted in immediate, recent, and long-term memory skills. These improvements, however, were not statistically significant. Short-term memory skills remain the most common long-term deficit secondary to severe brain injury. Within rehabilitation, strategies can be taught to compensate for these deficits. The skills necessary to learn these compensations are included in the areas of attention, thought organization, and higher-order language. Although early intervention does not appear to have a significant impact on memory skills, it significantly improves those skills necessary to compensate for that loss.

Overall improvements in cognitive, behavioral, language, and physical skills ultimately affect an individual's functional performance. Early, aggressive rehabilitation improves a patient's opportunity to return to independent function. As a result, in one study, higher percentages of patients were discharged home from a rehabilitation hospital versus an extended-care facility (94% versus 57%).[167]

Length of Stay and Disposition

The most consistently identified area of improvement resulting from early rehabilitation intervention is LOS. Changes in LOS have been reported in both acute care and rehabilitation hospitals. Within these class II studies, the timing of early rehabilitation varies. Comparisons were made between groups when rehabilitation was initiated in less than or greater than 35 days post injury (Cope and Hall,[196] Hall and Wright[192]), in less than or greater than 8 days (Morgan et al[191]), and in an average of 2 days versus 23 days post injury (Mackay et al[167]). One study evaluated LOS and other outcomes as it related to initiation of physical therapy services only.[166] All other studies included all three therapies (physical therapy, occupational therapy, and speech/language pathology).[167,191,192,196]

Significant reductions in length of stay were noted in all studies. Differences in acute care or trauma center lengths of stay are displayed in Figure 15–2. These differences varied from a low of 13% to a high of 63%. Without early rehabilitation, lengths of stay increased an average of 40%. Percentages for each study are displayed in Figure 15–3.

Some studies have also identified the effect of early rehabilitation on rehabilitation hospital LOS.[167,192,196] Statistically significant reductions were noted in all studies (Figure 15–4). Although variations in the number of days exist among studies, the percentage of reduction remained fairly consistent with the use of early intervention (Figure 15–5). These studies demonstrated that the use of early, aggressive therapy can reduce LOSs by at least 50%, as well as improve functional outcome.

Interestingly, in the data reviewed, acute hospital LOSs have increased, rather than decreased, over time. Differences in LOS can be attributed to uncontrolled factors, including CT results and severity of brain injury, other injuries, and secondary complications. In more recent years, factors such as infections (methicillin-resistant *Staphylococcus aureus* [MRSA], vancomycin-resistant enterococci [VRE]) and insurance and managed-care issues have complicated LOS issues.

TRANSFER PLANNING

Other aspects of health care that can affect patients are managed-care and insurance issues. The intent of present as well as future changes is to streamline health care costs without compromising patient care. Aggressive and early discharge planning becomes more crucial to hospitals as insurance companies and managed-care agencies become more stringent in providing medical coverage and benefits. Inpatient LOSs and coverage of specific services continue to be reduced in many plans. Discharge planning must begin immediately following admission. Acute care hospitals must anticipate the extended needs of the patient, often while the

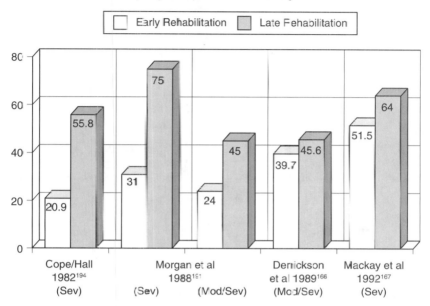

Figure 15–2 Differences in acute medical/surgical hospital lengths of stay with early versus late initiation of rehabilitation.

patient is still in the ICU. The immediate involvement of the hospital discharge planner helps to organize the anticipated needs of the patient and family and facilitate planning.

The inclusion of insurance company case managers in management and planning decisions is becoming more commonplace. Their presence, however, does not affect medical decisions and interventions. Those issues remain under the direct purview of the physician. Rather, the insurance company case manager interacts with the hospital discharge planner in providing input regarding a patient's medical coverage and options for continued services based on the team's recommendations.

Insurance companies often have negotiated contracts with specific hospitals and service providers. Fortunately, prehospital personnel continue to transport patients to the closest facility adequately equipped to provide the necessary care, sometimes resulting in admission to hospitals that do not have negotiated contracts with the patients' insurance companies. In these cases, the insurance company case manager will work with hospital personnel, including the discharge

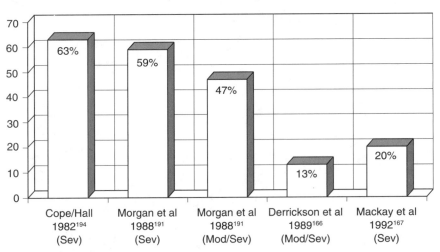

Figure 15–3 Reductions in acute medical/surgical hospital lengths of stay with the use of early rehabilitation intervention.

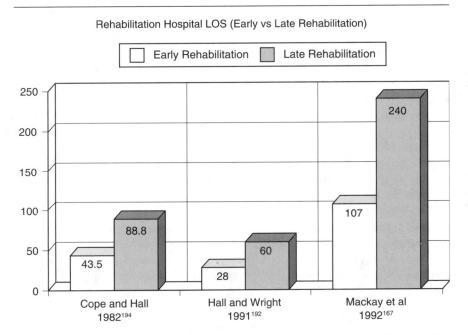

Figure 15–4 Differences in rehabilitation hospital lengths of stay with early versus late initiation of rehabilitation.

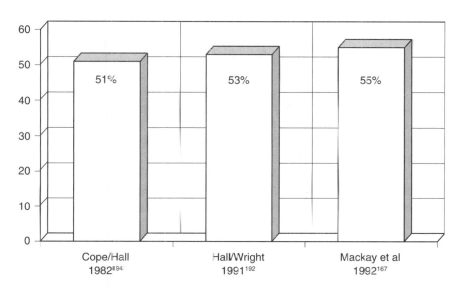

Reductions in Rehabilitation Hospital LOS with Early Rehabilitation Intervention

Figure 15–5 Reductions in rehabilitation hospital lengths of stay with the use of early rehabilitation intervention.

planner and physician, to negotiate terms for this admission or arrange transfer to another hospital when the patient is medically stable and ready for discharge from the ICU setting.

The discharge planner is instrumental in identifying the characteristics of an individual's insurance plan. Insurance companies have many different medical plans, dependent on the requested options of the purchaser. Some contracts involve the approval or denial of individual services, while others offer a flat rate for all services rendered. Identifying the specifics of a patient's insurance coverage is time consuming and often frustrating, but nonetheless invaluable in fostering a plan of care across the continuum of recovery.

Changes in health care coverage result in institutions' being unable to afford the luxury of extending LOSs until families make decisions or beds become available in rehabilitation or other extended-care facilities. Trauma centers are more frequently becoming part of health care systems that incorporate rehabilitation facilities into their service provisions due to the economics of the health care industry. Early and ongoing communication between medical and rehabilitation staff, discharge planners, and insurance representatives can prevent unnecessary extensions in LOSs while facilitating appropriate and timely transition of patients and families to a rehabilitation environment.

CONCLUSION

Attempts to highlight interventions that are proven to improve neurologic function are currently being initiated. Several medical and therapeutic interventions have already been identified in the literature. Currently, the primary medical interventions recommended include achieving adequate physiologic parameters (ie, ICP, CPP, BP), maintaining adequate nutrition, and decreasing complications such as electrolyte abnormalities, pneumonia, and sepsis. With continued drug trials, the use of pharmacologic intervention, both prehospital and in the hospital, holds great promise. A growing body of literature also demonstrates the benefits of early, aggressive rehabilitation and the use of organized multidisciplinary teams. These interventions have demonstrated a variety of benefits, including reduced LOSs (acute and rehabilitation), reduced complications, and improved functional outcomes.

These initiatives will become the forerunners of practice standards across the continuum of care for the treatment of persons with severe brain injury. The *Guidelines for the Mangement of Severe Head Injury*[197] is one such example. In 1994, a task force was formed from the Joint Section on Neurotrauma and Critical Care (American Association of Neurological Surgeons and Congress of Neurological Surgeons [AANS/CNS]) to develop scientific, evidence-based guidelines for acute management of severe brain injury. Those guidelines include 14 topics ranging from trauma systems and prehospital resuscitation to intensive care management. This document identifies standards, guidelines, and options within these 14 areas, based upon available, published class I, II, and III studies.

In 1987, the U.S. Department of Education's National Institute on Disability and Rehabilitation Research (NIDRR) supported the establishment of the Traumatic Brain Injury Model Systems (TBIMS) of Care.[198] This project, funded through 1997, is a prospective, longitudinal multicenter study focusing on development of model systems of care and examining the course of recovery and outcomes via a standardized national database. The four TBIMS centers are Medical College of Virginia (Richmond), Wayne State University/Rehabilitation Institute of Michigan (Detroit), the Institute for Rehabilitation and Research (Houston), and Santa Clara Valley Medical Center (San Jose). Each center provides a coordinated system of care from the emergency department through neurotrauma management, inpatient rehabilitation, and long-term interdisciplinary follow-up services. This endeavor is the first organized attempt to collect data on short- and long-term outcomes across a model continuum of care for persons with brain injury. Initial outcome data from the Traumatic Brain Injury Model Systems National Database were published in October 1996 in the *Journal of Head Trauma Rehabilitation.*[198]

Formalized early intervention programs rely on a unique combination of medical and rehabilitative therapies. In the future, more aggressive neuropharmacologic intervention will join with these therapies to improve the overall management approach with severe brain injury. Mounting evidence is accruing on the benefits of these types of programs. Increasing demands to improve outcomes and reduce costs will most likely give rise to continued substantiation of early intervention. The benefits of early formalized approaches to treatment are diverse. "This early team approach allows for better communication and servicing within the health care system and with the patient and family."[99(p203)] It allows an "opportunity for health care professionals to work more closely together."[199(p204)] It facilitates staff and family members to be more focused and more aware of the total care of the patient. Its primary benefits, however, are not limited to reductions in LOS or cost. More important, individually designed, formalized early intervention programs "improve a patient's functional outcome and ultimately quality of life."[200(p337)]

REFERENCES

1. Taskforce of Joint Section of Neurotrauma and Critical Care. *Guidelines for the Management of Severe Head Injury.* New York, NY: Brain Trauma Foundation; 1995.
2. Ropper AH. Introduction to critical care in neurology and neurosurgery. In: Ropper AH, ed. *Neurological and Neurosurgical Intensive Care.* New York, NY: Raven Press; 1993;3–9
3. Becker DP, Miller JD, Ward JD, Greenberg RP, et al. The outcome from severe head injury with early diagnosis and intensive management. *J Neurosurg.* 1977;47:491–502.
4. Marshall LF, Smith RW, Shapiro HM. The outcome with aggressive treatment in severe head injuries. Part I: the significance of intracranial pressure monitoring. *J Neurosurg.* 1979;50: 20–25.
5. Marshall LF. Treatment of brain swelling and brain edema in man. *Adv Neurol.* 1980;28:459–469.
6. Miller JD, Butterworth JF, Gudeman SK, Faulkner JE, et al. Further experience in the management of severe head injury. *J Neurosurg.* 1981;54:289–299.
7. Saul TG, Ducker TB. Effects of intracranial pressure monitoring and aggressive treatment on mortality in severe head injury. *J Neurosurg.* 1982;56:498–503.
8. Marshall LF, Marshall SB. Medical management of intracranial pressure. In: Cooper PR, ed. *Head Injury.* Baltimore, Md: Williams & Wilkins; 1986:177–196.
9. Marmarou A, Anderson JD, Eisenberg HM, et al. The traumatic coma data bank: monitoring of ICP. In: Hoff JT, Betz AL, eds. *Intracranial Pressure.* Vol 7. Berlin, Germany: Springer-Verlag; 1989;549–551.
10. Marmarou A, Anderson RL, Ward JD, et al. Impact of ICP instability and hypotension on outcome in patient with severe head trauma. *J Neurosurg.* 1991;75(suppl):S159–S166.
11. Chesnut RM, Marshall LF. The role of secondary brain injury in determining outcome from severe head injury. Paper presented in receipt of the Volvo Neurotrauma Award from the Neurotraumatology Section of the World Federation of Neurosurgical Societies; New Delhi, India; April 1989:596.
12. Woratyla SP, Morgan AS, Mackay L, Bernstein B, et al. Factors associated with early onset pneumonia in the severely brain injured patient. *Conn Med.* 1995;59:643–647.

13. Chesnut RM, Marshall LF, Klauber MR, Blunt BA, et al. The role of secondary brain injury in determining outcome from severe head injury. *J Trauma.* 1993;34:216–222.

14. Fearnside MR, Cook RJ, McDougall P, McNeil RJ. The Westmead Head Injury Project outcome in severe head injury: a comparative analysis of pre-hospital, clinical and CT variables. *Br J Neurosurg.* 1993;7:267–279.

15. Pietropaoli JA, Rogers FB, Shackford SR, Wald SL, et al. The deleterious effects of intraoperative hypotension on outcome in patients with severe head injuries. *J Trauma.* 1992;33:403–407.

16. Kohi YM, Mendelow AD, Teasdale GM, Allardice GM. Extracranial insults and outcome in patients with acute head injury-relationship to the Glasgow Coma Scale. *Injury.* 1984;16:25–29.

17. Miller JD, Becker DP. Secondary insults to the injured brain. J R *Coll Surg (Edinburgh).* 1982;27:292–298.

18. Jeffreys RV, Jones JJ. Avoidable factors contributing to the death of head injury patients in general hospital in Mersey region. *Lancet.* 1981;2:459–461.

19. Miller JD, Sweet RC, Narayan R, Becker DP. Early insults to the injured brain. *JAMA.* 1978;240:439–442.

20. Pigula FA, Wald SL, Shackford SR, Vane DW. The effect of hypotension and hypoxia on children with severe head injuries. *J Pediatr Surg.* 1993;28:310–314.

21. Fortune JB, Feustel PJ, Weigle CG, Popp AJ. Continuous measurement of jugular venous oxygen saturation in response to transient elevations of blood pressure in head-injured patients. *J Neurosurg.* 1994;80:461–468.

22. Clifton GL, Allen S, Barrodale P, Plenger P, et al. A phase II study of moderate hypothermia in severe brain injury. *J Neurotrauma.* 1993;10:263–271.

23. Marion DW, Obrist WD, Carlier PM, Penrod LE, et al. The use of moderate therapeutic hypothermia for patients with severe head injuries: a preliminary report. *J Neurosurg.* 1993;79:354–362.

24. Yoshida A, Shima T, Okada Y, et al. Outcome of patients with severe head injury: evaluation by cerebral perfusion pressure. In: *Recent Advances in Neurotramatology.* Nakamura N, Hashimoto T, Yasue M, eds. Hong Kong: Springer-Verlag; 1993:309–312.

25. Rosner MJ, Daughton S. Cerebral perfusion pressure management in head injury. *J Trauma.* 1990;30:933–940.

26. Marshall LF, Gautille T, Klauber MR, et al. The outcome of severe closed head injury. *J Neurosurg.* 1991;75:S28–S36.

27. Muizelaar JP, Marmarou A, Ward JD, Kontos HA, et al. Adverse effects of prolonged hyperventilation in patients with severe head injury: a randomized clinical trial. *J Neurosurg.* 1991;75:731–739.

28. Rapp RP, Young B, Twyman D, Bivins BA, et al. The favorable effect of early parenteral feeding on survival in head-injured patients. *J Neurosurg.* 1983;58:906–912.

29. Young B, Ott L, Twyman D, Norton J, et al. The effect of nutritional support on outcome from severe head injury. *J Neurosurg.* 1987;67:668–676.

30. Waters DC, Dechert R, Bartlett R. Metabolic studies in head injury patients: a preliminary report. *Surgery.* 1986;100:531–534.

31. Balzola F, Boggio Bertinet D, Solerio A, Rizzonato P, et al. Dietetic treatment with hypercaloric and hyperprotein intake in patients following severe brain injury. *J Neurosurg Sci.* 1980;24:131–140.

32. Rabb CH. Options for cerebral protection after penetrating head injury. *Neurosurg Clin North Am.* 1995;6:643–656.

33. Bullock R. Opportunities for neuroprotective drugs in clinical managment of head injury. *J Emerg Med.* 1993;11:23–30.

34. Hall ED. The role of oxygen radicals in traumatic injury: clinical implications. *J Emerg Med.* 1993;11:31–36.

35. Hayes RI, Jenkis LW, Lyeth BG. Neurochemical aspects of head injury: role of excitatory neurotransmission. *J Head Trauma Rehabil.* 1992;7:16–28.

36. Hilton G. Experimental neuroprotective agents: nursing challenge. *Dimens Crit Care Nurs.* 1995;14:181–188.

37. Boyeson MG, Harmon RL. Acute and postacute drug-induced effects on rate of behavioral recovery after brain injury. *J Head Trauma Rehabil.* 1994;9:78–90.

38. Mayer ML, Vylkicky L, Sernagor E. A physiologist's view of the NMDA receptor: an allosteric ion channel with multiple regulatory sites. *Drug Dev Res.* 1989;17:263–280.

39. Demopoulos HB, Flamm ES, Pietronigro DD, Seligman MC. The free radical pathology and the microcirculation in the major central nervous system disorders. *Acta Physiol Scand.* 1980;492:91–119.

40. Baker AJ, Moulton RJ, MacMillan VH, Shedden PM. Excitatory amino acids in cerebrospinal fluid following traumatic brain injury in humans. *J Neurosurg.* 1993;79:369–372.

41. Pickard JD, Czosnyka M. Management of raised intracranial pressure. *J Neurol Neurosurg Psychiatry.* 1993;56:845–858.

42. Choi D. Methods of antagonizing glutamate neurotoxicity. *Cerebrovasc Brain Metab Rev.* 1990;2:105–147.

43. Michikawa M, Lim KT, McLarnon JG, Kim SU. Oxygen radical-induced neurotoxicity in spinal cord neuron cultures. *J Neurosci Res.* 1994;37:62–70.

44. McIntosh TK, Vink R, Soares H, Hayes R, et al. Effects of the N-methyl-D-aspartate receptor blocker MK-801 on neurologic function after experimental brain injury. *J Neurotrauma.* 1989;6:247–259.

45. Faden AI, Demidiux P, Panter SS, Vink R. The role of excitatory amino acids and NMDA receptors in traumatic brain injury. *Science.* 1989;244:798–800.

46. Faden AI, Simon RP. A potential role for excitotoxins in the pathophysiology of spinal cord injury. *Ann Neurol.* 1988;23:623–626.

47. Boast CA, Gerhardt SC, Pastor G, Lehmann J, et al. The N-methyl-D-aspartate antagonists CGS 19755 and CPP reduce ischemic brain damage in gerbils. *Brain Res.* 1988;442:345–348.

48. Prince DA, Feeser HR. Dextromethorphan protects against cerebral infarction in a rat model of hypoxia-ischemia. *Neurosci Lett.* 1988;85:291–296.

49. Gill R, Foster AC, Woodruff GN. Systemic administration of MK-801 protects against ischemia-induced hippocampal neurodegeneration in the gerbil. *J Neurosci* 1987;7:3343–3349.

50. Nehls DG, Park CK, MacCormack AG, McCulloch J. The effects of N-methyl-D-aspartate blockade. *Brain Res.* 1990;511:271–279.

51. McCulloch J, Ozyurt E, Park CK, Nehls DG, et al. Glutamate receptor antagonists in experimental focal cerebral ischemia. *Acta Neurochir.* 1993;57(suppl):73–79.

52. Ozyurt E, Graham DI, Woodruff GN, McCulloch J. Protective effect of the glutamate antagonist, MK-801 in focal cerebral ischemia in the cat. *J Cereb Blood Flow Metab.* 1988;8:138–143.

53. Park CK, Nehls DG, Graham DI, Teasdale GM, et al. Focal cerebral ischemia in the cat: treatment with the glutamate antagonist MK-801 after induction of ischaemia. *J Cereb Blood Flow Metab.* 1988;8:757–762.

54. Davies J, Evans RH, Herrling PL, Jones AW, et al. CPP, a new potent and selective NMDA antagonist: depression of central neuron responses, affinity for [3H]D-AP5 binding sites on brain membranes and anticonvulsant activity. *Brain Res.* 1986;382:169–173.

55. Casey KF, McIntosh T. The role of novel pharmacotherapy in brain injury. *J Head Trauma Rehabil.* 1994;9:82–90.

56. Rod MR, Auer RN. Combination therapy with nimodipine and dizocilpine in a rat model of transient forebrain ischemia. *Stroke.* 1992;23:725–732.

57. Lyeth BG, Ray M, Hamm RJ, Schnabel J, et al. Post-injury scopolamine administration in experimental traumatic brain injury. *Brain Res.* 1992;569:281–286.

58. Smith DH, et al. An NMDA receptor associated glycine-site antagonist attentuates memory loss after experimental brain injury. *Neurosci Abstr.* 1990;11:779.

59. Manev H, Favaron M, DeErausquin G, Guidotti A, et al. Destabilization of ionized CA^{2+} homeostasis in excitatory amino acid neurotoxicity: antagonism by glycosphingolipids. *Cell Biol Int Rep.* 1990;14:3–14.

60. McIntosh TK, Vink R, Noble L, Yamakami I, et al. Traumatic brain injury in the rat: characterization of a lateral fluid-percussion model. *Neuroscience.* 1989;28:233–244.

61. Manev H, Favaron M, Guidotti A, Costa E. Delayed increase in CA^{2+} influx elicited by glutamate: role in neuronal death. *Mol Pharmacol.* 1989;36:106–112.

62. Gelmers HJ, Gorter K, deWeerdt CJ, Weizer HJ. A controlled trial of nimodipine in acute ischemic stroke. *N Engl J Med.* 1988;318:203–207.

63. Uematsu D, Araki N, Greenberg JH, Sladky J, et al. Combined therapy with nimodipine and MK-801 for protection of ischemia brain damage. *Neurology.* 1991;41:88–94.

64. Kostyuk PG, Tepikin AV. Calcium signals in nerve cells. *News Physiol Sci.* 1991;6:6–10.

65. A multicenter trial of the efficacy of nimodipine on outcome after severe head injury. European Study Group on Nimodipine in Severe Head Injury. *J Neurosurg.* 1994;80:797–804.

66. Teasdale G, Bailey I, Bell A, Gray J, et al. The effects of nimodipine on outcome after head injury: A prospective randomized controlled trial. *Acta Neurochir.* 1990;51:315–316.

67. Tettenborn D, Dycka J. Prevention and treatment of delayed ischemic dysfunction in patients with aneurysmal subarachnoid hemorrhage. *Stroke.* 1990;21(suppl 12):IV85–IV89.

68. Gilsbach JM. Nimodipine in the prevention of ischaemic deficits after aneurysmal subarachnoid hemorrhage. *Acta Neurochir.* 1988;45(suppl):41–50.

69. Jan M, Buchheit F, Tremoulet M. Therapeutic trial of intravenous nimodipine in patients with established cerebral vasospasm after rupture of intracranial aneurysms. *Neurosurgery.* 1988;23:154–157.

70. Laursen J, Jensen F, Mikkelsen E, Jakobsen P. Nimodipine treatment of subarachnoid hemorrhage. *Clin Neurol Neurosurg.* 1988;90:329–337.

71. Ohman J, Heiskanen O. Effect of nimodipine on the outcome of patients after aneurysmal subarachnoid hemorrhage and surgery. *J Neurosurg.* 1988;69:683–686.

72. Petruk KC, West M, Mohr G, Weir BK, et al. Nimodipine treatment in poor-grade patients: results of a multicenter double-blind placebo-controlled trial. *J Neurosurg.* 1988;68:505–517.

73. Phillipon J, Grob R, Dagreou F, Guggiari M, et al. Prevention of vasospasm in subarachnoid haemorrhage: a controlled study with nimodipine. *Acta Neurochir.* 1986;82:110–114.

74. Kostron H, Twerdy K, Stampfl G, Mohsenipour I, et al. Treatment of cerebral vasospasm with the calcium channel blocker nimodipine. *Neurol Res.* 1984;6:29–32.

75. Ljunggren B, Brandt L, Save and H, Nilsson PE, et al. Outcome in 60 consecutive patients treated with early aneurysm operation and intravenous nimodipine. *J Neurosurg.* 1984;61: 864–873.

76. Allen GS, Ahn HS, Preziosi TJ, Battye R, et al. Cerebral arterial spasm: a controlled trial of nimodipine in patients with subarachnoid hemorrhage. *N Engl J Med.* 1983;308:619–624.

77. Morgan AS. The use of nimodipine as adjuvant therapy for brain injury. Unpublished manuscript. 1995.

78. Kontos HA, Wei EP. Superoxide production in experimental brain injury. *J Neurosurg.* 1986;64:803–807.

79. Muizelaar JP, Marmarou A, Young HF, Choi SC, et al. Improving outcome of severe head injury with oxygen radical scavenger polyethylene glycol-conjugated superoxide dismutase: a Phase II trial. *J Neurosurg.* 1993;78:375–382.

80. Kontos HA. Oxygen radicals in experimental brain injury. In: Hoff JT, Betz AL, eds. *Intracranial Pressure.* Vol 7. Berlin, Germany: Springer-Verlag; 1989:787–798.

81. Levasseur JE, Patterson JL Jr, Ghatak NR, Kontos HA, et al. Combined effect of respirator-induced ventilation and superoxide dismutase in experimental brain injury. *J Neurosurg.* 1989;71:573–577

82. Zimmerman RS, Muizelaar JP, Wei EP, et al. Reduction of intracranial hypertension with free radical scavengers. In: Hoff JT Betz AL, eds. *Intracranial Pressure.* Vol 7. Berlin, Germany: Springer-Verlag. 1989:804–805.

83. Wei EP, Kontose HA, Dietrich WD, Povlishock JT, et al. Inhibition by free radical scavengers and by cyclooxygenase inhibitors of pial arteriolar abnormalities from concussive brain injury in cats. *Circ Res.* 1981;48:95–103

84. Haun SE, Kirsch JR, Helfaer MA, Kubos KL, et al. Polyethylene glycol-conjugated superoxide dismutase fails to augment brain superoxide dismutase activity in piglets. *Stroke.* 1991;22: 655–659.

85. Marmarou A, Anderson RL, Ward JD, et al. Impact of ICP stability and hypotension on outcome in patients with severe head trauma. *J Neurosurg.* 1991;75:S59–S66.

86. Imaizumi S, Woolworth V, Fishman RA, Chan PH. Liposome-entrapped superoxide dismutase reduces cerebral infarction in cerebral ischemia in rats. *Stroke.* 1990;21:1312–1317.

87. Davis RJ, Bulkley GB, Traystman RJ. Role of oxygen free radicals in focal brain ischemia. In Tomita M, Saunda T, Naritomi F, et al, eds. *Cerebral Hyperemia and Ischemia: From the Standpoint of Cerebral Blood Volume.* Amsterdam, the Netherlands: Excerpta Medica; 1988:151–156.

88. Snelling LK, Ackerman AD, Dean JM, et al. The effects of superoxide dismutase on neurologic recovery (cerebral blood flow and evoked potentials) following global cerebral ischemia. *Anesthesiology.* 1987;67:A153.

89. Muizelaar JP. Cerebral ischemia-reperfusion injury after severe head injury and its possible treatment with polyethyleneglycol-superoxide dismutase. *Ann Emerg Med.* 1993;22:1014–1021.

90. Chan PH, Epstein CJ, Kinochi F, et al. Role of superoxide dismutase in ischemia brain injury: reduction of edema and infarction in transgenic mice following focal cerebral ischeia. In: Kogure K, Hossman KA, Siesjo BK, eds. *Progress in Brain Research.* Amsterdam, the Netherlands: Elsevier Science; 1993.

91. Chan PH. Antioxidant-dependent amelioration of brain injury: role of CuZn-superoxide dismutase. *J Neurotrauma.* 1992 2(suppl):S417–S423.

92. Floyd RA, Carney J. Free radical damage to protein and DNA: mechanisms involved and relevant observations on brain undergoing oxidative stress. *Ann Neurol.* 1992;32(suppl):S22–S27.

93. Kontos HA. Oxygen radicals in CNS damage. *Chem Biol.* 1989;72:229–255.

94. Ginsberg MD, Watson BD, Busto R, Yoshida S, et al. Peroxidative damage to cell membranes following cerebral ischemia: a cause of ischemic brain injury? *Neurochem Pathol.* 1988;9:171–193.

95. Chan PH, Longar S, Fishman RA. Protective effects of liposome-entrapped superoxide dismutase on posttraumatic brain edema. *Ann Neurol.* 1987;21:540–547.

96. Kontos HA, Wei EP. Superoxide production in experimental brain injury. *J Neurosurg.* 1986;64:803–807.

97. Watson BD, Busto R, Goldberg WJ, Santiso M, et al. Lipid peroxidation in vivo induced by reversible global ischemia in rat brain. *J Neurochem.* 1984;42:268–274.

98. Hall ED. The neuroprotective pharmacology of methylprednisolone. *J Neurosurg.* 1992;76:13–22.

99. Hall ED, Braughler JM, McCall JM. New pharmacological treatment of acute spinal cord trauma. *J Neurotrauma.* 1988;5:81–89.

100. Hall ED, Yokers PA, McCall JM, Braughler JM. Effect of the 21-aminosteroid U74006F on experimental head injury in mice. *J Neurosurg.* 1988;68:456–461.

101. Braughler JM, Pregenzer JF, Chase RL, Duncan LA, et al. Novel 21-aminosteroids as potent inhibitors of iron-dependent lipid peroxidation. *J Biol Chem.* 1987;262:1438–1440.

102. Francel PC, Long BA, Malik JM, Tribble C, et al. Limiting ischemic spinal cord injury using a free radical scavenger 21-aminosteroid and/or cerebrospinal fluid drainage. *J Neurosurg.* 1993;79:742–751.

103. Sanada T, Nakamura T, Nishmura M, Isayama K, et al. Effect of U74006 on neurological function and brain edema after fluid percussion injury in rats. *J Neurotrauma.* 1993;10:65–71.

104. McIntosh TK, Thomas M, Smith D, Banbury M. The novel 21-aminosteroid U74006F attenuates cerebral edema and improves survival after brain injury in the rat. *J Neurotrauma.* 1992;9:33–46.

105. Sato PH, Hall ED. Tirilazad mesylate protects vitamin C and E in brain ischemia-reperfusion injury. *J Neurochem.* 1992;58:2263–2268.

106. Hall ED, Pazara KE, Braugler JM. Effects of tirilazad mesylate on postischemic brain lipid peroxidation and recovery of extracellular calcium in gerbils. *Stroke.* 1991;22:361–366.

107. Braughler J, Hall ED, Jacobsen E, et al. The 21-aminosteroids: potent inhibitors of lipid peroxidation for the treatment of central nervous system trauma and ischemia. *Drugs Future.* 1989;14:143–152.

108. Natale JE, Schott RJ, Hall ED, Braughler JM, et al. Effect of the 21-aminosteroid U74006F after cardiopulmonary arrest in dogs. *Stroke.* 1988;19:1371–1378.

109. Helfaer MA, Kirsch JR, Hurn PD, Blizzard KK, et al. Tirilazad mesylate does not improve early cerebral metabolic recovery following compression ischemia in dogs. *Stroke.* 1992;23:1479–1486.

110. Xue D, Slivka A, Buchan AM. Tirilazad reduces cortical infarction after transient but not permanent focal cerebral ischemia in rats. *Stroke.* 1992;23:894–899.

111. Clark WM, Hazel JS, Coull BM. Lazaroids: CNS pharmacology and current research. *Drugs.* 1995;50:971–983.

112. Kaplan AP, Silverberg M, Ghebrehiwet B, Atkins P, et al. The kallikrein-kinin system in inflammation. *Adv Exp Med Biol.* 1989;247A:125–136.

113. Aksoy MO, Harakal C, Smith JB, Stewart GJ, et al. Mediation of bradykinin-induced contraction in canine veins via thromboxane/prostaglandin endoperoxide receptor activation. *Br J Pharmacol*. 1990;99:461–466.

114. Dixon BS, Breckon R, Fortune J, Vavrek RJ, et al. Effects of kinins on cultured arterial smooth muscle. *Am J Physiol*. 1990;258:C299–C308.

115. Francel PC, Keefer JF, Dawson G. Bradykinin analogs antagonize bradykinin-induced second messenger production in a sensory neuron cell lines. *Mol Pharmacol*. 1989;35:34–38.

116. Francel PC. Bradykinin and neuronal injury. *J Neurotrauma*. 1992;9:S27–S45.

117. Hendrick EB. The use of hypothermia in severe head injuries in childhood. *Arch Surg*. 1959;79:362–364.

118. Sedzimir CB. Therapeutic hypothermia in cases of head injury. *J Neurosurg*. 1959;16:407–414.

119. Lazorthes G, Campan L. Hypothermia in the treatment of craniocerebral traumatism. *J Neurosurg*. 1958;15:162–167.

120. Fay T. Observations on general refrigeration in cases of severe cerebral trauma. *Assoc Res Nerv Ment Dis Proc*. 1943;24:611–619.

121. Fay T. Observations on prolonged human refrigeration. *NY State J Med*. 1940;15:1351–1353.

122. Clifton GL, Jiang JY, Lyeth BG, Jenkins LW, et al. Marked protection by moderate hypothermia after experimental traumatic brain injury. *J Cereb Blood Flow Metab*. 1991;11:114–121.

123. Cold GE. Cerebral blood flow in acute head injury: the regulation of cerebral blood flow and metabolism during the acute phase of head injury, and its significance for therapy. *Acta Neurochir*. 1990;49(supp.):1–64.

124. Chopp M, Knight R, Tidwell CD, Helpern JA, et al. The metabolic effects of mild hypothermia on global cerebral ischemia and recirculation in the cat: comparison to normothermia and hypothermia. *J Cereb Blood Flow Metab*. 1989;9:141–148.

125. Ward JD, Becker DP, Miller JD, Choi SC, et al. Failure of prophylactic barbiturate coma in the treatment of severe head injury. *J Neurosurg*. 1985;62:383–388.

126. Berntman L, Welsh FA, Harp JR. Cerebral protective effect of low-grade hypothermia. *Anesthesiology*. 1981;55:495–498.

127. Steen PA, Soule EH, Michenfelder JD. Detrimental effect of prolonged hypothermia in cats and monkeys with and without regional cerebral ischemia. *Stroke*. 1979;10:522–529.

128. Shapiro HM, Wyte SR, Loeser J. Barbiturate-augmented hypothermia for reduction of persistent intracranial hypertension. *J Neurosurg*. 1974;40:90–100.

129. Resnick DK, Marion DW, Darby JM. The effect of hypothermia on the incidence of delayed traumatic intracerebral hemorrhage. *Neurosurgery*. 1994;34:255–256.

130. Sterz F, Safar P, Tisherman S, Radovsky A, et al. Mild hypothermia cardiopulmonary resuscitation improves outcome after prolonged cardiac arrest in dogs. *Crit Care Med*. 1991;19:379–389.

131. Kader A, Frazzini VI, Baker CJ, Solomon RA, et al. Effect of mild hypothermia on nitric oxide synthesis during focal cerebral ischemia. *Neurosurgery*. 1994;35:272–277.

132. Goto Y, Kassell NF, Hiramatsu K, Scleau SW, et al. Effects of intraischemic hypothermia on cerebral damage in a model of reversible focal ischemia. *Neurosurgery*. 1993;32:980–984.

133. Xue D, Huang ZG, Smith KE, Buchan AM, et al. Immediate or delayed mild hypothermia prevents focal cerebral infarction. *Brain Res*. 1992;587:66–72.

134. Lundgren J, Smith ML, Siesjo BK. Influence of moderate hypothermia on ischemic brain damage incurred under hyperglycemic conditions. *Exp Brain Res*. 1991;84:91–101.

135. Minamisawa H, Smith ML, Siesjo BK. The effect of mild hyperthermia and hypothermia on brain damage following 5, 10, and 15 minutes of forebrain ischemia. *Ann Neurol.* 1990;28: 26–33.

136. Astrup J. Energy-requiring cell functions in the ischemic brain: their critical supply for possible inhibition in protective therapy. *J Neurosurg.* 1982;56:482–497.

137. Marion DN, White MJ. Treatment of experimental brain injury with moderate hypothermia and 21-aminosteroids. *J Neurotrauma.* 1996;13:139–142.

138. Marion DW, Obrist WD, Carlier PM, Penrod LE, et al. The use of moderate therapeutic hypothermia for patients with severe head injuries: a preliminary report. *J Neurosurg.* 1993;79: 354–362.

139. Shiozaki T, Sugimoto H, Taneda M, Yoshida H, et al. Effect of mild hypothermia on uncontrollable intracranial hypertension after severe head injury. *J Neurosurg.* 1993;79:363–368.

140. Clifton GL, Allen S, Barrodale P, et al. A phase II study of moderate hypothermia in severe brain injury. *J Neurotrauma.* 1993;10:263–271.

141. Marion DW, Penrod LE, Kelsey SF. Treatment of traumatic brain injury with moderate hypothermia. *N Engl J Med.* 1997;336:540–546.

142. Coimbra C, Wieloch T. Moderate hypothermia mitigates neuronal damage in the rat brain when initiated several hours following transient cerebral ischemia. *Acta Neuropathol (Berlin).* 1994;87:325–331.

143. Pomeranz S, Safar P, Radovsky A, Tisherman SA, et al. The effect of resuscitative moderate hypothermia following epidural brain compression on cerebral damage in a canine outcome model. *J Neurosurg.* 1993;79:241–251.

144. Kader A, Brisman MH, Maraire N, Huh JT, et al. The effect of mild hypothermia on permanent focal ischemia in the rat. *Neurosurgery.* 1992;31:1056–1060.

145. Busto R, Globus MY, Dietrich WD, Martinez E, et al. Effect of mild hypothermia on ischemia-induced release of neurotransmitters and free fatty acids in rat brain. *Stroke.* 1989;20:904–910.

146. Michenfelder JD, Van Dyke RA, Theye RA. The effects of anesthetic agents and techniques on canine cerebral ATP and lactate levels. *Anesthesiology.* 1970;33:315–321.

147. Hagerdal M, Harp J, Nilsson L, Siesjo BK. The effect of induced hypothermia upon oxygen consumption in the rat brain. *J Neurochem.* 1975;24:311–316.

148. Rosomoff HL, Holaday DA. Cerebral blood flow and cerebral oxygen consumption during hypothermia. *Am J Physiol.* 1954;179:85–88.

149. Clifton GL, Hayes RL, Levin HS, Michel ME, et al. Outcome measures for clinical trials involving traumatically brain-injured patients: report of a conference. *Neurosurgery.* 1992;31: 975–978.

150. Cervelli L, Berrol S. *Description of a Model Care System: Head Injury Rehabilitation Project. Vol 1. Report to the National Institute for Handicapped Research (Project 13-P-S9156/9).* San Jose, Calif: Institute for Medical Research at Santa Clara Valley Medical Center; 1982.

151. Heist KK. The demand for trauma rehabilitation. In: Cardona VD, Hurn PD, Mason PJ, Scanlon A, et al. eds. *Trauma Nursing: From Resuscitation through Rehabilitation.* 2nd ed. Philadelphia, Pa: WB Saunders Co; 1994:363–379.

152. Zasler ND, Kreutzer JS, Taylor D. Coma stimulation and coma recovery: a critical review. *Neurorehabilitation.* 1991;1:33–40.

153. Wells JD, Nicosia S. The effects of multidisciplinary team care for acute spinal cord injury patients. *J Am Paraplegia Soc.* 1993;16:23–29.

154. Oakes DD, Wilmot CB, Hall KM, Sherck JP. Benefits of early admission to a comprehensive trauma center for patients with spinal cord injury. *Arch Phys Med Rehabil.* 1990;71:637–643.

155. DeVivo MJ, Kartus PL, Stover SL, Fine PR. Benefits of early admission to an organised spinal cord injury care system. *Paraplegia.* 1990;28:545–555.

156. Rinehart ME. Early mobilization in acute spinal cord injury: a collaborative approach. *Crit Care Nurs Clin North Am.* 1990;2:399–405.

157. Franz SI. On the functions of the cerebrum: the frontal lobes in relation to the production and retention of simple sensory-motor habits. *Am J Physiol.* 1902;8:1–22.

158. Chow KL, Stewart DL. Reversal of structural and functional effects of long-term visual deprivation in cats. *Exp Neurol.* 1972;34:409–433.

159. Yu J. Functional recovery with and without training following brain damage in experimental animals: a review. *Arch Phys Med Rehabil.* 1976;57:38–41.

160. Rosenzweig MR. Animals models for effects of brain lesions and for rehabilitation. In: Bach-y-Rita P, ed. *Recovery of Function: Theoretical Considerations for Brain Injury Rehabilitation.* Bern, Germany: Hans Huber Publishers; 1980:127–172.

161. Black P, Markowitz RS, Cianci S. Recovery of motor function after lesions in motor cortex of monkeys. *Ciba Found Symp.* 1975;34:65–83.

162. Wall PD, Egger MD. Formation of new connexions in adult rat brains after partial deafferentation. *Nature.* 1971;232:542–545.

163. Mackenzie C, Ciesla N, Imle PC, et al. *Chest Physiotherapy in the Intensive Care Unit.* Baltimore, Md: Williams & Wilkins; 1981.

164. Kottke FJ. Therapeutic exercise to maintain mobility. In: Kottke FJ, Stillwell GK, Lehman JF, eds. *Krusen's Handbook of Physical Medicine and Rehabilitation.* 3rd ed. Philadelphia, Pa: WB Saunders Co; 1982.

165. Cherry DB. Review of physical therapy alternatives for reducing muscle contracture. *Phys Ther.* 1980;60:877–881.

166. Derrickson JG, Ciesla N, Matello P. A comparison of acute medical therapeutic management on the functional outcome of brain-injured patients. *APTA (Neurol Rep).* 1989;13:10–12.

167. Mackay LE, Bernstein BA, Chapman PE, Morgan AS, et al. Early intervention in severe head injury: long-term benefits of a formalized program. *Arch Phys Med Rehabil.* 1992;73:635–641.

168. Powell JN, Chapman P. The impact of early orthopedic management on patients with traumatic brain injury. *J Head Trauma Rehabil.* 1994;9:57–66.

169. Narayan RK, Kishore PRS, Becker DP, Ward JD, et al. Intracranial pressure: to monitor or not to monitor? A review of our experience with severe head injury. *J Neurosurg.* 1982;56:650–659.

170. Feldman Z, Reichenthal E. Intracranial pressure monitoring. *J Neurosurg.* 1994;81:329–330. Letter to the editor.

171. Rogers RC. Heterotopic calcification in severe head injury: a preventive programme. *Brain Inj.* 1988;2:169–173.

172. Kalisky Z, Morrison DP, Meyers CA, Von Laufen A. Medical problems encountered during rehabilitation of patients with head injury. *Arch Phys Med Rehabil.* 1985;66:25–29.

173. Garland DE, Blum CE, Waters RL. Periarticular heterotopic ossification in head-injured adults: incidence and location. *J Bone Joint Surg (Am).* 1980;62:1143–1146.

174. Citta-Pietrolungo TJ, Alexander MA, Steg NL. Early detection of heterotopic ossification in young patients with traumatic brain injury. *Arch Phys Med Rehabil.* 1992;73:258–262.

175. Lehmkuhl LD, Thoi LL, Baize C, Kelley CJ, et al. Multimodality treatment of joint contractures in patients with severe brain injury: cost, effectiveness, and integration of therapies in the application of serial/inhibitive casts. *J Head Trauma Rehabil.* 1990;5:23–42.

176. Sullivan T, Connie TA, Goodman M, Mackie T. Serial casting to prevent equinus in acute traumatic head injury. *Physiother Can.* 1988;40:346–350.

177. Booth BJ, Doyle M, Montgomery J. Serial casting for the management of spasticity in the head-injured adult. *Phys Ther.* 1983;63:1960–1966.

178. Murdock K, Ciesla N. The effect of serial casting on intracranial pressure. Presented at Fourth Conference of the International Association for the Study of Traumatic Brain Injury; September 25, 1994; St. Louis, Mo.

179. Cameron ID, Lyle DM, Quine S. Accelerated rehabilitation after proximal femoral fracture: a randomized controlled trial. *Disabil Rehabil.* 1993;15:29–34.

180. Eiff MP, Smith AT, Smith GE. Early mobilization versus immobilization in the treatment of lateral ankle sprains. *Am J Sports Med.* 1994;22:83–88.

181. Riemer BL, Butterfield SL, Diamond DL, Young JC, et al. Acute mortality associated with injuries to the pelvic ring: the role of early patient mobilization and external fixation. *J Trauma.* 1993;35:671–675.

182. Collins DC. Management and rehabilitation of distal radius fractures. *Orthop Clin North Am.* 1993;24:365–378.

183. Clifton GL, Robertson CS, Choi SC. Assessment of nutritional requirements of head-injured patients. *J Neurosurg.* 1986;64:895–901.

184. Logeman JA, Pepe J, Mackay LE. Disorders of nutrition and swallowing: intervention strategies in the trauma center. *J Head Trauma Rehabil.* 1994;9:43–56.

185. Clifton GL, Robertson CS, Choi SC. Assessment of nutritinal requirements of head-injured patients. *J Neurosurg.* 1986;64:895–901.

186. Hsieh AH, Bishop MJ, Kubilis PS, Newell DW, et al. Pneumonia following closed head injury. *Am Rev Respir Dis.* 1992;146:290–294.

187. Frost EA. Respiratory problems associated with head trauma. *Neurosurgery.* 1977;1:300–306.

188. Rodriguez JL, Gibbons KJ, Bitzer LG, Dechert RE, et al. Pneumonia: incidence, risk factors, and outcome in injured patients. *J Trauma.* 1991;31:907–912.

189. Helling TS, Evans LL, Fowler DL, Hays LV, et al. Infectious complications in patients with severe head injury. *J Trauma.* 1988;28:1575–1577.

190. Hagen C. Language disorders secondary to closed head injury: diagnosis and treatment. *Top Lang Disord.* 1981;1:73–87.

191. Morgan AS, Chapman P, Tokarski L. Improved care of the traumatically brain injured. Presented at First Annual Conference of Eastern Association for Surgery of Trauma; January 15, 1988; Longboat Key, Fla.

192. Hall K, Wright J. The cost versus benefit of rehabilitation in traumatic brain injury. Presented at 11th Annual Southwest Brain Injury Symposium; January 18, 1993; Santa Barbara, Calif.

193. Rappaport M, Hall KM, Hopkins HK, Belleza T, et al. Disability rating scale for severe head trauma patients: coma to community. *Arch Phys Med Rehabil.* 1982;63:118–123.

194. Hall K, Cope DN, Rappaport M. Glasgow outcome scale and disability rating scale: comparative usefulness in following recovery on traumatic head injury. *Arch Phys Med Rehabil.* 1985;66:35–37.

195. Cope DN. Social Status Outcome Scale. Head Trauma Rehabilitation Project. Vol I. Report to the National Institute for Handicapped Research (Project 13-P-S9156/9). San Jose, Calif: Institute for Medical Research at Santa Clara Valley Medical Center; 1982.

196. Cope DN, Hall K. Head injury rehabilitation: benefit of early intervention. *Arch Phys Med Rehabil.* 1982;63:433–437.

197. Bullock R, Chesnut RM, Clifton G, et al. Guidelines for the management of severe head injury. *J Neurotrauma.* 1996;13:639–734.

198. Harrison-Felix C, Newton N, Hall K, Kreutzer J. Descriptive findings from the Traumatic Brain Injury Model Systems National Database. *J Head Trauma Rehabil.* 1996;11:5

199. Hall M, Brandys C, Yetman L. Multidisciplinary approaches to management of acute head injury. *J Neurosci Nurs.* 1992;24:159–204.

200. Sosnowski C, Ustik M. Early intervention: coma stimulation in the intensive care unit. *J Neurosci Nurs.* 1994;26:336–341.

Index

A

Abdominal injury, 260–265
  computed tomography, 263
  diagnosis, 261–263
  diagnostic peritoneal lavage, 262
  traumatic brain injury, treatment
    priority, 263–265
  ultrasonography, 262–263
Abducens nerve, 136, 145
  components, 138
  cortical and other connections, 145
  functions, 138
  injury diagnosis, 162
  injury mechanism, 162
  subdivisions and pathways, 145
Accessory nerve, 136, 156–157
  components, 139
  cortical and subcortical
    connections, 156–157
  functions, 139, 156
  injury diagnosis, 166
  injury management, 166
  subdivisions and pathways, 156
Acetylcholine, 499
Acoustic reflex testing, 487
Adult respiratory distress syndrome,
  364–372

exudative phase, 368
fibrotic phase, 368
patients at risk, 365–367
pharmacologic treatment, 371–372
physiologic alterations leading to,
  367–368
proliferative phase, 368
pulmonary dysfunction, 365
pulmonary mechanics, 369–370
pulmonary pathology, 368–369,
  370
sepsis syndrome, 365–366
ventilation, 370–371
Advanced life support, 13
Afferent fiber, 81
Agitation, pharmacologic
  management, 512–515
Air bag, 8–9
Air flow bed, 204–207
Airway, documentation, 184
Alcohol, documentation, 191–192
Alternating air flow bed, 204–207
Amantadine, 509–510
Ambient-air arterial blood gas,
  normal, 333–334
American College of Emergency
  Physicians, 5

American College of Surgeons'
  Committee on Trauma, 5
Amygdala, 101
Anger, 542, 543–544
Anterior cerebral artery, 106
Anterior cord syndrome, 227
Antibiotics, pneumonia, 351
Anticatecholaminergic drug, 507–511
Anticholinergic drug, 506–507
Anxiety, 542–543
Aortic dissection, 258–259
Arachnoid mater, 85
Arrhythmia, 419–420
Arterial line, 200–201
  precautions, 195
  purpose, 195
Artificial ventilation, 342–349
Aspiration pneumonia, 351
Astrocyte, 83–84
Auditory cortex, 92, 93, 95
Auditory pathways, 151
Auditory perception, 483–499
Autonomic disturbance,
  pharmacologic management, 504,
  518–519
Axon, 81

B

Barbiturate, intracranial pressure,
  116–117
Basal ganglia, 90
Basic life support, 12–13
Bed, 204–207
Benzodiazepine, 507
Beta blocker, 503–504
Bicycle, 4
Bicycle helmet, 9–10
Bicycle injury, documentation,
  181
Blood gas physiology, 333–334

Blunt injury to carotid artery,
  171–173
Bouton, 83
Bradykinin, 577–578
Brain
  arterial blood supply, 106–107
  blood supply, 106–108
  cellular anatomy, 80–85
  gross anatomy, 85–106
  normal pH, 110
  pathophysiology, 110–112
    dynamics, 110–111
    treatment, 111–112
  physiology, 108–110
  venous drainage, 107–108
  vertebral arterial system, 107
Brain abscess, 430–432
Brain death, 210–211
Brain Injury Association, vii
Brainstem, 101–103
Brainstem auditory evoked-potential
  testing, hearing, 494–497
Breathing
  documentation, 184
  mechanics, 332–333
Brodmann's areas, 91
Bromocriptine, 511
Bronchodilator therapy, 347–348
Brown-Séquard syndrome, 226–227

C

Calcium, 110, 505–506
Carbamazepine, 503–504
Carbidopa, 510
Cardiac monitor
  precautions, 195
  purpose, 195
Cardiovascular trauma, 250–259
Cast, 290–291
Catechol, 508

Catecholaminergic drug, 507–511
Catheter-related infection, 422–424
Cauda equina–corus medullaris
   syndrome, 227
Caudate nucleus, 90
Cell body, 80
Cellular anatomy, 80–85
Central cord syndrome, 226
Central pontine myelinolysis, 415
Central spinal fluid, 96–98
Central sulcus, 89
Central venous pressure line, 201
   precautions, 195
   purpose, 195
Cerebellum, 104–106
Cerebral blood flow, 108–110
   bedside cerebral blood flow
      monitoring, 122–123
Cerebral cortex, 90
   Brodmann's areas, 91
   motor areas, 92–94
   organization, 91–92
   psychological areas, 95–96
   somatosensory areas, 94
Cerebral dominance, 96
Cerebral hemisphere, 86
Cerebral perfusion pressure, 110
Cerebral vascular resistance, 108–110
Cerebrum, 86–98
   divisions, 87–90
   lobes, 88–90
Cervical spinal cord injury,
   occupational therapy, 325
Chemical paralysis, 289–290
Chest physiotherapy, 347–348
Chest tube, 202–203
   precautions, 196
   purpose, 196
Chest wall, 326
Cholinergic drug, 506–507
Cimetidine, 503–504

Cingulate gyrus, 89, 101
Cingulate sulcus, 89
Cingulum, 101
Circle of Willis, 107
Circulation, documentation, 184–185
Cisapride, 503–504
Claustrum, 90
Cognition, 584–585
Coma stimulation program, 579
Communication, traumatic brain
   injury team, 74–75
Complication, 67–68
Continuing education, 52
Continuous jugular venous oximetry,
   intracranial pressure, 121–122
Contusion, 125–126
Cooling blanket, 209
   precautions, 197
   purpose, 197
Coping, 539
Cortical lesion
   area 1, 95
   area 2, 95
   area 3, 95
   area 4, 94
   area 6, 94
Corticotropin-releasing hormone, 100
Cost containment, trauma center,
   32–33
Cranial nerve, 104–105. *See also*
   Specific type
   anatomy, 135–159
   eye, potential impairments, 313
   physiology, 135–159
Cranial nerve injury
   diagnosis, 159–166
   management, 159–166
Crisis
   characterized, 531–532
   classified, 532
   developmental phases, 533

factors, 533–535
family
    anger, 542, 543–544
    anxiety, 542–543
    assessment, 535–538
    being with patient, 547–550,
        551–555
    children and siblings, 558
    coping, 545
    crisis intervention, 530–562
    cultural diversity, 558–561
    culturally sensitive guidelines,
        560, 561
    denial, 542, 543
    family guidelines for interaction
        with patients, 551–555
    family needs, 538, 540–541,
        545–558
    feeling helpful and needed,
        550–556
    grief, 544
    hope, 542
    information needs, 546–548,
        549–550, 551, 555
    intervention, 536, 538–545
    patient information sheet, 556,
        557
    phases of recovery, 539–545
    recognizing own personal needs,
        556–558
    reconciliation, 544–545
    remorse, 544
    support groups and advocacy
        associations, 547, 566–571
    historical development of crisis
        theory, 532–533
    paradigm, 533, 534
Critical care
    audiological issues, 483–499
    rehabilitation
        animal studies, 581

        benefits, 579–585
        benefits of combining, 572–591
        cognition, 584–585
        disposition, 586
        early-intervention program,
            579–580
        length of stay, 586, 587, 588, 589
        level of functioning, 584–585
        medical benefits, 584
        physical/motor skills, 582–584
        transfer planning, 586–589
    team-focused intervention, 56–76
Critical care staff, cultural diversity,
    559
Cultural diversity, 558–561
    critical care staff, 559
    decision making, 559–560
    illness, 559

                        D
Dead space ventilation, 333
Decision making, cultural diversity,
    559–560
Decubitus ulcer, 425–426
Decussation of the pyramids, 103
Deep-venous thrombosis, 372–378
    diagnosis, 375–378
    Doppler ultrasonography, 376
    duplex ultrasonography, 376–377
    features, 373
    heparin, 374–375
    125I-fibrinogen leg scan, 377
    impedance plethysmography, 376
    incidence, 373
    management, 378
    prophylactic therapy, 374–375
    radiographic methods, 377
    risk, 373
    stasis, 374
Dendrite, 81

Denial, 542, 543
Depressed skull fracture, 125, 127
Dextroamphetamine, 511
Diaphragmatic injury, 259
Diaphragmatic rupture, 259
Diencephalon, 85, 98–100
Diffuse axonal injury, 126–127
Disease, defined, 559
Diuretic, intracranial pressure, 116
Dobhoff tube
  precautions, 196
  purpose, 196
Documentation, 68, 69, 75–76,
  177–194
  airway, 184
  alcohol, 191–192
  bicycle injury, 181
  breathing, 184
  circulation, 184–185
  drug usage, 191–192
  emergency department, 183–193
    report, 183–187
  EMS run sheet, 181–183
  intensive care, 183
  mechanism of injury, 178–181
  medical history, 193–194
  medication, 192–193
  motor vehicle collision, 179–180
    frontal collision, 179–180
    lateral collision, 180
    rollover collision, 180
  motorcycle collision, 180–181
  neurological assessment, 188–189
  orthopaedic injury, 190–191
  patient status, 181–193
  pedestrian injury, 181
  spinal injury, 189–190
Dopamine, 507–509
Doppler ultrasonography,
  deep-venous thrombosis, 376
Drug usage, documentation, 191–192

Duplex ultrasonography, deep-venous
  thrombosis, 376–377
Dura mater, 85
Dural venous sinus, 85
Dysconjugate gaze, 318, 319
Dysphagia, 469–471

E

Ear, mechanisms of damage, 483–486
Early-onset pneumonia, 351–352
Edema, 298
Education program, rehabilitation
  staff, 580
Efferent fiber, 81
Electrocardiogram, 199–200
Electrolyte abnormality, 413–417
Emergency department,
  documentation, 183–193
  report, 183–187
Emergency medical technician, 12
Emotional homeostasis, 533
Empyema, 432–433
EMS run sheet, 181–183
Endotracheal intubation, 336–338
  problems, 338
Endotracheal suctioning, 347
Enteral nutrition, 406–411
  complications, 410–411
  enteral access devices, 406–410
Epidural hematoma, 124, 125
Epinephrine, 507–509
Equipment
  intensive care unit, 194–207
  orthopaedic equipment, 203–204
  unstable patient, 207–211
    neurological status, 209–211
Esophageal injury, 257
Evoked-potential testing, hearing,
  assessment of neurologic integrity,
  495–497

Excitatory amino acid, 574–575
External drain, 202–203
External fixator, 203–204
Eye
    autonomic innervation, 143,
        145–146
        cortical and subcortical
            connections, 146
        functions, 145–146
        subdivisions and pathways, 146
    cranial nerve, potential
        impairments, 313
    reflexes, 143, 145–146
        cortical and subcortical
            connections, 146
        functions, 145–146
        subdivisions and pathways, 146

F

Facial nerve, 136, 148–151
    components, 138
    cortical and subcortical
        connections, 150–151
    diagnostic tests, 163–164
    electrical stimulation, 163–164
    functions, 138, 148
    imaging studies, 164
    subdivisions and pathways,
        148–150
    treatment, 164–165
Falx cerebelli, 85
Falx cerebri, 85
Family, vii, 300
    crisis
        anger, 542, 543–544
        anxiety, 542–543
        assessment, 535–538
        being with patient, 547–550,
            551–555
        children and siblings, 558

coping, 545
cultural diversity, 558–561
culturally sensitive guidelines,
    560, 561
denial, 542, 543
family guidelines for interaction
    with patients, 551–555
family needs, 538, 540, 541,
    545–558
feeling helpful and needed,
    550
grief, 544
hope, 542
information needs, 546–547, 548,
    549–550, 551–555
intervention, 530–560, 536,
    538–545
patient information sheet, 556,
    557
phases of recovery, 539–545
recognizing own personal needs,
    556–558
reconciliation, 544–545
remorse, 544
support groups and advocacy
    associations, 547, 566–571
occupational therapy, 333–334
transactional patterns, 530
Fat embolism syndrome, 247–249
Fecal collection bag
    precautions, 197
    purpose, 197
Femoral shaft fracture, 245
Firearms, 2–3, 10–12
    cost, 4
    suicide, 2–3
Firm-surface rotating bed, 206
Flail chest, 254–255
Flowsheet, 68, 69, 75–76
Follicle-stimulating hormone, 100
Forebrain, 85

Free radical, 505–506
Frontal lobe, 87
Functional outcome, regionalized
    trauma system, 22–29

G

Gamma-aminobutyric acid, 507
Gastrointestinal disturbance,
    pharmacologic management, 504,
    517–518
Gastrostomy tube
    precautions, 195
    purpose, 196
Glasgow Coma Score
    components, 65
    scoring, 65
Globus pallidus, 90
Glossopharyngeal nerve, 136,
    153–155
    central connections, 154
    components, 138
    cortical and subcortical
        connections, 155
    functions, 138, 153
    injury diagnosis, 166
    injury management, 166
    subdivisions and pathways,
        153–155
Glutamate, 505
    intracranial pressure, 119
Gonadotropin-releasing hormone, 100
Gray matter, 81–82
Grief, 533, 544
Growth hormone-releasing hormone,
    100
Gun control, 11

H

Health care reform, regionalized
    trauma system, 31–33

Hearing
    acoustic reflex testing, 493
    audiologic referral flowchart, 484,
        485
    brainstem auditory
        evoked-potential testing,
        494–497
    chart review, 486–487
    evoked-potential testing,
        assessment of neurologic
        integrity, 495–497
    hearing acuity assessment, 490–497
    otoacoustic emissions testing,
        493–494
    patient selection, 483–486
    pure tone audiogram, 490–492
    skull fracture, 486
    skull vault fracture, 484
    test methodology, 488–490
    test rationale, 487–488
    transverse temporal bone fracture,
        485
    tympanometry, 492–493
Helmet. *See* Specific type
Hematoma, 123–125, 126
Hemodynamic monitor, 199–202
Heparin, deep-venous thrombosis,
    374–375
High-frequency jet ventilation, 344
Hindbrain, 85
Hip dislocation, 245
Hippocampus, 101
Hope, 542
Hypercatabolism, 400–401, 402
Hypermetabolism, 396–400, 505
Hypernatremia, 415–416
Hypertension, 417–419
Hyperventilation, intracranial
    pressure, 114–115
Hypoglossal nerve, 136, 157–159
    components, 139

cortical and subcortical
    connections, 159
  functions, 139
  injury diagnosis, 166
  injury management, 166
  subdivisions and pathways, 159
Hyponatremia, 413, 414–415
Hypotension, 573
Hypothalamic sulcus, 99
Hypothalamus, 98–100
Hypothermia, 578–579
  intracranial pressure, 117–118
Hypoxia, 573

I

Illness
  cultural diversity, 559
  defined, 559
Immunosuppression, 402–403
Impedance plethysmography,
    deep-venous thrombosis, 376
Independent lung ventilation,
    344–345
Infection, occupational therapy,
    331–332
Inferior frontal gyrus, 87
Insula, 89, 101
Intensive care unit
  documentation, 183
  equipment, 194–207
  monitoring, normative values, 194
  occupational therapy, equipment,
    306–307
  physical therapy, 271–301
    active movement, 278
    assessment, 272–280
    benefits of multidisciplinary
      treatment sessions, 280–281
    cast, 290–291
    chemical paralysis, 289–290

cognitive level, 279–280
complications, 297–300
direct assessment, 275–280
edema, 298
equipment, 273–275
eye movement, 278
family, 300
level of alertness, 281–284
multidisciplinary input, 272–273
normal motor control, 291–296
normalization of tone, 284–287,
    288
orientation, 281–284
orthopaedic injuries, 297–298
pain stimulus, 278–279
patient observation, 275
posturing, 276–277
primary areas of focus, 280, 281
pulmonary complications,
    298–299
range of motion, 277–278
range of motion maintenance,
    287–291
skin integrity, 296–297
spinal injuries, 297–298
splint, 290–291
treatment, 280–297
speech/language pathology,
    444–477
alertness, 447–448
arousal, 447–448
assessment, 447–450
cognition, 447–448
cognition/language, 454–455
communicative intent, 455–458
electronic technology, 457–458
equipment, 445
family, 475–476
formal assessment tools,
    451–452
monitoring device, 445

movement, 450
oral-motor responses, 449–450
patient observation, 446–447
Rancho Los Amigos Scale of
Cognitive Functioning, 452
responsiveness/interaction with
the environment, 454
role, 444
swallowing, 468–475
talking tracheostomy tube,
464–465
tracheostomy speaking valve,
465–468
tracheostomy tube, 460–464
treatment, 451–458
visual responses, 449
vocal communication options,
464–468
vocal cords, 458–468
technology, 194–207
Internal carotid artery, 106
blunt injury, 171–173
Intracerebral hematoma, 124–125,
126
Intracranial hypertension, 112–123
management, 114–123
pathology, 112–114
technology, 120–123
treatment, 114–123
Intracranial pressure
barbiturate, 116–117
bedside cerebral blood flow
monitoring, 122–123
cerebrospinal fluid drainage, 116
continuous jugular venous
oximetry, 121–122
diuretic, 116
glutamate, 119
head elevation, 116
hyperventilation, 114–115
hypothermia, 117–118

management, 114–123
mannitol, 115–116
monitoring, 66–67, 120–121
precautions, 195
purpose, 195
pathology, 112–114
posttraumatic seizure, 118–119
management, 118–119
steroid, 119–120
technology, 120–123
transcranial Doppler
ultrasonography, 121
treatment, 114–123
Intravenous line, 201–202

J

Jejunostomy tube
precautions, 196
purpose, 196
Jet ventilator, 208–209

K

Knee injury, 246

L

Language neural circuit, 92, 95
Length of stay, 586, 587, 588, 589
Level of functioning, 584–585
Levodopa, 509, 510
Limbic system, 100–101
Lipid peroxidation, 576–577
Lithium, 503–504
Long circumferential artery, 107
Lower extremity
compartment syndrome, 246–247
mangled extremity, 247
Lower extremity fracture, long bone
fracture, 244–250

operative fixation timing, 249–250
Lung
  bacterial interference, 350
  pulmonary defense system, 350
Lung abscess, 358–359
Lung ventilation-perfusion scan,
  pulmonary embolism, 380, 381
Luteinizing hormone-releasing
  hormone, 100

M

Mammillary body, 101
Mandibular nerve, 147
Mannitol, intracranial pressure,
  115–116
Mattress, 205–206
Mattress pad, 205, 207
Maturational crisis, 532
Maxillary nerve, 147
Maxillofacial injury, 166–171
  management, 167–161
  radiology, 169–170
  repair timing, 170–171
Mechanism of injury, documentation,
  178–181
Medial nucleus, 99
Medical history, documentation,
  193–194
Medical record, 177–194
Medication, documentation, 192–193
Medulla oblongata, 102–103
Meninges, 85
Meningitis, 428–430
Mesencephalon, 85, 101–102
Metoclopramide, 503–504
Microglia, 84–85
Midbrain, 85
Middle cerebral artery, 106
Middle frontal gyrus, 87
Minute ventilation, 327

Monitoring, ventilation, 345–346
Mortality, traumatic brain injury, 1
Motor cortex, 92–94
Motor vehicle collision,
  documentation, 179–180
  frontal collision, 179–180
  lateral collision, 180
  rollover collision, 180
Motorcycle, 4
Motorcycle collision, documentation,
  180–181
Motorcycle helmet, 9
Musculoskeletal injury, 236–250
Myelin, 82
Myelin sheath, 81
Myocardial contusion, 257–258
Myocardial injury, 419
Myogenic autoregulation, 110

N

Nasogastric tube, 202
  precautions, 196
  purpose, 196
Nasotracheal intubation, 337,
  338
  problems, 338
Nerve fiber, 81, 82
Neuroanatomy, overview, 80–106
Neurogenic diabetes insipidus,
  416–417
Neurogenic pulmonary edema,
  360–364
  incidence, 362–363
  pathophysiology, 360–362
  signs and symptoms, 363
  treatment, 363–364
Neuroglia, 83
Neurologic assessment, 65–66
Neurological assessment,
  documentation, 188–189
Neurological monitoring, 202

Neurological status, 209–211
Neuromuscular function,
    occupational therapy, 320–325
Neuron, 80–81
    axonal portion, 82
    intracellular structures, 81
Neurotransmitter
    acute stage of recovery, 504–506
    postacute stage of recovery, 506
    role, 504–506
Node of Ranvier, 82
Norepinephrine, 507–509
Nosocomial infection, 420–433
Nosocomial sinusitis, 426–428
Nursing, traumatic brain injury team
    airway and breathing, 63–64
    circulation, 64
    complication, 67–68
    contributions, 63–71
    documentation, 68, 69, 75–76
    flowsheet, 68, 69, 75–76
    Glasgow Coma Score, 65
    initial assessment, 63
    intracranial pressure monitoring,
        66–67
    neurologic assessment, 65–66
    paralysis, 67
    psychosocial issues, 68–69
    role, 63–71
    sedation, 67
    stabilization, 63
    trauma nurse coordinator,
        69–71
Nutritional support, 207, 403–413,
    573–574
    caloric requirement, 404–405
    enteral nutrition, 406–411
    outcome, 411–413
    parenteral nutrition, 405–406
    protein requirement, 405
    requirements, 404–405

O

Occipital lobe, 88, 89
Occupational therapy, 304–328
    assessment, 305
        cognitive assessment, 315
        motor control, 309
        multidisciplinary input, 305–306
        posturing, 310–311
        purposeful on-command
            movement, 311–312
        range of motion, 311
        response to auditory stimulation,
            308
        response to kinesthetic
            stimulation, 308
        response to painful stimuli, 308
        response to proprioceptive
            stimulation, 308
        response to tactile stimulation,
            308
        response to visual stimulation,
            308
        tone, 310–311
        visual-motor assessment,
            312–315
    cervical spinal cord injury, 325
    complications, 325–326
    direct assessment, 307–315
    family, 327–328
    goals, 315–316, 317
    infection, 325–326
    intensive care unit, equipment,
        306–307
    neuromuscular function,
        320–325
    observation, 307
    oculomotor function, 319–320
    role, 304
    treatment, 316–317
        alertness, 317–319
        arousal, 317–319

benefits of multidisciplinary
treatment sessions, 316
orientation, 317–319
Oculomotor function, occupational
therapy, 319–320
Oculomotor nerve, 136, 144
components, 138
cortical and other connections, 144
functions, 138
injury diagnosis, 161
injury management, 161
subdivisions and pathways, 144
Olfactory nerve, 136, 137–140, 141
components, 138
cortical and other connections, 140
function, 137, 138
injury diagnosis, 159–160
injury management, 159–160
subdivisions and pathways,
137–140, 141
Oligodendroglia, 81, 84
Olive, 103
Ophthalmic nerve, 147
Optic nerve, 136, 138, 140–142
components, 138
cortical and other connections, 142,
143
functions, 138, 140–142
injury diagnosis, 160–161
injury management, 160–161
subdivisions and pathways, 141,
142
Orthopaedic equipment, 203–204
Orthopaedic injury, documentation,
190–191
Otoacoustic emissions testing,
593–594
Oxygen, 332–333
cerebral oxygen delivery and
consumption normal values, 109
Oxygen free radical, 576

Oxyhemoglobin dissociation curve,
334, 335

P

Parahippocampal gyrus, 101
Paralysis, 67
Paramedian artery, 107
Paramedic, 12
Paraventricular nucleus, 100
Parenchymal pulmonary injury,
255–256
Parenteral nutrition, 405–406
Parietal lobe, 88, 89
Patient data, 177–194
Patient status, documentation,
181–193
Pedestrian injury, documentation, 181
Pelvic anatomy, 236–237
Pelvic fracture, 236–244
classification, 237–240
coexisting injuries, 240–241
management, 241–244
Percutaneous dilational tracheostomy,
339–342
Periosteum, 85
Pharmacologic management,
503–521
agitation, 512–515
autonomic disturbance, 504,
518–519
future medical advances, 574–579
gastrointestinal disturbance, 504,
517–518
restlessness, 512–515
seizure prophylaxis, 504,
515–517
spasticity, 504, 519–521
Phenytoin, 503–504
Physiatrist, traumatic brain injury
team, 71

Physical therapy
  intensive care unit, 271–301
    active movement, 278
    assessment, 272–280
    benefits of multidisciplinary
      treatment sessions, 280–281
    cast, 290–291
    chemical paralysis, 289–290
    cognitive level, 279–280
    complications, 297–300
    direct assessment, 275–280
    edema, 298
    equipment, 273–275
    eye movement, 278
    family, 300
    level of alertness, 281–284
    multidisciplinary input, 272–273
    normal motor control, 291–296
    normalization of tone, 284–287,
      288
    orientation, 281–284
    orthopaedic injuries, 297–298
    pain stimulus, 278–279
    patient observation, 275
    posturing, 276–277
    primary areas of focus, 280, 281
    pulmonary complications,
      298–299
    range of motion, 277–278
    range of motion maintenance,
      287–291
    skin integrity, 296–297
    spinal injuries, 297–298
    splint, 290–291
    treatment, 280–297
  sensorimotor integration, 326–327
Physician support, trauma center, 32
Pia mater, 85
Pleural injury, 253–254
Pneumonia, 349–355
  antibiotics, 351

diagnosis, 352–354
early-onset pneumonia, 351–352
pulmonary defense, 350
signs and symptoms, 352
susceptibility, 350–351
treatment, 354–355
ventilation, 351
Pons, 102
Positive-pressure ventilation, 343
Posttraumatic seizure, intracranial
  pressure, 118–119
  management, 118–119
Posturing, 276–277
Potassium, 110
Precentral gyrus, 87
Prehospital care, 12–13
  advanced life support, 13
  basic life support, 12–13
Premotor cortex, 93
Preoptic nucleus, 99
Prevention, 7–12, 51
Primary motor cortex, 93
Primary prevention, 7–12
Prolactin inhibitory factor, 100
Prophylactic hyperventilation, 573
Propofol, 503–504
Prosencephalon, 85
Protein requirement, 405
Proximal femur fracture, 245
Psychosocial issues, 68–69
Public education, 51
Pulmonary angiogram, pulmonary
  embolism, 380–382
Pulmonary embolism, 378–383
  diagnosis, 379–382
  lung ventilation-perfusion scan,
    380, 381
  management, 379–383
  pulmonary angiogram, 380–382
Pulmonary empyema, 355–357, 358
Pulmonary function, 331–349

Pulmonary infection, 416
Pulse oximeter
    precautions, 197
    purpose, 197
Pure tone audiogram, 490–492
Putamen, 90

Q

Quality improvement, 50–51

R

Race, traumatic brain injury, 4–5
Range of motion, 277–278
Reconciliation, 544–545
Regionalized trauma system
    components, 29
    current status, 29–30
    economic status, 31–33
    effectiveness, 23–28
    functional outcome, 22–29
    health care reform, 31–33
    impact, 20–22
Rehabilitation
    critical care
        animal studies, 581
        benefits, 579–585
        benefits of combining, 572–591
        cognition, 584–585
        disposition, 586
        early-intervention program,
            579–580
        length of stay, 586, 587, 588, 589
        level of functioning, 584–585
        medical benefits, 584
        physical/motor skills, 582–584
        transfer planning, 586–589
    trauma center, 16–20
Rehabilitation staff, education
    program, 580

Reimbursement, trauma care, 31–32
Remorse, 544
Resources for Optimal Care of the
    Injured Patient, 13, 16–17
Respiration, normal respiratory
    control, 331–333
Respiratory insufficiency,
    assessment, 334–336
Respiratory management, 331–395
    methods, 336–349
    pulmonary complications, 349–383
Respiratory rate, 333
Respiratory support, 331–349
Restlessness, pharmacologic
    management, 512–515
Rhomboencephalon, 85
Rotating air flow bed, 204–206

S

Safety belt, 7–8
Secondary medical prevention,
    benefits, 572–574
Sedation, 67
Seizure prophylaxis, pharmacologic
    management, 504, 515–517
Sensorimotor integration, physical
    therapy, 332–333
Sensory stimulation program, 579
Sepsis syndrome, adult respiratory
    distress syndrome, 365–366
Septum pellucidum, 101
Serotonergic drug, 511–512
Short circumferential artery, 107
Situational crisis, 526
Skin integrity, 296–297
Skull fracture, hearing loss, 486
Skull vault fracture, hearing, 484
Social worker, traumatic brain injury
    team, 72–73
Sodium, 110

Somatosensory cortex, 94–95
Somatostatin, 100
Spasticity, pharmacologic
   management, 504, 519–521
Speech/language pathology, intensive
   care unit, 444–477
   alertness, 447–448
   arousal, 447–448
   assessment, 447–450
   cognition, 447–448
   cognition/language, 454–455
   communicative intent, 455–458
   electronic technology, 457–458
   equipment, 444
   family, 474–475
   formal assessment tools, 451–452
   monitoring device, 445
   movement, 450
   oral-motor responses, 449–450
   patient observation, 446–447
   responsiveness/interaction with the
     environment, 454
   role, 444
   swallowing, 468–475
   talking tracheostomy tube, 464–465
   tracheostomy speaking valve,
     465–468
   tracheostomy tube, 460–464
   treatment, 451–458
   visual responses, 449
   vocal communication options,
     464–468
   vocal cords, 458–468
Spinal cord injury, 215–236
   classification, 223–226
   complete vs. incomplete, 224
   functional classification, 224–226
   initial evaluation, 217–218
   mechanism, 218–222
   neurologic level of injury,
     223–224, 225

   pharmacologic therapy, 228–229
   secondary, 227–228
   skeletal level of injury, 223
   spinal cord syndromes, 226–227
   traumatic brain injury
     intensive care unit management,
       234–236
     surgical management, 229–230
     treatment, 230–233
     type, 218–222
Spinal injury, documentation,
   189–190
Spinal shock, 227
Splint, 290–291
Staff education
   rehabilitation staff, 580
   traumatic brain injury team, 75
Statutory conduction, 82
Steroid, intracranial pressure,
   119–120
Striate artery, 106
Subarachnoid hemorrhage, 126
Subarachnoid space, 85
Subdural hematoma, 123–124
Sucralfate, 503–504
Suicide, firearms, 2–3
Superior frontal gyrus, 87
Superoptic nucleus, 99
Supplementary motor area, 93
Swallowing disorder, 468–475
   bedside assessment and
     observation, 471–472
   dysphagia, 469–471
   oral feeding initiation, 474–475
   timing of swallowing assessment,
     471
   tracheostomy, 472–473
   ventilator, 473–474
Swan-Ganz catheter, 208
   precautions, 195
   purpose, 195

Synapse, 81
Synaptic cleft, 83
Synaptic vesicle, 83
Syndrome of inappropriate release of
    antidiuretic hormone, 413, 414

T

Talking tracheostomy tube, 464–465
Team-focused intervention, 56–76
Tectum, 102
Tegmentum, 102
Telencephalon, 85
Temperature probe
    precautions, 197
    purpose, 197
Temporal lobe, 88, 89
Thalamus, 98
Thoracic empyema, 355–357, 358
    clinical picture, 356
    treatment, 356–357
Thoracic trauma, 250–259
Thyrotropin-releasing hormone,
    100
Tibial fracture, 246
Tidal volume, 333
Topographic testing, 163
Tracheobronchial injury, 256–257
Tracheostomy, 339–342
    percutaneous dilational
        tracheostomy, 339–342
    swallowing disorder, 472–473
    timing, 339
Tracheostomy speaking valve,
    465–468
Tracheostomy tube, 460–464
Traction, 203
Transcranial Doppler
    ultrasonography, intracranial
        pressure, 121
Transfer planning, 586–589

Transverse temporal bone fracture,
    hearing, 485
Trauma care
    evolution, 5–7
    reimbursement, 31–32
    three-dimensional model, 6
Trauma Care Systems Planning and
    Development Act, 6
Trauma center, 13–20
    cost containment, 32–33
    guidelines, 14–16
    Level I, 14
        capabilities, 46–50
        clinical capabilities, 45–46
        continuing education, 52
        desirable characteristics, 45–55
        essential characteristics, 45–55
        facilities, 46–50
        guidelines, 14
        hospital organization, 45
        organ procurement activity, 52
        outreach program, 51
        prevention, 51
        public education, 51
        quality improvement, 50–51
        rehabilitation services
            characteristics, 19
        resources, 46–50
        transfer agreements, 52
        trauma research program, 51–52
        trauma service support personnel,
            52
    Level II, 14–15
        capabilities, 46–50
        clinical capabilities, 45–46
        continuing education, 52
        desirable characteristics, 45–55
        essential characteristics, 45–55
        facilities, 46–50
        guidelines, 14–15
        hospital organization, 45

organ procurement activity, 52
outreach program, 51
prevention, 51
public education, 51
quality improvement, 50–51
resources, 46–50
transfer agreements, 52
trauma research program, 51–52
trauma service support personnel,
  52
Level III, 15
  capabilities, 46–50
  clinical capabilities, 45–46
  continuing education, 52
  desirable characteristics, 45–55
  essential characteristics, 45–55
  facilities, 46–50
  guidelines, 15
  hospital organization, 45
  organ procurement activity, 52
  outreach program, 51
  prevention, 51
  public education, 51
  quality improvement, 50–51
  resources, 46–50
  transfer agreements, 52
  trauma research program, 51–52
  trauma service support personnel,
    52
Level IV, 15–16
  capabilities, 46–50
  clinical capabilities, 45–46
  continuing education, 52
  desirable characteristics, 45–55
  essential characteristics, 45–55
  facilities, 46–50
  guidelines, 15–16
  hospital organization, 45
  organ procurement activity, 52
  outreach program, 51
  prevention, 51

public education, 51
quality improvement, 50–51
resources, 46–50
transfer agreements, 52
trauma research program, 51–52
trauma service support personnel,
  52
physician support, 32
rehabilitation, 16–20
Trauma nurse coordinator, 69–71
Traumatic brain injury
  abdominal injury, treatment
    priority, 263–265
  associated injury, 215–265
  blunt force, 486
  cardiovascular complications,
    417–420
  epidemiology, 1–5
  external causes, 2, 3
  family guidelines for interaction
    with patients, 551–555
  future medical advances, 574–579
  hearing loss prevalence, 484
  incidence
    age, 1–2
    gender, 1–2
  mechanisms of injury, 4
  metabolic response, 396–434
    acute-phase response, 401–402
  mortality, 1
  pharmacologic management,
    503–521
  previous social maladjustment, 535
  pulmonary complications, 349–383
  race, 4–5
  spinal cord injury
    intensive care unit management,
      234–236
    surgical management, 229–230
  support groups and advocacy
    associations, 547, 565–571

treatment, 111–112
vs. other forms of trauma, 5
Traumatic brain injury team, 56–76
    benefits, 58–59
    communication, 74–75
    constellations, 59–63
    effectiveness, 73–76
    functional components, 74, 75
    interdisciplinary approach, 56
    members, 59–73
    multidisciplinary approach, 56
    nursing
        airway and breathing, 63–64
        circulation, 64
        complication, 67–68
        contributions, 63–71
        documentation, 68, 69, 75–76
        flowsheet, 68, 69, 75–76
        Glasgow Coma Score, 65
        initial assessment, 63
        intracranial pressure monitoring,
            66–67
        neurologic assessment, 65–66
        paralysis, 67
        psychosocial issues, 68–69
        role, 63–71
        sedation, 67
        stabilization, 63
        trauma nurse coordinator, 69–71
    organization, 57–58
    physiatrist, 71
    social worker, 72–73
    staff education, 75
    structural components, 74, 75
    transdisciplinary approach,
        56–57
Trazodone, 511–512
Trigeminal nerve, 136, 146–148
    components, 138
    cortical and subcortical
        connections, 148

functions, 138
injury diagnosis, 162
injury mechanism, 162
subdivisions and pathways,
    147–148
Trochlear nerve, 136, 144–145
    functions, 138, 144
    injury diagnosis, 162
    injury mechanism, 162
    subdivisions and pathways, 145
Turning frame, 205, 207
Tympanometry, 492–493

U

Upper airway, 332
    management, 336–337
Urinary catheter, 203
    precautions, 197
    purpose, 197
Urinary tract infection, 421–422

V

Vagus nerve, 136, 155–156
    central connections, 154
    components, 138
    cortical and subcortical
        connections, 156
    functions, 138, 155
    injury diagnosis, 166
    injury management, 166
    subdivisions and pathways,
        155–156
Valproic acid, 503–504
Ventilation, 342–343. See also
    Specific type
    complications, 343
    goals, 342–343
    manual calculations for physiologic
        variables, 345–346

monitoring, 345–346
pneumonia, 351
weaning, 348–349
Ventilator, 198–199
   control or phase variables,
      343
   precautions, 196
   purpose, 196
   swallowing disorder, 473–474
Ventilator tube
   precautions, 196
   purpose, 196
Ventricle, 96–98
Vestibulocochlear nerve, 136,
   151–153
   components, 138

cortical and subcortical
   connections, 152–153
functions, 138, 151–152
injury diagnosis, 165–166
injury management, 165–166
subdivisions and pathways, 152
Violence, 2–3, 10–12
Visual cortex, 91, 95
Vocal cords, 458–468

W

Weapon-Related Injury Surveillance
   System, 12
White matter, 81
Wound infection, 424–425